GW00367222

WITHDRAWN

Handbook of PLAB

Second Edition

Kunal Goyal MBBS MRCP
Specialist Registrar
West Midlands Deanery, UK

Seema Mittal MBBS
Senior House Officer
Manchester

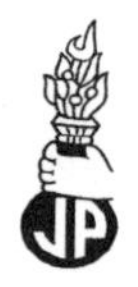

JAYPEE BROTHERS
MEDICAL PUBLISHERS (P) LTD
New Delhi

Published by

Jitendar P Vij
Jaypee Brothers Medical Publishers (P) Ltd
EMCA House, 23/23B Ansari Road, Daryaganj
New Delhi 110 002, India
Phones: 23272143, 23272703, 23282021, 23245672, 23245683
Fax: 011-23276490 e-mail: jpmedpub@del2.vsnl.net.in
Visit our website: http://www.jpbros.20m.com

Branches

- 202 Batavia Chambers, 8 Kumara Kruppa Road, Kumara Park East, **Bangalore** 560 001, Phones: 2285971, 2382956 Tele Fax: 2281761 e-mail: jaypeebc@bgl.vsnl.net.in
- 282 IIIrd Floor, Khaleel Shirazi Estate, Fountain Plaza Pantheon Road, **Chennai** 600 008, Phone: 28262665 Fax: 28262331 e-mail: jpmedpub@md3.vsnl.net.in
- 4-2-1067/1-3, Ist Floor, Balaji Building, Ramkote Cross Road, **Hyderabad** 500 095, Phones: 55610020, 24758498 Fax: 24758499 e-mail: jpmedpub@rediffmail.com
- 1A Indian Mirror Street, Wellington Square **Kolkata** 700 013, Phone: 22451926 Fax: 22456075 e-mail: jpbcal@cal.vsnl.net.in
- 106 Amit Industrial Estate, 61 Dr SS Rao Road, Near MGM Hospital Parel, **Mumbai** 400 012 , Phones: 24124863, 24104532 Fax: 24160828 e-mail: jpmedpub@bom7.vsnl.net.in

Handbook of PLAB

First Edition: 2001
Second Edition: **2003**

ISBN 81-8061-190-6

Typeset at JPBMP typesetting unit
Printed at Gopsons Papers Ltd., Noida

Preface to the First Edition

Handbook of PLAB is an effort to provide its readers an understanding of the new pattern of this examination from the year 2000. It is the first book of its kind wherein the author has tried his best to make it easily readable and easy to follow. It incorporates about 3500 extended matching questions (EMQs) covering all the major topics. More stress has been laid on the topics which are rendered important from the point of view of the PLAB examination. First timers (beginner aspirants) as well as those who have been preparing already will find the Handbook equally useful. The author is quite hopeful that the latter will find it of immense use for revision and refresh whatever they have read before.

The author got the idea of writing the book when he along with his friends and colleagues was preparing for the PLAB examination. This new pattern examination was totally new so the author and his friends had to face a new unknown challenge hence they felt the need of such a book all the more. This book has been written with the first hand experience gained by the author himself.

Learning can be self or from the experience of others. The author was not lucky enough to learn from the experience of others so he had to venture himself in the blind alleys. However, the experience had been quite useful and hence this book. The author is quite hopeful that it will meet the needs of the students in their preparation of the PLAB. Candid comments from the readers are most welcome.

Kunal Goyal

Acknowledgements

We owe my heartfelt gratitude to:

My brother, Amit, whose unconditional support and inspiration has helped me to reach where I an today.

Our parents who have stood by me at all times.

All the well wishers for all their support and assistance.

Mr JP Vij, Chairman and Managing Director of M/s Jaypee Brothers Medical Publishers (P) Ltd., and his team of dedicated staff for their untiring efforts.

Preface to the Second Edition

The huge success of the first edition filled me with enthusiasm, to work hard to update the book. When I first wrote the book, being the first one in the field, just after first exam based on new pattern, I do realize it had questions, which were difficult and not really suitable for PLAB.

Over time, we have learnt more about GMC questioning style and topics of interest and importance. We have tried our best to add on the relevant questions and change the previous ones to make this book an essential read for all PLAB aspirants. First time (beginner aspirants) as well as those who have been prepairing already will find the handbook equally useful. We are quite hopeful that the latter will find it of immense use for revision and refresh whatever they have read before.

I do hope all of you enjoy the book, as much as we did revising it. We are as always open to candid comments from our readers.

Kunal Goyal
Seema Mittal

Contents

Introduction

WHAT **PLAB** STANDS FOR–PLAB means The Professional and Linguistic Assessments Board.

WHY TAKE THE PLAB TEST

If an overseas–qualified doctor wants to practice in the UK under supervision in approved training posts, he/she needs to have been granted limited registration by the General Medical Council (GMC). To get this limited registration, you have to satisfy the GMC that you have the knowledge and skills which are necessary for medical practice in the United Kingdom (UK), and one of the ways of doing this is by passing the PLAB test.

WHAT HAPPENS AFTER PLAB TEST

Passing the PLAB test will not guarantee any offer of a job and one should be aware that there are fewer vacancies in some specialized fields than others. Additionally most of us find that there is delay of several weeks, possibly months, between passing the tests and getting a job.

Having said that, I should also tell that most of the candidates are successful in securing the desired jobs before their patience gets exhausted and only a few come back without a job. As a matter of fact, getting the first job is the most difficult step as after that, the things usually get easier. All this information, is not to discourage you but help you to make the right decision. If anyone decides to take this exam, maximum help shall be rendered by this book.

QUALIFICATION AND EXPERIENCE TO ENTER THE PLAB TEST

1. A primary medical qualification accepted for limited registration, which for example in India is degree of MBBS. Other acceptable qualifications include those listed in the world direc-

tory of medical schools published by the World Health Organization.

2. One year of clinical experience from teaching hospitals or other hospitals approved by the medical registration authorities in the appropriate country, e.g. the one-year internship program in India.

   One can take the PLAB test without this experience of one year, but this could prove as a disadvantage because the exam is at the Senior House Officer (SHO) level, where the knowledge of clinical experience would have come handy and moreover, the GMC requires you to have this experience before getting you the limited registration even after passing the test.

   For those of you who do not want to waste any time after internship, can take this exam somewhere in-between their internship program.

3. For applying for the PLAB test, you should have proved your linguistic capabilities with English as a language and for this you need to take IELTS tests. The minimum score for qualification in speaking: 7.0, listening: 6.0, academic reading: 6.0, academic writing: 6.0 and overall: 7.0.

The IELTS test score is valid for two years from the date of declaration of result to the time you appear for your PLAB part I exam.

WHAT IT WILL COST

• The fee for taking part I	145 pound sterlings
• The fee for taking part II	430 pound sterlings
• The fee for checking your original documents when you apply for limited registration	100 pound sterlings
• Air ticket (Return)	500 pound sterlings
• Others	300 pound sterlings

ABOUT THE PLAB TEST ITSELF

This test refers to the whole PLAB test which is in two parts.

PART I

An extended matching questions (EMQs) examination. The emphasis of this examination is on the clinical management and science as applied to clinical problems. It is confined to core knowledge, skills and attitudes relating to conditions management seen by SHO's, the generic management of life-threatening situations and rarer, but important problems.

The examination paper will contain 200 questions divided into a number of themes. It will last 3 hours. As per the GMC information the picture tests, clinical problem solving questions will no more be asked, but it is very difficult to say and hard to believe that there will be no pictures in any form in the exam. As for the July 2000 exam, there were no questions based on pictures.

Syllabus (as outlined by the GMC in their information brochure).

Part I Assesses the ability to apply knowledge to the care of patients. The subject matter is defined in terms of the skill and of the content.

Skills Four groups of skills will be tested in approximately equal proportions:

a. Diagnosis: Given the important facts about a patient (such as age, sex, and nature of presenting symptoms, duration of symptoms) you are asked to select the most likely diagnosis from a range of possibilities.
b. Investigations: This may refer to the selection or the interpretation of diagnostic tests. Given the important facts about a patient, you will be asked to select the investigation, which is most likely to provide the key to the diagnosis. Alternatively, you may be given the findings of investigations and asked to relate these to a patient's condition or to choose the most appropriate next course of action.
c. Management: Given the important facts about a patient's condition, you will be asked to choose from a range of possibilities the most suitable course of treatment. In the case of medical treatments, you will be asked to choose the correct drug therapy and will be expected to know about side effects.
d. Others: these may include:
    i. Explanation of disease process: The natural history of disease will be tested with reference to basic physiology and pathology.

ii. Legal/ethical: You are expected to know the major legal and ethical principles set out in the GMC publication duties of a doctor.
iii. Practice of evidence based medicine: Questions on diagnosis, investigations and management may draw upon recent evidence published in peer-reviewed journals. In addition, there may be questions on the principles and practice of evidence-based medicine.
iv. Understanding of Epidemiology: You may be tested on the principles of epidemiology, and on the prevalence of important diseases in the UK.
v. Health promotion: The prevention of disease through health promotion and knowledge of risk factors.
vi. Awareness of multicultural society: You may be tested on your appreciation of the impact of the practice of medicine of the health beliefs and cultural values of the major cultural groups represented in the UK population.
vii. Application of scientific understanding to medicine.

CONTENTS

The content to be tested is, for the most part, defined in terms of patient presentations. Where appropriate, the presentation may be either acute or chronic. Questions in part I will begin with a title which specifies both the skill and the content, for example, the management of varicose veins.

You will be expected to know about conditions that are common or important in the United Kingdom for all of the systems outlined below. Examples of the cases that may be asked about are given under each heading and may appear under more than one heading.

These examples are for illustration and the list is not exhaustive. Other similar conditions might appear in the examination.

a. Accident and emergency medicine (to include trauma and burns)

   Examples: Abdominal injuries, abdominal pain, back pain, bites and stings, breathlessness/wheeze, bruising and purpura, burns, chest pain, collapse, coma, convulsions, diabetes, epilepsy, eye problems, fractures, dislocations, head injury, loss of consciousness, non-accidental injury, sprains and strains, testicular pain.

b. Blood (to include coagulation defects)

Examples: Allergy aneurysm, chest pain, deep vein thrombosis (DVT), diagnosis and management of hypertension, heart failure, ischemic limbs, myocardial infarction, myocardial ischemia, stroke, varicose veins.

c. Cardiovascular system (to include heart and blood vessels and blood pressure)

Examples: Aortic aneurysm, chest pain, and deep vein thrombosis (DVT), diagnosis and management of hypertension, heart failure,ischemic limbs, myocardial infarction, myocardial-ischemia, stroke, varicose veins.

d. Dermatology, allergy, immunology and infectious diseases.

Examples: Allergy, fever and rashes, influenza/pneumonia, meningitis, skin cancers.

e. ENT and eyes

Examples: Earache, hearing problems, hoarseness, difficulty in swallowing, glaucoma, 'red eyes', sudden visual loss.

f. Female reproductive system (to include obstetrics, gynecology and breast)

Examples: Abortion/sterilization, breast lump, contraception, infertility, menstrual disorders, menopausal symptoms, normal pregnancy, post-natal problems, pregnancy complications, vaginal disorders.

g. Gastrointestinal tract, liver and biliary system and nutrition

Examples: Abdominal pain, constipation, diarrhea, and difficulty in swallowing, digestive disorders, gastrointestinal bleeding, jaundice, rectal bleeding/pain, vomiting, weight problems.

h. Metabolism, endocrinology and diabetes

Examples: Diabetes mellitus, thyroid disorders, weight problems.

i. Nervous system (both medical and surgical)

Examples: Coma, convulsions, dementia, epilepsy, eye problems, headache, loss of consciousness, vertigo.

j. Orthopaedics and rheumatology

Examples: Alcohol abuse, anxiety, assessing suicidial risk, dementia depression, drug abuse, overdoses and self harm, panic attacks, post-natal problems.

k. Psychiatry (to include substance abuse)

Examples: Hematuria, renal and ureteric calculi, renal failure, sexual health, testicular pain, and urinary infections.

l. Renal system (to include urinary tract and genitourinary medicine)

Examples: Hematuria, renal and urteric calculi, renal failure, sexual health, testicular pain, urinary infections.

m. Respiratory system.

Examples: Asthma, breathlessness/wheeze, cough, hemoptysis, hoarseness, and influenza/pneumonia.

n. Disorders of childhood (to include non-accidental injury and child sexual abuse; fetal medicine; growth and development)

Examples: Abdominal pain, asthma, child development, childhood illness, earache, epilepsy, eye problems, fever and rashes, joint pain/swelling, loss of consciousness, meningitis, non-accidental injury, testicular pain, urinary disorders.

o. Disorders of the elderly (to include palliative care)

Examples: Breathlessness, chest pain, constipation, dementia, depression, diabetes, diarrhea, digestive disorders, headache, hearing problems, influenza/pneumonia, jaundice, joint pain/swelling, loss of consciousness, pain relief, terminal care, trauma, urinary disorders, vaginal disorders, varicose veins, vertigo, vomiting.

p. Peri-operative management

Examples: Pain relief, shock.

How to Approach the Extended Matching Questions Examination

The examination paper will contain 200 questions in the extended matching format, divided into a number of theme.

Each theme has a heading which tells you what the questions are about, in terms both of the clinical problem area (e.g. chronic joint pain) and the skill required (e.g. diagnosis).

Within each theme there are several numbered items, usually between four and six. These are the questions—the problems you have to solve. These are examples below.

Begin by reading carefully the instruction which preceded the numbered items. The instruction is very similar throughout the paper and typically reads 'For each scenario below, choose the SINGLE most discrimination investigation from the above list of options. Each option may be used once, more than once or not at all.'

Consider each of the numbered items and decide what you think the answer is. You should then look for that answer in the list of options (each of which is identified by a letter of the alphabet). If you cannot find the answer in the list you have thought of, you should look for the option which, in your opinion, is the best answer to the problem posed.

For each numbered item, you must choose ONE, and only, of the option. You may feel that there are several possible answers to an item, but you must choose the one most likely from the option list. *If you enter more than one answer on the answer sheet you will gain no mark* for the question even though you may have given the right answer along with one or more wrong ones.

In each theme there are more option than items, so not all the options will be used as answer. This is why the instruction says that some options may not be used at all.

A given option may provide the answer to more than one item. For example, there might be two items which contain descriptions of patients, and the most likely diagnosis could be the same in both instances. In these cases, the option would be used more than once.

You will be awarded one mark for each item answered correctly. Marks are not deducted for incorrect answers nor for failure to answer. You should, therefore, attempt all items.

PART II

You may only enter part II of the test when you have passed part I. You have to take part II within 2 years of passing part I. This test is set at the following standard:

A candidate's command on English language and professional knowledge and skill must be shown to be sufficient for him or her to undertake safety, employment at first year Senior House Officer level in a British hospital.

This test is a 14 station Objective Structured Clinical Examination (OSCE).

The syllabus and format of this test as given in the GMC information brochure:

The Objective Structured Clinical Examination (OSCE)

Aim

1. The aim of the OSCE is to test your clinical and communication skills. It is designed so that an examiner can observe you putting these skills into practice.

Overall format

2. When you enter the examination, you find a series of 14 booths, known as 'station'. Each station requires you to undertake a particular task. Some tasks will involve talking to or examining patients, some will involve demonstrating a procedure on an anatomical model. Detail of the tasks are explained below under 'Content'.
3. There will also be two rest stations in the circuit. At some tests one of these two stations will contain instruction asking you to perform certain tasks as if you were at a real station. These are pilot stations and the results will not count towards your overall OSCE grades.
4. You will be required to top perform all tasks. You will be told the number of the station at which you should begin when you enter the examination room. Each task will last five minutes.
5. Your instruction will be posted outside the station. You should read these instructions carefully to ensure that you follow them exactly. An example might be:
   'Mr McKenzie has been referred to you in a rheumatology clinic because he has joint pains. Please take a short history to establish supportive for a differential diagnosis.
6. A bell will ring. You may then enter the station. There will be an examiner in each station. However, unlike in the oral examination, you will not be required to have a conversation with the examiner; you should only direct your remarks to him or her if the instructions specifically ask you to do so. You should undertake the task as instructed. A bell will ring after four minutes 30 seconds to warn you that you are nearly out of time. Another bell will ring when the five minutes are up. At this point you must stop immediately and go and wait outside the next station. If you finish before the end, you must wait inside the station but you should not speak to the examiner or to the patient during this time.

7. You will wait outside the next station for minute. During this time you should read the instructions for the tasks in this station. After one minute, a bell will ring. You should then enter the station and undertake the task as instructed.
8. You should continue in this way until you have completed all 14 tasks. You will then have finished the OSCE.

Content of the station

9. Each station consists of a scenario. An examiner will be present and will observe you at work.
10. The scenario could be drawn from any medical speciality appropriate to a Senior House Officer (SHO).
11. Although the tasks you will be instructed to do will not necessarily be tested in the order given here. Under each skill area, you will find some examples. Please note that these are *only examples;* other topics will be tested.

m History Taking

Your candidate instructions will set the scene. You will be asked to take a history from an actor pretending to be a patient (a stimulated patient). The actor will have been given all the necessary information to be able to answer your questions accurately. You should treat him or her as you would a real patient.

m Examination Skills

You will be asked to examine a particular part of the body. You may have to examine a stimulated or real patient or perform the examination on an anatomical model. Although you should talk to the patient as you would to a patient in real life. You should only take a history or give a diagnosis if the instructors require you to do so. You may be asked to explain your actions to the examiner as you go along.

Examples: Breast examination, cardiovascular examination, examination of abdomen, hip examination, knee examination.

m Practical Skills/Use of Equipment

This is to assess some of the practical skills an SHO needs. The stations concerned will normally involve anatomical models rather than patients.

Examples: IV cannulation, cervical smear, suturing, blood pressure.

Emergency Management

These stations will test whether you know what to do in an emergency situation. You may have to explain what you are doing to the patient or to the examiner. Your instructions will make this clear.

Examples: Resuscitation skills.

m Communication Skills

There will be a communication skill element in most stations. However, in some stations this skill will be the principal skill tested. Areas tested may include interviewing (including appropriate questioning, active listening, explaining clearly, checking understanding) and building rapport (including showing empathy and respect, sensitivity to other's emotions and copying with strong emotions in others).

Examples: Instructions for discharge from hospital, explaining treatment, consent for autopsy, ectopic pregnancy explanation.

VENUE FOR EXAMINATIONS

You can take part I of the test in:

- The UK (Birmingham, Edinburgh, Glasgow, London).
- Bangladesh (Dhaka).
- Egypt (Cairo).
- India (Kolkata, Chennai, New Delhi, Mumbai).
- Pakistan (Islamabad, Karachi).
- Sri Lanka (Colombo).

Part II of the test is available in London, Edinburgh, Leeds and Liverpool.

Details of dates are set out by the GMC at regular intervals the candidates are advised to get in contact with the office of the nearest British Council Divisions.

NOTIFICATION OF RESULTS

The part I paper is marked by Computer. At the end of the part I test, you will be told the date on which your results will be available. Usually it takes about 4 weeks for the declaration of results.

For part II, you will be given grades for each station. However, the overall result of the examination is either pass or fail and this result is usually sent out 2 weeks after the date of the examination.

ANNEX

Contacts

Before you take the PLAB Test
Routes to Limited registration and Qualifications needed

General Medical Council

Address:	
178 Great Portland Street	First Application Service
London	Tel: 44 207 915 3481
United Kingdom	Fax: 44 207 915 3558
W1N 6JE	E-mail: firstcontact@gmc-uk.org

Job Opportunities in the UK

The British Council National
Advice Centre

Address:	
Bridgewater House	
58 Whitworth Street	Tel: 44 161 957 7218
Manchester, United Kingdom	Fax: 44 161 957 7029
M1 6BB	E-mail: ed@britcoun.org

The IELTS Test

The British Council National
Advice Centre

Address:	
Bridgewater House	
58 Whitworth Street	Tel: 44 161 957 7218
Manchester, United Kingdom	Fax: 44 161 957 7029
M1 6BB	E-mail: ed@britcoun.org

Taking the test

The United Kingdom

The General Medical Council
PLAB Test Section

Address:	Name: Candidate Services
178 Great Portland Street	Tel: 44 207 915 3727
London	Fax: 44 207 915 3565
W1N 6JE	E-mail: plab@gmc-uk.org

India

Examination Services Manager
New Delhi

Address:	Name: Sanjay Patro
British High Commission	Tel: 91–3710111/37 10555
British Council Division	Fax: 91–3710 717
17 Kasturba Gandhi Marg	E-mail: sanjay.patro@in.
New Delhi 110 001	britishcouncil.org

Examination Services Manager
Chennai

Address:	Name: Nirupa Fernandez
British Deputy High Commission	Tel: 91-44-852-5002
British Council Division	Fax: 91-44-852-3234
737 Anna Salai	E-mail: Nirupa.fernan
Chennai 600 002	
dez@in.britishcouncil.org	

Examination Services Manager
Kolkata

Address:	Name: Suchitra Mukherjee
British Deputy Commission	Tel: 91-33-282-9108/9144
British Council Division	Fax: 91-33-282-4808
5 Shakespeare Sarani	E-mail:Suchitra.mukherjee@in.
Calcutta 700 071	britishcouncil.org

Examination Services Manager
Mumbai

Address:
British Deputy High Commission

British Council Division	Name: Kamal Taraparevala
Mittal Tower 'C' Wing	Tel: 91-22-222-3560
Nariman Point	Fax: 91-22-285-2024

Mumbai 400 021
E-mail: kamaltaraparevala@in.britishcouncil.org

Pakistan

Examination Services Manager
Karachi

Address:	Name: Irum Fawad
The British Council	Tel: 92 21 5670391-7
20 Bleak House Road	Fax: 92 21 5682694

Near Cant's Station
E-mail: Irum.Fawad@bc-karachi.bcouncil.org
(PO Box 10410)
Karachi

Examination Services Manager
Islamabad

Address:
The British Council
Block 14
Civic Centre
G – 6
E-mail: Shahnaz.Farooq@bc-islamabad.
Islamabad

Name: Shahnaz Farooq
Tel: 92 51 111 424 424
Fax: 92 51 27 6683

Bangladesh

Examination Services Manager
Dhaka

Address:
The British Council
5 Fuller Road
PO Box 161
E-mail: srahman@TheBritishCouncil.net
Dhaka – 1000

Name: Saidur rahman
Tel: 880 2 868905-7
Fax: 880 2 863375

Sri Lanka

Examination Services Manager
Colombo

Address:
The British Council
49 Alfred Gardens
E-mail: ethel.nanayakkara@britcoun.lk
(PO Box 753) Colombo 3
Sri Lanka

Name: Ethel Nanayakkara
Tel: 94 1 581171
Fax: 94 1 587079

RECOMMENDED BOOKS

Medicine

- Davidson or Kumar Clarke should form the basic textbook to prepare for medicine. There is no need to try and go through both of these books. A candidate should be thorough with either of the two books.
- "Oxford Handbook of Clinical Medicine" is a must book to read.
- "Oxford Handbook of Clinical Specifications" is also a must book to read.
- "Lecture Notes on Clinical Medicine". This book is optional. You may briefly go through this book. You do not have to read this book thoroughly if you have done the above reading for medicine.
- "French Index of Differential Diagnosis" is a good book if time permits.

Surgery

- "Lecture Notes on Surgery" is a good book to get a broader view of general surgery.
- Oxford handbooks contribute good supplementary reading, especially the "Oxford Handbook of Clinical Medicine".
- Orthopedics is well covered in the "Oxford Handbook of Clinical Specialties", but if time allows one should also read "Lecture Notes on Orthopedics".
- Love and Bailey can be referred to for selected important topics, e.g. Breast disease, thyroid disease or vascular diseases.

Obstetrics and Gynecology

- "Ten Teachers" is the one, which is commonly referred to by most of the students.
- "Lecture Notes on Obstetrics and Gynecology" can be another option but these subjects are also very well covered in the "Oxford Handbook of Clinical Specialties".

ENT and Ophthalmology

- "Oxford Handbook of Clinical Specialties" does contain ENT and Ophthalmology. ENT and Ophthalmology constitutes a

very small portion of the PLAB test. The small coverage of this topic in this book is quite adequate to prepare for the PLAB test.
- "Lecture Notes in ENT and Ophthalmology" can be referred to for some selected important topics.

Pediatrics

Oxford handbooks cover this subject adequately, but "Essential Paediatrics" by David Hull can be referred for important topics.

Dermatology

Davidson has covered Dermatology adequately, but you may refer to the Oxford handbook and for some of the very important topics please go through "Lecture Notes in Dermatology".

Most of the information, given above has been taken from the GMC brochure and also what the author feels about to this examination. As the regulations of the test are liable to changes the candidate is advised to be appraised of the latest information by directly contacting the GMC or the British Council Divisions. Although, everything has been written for the candidate's utmost benefit, but the author takes no responsibility for the content of this information.

The author wishes the candidate happy reading and smooth sailing through this exam.

One

Cardiovascular System

THEME: 1
INTERPRETATION OF PULSE RATE

Options

a. Regular fast palpitations.
b. Regular slow palpitations.
c. Irregular fast palpitations.
d. Dropped beats
e. Regular and pounding.

For each of the situations/conditions given below, choose the one most appropriate/discriminatory option from above. The options may be used once, more than once, or not at all.

Questions

1. Pulsus bigeminus.
2. Anxiety.
3. Atrial fibrillation.
4. Atrial ectopics.
5. Atrial flutter.
6. Patient on beta blockers.

THEME: 2
DIAGNOSIS OF APEX BEAT

Options

a. Undisplaced, tapping apex.
b. Displaced, forceful apex.
c. Undisplaced, heaving apex.
d. Displaced, hyperdynamic apex.
e. Dyskinetic.
f. Double impluse.

For each of the situations/conditions given below, choose the one most appropriate/discriminatory option from above. The options may be used once, more than once, or not at all.

Questions

7. Aortic stenosis.
8. Mitral stenosis
9. Anterior wall myocardial infarction (MI)
10. Aortic regurgitation.
11. Cardiomyopathy.
12. Mitral regurgitation.

THEME: 3
TYPES OF PERIPHERAL PULSES

Options

a. Aortic stenosis.
b. Severe aortic regurgitation.
c. Dilated cardiomyopathy.
d. Toxic myocarditis.
e. Pericarditis.
f. Atrio-ventricular block.
g. Liver failure.

For each of the situations/conditions given below, choose the one most appropriate/discriminatory option from above. The options may be used once, more than once, or not at all.

Questions

13. Pulsus paradoxus.
14. Anacrotic pulse.
15. Pulsus parvus et tardus.
16. Plateau pulse.
17. Pulsus alternans.
18. Bounding pulse.
19. Dicrotic pulse.
20. Pulsus bisferiens.
21. Pulsus bigeminus.

THEME: 4
INTERPRETATION OF JVP

Options

a. Raised JVP with normal waveform.
b. Raised JVP with absent pulsation.
c. Large 'a' wave.
d. Cannon wave.
e. Systolic 'cv' waves.
f. Deep 'y' descent.
g. Absent a wave

For each of the situations/conditions given below, choose the one most appropriate/discriminatory option from above. The options may be used once, more than once, or not at all.

Questions

22. Tricuspid stenosis.
23. Tricuspid regurgitation.
24. Constrictive pericarditis.
25. SVC obstruction.
26. Pulmonary hypertension.
27. Atrial flutter.
28. Atrial fibrillation.

THEME: 5
ECG – ABNORMALITIES

Options

a. ST depression and inverted T–wave in V5–6.
b. Small T waves, prominent 'V' waves, ventricular bigemini.
c. Tall tended T waves, ST segment depression.
d. Short QT interval.
e. Prolonged QT interval.
f. ST elevation.
g. Saddle shaped 'ST' in all leads except aVR.
h. 'V' wave.
i. Delta wave.
j 'J' wave.

For each of the situations/conditions given below choose the one most appropriate/discriminatory option from above. The options may be used once, more than once, or not at all.

Questions

29. WPW syndrome.
30. Hypokalemia.
31. Hypothermia.
32. Hyperkalemia.
33. Hypercalcemia.
34. Digoxin toxicity.
35. Myocardial infarction.
36. Acute pericarditis.

THEME: 6
ECG INTERPRETATION

Options

a. Hypothermia
b. Pyrexia
c. RA hypertrophy
d. LA hypertrophy
e. RVH
f. LVH
g. Conduct defect
h. MI
i. IHD
j. Pulmonary hypertension
k. Myocarditis
l. Rheumatic heart disease
m. Potassium excess
n. Hypothyroidism

For each of the situations/conditions given below, choose the one most appropriate/discriminatory option from above. The option may be used once, more than once, or not at all.

Questions

37. A teenage boy with dyspnoea and chest pain is brought into A&E. He has a history of rheumatic fever. An ECG demonstrates LAH and LVH. It also demonstrates Q waves and raised ST segments.
38. An elderly woman is found unconscious at home. An ECG demonstrates sinus bradycardia, J waves, ST depression and flattened T waves.
39. A patients ECG shows a biphasic P wave.
40. A patients ECG shows T waves inversion and ST depression.
41. A 35-year-old woman complains of tiredness and malaise. Her T waves are widespread and deep.

THEME: 7
INTERPRETATION OF ABNORMAL ECG

Options

a. Hypokalemia
b. Hyperkalemia
c. Hypocalcemia
d. Hypercalcemia
e. Myocardial ischaemia
f. Inferior MI
g. Acute pulmonary embolism
h. Acute pericarditis
i. Atrial fibrillation
j. Myxoedema
k. Digitalis intoxication
l. Inferolateral MI

For each of the situations/conditions given below, choose the one most appropriate/discriminatory option from above. The option may be used once, more than once, or not at all.

Questions

42. A 60-year-old woman taking frusemide is noted to have U waves in V3 and V4.

43. A 50-year-old man presents with fever and chest pain. He has a history of angina. His ECG reveals concave elevations of the ST segments in leads II, V5 and V6.
44. A 55-year-old presents with chest pain and dyspnoea. His ECG reveals Q waves in leads III and aVF and inverted T waves in leads V1-3.
45. A 55-year-old woman who has undergone thyroidectomy is noted to have an ECG with a QT interval of 0.5 sec.
46. A 60-year-old woman presents with hoarseness. She is a smoker and is on prozac. Her pulse rate is 44/min and the ECG is noted for sinus bradycardia and reduced amplitude of P, QRS and T waves in all leads.

THEME: 8
INTERPRETATION OF ECG

Options

a. RBBB
b. Second degree block
c. Hyperkalemia
d. *PTE*
e. Sinus arrhythmia
f. Anterior MI
g. LBBB
h. WPW syndrome
i. Complete heart block
j. 1st degree block
k. 2nd degree block (mobitz type 2)

For each of the situations/conditions given below, choose the one most appropriate/discriminatory option from above. The option may be used once, more than once, or not at all.

Questions

47. Progressive lengthening of PR interval with one non-conduncted beat.
48. Constant PR interval but one P wave is not followed by a QRS complex.

49. One P wave per QRS complex, constant PR interval and progressive beat to beat change in the RR interval.
50. Dominant R in V1 and inverted T in the anterior chest leads.
51. Peaked P waves, right axis deviation, inverted T waves in leads V1 to V3 and tall R waves in V1.
52. Dominant R waves in V1, inverted T waves in leads V1-3 and deep S waves in V6.

THEME: 9
INTERPRETATION OF ECG ABNORMALITIES

Options

a. Pulmonary embolism
b. Angina
c. Hyperkalemia
d. Hypokalemia
e. Hypothyroidism
f. Hypothermia
g. Hypocalcemia
h. Hypercalcemia
i. Hypertension with LVH
j. Acute pericarditis
k. Severe pneumonia
l. Pericardial effusion

For each of the situations/conditions given below, choose the one most appropriate/discriminatory option from above. The option may be used once, more than once, or not at all.

Questions

53. J waves, bradycardia and first degree heart block.
54. Prolonged QT, all ST segments elevated and show characteristic saddle shape.
55. Shortened QT interval.
56. Tall QRS complexes with LVH pattern
57. Atrial fibrillation, self-resolving.

THEME: 10
DIAGNOSIS OF CHEST PAIN

Options

a. Anxiety
b. Massive pulmonary embolism
c. Pulmonary HTN
d. Pulmonary infarction
e. Pneumothorax
f. IHD
g. Dissecting aneurysm
h. Chylothorax
i. Oesophagitis
j. MI
k. Carcinoma
l. Asthma
m. Pneumonia
n. Dry pleurisy

For each of the situations/conditions given below, choose the one most appropriate/discriminatory option from above. The option may be used once, more than once, or not at all.

Questions

58. A 48-year-old man complains of chest pain. He describes it as gripping and crushing and involving whole chest. He says he has had to give up exercise because it aggravates the pain and makes both hands numb.
59. A middle-aged lady complains of chest pain, breathlessness and fainting. On examination there is a prominent a wave in JVP, a right ventricular heave and a loud P2.
60. A 53-year-old man is brought to A&E with crushing chest pain and pallor. He cannot breathe and his heart is racing. His sputum is blood stained; he has a pleural rub and pyrexia.
61. A young man brought to hospital in a state of collapse. He was at his desk saw the value of his stocks fall and felt a constricting pain in the chest. A few moments later he woke up in the ambulance.

62. A 50-year-old lady complains of chest pain radiating across the chest. She says her muscles are very tender. Breathing aggravates the pain and coughing brings tears to her eyes. She thinks she has had a heart attack.

THEME: 11
DIAGNOSIS OF CHEST COMPLAINTS

Options

a. Bronchogenic carcinoma
b. Cushing's disease
c. Hyperparathyroidism
d. Diabetes mellitus
e. Steroid abuse
f. Coarctation of the aorta
g. Conn's syndrome
h. Acromegaly
i. Alcoholism
j. PAN
k. Systemic sclerosis
l. Essential hypertension
m. Chronic pyelonephritis
n. Insulinoma

For each of the situations/conditions given below, choose the one most appropriate/discriminatory option from above. The option may be used once, more than once, or not at all.

Questions

63. A 38-year-old woman complains of feeling bloated and recurrent chest infections. She says she bruises easily and has missed periods. On examination you find her BP to be high.
64. A 40-year-old man presents with sweating, headaches and hypertension. He also complains of joint pain muscle weakness and numbness in both hands. Over the past few months he has become increasingly breathless and his ankles have swollen up.

65. A 48-year-old woman presents with fever, malaise, weight loss and joint pains. She has high blood pressure and large feet. She complains of persistent chest pain. She has purpuric rash and skin nodules.
66. A middle-aged man presents with abdominal pain and bone pain. He has hypertension and a recent history of recurrent renal stones.
67. At a routine health check up you carry out a fundoscopy on an apparently healthy man. You find he has an arteriolar narrowing and tortuosity and an increased light reflex.

THEME: 12
DIAGNOSIS OF HEART CONDITIONS

Options

a. Anterolateral MI
b. LVF
c. AF
d. Acute pulmonary embolism
e. Acute pericarditis
f. Mitral stenosis
g. RVF
h. Hypokalemia
i. Hypocalcemia
j. Aortic regurgitation
k. Inferolateral MI

For each of the situations/conditions given below, choose the one most appropriate/discriminatory option from above. The option may be used once, more than once, or not at all.

Questions

68 A 60-year-old man presents with chest pain radiating down his left arm. His 12 lead ECG shows Q waves in II, III and aVF with T wave changes in V5 and V6.
69. A 50-year-old woman presents with a fast heart rate with an irregular rhythm. There are no P waves on the ECG.

She states that she has lost weight recently and is nervous. She also suffers from palpitations.

70. On auscultation a patients is noted to have a rumbling diastolic murmur at the apex. The murmur is accentuated during exercise.
71. A 60-year-old man on digitalis and diuretics presents with a raised JVP, hepatomegaly, ankle and sacral oedema.

THEME: 13
DIAGNOSIS OF CHEST PAIN

Options

a. Pneumothorax.
b. Aortic dissection.
c. Lobar pneumonia.
d. Pulmonary embolism.
e. Postherpetic neuralgia.
f. Myocardial infarction.
g. Trauma.
h. Peptic ulcer.
i. Pericarditis.
j. Hypertrophic cardiomyopathy.
k. Esophageal reflux.
l. Cervical disc disease.
m. Costochondritis.
n. Breast disease.
o. Esophageal spasm.

For each of the situations/conditions given below choose the one most appropriate/discriminatory option from above. The options may be used once, more than once, or not at all.

Questions

72. A collapsed 34-year-old male patient is brought to the emergency room. He was playing basketball, when he complained of severe chest pain and collapsed. On examination is drowsy but arousable. Pulse 126/min regular and not palpable on the left radial/brachial artery. ECG and chest X-ray normal.

73. A 48-year-old heavy smoker complains of severe chest pain radiating to the left shoulder of 30 minutes duration. He has had previous episodes on walking up hill. On examination he is sweating, has a pulse of 98/min, BP 150/90 mm Hg and normal heart sounds. ECG is still awaited.
74. A 21-year-old student became suddenly breathless and had left sided chest pain during a cycling trip.
75. A well built young man has recurrent chest pain. On examination he has jerky pulse and a soft systolic murmur.
76. Localized, sharp pain exacerbated by coughing and respiration.
77. Pain following or accompanying eating and increased by bending, hot drinks or lying supine.
78. Central chest pain radiating to jaw and associated with excitement and feeling of impending doom.
79. Central chest pain radiating to back and lower limb pulses not felt.
80. A 75-year-old lady is on her seventh postoperation day after a hip replacement surgery and suddenly complains of chest pain and is breathless. Pulse is 102/min, BP 100/60 mm Hg. Blood gases done have the following results pH 7.35, PaO_2 8.2 kPa, $PaCO_2$ 4.2 kPa.
81. A 45-year-old smoker comes with a stabbing left sided chest pain of 6 hours duration. He is anxious breathing at the left base.

THEME: 14
DIFFERENTIAL DIAGNOSIS OF ANGINA

Options

a. Unstable angina
b. Stable angina
c. Syndrome X
d. Myocardial infection
e. Pericarditis
f. Peptic ulcer disease
g. Arrhythmia

h. Spontaneous pneumothorax
i. Acute cholecystitis
j. Chronic cholecystitis
k. Pneumonia

For each of the situations/conditions given below, choose the one most appropriate/discriminatory option from above. The options may be used once, more than once, or not at all.

Questions

82. An obese 34-year-old man complains of epigastric pain, which seems to be exacerbated by eating his favourite meal, fish and chips. He get temporary relief when hungry.
83. An obese 45-year-old man complains of recurring chest pain which radiates to his neck lasting 20 minutes. It coincides with his weekly executive board meetings.
84. An obese 29-year-old woman complains of cough of two weeks and right upper quadrant pain. She is mildly febrile. There was no abdominal tenderness on examination.

THEME: 15
DIAGNOSIS OF CHEST PAIN

Options

a. Atrial fibrillation
b. Angina pectoris
c. Reflux oesophagitis
d. Peptic ulcer
e. Oesophageal carcinoma
f. Asthma
g. Bornholm's disease
h. MI
i. Tuberculosis
j. Pneumonia
k. Spontaneous pneumothorax
l. Dissecting aneurysm
m. Pulmonary embolism
n. Pleurisy

For each of the situations/conditions given below, choose the one most appropriate/discriminatory option from above. The option may be used once, more than once, or not at all.

Questions

85. A middle-aged woman with sedentary habits has chest pain aggravated by breathing and coughing. She has a slight fever. 2 months ago she had pneumonia but recovered fully.
86. A short overweight middle-aged woman complains of chest pain below her sternum. The pain is worse at night and always starts up after meals.
87. A 48-year-old man presents with acute chest pain in the substernal area. The pain radiates to the neck and arm. He says that the pain also goes through to the back.
88. A 62-year-old housewife complains of central chest pain after a heavy meal. The pain goes to her back, she says and her fingertips on left hand are numb. Her serum transaminase and LDH are normal.
89. A young asthmatic comes to you with chest pain of sudden onset. The pain is on the lower left side. He says the pain followed a bout of coughing and has left him breathless.

THEME: 16
CAUSES OF CHEST PAIN

Options

a. Dissecting aortic aneurysm
b. Myocardial infarction
c. Angina pectoris
d. Pericarditis
e. Pulmonary embolism
f. Costochondritis
g. Gastroesophageal reflux disease
h. Spontaneous pneumothorax
i. Mediastinitis
j. Enlarging aortic aneurysm

k. Tension pneumothorax
l. Pleurisy

For each of the situations/conditions given below, choose the one most appropriate/discriminatory option from above. The option may be used once, more than once, or not at all.

Questions

90. A 55-year-old man presents with sudden onset of severe central chest pain radiating to the back. Peripheral pulses are absent. There are no ECG changes. The CXR shows a widened mediastinum.
91. A 20-year-old man recently returned from a holiday in the caribbean presents with a left sided chest discomfort and dyspnoea. On CXR there is a small area devoid of lung markings in the apex of the left lung.
92. A 50-year-old man recently back from business trip in Hong Kong presents with sudden onset of breathlessness haemoptysis and chest pain. He is bought to A&E in shock. His CXR is normal. The ECG shows sinus tachycardia.
93. A 40-year-old man presents with a central crushing chest pain that radiates to the jaw. The pain occurred while jogging. The pain was relieved by rest. The ECG is normal.
94. A 50-year-old woman with ovarian cancer presents with right-sided chest pain. The CXR shows obliteration of the right costophrenic angle.

THEME: 17
INVESTIGATION OF CHEST PAIN

Options

a. Rectal examination, faecal occult blood test
b. ECG
c. Arterial blood gases
d. V/Q scan
e. Treadmill exercise test
f. Seek immediate expert advice
g. Endoscopy
h. CXR

i. Sputum culture
j. Bronchoscopy
k. 2 min hyperventilation
l. Coronary angiography

For each of the situations/conditions given below, choose the one most appropriate/discriminatory option from above. The option may be used once, more than once, or not at all.

Questions

95. A 50-year-old man complains of intermittent exert ional chest pain radiating to the jaw and left shoulder, relieved by rest. The ECG is normal. Eating can also precipitate his symptoms.
96. A 44-year-old diabetic develops central crushing chest pain lasting over 30 min and associated with nausea and vomiting.
97. Epigastric pain and anaemia in a 50-year-old overweight woman on treatment for joint disease.
98. A 20-year-old man presents with sudden onset of pleuritic chest pain and dyspnoea. He is 182 cm tall and has smoked for 6 years. There is no other medical history.
99. A 58-year-old chronically hypertensive man is admitted with shearing central chest pain radiating through to the interscapular region.

THEME: 18
DIAGNOSIS OF CARDIAC LESIONS

Options

a. Mitral stenosis
b. ASD
c. Tetralogy of Fallot
d. Aortic stenosis
e. HOCM
f. Mitral regurgitation
g. Tricuspid stenosis
h. Aortic regurgitation
i. Tricuspid regurgitation

j. Pulmonary stenosis
k. VSD

For each of the situations/conditions given below, choose the one most appropriate/discriminatory option from above. The option may be used once, more than once, or not at all.

Questions

100. Slow rising pulse, prominent left ventricular impulse, ejection systolic murmur and fourth heart sound.
101. Bounding carotid pulse, laterally displaced apex, ejection systolic murmur, early diastolic murmur and 3rd heart sound.
102. Jerky carotid pulse, dominant 'a' wave in the JVP, double apical impulse, ejection systolic murmur at the base and PSM at the apex.
103. Elevated JVP, early diastolic opening snap MDM at the apex and loud S1.
104. Elevated JVP displaced apex, PSM at the apex and 3rd heart sound.
105. Loud PSM at the left lower sternal area. Mid-diastolic flow murmur at the apex and loud S2.

THEME: 19
MANAGEMENT OF CHEST PAIN

Options

a. Sympathy
b. Diazepam
c. Anxiolytics
d. Pericardial tap
e. Pericardial resection
f. Frusemide
g. Aspirin
h. Diamorphine
i. Antibiotics
j. Lobectomy
k. Incision and drainage

l. Radiotherapy
m. Antiemetics
n. Chest X-ray

For each of the situations/conditions given below, choose the one most appropriate/discriminatory option from above. The option may be used once, more than once, or not at all.

Questions

106. A young officer complains of palpitation for 2 months. He says that when he mounts stairs he can feel his heart beating. His health history is unremarkable.
107. A 40-year-old man complains of swollen legs and breathlessness. Examination reveals hepatosplenomegaly. CXR shows a normal but dense heart shadow and clear lung fields.
108. A middle-aged man complains of severe chest pain radiating to the neck. The pain came on after dinner as he was retiring for the night. His wife called out a locum at 3 am.
109. An elderly housewife was operating on for gallstones and at operation a gangrenous gallbladder was removed. A couple of days later she complained of nausea and feeling unwell.
110. A 60-year-old warehouse man has been acutely breathless for last week. He is a smoker and has a chronic productive cough for last 14 years.

THEME: 20
MANAGEMENT OF ACUTE CHEST PAIN

Options

a. Glyceryl trinitrate (0.5 mg) Sublingually
b. IV 50 ml of 50% dextrose
c. High flow O_2 and Ramipril 2.5 mg 12 hr PO
d. High flow O_2 10 mg IV morphine –anticoagulation
e. Crossmatch blood and inform surgeons
f. Insert a 16 G cannula in second intercostal space

g. IV heparin 5000-10,000 i.u over 5 min.
h. Underwater seal drainage
i. 10 mg IV diamorphine
j. Nifedipine

For each of the situations/conditions given below, choose the one most appropriate/discriminatory option from above. The options may be used once, more than once, or not at all.

Questions

111. A tall young woman developed sharp pain on one side of his chest two days ago. Since then he has been short of breath on exertion.
112. After a heavy bout of drinking a 56-year-old man vomits several times and develops chest pain. When you examine him , he has a crackling feeling under the skin around his neck.
113. A 23-year-old woman on the oral contraceptive pill suddenly gets tightness in her chest and becomes very breathless.
114. A 30-year-old man with Marfan's syndrome has sudden central chest pain going through to the back.
115. A 57-year-old man develops crushing pain in the chest associated with nausea and profuse sweating. The pain is still present when he arrives in hospital an hour later.

THEME: 21
DIAGNOSTIC TEST FOR PATIENT PRESENTING WITH CHEST PAIN

Options

a. Abdominal ultrasound
b. Blood culture
c. Bronchoscopy
d. Cardiac enzymes
e. Chest X-ray
f. Computed tomography (CT)
g. Electrocardiogram

h. Full blood count
i. Lumbar puncture
j. Oesophago-gastro-duodenoscopy
k. Ventilation/Perfusion scan

For each of the situations/conditions given below, choose the one most appropriate/discriminatory option from above. The options may be used once, more than once, or not at all.

Questions

116. A 68-year-old man has had malaise for five days and fever for two days. He has a cough and you find dullness at the left lung base.
117. A 50-year-old woman returned by air to the UK from Australia. Three days later she presents with sharp chest pain and breathlessness. Her chest X-ray and ECG are normal.
118. A tall, thin, young man presents with a sudden pain in the chest and left shoulder and breathlessness while cycling.
119. A 45-year-old manual worker presents with a two hour history of chest pain radiating into left arm. His ECG is normal.
120. A 52-year-old obese man has had episodic anterior chest pain, particularly at night, for three weeks. Chest X-ray and ECG are normal.

THEME: 22
INVESTIGATIONS

Options

a. Coronary angiography.
b. Stress test.
c. Chest X-ray in deep expiration.
d. Ventilation-perfusion scan.
e. Blood culture.
f. Upper GI endoscopy.

For each of the situations/conditions given below choose the one most appropriate/discriminatory option from above. The options may be used once, more than once, or not at all.

Questions

121. A relapsed ovarian cancer patient with poor mobility complains of subacute onset of breathlessness and chest pain.
122. A 14-year-old tall girl complains of severe chest pain and breathlessness.
123. Uncomplicated anterior wall myocardial infarction now asymptomatic, has come for review after 6 weeks prior to return to work in a clerical capacity.
124. A 45-year-old male with an anterior wall infarction, thrombolysed three days ago develops chest pain and an irregular pulse on the third day in intensive care not responding to nitrates.

THEME: 23
MATCH THE PATHOPHYSICAL FEATURES WITH THE CONGENITAL DEFECTS BELOW

Options

a. Hypoplastic left heart syndrome.
b. Persistent truncus arteriosus.
c. Tricuspid atresia.
d. Pulmonary atresia with VSD.
e. Critical aortic stenosis.

For each of the situations/conditions given below, choose the one most appropriate/discriminatory option from above. The options may be used once, more than once, or not at all.

Questions

125. An obligatory right to left atrial shunt.
126. Symptoms are primarily related to pulmonary vascular resistance and size of pulmonary arteries.
127. Ductus dependent systemic flow with an obligatory left to right atrial shunt.
128. Ductus dependent pulmonary flow with an obligatory right to left ventricular shunt.

THEME: 24

MATCH THE FOLLOWING X-RAY FINDINGS WITH CONGENITAL HEART DISEASE

Options

a. Snowman sign.
b. Egg-shaped heart.
c. "3" sign.
d. Convex left heart border.
e. Boot-shaped heart.

For each of the situations/conditions given below, choose the one most appropriate/discriminatory option from above. The options may be used once, more than once, or not at all.

Questions

129. Coarctation of aorta.
130. Tetralogy of Fallot.
131. Dextra position of great vessels.
132. Levo-transposition of the great arteries.
133. Total anomalous pulmonary venous return.

THEME: 25

DIAGNOSIS OF CHEST COMPLAINTS

Options

a. Anxiety
b. MI
c. Pulmonary embolism
d. Aortic dissection
e. Angina
f. Herpes
g. Tabes dorsalis
h. Lung infarct
i. Pleurisy
j. Myocarditis
k. Oesophagitis
l. Peptic ulcer

m. Cholecystitis
n. Pancreatitis

For each of the situations/conditions given below, choose the one most appropriate/discriminatory option from above. The option may be used once, more than once, or not at all.

Questions

134. A 40-year-old woman complains of pain aggravated by breathing. She sits up erect and is reluctant to breathe. On examination the lung fields are clear and you find tenderness in region to the left of sternum.
135. Following streptococcal sore throat infection, a middle-aged man develops acute chest pain with breathlessness and pallor. His heart rate is rapid and irregular. His cardiac enzymes are normal.
136. A young woman complains of acute chest pain. It is stabbing and makes her breathless. It involves her whole chest and lips and feet have gone numb.
137. A 52-year-old man drives himself to A&E with an acute stabbing pain. He has had the pain for more than half an hour and is in extreme distress. He is pale and sweaty and he vomits.
138. A 33-year-old woman complains of chest pain radiating through to the back. She is overweight and decided to come in after taking a cup of hot tea, which brought on the chest pain. She says it is worse on leaning forward.

THEME: 26
DIAGNOSIS OF CHEST PAIN

Options

a. Dissecting aortic aneurysm
b. Dressler's syndrome
c. Boerhaave's syndrome
d. Ventricular aneurysm
e. Pulmonary embolism
f. Kawasaki's disease
g. HOCM

h. Pneumothorax
i. Right ventricular infarction
j. Cardiac neurosis
k. Reflux oesophagitis

For each of the situations/conditions given below, choose the one most appropriate/discriminatory option from above. The option may be used once, more than once, or not at all.

Questions

139. A 56-year-old man had been operated for fracture neck femur. Six days later he complained of dyspnoea at rest and chest pain. ECG showed sinus tachycardia and right axis deviation.
140. A 55-year-old porter collapsed while bending. On admission he regained consciousness but started to vomit, was sweating profusely and complained of chest pain. CXR showed widened mediastinum.
141. A 69-year-old man is admitted with severe epigastric pain and sweating. Over the last few weeks he has suffered from chest pain and shortness of breath on moderate exercise. On examination his JVP is 10 cm above the sternal angle, pulse 65/min and BP 115/65 and there is bilateral ankle oedema.
142. A 45-year-old alcoholic is admitted to A&E with severe retrosternal pain and shortness of breath. The pain is constant and radiates to the neck and interscapular region. On examination his pulse is 120/min, BP is 90/60 and left lung base is dull on percussion.
143. A 25-year-old man presents with shortness of breath and chest tightness. His father had collapsed and died suddenly when he was 33. On examination the cardiac apex is double and with S4 and a late systolic murmur.
144. A 28-year-old man presented to A&E with severe tightness of chest, which was worse on exercise. He had a strong history of MI. On examination his temperature was 37.8. Pulse 90 and BP 130/80. Apex was normal. Cervical lymphadenopathy, erythematous buccal cavity and polymorphous rash.

THEME: 27
DIAGNOSIS OF CHEST PAIN

Options

a. Angina pectoris
b. Acute MI
c. Bronchiectasis
d. Hiatus hernia
e. Pneumonia
f. Pulmonary embolism
g. Pleural effusion
h. Tension pneumothorax
i. Lung fibrosis
j. Reflux oesophagitis
k. Spontaneous pneumothorax
l. Aortic dissection
m. Possible malignancy

For each of the situations/conditions given below, choose the one most appropriate/discriminatory option from above. The option may be used once, more than once, or not at all.

Questions

145. A 65-year-old man has had generalised weakness for a week and fever for past 3 days. He has had a cough and on examination you find stony dullness at the right lung base.
146. A 50-year-old woman returned by flight to UK from Paris. 3 days later she presents to A and E with central chest pain and breathlessness. Her CXR and ECG are normal.
147. A tall thin 35-year-old man with sudden chest pain radiating to the left shoulder and breathlessness while cycling.
148. A 50-year-old porter presents with a 3 hours history of chest pain radiating into the left arm. His ECG is normal.
149. A 50-year-old obese man has had episodic anterior chest pain; particularly at night for 2 weeks CXR and ECG are normal.

THEME: 28
DIAGNOSIS OF CHEST PAIN

Options

a. Acute pancreatitis
b. Angina pectoris
c. Aortic dissection
d. Trigeminal neuralgia
e. Herpes zoster
f. Lobar pneumonia
g. Ruptured oesophagus
h. Herpes simplex
i. Acute MI
j. Spontaneous pneumothorax
k. Acute cholecystitis
l. Bornholm disease
m. Tietze's syndrome
n. Oesophageal spasm
o. Fracture rib

For each of the situations/conditions given below, choose the one most appropriate/discriminatory option from above. The option may be used once, more than once, or not at all.

Questions

150. A 24-year-old man develops acute pain on the right side of the chest radiating to the right shoulder associated with fever. She has vomiting and has mild yellowing of the skin
151. A tall young man developed chest pain in the right hemithorax following RTA. On palpitation this area is tender. A CXR shows no lung injury.
152. A 22-year-old male prostitute develops severe chest pain. The area of chest pain corresponds to an area with an erythematous rash.
153. A 70-year-old man develops crushing central pain associated with nausea and profuse sweating radiating to the neck. By the time he gets to the hospital the pain has gone.

154. Minutes after upper GI endoscopy, a 56-year-old man develops chest pain. On examination he has a crackling feeling under the skin around his upper chest and neck.

THEME: 29
DIAGNOSIS OF CHEST COMPLAINTS

Options

a. Uraemia
b. Dressler's syndrome
c. Pneumonia
d. Acute myocarditis
e. Left atrial myxoma
f. Obstructive cardiomyopathy
g. Congestive cardiomyopathy
h. MI
i. Pericardial effusion
j. Constrictive pericarditis
k. Pericarditis
l. SLE
m. Endocarditis
n. Bacteremia

For each of the situations/conditions given below, choose the one most appropriate/discriminatory option from above. The option may be used once, more than once, or not at all.

Questions

155. A middle-aged man presents with variable heart murmur. He also complains of fever, malaise and night sweats. On examination you find clubbing and splenomegaly.
156. A 43-year-old woman presents with fever and weight loss. She is pale and her spleen is enlarged. Her fingers are mildly clubbed with painful lesions on the pulps. She is breathless.
157. A young man presents with dyspnoea especially at nights and wheeze. He is exhausted and coughs. His sputum is frothy and contains blood. ECHO shows the heart to be globular in shape and contracting poorly.

158. A young man present with dyspnoea, chest pain, fainting spells and palpitations. On auscultation you find a jerky pulse and a late systolic murmur. ECHO demonstrates asymmetrical septal hypertrophy.
159. A 62-year-old man presents with sharp chest pain. He has had it for 3 days and it radiates down into his abdomen. Breathing deeply and coughing aggravate it. On auscultation of the chest you hear a scratching sound.

THEME: 30
INVESTIGATIONS OF CHEST PAIN

Options

a. Chest X-ray
b. Exercise ECG
c. ECHO
d. Gastroscopy
e. Oesophagoscopy
f. CT scan
g. ECG
h. Pulmonary angiography
i. Cardiac catheterization
j. Indirect laryngoscopy

For each of the situations/conditions given below, choose the one most appropriate/discriminatory option from above. The option may be used once, more than once, or not at all.

Questions

160. A 30-year-old obese man complains of retrosternal chest pain worse at night and after meals.
161. A 34-year-old man presents with a history of chest pain radiating to the jaw, brought on by exercise and relieved by rest.
162. A 67-year-old woman presents with a 2 hours history of chest pain radiating to the left shoulder. She is sweating and feels sick.
163. A tall young man presents with history of sudden chest pain radiating to the.back and the interscapular area.

THEME: 31
DIAGNOSIS OF CARDIOVASCULAR DISEASES IN CHILDREN

Options

a. Kawasaki disease
b. Hereditary angioedema
c. Congenital nephrotic syndrome
d. Myocarditis
e. Pericarditis
f. Primary pulmonary HTN
g. Still's disease
h. Acute rheumatic fever
i. Congestive heart failure
j. Toxic synovitis
k. Aortic stenosis
l. SLE
m. Paroxysmal atrial tachycardia
n. Mitral stenosis

For each of the situations/conditions given below, choose the one most appropriate/discriminatory option from above. The option may be used once, more than once, or not at all.

Questions

164. A 10-year-old boy presents with stridor. He has a history of recurrent swelling of the hands and feet with abdominal pain and diarrhoea. His sister also suffers from similar attacks.
165. A 6-year-old girl presents with spiking fevers. On examination she has spindle-shaped swellings of her finger joints.
166. A 12-year-old boy presents with polyarthritis and abdominal pain. He had a sore throat a week ago. On examination he is noted to have an early blowing diastolic murmur at the left sternal edge.
167. A 10-year-old boy presents to casualty following a seizure while at the gym. On examination he has a loud systolic ejection murmur with a thrill.

168. A 12-year-old girl presents with pallor, dyspnoea and a PR of 190. She is noted to have cardiomegaly and hepatomegaly.

THEME: 32
DIAGNOSIS OF CONGENITAL HEART DISEASE

Options

a. ASD
b. Ebstein's anomaly
c. Congenital pulmonary stenosis
d. VSD
e. PDA
f. HOCM
g. Fallot's tetralogy
h. Coarctation of aorta and bicuspid aortic valve
i. Dextrocardia
j. Transposition of great arteries
k. Congenital aortic stenosis

For each of the situations/conditions given below, choose the one most appropriate/discriminatory option from above. The option may be used once, more than once, or not at all.

Questions

169. A 27-year-old woman presented with headache. On examination her BP was 165/115 mmHg, pulse 90 and there was ejection systolic murmur all over the precordium and back.
170. A 39-year-old man presented with progressive breathlessness and palpitations. On examination the JVP was elevated with a prominent 'a' wave and there was a pulmonary ejection systolic murmur. ECG showed a RBBB with large P waves.
171. A 12-year-old boy with a history of recurrent chest infections presented with worsening shortness of breath. On examination there was systolic thrill at the left lower sternal edge, PSM and accentuated S2.

172. A 21-year-old man presented with worsening shortness of breath. He had been told that he had a murmur since he was a child. On examination there was a continuous murmur and the pulse was bounding.
173. A 5-year-old boy was referred for poor growth and worsening shortness of breath. On examination he was cyanosed and there was clubbing. There was an ESM single S1 and parasternal heave. CXR showed RVH and a small pulmonary artery.
174. An infant was referred for heart failure and cyanosis. On examination there was elevated JVP, hepatomegaly, PSM at the lower left sternal edge and S3. CXR showed a large globular heart. ECG showed RBBB.

THEME: 33
DIAGNOSIS OF CARDIOVASCULAR DISEASE

Options

a. AR
b. Mitral stenosis
c. MR
d. AS
e. Atrial myxoma
f. TR
g. PS
h. ASD
i. VSD
j. Fallot's tetralogy
k. PDA
l. Coarctation of aorta
m. Eisenmenger's syndrome

For each of the situations/conditions given below, choose the one most appropriate/discriminatory option from above. The option may be used once, more than once, or not at all.

Questions

175. A 35-year-old pregnant woman presents to her GP for her first prenatal check up. He notes that her BP differs in both arms and is lower in the legs.

176. A 13-year-old boy presents with dyspnoea and a short stature. He is noted to have finger clubbing. His CXR reveals a boot-shaped heart and a large aorta.
177. A preterm baby presents with tachypnea and expiratory grunting. The baby is noted to have a continuous machinery murmur in the 2nd intercostal space.
178. A 33-year-old woman with Marfan's syndrome is noted to have a fixed wide splitting of S2. The ECG shows partial RBBB and right axis deviation and RVH.
179. A 40-year-old drug addict is noted to have a PSM at the bottom of the sternum. Giant 'cv' waves are presented in the JVP.

THEME: 34
CLINICAL DIAGNOSIS OF HEART DISEASE

Options

a. Atrial septal defect.
b. Ventricular septal defect.
c. Coarctation of aorta.
d. Mitral stenosis.
e. Aortic regurgitation.
f. Eisenmenger's syndrome.
g. Infective endocarditis.
h. Hypertensive heart failure.
i. Cardiomyopathy.
j. Patent ductus arteriosus.
k. Ebsteins anomaly.

For each of the situations/conditions given below choose the one most appropriate/discriminatory option from above. The options may be used once, more than once, or not at all.

Questions

180. A 20-year-old male with pulse 100/min regular, BP 130/80 mm Hg, JVP raised, cyanosis and parasternal heave present. Midsystolic murmur is heard in left second intercostal space. S2 is widely split and fixed.
181. 30-year-old male with pulse 90/min, BP 160/60 mm Hg, JVP normal. Apex is in the left 6th intercostal space.

182. 10-year-old male with pulse 80/min regular, BP 110/80 mm Hg, JVP normal. Apex is felt in the left 5th IC space and a parasternal murmur heard at lower parasternal area with systolic thrill.
183. Chronic alcoholic with history of breathlessness on exertion. On examination edema of legs present, JVP raised, BP 130/86 mm Hg. Apical impulse felt in left 6th intercostal space. Grade II systolic murmur could be heard.
184. Quintuple cardiac cadence on auscultation.
185. Continous murmur.

THEME: 35
DIAGNOSIS OF CARDIOVASCULAR DISEASE

Options

a. Angina pectoris
b. Aortic stenosis
c. Tricuspid regurgitation
d. Aortic regurgitation
e. MI
f. Acute pericarditis
g. HOCM
h. MR
i. Congestive cardiomyopathy
j. MS
k. Restrictive cardiomyopathy
l. Constrictive pericarditis
m. Dressler's syndrome

For each of the situations/conditions given below, choose the one most appropriate/discriminatory option from above. The option may be used once, more than once, or not at all.

Questions

186. A 40-year-old man presents with inspiratory chest pain 2 months after heart attack. On examination a friction rub is heard. ECG shows global ST elevation.
187. A 35-year-old IV drug abuser presents with a right upper quadrant abdominal pain. On examination he has periph-

eral oedema, ascites and a pulsatile liver. On auscultation he has holosystolic murmur along the left sternal border.

188. A 30-year-old man presents with chest pain and feeling faint. On examination he has PSM and a S4. ECG shows LVH. Echo shows septal hypertrophy and abnormal mitral valve motion.
189. A 40-year-old woman with Marfan's syndrome presents with shortness of breath, fainting spells and pounding of the heart. On examination she is noted to have capillary pulsation in the nail bed and pistol shot femoral pulses.
190. A 40-year-old presents after fainting during a workout in the gym. On auscultation he has a harsh midsystolic murmur in the aortic area radiating to the carotids.

THEME: 36
INVESTIGATIONS OF HEART DISEASE

Options

a. Doppler echocardiography.
b. Time motion/two-dimensional echocardiography.
c. Phonocardiography.
d. Chest roentgenography.
e. Chest fluoroscopy.
f. 24-hour ambulatory ECG monitoring.
g. Transtelephonic ECG telemetry.
h. Electrophysiologic stimulation/monitoring with intracar diac catheter techniques.
i. Esophageal electrocardiography.
j. His bundle electrocardiography.
k. ECG signal averaging.

For each of the situations/conditions given below, choose the one most appropriate/discriminatory option from above. The options may be used once, more than once, or not at all.

Questions

191. A febrile patient with a new high-frequency diastolic decrescendo murmur at the lower left sternal border.

192. A patient with an enlarged area of precordial dullness to percussion.
193. A 46-year-old patient with an undetermined degree of aortic stenosis.
194. A patient with suspected intracardiac calcification.
195. A patient with a strong family history of hypertrophic cardiomyopathy and sudden death.
196. An asymptomatic patient with severe aortic regurgitation who is seen for annual follow-up examination.
197. A patient with daily bouts of palpitations lasting 1-3 minutes.
198. An elderly patient who is being treated with digoxin for shortness of breath develops episodic dizziness and presyncope. A 12-lead ECG shows RBBB and an axis of minus 70 degrees. On subsequent bedside monitoring in the hospital, there is 2:1 AV block with an atrial rate of 100 per minute.
199. A patient with a narrow QRS tachycardia that is regular at a rate of 150 per minute. There is no response to vagal interventions, and a 12-lead ECG fails to define atrial activity.
200. A patient with rare (1 – 2 times per month) bouts of rapid heart action lasting 1 – 3 minutes.
201. A patient with a wide (0.14 second) QRS tachycardia at 136 per minute. There is a 1:1 relationship between the P and QRS waves.
202. A patient with WPW syndrome and three bouts of rapid heart action over the past one year, each associated with syncope.

THEME: 37
TREATMENT OF CARDIAC CONDITIONS

Options

a. Anticoagulation and digitalisation
b. GTN
c. Propanolol
d. Adrenaline
e. Lignocaine

f. DC cardioversion
g. Atropine
h. Check digoxin level
i. Start dopamine
j. IV frusemide
k. Carotid sinus massage

For each of the situations/conditions given below, choose the one most appropriate/discriminatory option from above. The option may be used once, more than once, or not at all.

Questions

203. A 50-year-old man presents with shortness of breath. His pulse is irregularly irregular. The CXR shows cardiomegaly and left atrial enlargement. ECG shows absent P waves.
204. A 60-year-old man is on verapamil for HTN and digoxin for atrial fibrillation. He is listed for herniorrhaphy. His preoperative ECG shows inverted P waves after QRS complex and a regular rhythm. He is asymptomatic.
205. A 70-year-old patient in ITU suddenly looses consciousness. His ECG shows VT.
206. A 40-year-old man admitted for acute MI suddenly drops his BP to 70/45. He has bilateral rales on auscultation.
207. A 50-year-old man in ITU is noted to have paroxysmal SVT on his ECG monitor.

THEME: 38
TREATMENT OF CARDIAC CONDITIONS

Options

a. Oxygen morphine and streptokinase
b. CABG
c. Angioplasty
d. Intra-aortic balloon angioplasty
e. Swan Ganz catheter
f. Defibrillation
g. Oxygen IV frusemide, morphine GTN
h. GTN tablet and atenolol
i. GTN and nifedepine

For each of the situations/conditions given below, choose the one most appropriate/discriminatory option from above. The option may be used once, more than once, or not at all.

Questions

208. A 40-year-old man has severe mitral valve regurgitation and is unable to maintain an adequate cardiac output. He is awaiting a valve replacement.
209. A 50-year-old man presents with dyspnoea and tachycardia. He has bilateral rales on auscultation. He has a history of IHD. CXR shows cardiomegaly and pulmonary oedema.
210. A 60-year-old man complains of chest pain after jogging. He takes ventolin inhaler for his asthma. ECG shows ST segment depression.
211. A 55-year-old man with frequent episodes of angina now complains that the pain is no longer alleviated by rest or with GTN. Coronary angiogram shows left main stem obstruction.
212. A 60-year-old man complains of severe excruciating chest pain at rest. He is diaphoretic and nauseated. The ECG shows Q waves and ST elevation in leads II, aVL and I.

THEME: 39
CAUSES OF SYNCOPE

Options

a. Vasovagal attack.
b. Prolonged QT on ECG.
c. Aortic stenosis.
d. Pulmonary embolism.
e. Left atrial myxoma.
f. Eisenmenger's complex.
g. Carotid sinus syndrome.
h. Pacemaker malfunction.
i. Third degree heart block.
j. Ethanol.

For each of the situations/conditions given below, choose the one most appropriate/discriminatory option from above. The options may be used once, more than once, or not at all.

Questions

213. On physical examination, the patient is found to have a diastolic "plop" of variable intensity and timing.
214. A 22-year-old male is brought to the emergency room after "passing out" at his construction job.
215. A 45-year-old woman presents with chest pain following syncope; physical examination reveals a pansystolic murmur.

THEME: 40
CAUSES OF SHOCK

Options

a. Pulmonary embolism
b. Myocardial ischaemia
c. Cardiac tamponade
d. Trauma
e. Burns
f. Sepsis
g. Anaphylaxis
h. Major surgery
i. Ruptured aortic aneurysm
j. Ectopic pregnancy
k. Addisonian crisis
l. Hypothyroidsim
m. Acute pancreatitis

For each of the situations/conditions given below, choose the one most appropriate/discriminatory option from above. The option may be used once, more than once, or not at all.

Questions

216. A 50-year-old man arrives to the casualty in shock. His BP is 80/50, his heart sounds are muffled. His JVP is noted to increase with inspiration.

217. A 30-year-old woman presents to casualty with severe abdominal pain, vomiting and shock. She is noted to have stridor. Her lips are swollen and blue.
218. A 55-year-old man presents to casualty with severe abdominal pain vomiting and shock. The pain is in the upper abdomen and radiates to the back. He takes diuretics. The abdomen is rigid and the X-ray shows absent psoas shadow.
219. A 40-year-old woman presents to casualty in shock with continuous abdominal pain radiating to the back. The abdomen is rigid with an expansive abdominal mass.
220. A 35-year-old woman presents to casualty in shock with a BP of 80/50 and tachycardia. She is confused and weak. Her husband states that she forgot to take her prednisolone tablets with her on holiday and has missed several doses.

THEME: 41
HEART SOUND AND MURMURS

Options

a. Mitral stenosis.
b. Mitral regurgitation.
c. Atrial fibrillation.
d. Aortic stenosis.
e. Aortic regurgitation.
f. Pulmonary stenosis.
g. Pulmonary regurgitation.
h. Pulmonary embolism.

For each of the situations/conditions given below, choose the one most appropriate/discriminatory option from above. The options may be used once, more than once, or not at all.

Questions

221. Soft S_1, loud S_3, pansystolic murmur at apex radiating to axilla, Valsalva maneuver makes the murmur softer.
222. High pitched early diastolic murmur. On general examination, patient has collapsing pulse.

223. Loud S_1, rumbling mid-diastolic murmur with presystolic accentuation. Exercise brings out the murmur.
224. Summation gallop rhythm.
225. Loud P_2.
226. Reverse S_2 split with ejection systolic murmur.
227. No murmur heard.

THEME: 42
CLINICAL SIGNS OF STRUCTURAL HEART DISEASE

Options

a. AS
b. AR
c. MS
d. MI
e. TR
f. HOCM
g. ASD
h. VSD
i. PDA
j. MVP
k. PS
l. Left ventricular aneurysm
m. Aortic sclerosis
n. TS

For each of the situations/conditions given below, choose the one most appropriate/discriminatory option from above. The option may be used once, more than once, or not at all.

Questions

228. Harsh pansystolic murmur loudest at left lower sternal border and inaudible at apex. The apex is not displaced.
229. There is soft systolic murmur at the apex radiating to the axilla.
230. Low rising pulse and undisplaced apex, which is heaving in character. There ESM heard best at the intercostals space that does not radiate.

231. The pulse is regular and jerky in character. The cardiac impulse is hyperdynamic and not displaced. There is mid-systolic murmur with no ejection click loudest at the left sternal edge.
232. There is continuous machinery like murmur throught out the systole and diastole. The patient is clubbed and cyanosed.

THEME: 43
DIAGNOSIS OF DIASTOLIC MURMURS

Options

a. Early diastolic murmur.
b. Mid-diastolic murmur.
c. Late diastolic murmur.
d. Pandiastolic murmur.

For each of the situations/conditions given below, choose the one most appropriate/discriminatory option from above. The options may be used once, more than once, or not at all.

Questions

233. Carey-Coombs murmur.
234. Graham Steell murmur.
235. Austin Flint murmur.

THEME: 44
DIAGNOSIS OF HEART DISEASE

Options

a. Cardiac tamponade.
b. Constrictive pericarditis.
c. Restrictive cardiomyopathy.
d. Right ventricle myocardial infarction (RVMI).

For each of the situations/conditions given below, choose the one most appropriate/discriminatory option from above. The options may be used once, more than once, or not at all.

Questions

236. Prominent "y" descent of neck veins, Kussmaul's sign, low voltage on ECG.
237. Pulsus paradoxus, low ECG voltage, negative Kussmaul's sign.
238. Elevated neck veins, abnormal ECG, third heart sound (S_3) present.
239. Electrical alterans on ECG.
240. Pericardial knock.
241. No pulsus paradoxus, prominent "x" descent of neck veins, no Kussmaul's sign.

THEME: 45
TREATMENT OF ARRHYTHMIAS

Options

a. Fleicanide
b. Amiodarone
c. Chloroquine
d. Digoxin
e. Temporary pacing
f. Permanent pacing
g. DC cardioversion
h. Lignocaine
i. Reassurance
j. Nifedipine and glyceryl trinitrate
k. Warfarin
l. 5 ml of a 1:1000 solution of adrenaline
m. Atropine

For each of the situations/conditions given below, choose the one most appropriate/discriminatory option from above. The options may be used once, more than once, or not at all.

Questions

242. A 20-year-old officer worker gets palpitations when ever he walks a flight of several stairs to work.

243. A 55-year-old man complains of chest pain. His blood pressure is 145/92 mmHg. His pulse is irregularly irregular.
244. A 55-year-old man presents with dyspnoea and chest pain. He is found to have a broad complex tachycardia on ECG.
245. A 69-year-old man found to have a pulse rate of 60 beats/min and complains of chest pain and breathlessness. Drug treatment is no help.
246. A 65-year-old man is complaining of chest pain. He has had previous episodes of severe bradycardia, cardiac arrest, and supraventricular tachycardias alternating with asystole.
247. Useful for the conversion a supraventricular tachycardia to sinus rythmn, if done synchronous with the QRS complex.
248. A 45-year-old man presents with dyspnoea and chest pain. The ECG shows a short PR interval and wide QRS which begins with a "slurred" upstroke (delta wave).

THEME: 46
TREATMENT OF ARRHYTHMIAS

Options

a. Atropine 1 mg IV
b. Precordial thump
c. CPR until defibrillator is available
d. CPR adrenaline 1:1000 IV push
e. Transvenous pacemaker
f. Defibrillation
g. External pacemaker
h. Oxygen 4 lit/min
i. Lignocaine
j. Morphine IM

For each of the situations/conditions given below, choose the one most appropriate/discriminatory option from above. The option may be used once, more than once, or not at all.

Questions

249. A 60-year-old man presents with chest pain and shortness of breath. His ECG shows sinus bradycardia of 45/min.
250. A 55-year-old woman is noted to have a slow heart rate. She is asymptomatic. ECG shows no relation between atrial and ventricular activity. The ventricular rhythm is 40/min with wide QRS.
251. A 60-year-old man collapses on the street. The event is unwitnessed. He has no pulse.
252. A 30-year-old man involved in RTA is found unconscious at the scene. He is breathing spontaneously. In A&E the ECG monitor show irregular rhythm and no P, QRS, ST or T waves. The rate is rapid.
253. A 50-year-old man presents to casualty with severe chest pain. He has history of angina. The pain is not relieved with GTN. His BP is 120/70 with a pulse rate of 100. His ECG shows regular sinus rhythm.

THEME: 47
TREATMENT OF ARRHYTHMIAS

Options

a. Carotid sinus massage
b. Adenosine
c. Verapamil
d. Sotalol
e. Amiodarone
f. Digoxin
g. Lignocaine
h. $CaCl_2$
i. Flecainide
j. Disopyramide
k. Elective DC cardioversion
l. Emergency DC version

For each of the situations/conditions given below, choose the one most appropriate/discriminatory option from above. The option may be used once, more than once, or not at all.

Questions

254. A 30-year-old woman has a 6-month history of palpitations. Her resting ECG shows shortened PR interval and delta waves. Holter monitoring shows evidence of paroxysmal SVT.
255. A 50-year-old man was admitted with an acute anterior MI earlier in the day. 2 hrs after thrombolysis with tPA he suddenly complains of feeling faint. His pulse is 140/min and BP is 90/40 mmHg. Cardiac monitor shows long-term of VT.
256. A 24-year-old woman presents to casualty complaining of dizziness. Her ECG shows re-entrant tachycardia. She had one similar episode in the past which stopped spontaneously and she is on no medication. She is 31 weeks pregnant.
257. A 70-year-old man has collapsed on surgical ward following a left hemicolectomy. He has a very weak carotid pulse. His BP is unrecordable. Cardiac monitor shows broad complex tachycardia with a rate of 160/min.
258. A 60-year-old man has chronic renal failure, which is treated with CAPD. Her has a low-grade fever and abdominal pain for last 2 days and he has noticed that the dialysate is cloudy after exchange. He suddenly becomes unwell with broad complex tachycardia. His BP is 80/50 mmHg.

THEME: 48
DIAGNOSIS OF HYPERTENSION

Options

a. Cushing's disease
b. Conn's syndrome
c. Pheochromocytoma
d. Essential hypertension
e. Renal artery stenosis
f. Polycystic kidney disease
g. Coarctation of aorta

For each of the situations/conditions given below, choose the one most appropriate/discriminatory option from above. The options may be used once, more than once, or not at all.

Questions

259. An obese 34-year-old woman presents with excessive facial hair, a blood pressure of 150/95 mmHg and abdominal striae.
260. A 23-year-old man presents with a chronic headache. His blood pressure is 145/90 mmHg. He is found to have femoral delay.
261. An elderly man has three readings of blood pressure of 160/100 mmHg. He is otherwise well.
262. A 34-year-old man presents with haematuria. His blood pressure is found to be 145/100 mm Hg. His father died from chronic renal failure.
263. A 34-year-old woman presents with intermittent flushing, palpitations and headache.
264. A 45-year known hypertensive is found to have a bruit in the abdomen.

THEME: 49
CAUSES OF HYPERTENSION

Options

a. Essential hypertension
b. Renal artery stenosis
c. Polycystic kidney disease
d. Phaeochromocytoma
e. Cushing's syndrome
f. Conn's syndrome
g. Acromegaly
h. Coarctation of aorta
i. Hydronephrosis
j. White coat hypertension
k. Drug induced.

For each of the situations/conditions given below, choose the one most appropriate/discriminatory option from above. The option may be used once, more than once, or not at all.

Questions

265. A 60-year-old male smoker has a lone history of hypertension and angina. Four weeks ago he was started on Captopril by his GP. His creatinine has increased from 100 to 300 during that time. Renal US shows one kidney larger than other.
266. A 40-year-old woman has high blood pressure despite treatment with bendrofluazide and atenolol. Blood test shows sodium 140 mmol. Potassium 3 mmol urea 6 mmol/l. His bendrofluazide is stopped and he is prescribed potassium, supplements but 2 weeks later his K^+ is still 3 mmol/l. Plasma renin activity is low.
267. A 40-year-old woman is hypertensive and says she has been putting on weight. On examination she is centrally obese and has a moon face. There are purple striae on her abdomen. She has glycosuria.
268. A 40-year-old man is hypertensive and complains that he is putting on weight. On examination he has a prominent jaw and brow. And is sweaty. He has large hands and feet. He has glycosuria.
269. A 40-year-old woman with a history of neurofibromatosis has erratic blood pressure readings as high as 220/120 and normal sometimes. She also complains of intermittent headaches, sweating and palpitations.
270. An 18-year-old girl attends family planning clinic having recently started contraception. On examination she has a systolic murmur and weak foot impulses.

THEME: 50
CAUSES OF HYPERTENSION

Options

a. Coarctation of aorta
b. Cushing's syndrome
c. Phaeochromocytoma
d. Conn's syndrome
e. Polyarteritis nodosa
f. Polycystic kidney disease

g. Acromegaly
h. Pre-eclampsia
i. Essential hypertension
j. Renal artery stenosis
k. Chronic glomerulonephritis

For each of the situations/conditions given below, choose the one most appropriate/discriminatory option from above. The option may be used once, more than once, or not at all.

Questions

271. A 45-year-old woman presents with hypertension and confusion. She is noted to have truncal obesity, proximal muscle weakness and osteoporosis.
272. A 40-year-old man presents with hypertension and tingling in his finger. He is noted to have an enlarged tongue and prognathism. His glucose tolerance curve is diabetic.
273. A 42-year-old woman with disportionately long limbs presents with hypertension. Her BP is different in both arms and in the legs.
274. A 40-year-old man post-thyroidectomy for medullary carcinoma presents with hypertension and complains of palpitations and attacks of severe headaches. He is noted to have glycosuria.
275. A 50-year-old man presents with hypertension, haematuria and abdominal pain. A large kidney is palpated on examination.

THEME: 51
INVESTIGATIONS FOR HYPERTENSION

Options

a. Echocardiography.
b. Urinary VMA.
c. Renal angiography.
d. Pregnancy test.
e. 24 hour urinary cortisol.
f. Renal ultrasound.
g. CT scan brain.
h. ECG.

For each of the situations/conditions given below, choose the one most appropriate/discriminatory option from above. The options may be used once, more than once, or not at all.

Questions

276. A 45-year-old male presents with headaches. On examination he has coarse features, large and sweaty palms, a large jaw and a blood pressure of 180/100 mmHg.
277. An obese 55-year-old lady is diagnosed to have hypertension. Her investigations reveal she has an impaired glucose tolerance and potassium of 3.1 mmol/lit. She is not on any medication.
278. A 38-year-old male patient presented with headaches. He was found to have resistant hypertension and a CT scan of the abdomen that showed a retroperitoneal mass in the para-aortic region.
279. A 32-year-old female presented with LVF, papilloedema and a BP of 212/120 mm Hg not controlled on beta blockers, she has been taking for a month she has a family history of hypertension and her father died of a CVA at the age of 42.

THEME: 52
TREATMENT OF HYPERTENSION

Options

a. Thiazide diuretic
b. Beta blocker
c. Calcium channel blocker
d. ACE inhibitor
e. Alpha blocker
f. Angiotensin II receptor blocker
g. Moxonidine
h. Hydralazine
i. Methyldopa
j. Labetolol
k. Sodium nitroprusside

For each of the situations/conditions given below, choose the one most appropriate/discriminatory option from above. The option may be used once, more than once, or not at all.

Questions

280. A 50-year-old woman has hypertension and mild asthma with no other medical problems. Mean BP is 170/95 mmHg.
281. A 60-year-old man with claudication is already on bendrofluazide and remains hypertensive.
282. A 40-year-old man with diabetes, proteinuria and hypertension.
283. A 30-year-old woman who has developed hypertension early in her first pregnancy. She does not have any proteinuria or oedema.
284. A 45-year-old man has collapsed. He has papilloedema and multiple haemorrhages on fundoscopy. He has proteinuria. CT brain is normal. BP is 250/140 mmHg.
285. A 30-year-old man with hypertension was started on enalapril but has developed a dry cough and refuses to take the drug anymore. He is otherwise well and on no other medications.

THEME: 53
TREATMENT OF HYPERTENSION

Options

a. Atenolol
b. Bendrofluazide
c. Frusemide
d. Methyldopa
e. Amlodepine
f. Nigedopine
g. Hydralazine
h. Captopril
i. Sodium nitroprusside
j. Lisinopril
k. Non-drug treatment

For each of the situations/conditions given below, choose the one most appropriate/discriminatory option from above. The option may be used once, more than once, or not at all.

Questions

286. A 60-year-old man presents with BP of 165/95 mmHg. He is asymptomatic and all his investigations are normal.
287. A 50-year-old diabetic presents with a BP of 175/ 110 mmHg. His BP is consistently high on subsequent visits despite conservative measures. His blood tests are normal.
288. A 45-year-old asthmatic presents with BP of 180/120. All underlying causes have been excluded.
289. A 54-year-old man is brought to A&E complaining of severe headaches. On arrival he has a seizure. His BP was 220/150 and on fundoscopy there is papilloedema.
290. A 65-year-old man on atenolol 100 mg OD continues to have a diastolic BP of 115. He also takes allopurinol. A second drug is recommended.

THEME: 54
HEART DISEASES AND ASSOCIATED MALFORMATION

Options

a. Aortic stenosis.
b. Coarctation of the aorta.
c. Atrioventricular canal.
d. Pulmonary valve stenosis.
e. Patent ductus arteriosus.

For each of the situations/conditions given below, choose the one most appropriate/discriminatory option from above. The options may be used once, more than once, or not at all.

Questions

291. An infant with hypotonia, brachydactyly and trisomy for a small acrocentric autosome.

292. A 10-year-old boy who has hypertelorism, downward eye slant, mental retardation, pectus excavatum and a webbed neck.
293. A 15-year-old girl who has webbed neck, cubitus valgus, gonadal dysgenesis short, normal intelligence and 45 chromosomes as a newborn, she was noticed to have pedal edema.
294. A 20-year-old man who has coarse thickened lips, stellate iris, and mental retardation; he has a history of neonatal hypercalcemia.

THEME: 55
CAUSES OF INFECTIVE ENDOCARDITIS

Options

a. *Staphylococcus epidermidis.*
b. *Streptococcus viridans.*
c. *Staphylococcus aureus.*
d. *Streptococcus bovis.*

For each of the situations/conditions given below, choose the one most appropriate/discriminatory option from above. The options may be used once, more than once, or not at all.

Questions

295. Most Common causative agent.
296. Associated with colonic carcinoma.
297. Acute endocarditis.
298. In IV drug abuser.
299. In a patient with prosthetic value on 6th postoperation day.
300. In a patient with prior history of valvular disease.

THEME: 56
MANAGEMENT OF PATIENT ON DIGOXIN THERAPY

Options

a. Continue digoxin therapy unchanged.
b. Increase the dose of digoxin.
c. Decrease or hold further doses of digoxin.

d. Change to digitalis preparation.
e. Add propranolol or verapamil to the regimen.

For each of the situations/conditions given below, choose the one most appropriate/discriminatory option from above. The options may be used once, more than once, or not at all.

Questions

301. A 45-year-old woman who has known rheumatic heart disease, paroxysmal atrial fibrillation and chronic frusemide therapy; she returns with a new onset of nausea. Potassium level is 3.0 mEq/L. Electrocardiogram shows a regular atrial rate of 140 per minute with a 2.1 ventricular response.
302. A 49-year-old who has chronic atrial fibrillation and normal ventricular function; ventricular rate is 140 per minute and irregularly irregular. Digoxin level is 0.3 ng/ml.
303. A 65-year-old man who has mitral regurgitation, an ejection fraction of 70 percent and chronic atrial fibrillation; ventricular response is 130 per minute and irregularly irregular. Electrolytes are normal, digoxin level 2.1 ng/ml.
304. A 65-year-old woman who has chronic atrial fibrillation due to coronary artery disease with compensated congestive heart failure. She has mild exertional dyspnea but is comfortable at rest. Heart rate is 82 per minute at rest, increasing to 98 per minute when climbing one flight of stairs. Ventricular response is irregularly irregular. Digoxin level is 1.5 ng/ml.

THEME: 57
MANAGEMENT OF RHEUMATIC HEART DISEASE

Options

a. Commissurotomy of the value.
b. Prosthetic tissue valve replacement.
c. Prosthetic mechanical valve replacement.
d. Institution of indicated medical management; deferment of surgery.

For each of the situations/conditions given below, choose the one most appropriate/discriminatory option from above. The options may be used once, more than once, or not at all.

Questions

305. A 14-year-old boy with aortic stenosis who is asymptomatic. Cardiac catheterization shows no aortic valve calcification; valve area is 0.4 cm^2/m^2.
306. A 24-year-old man who has calcific aortic stenosis and a calculated valve area of 0.5 cm^2/m^2.
307. A 28-year-old woman in normal sinus rhythm who has moderate pulmonary hypertension and mitral stenosis. Cardiac catheterization shows that the mitral valve area is 0.7 cm^2, no valvular calcification is noted. The patient receives diuretics and continues to have orthopnea and dyspnea during mild exertion.
308. A 52-year-old woman with chronic atrial fibrillation who receives digoxin therapy and has well-controlled ventricular response. She is dyspnoeic during ordinary activities. Cardiac catheterization shows mild mitral stenosis and 3+ mitral regurgitation; the ejection fraction is 46 percent and the A– Vo_2 difference is 7.2 ml/dl. There is moderate pulmonary hypertension.
309. A 64-year-old man with long-standing aortic regurgitation who suffers primarily from fatigue. Cardiac catheterization shows 4+ aortic regurgitation, mild elevation in left atrial and pulmonary artery pressures and an A – VO_2 difference of 6.2 ml/dl. The ejection fraction is 42 percent. The patient has a history of diverticulosis with gastrointestinal bleeding, the precise site of bleeding has never been documented, despite extensive evaluation.

Two

Respiratory Diseases

THEME: 1
DIAGNOSTIC IMPORTANCE OF SPUTUM EXAMINATION

Options

a. Green or yellow.
b. Rusty.
c. Thin, white, mucoid.
d. Thick and sticky.
e. Large amount, watery.
f. Red current jelly.
g. Large amount, purulent and offensive.
h. Pink and frothy.

For each of the situations/conditions given below, choose the one most appropriate/discriminatory option from above. The options may be used once, more than once, or not at all.

Questions

1. Left ventricular failure.
2. Lung abscess.
3. Alveolar cell carcinoma.
4. Bronchial asthma.
5. Lobar pneumonia.
6. Bacterial infection.
7. Bronchogenic carcinoma.

THEME: 2
DIAGNOSIS OF CHRONIC COUGH

Options

a. Pulmonary embolism

b. Bronchial asthma
c. Bronchogenic carcinoma
d. Tuberculosis
e. Bronchitis
f. Fibrosing alveolitis
g. Heart failure
h. Pickwickian syndrome
i. Respiratory failure
j. Rheumatoid lung
k. Pneumonia
l. Rheumatic heart disease
m. Emphysema
n. Pneumothorax

For each of the situations/conditions given below, choose the one most appropriate/discriminatory option from above. The options may be used once, more than once, or not at all.

Questions

8. A 30-year-old accountant presents with a chronic cough, dyspnoea and wheezing. He produces copious sputum. His arterial carbon dioxide is low and his arterial oxygen is normal.
9. A 50-year-old smoker with chronic cough and copious yellow sputum presents in a state of agitation. He is confused. His pulse is bounding. He has a terrible headache and you find papilloedema on fundus examination.
10. A young woman complains of wheeze, dyspnoea and cough. She cannot sleep at night because of her chronic cough. She and her mother love animals and together they have 14 cats. Her peak flow is normal but her chest X-ray suggests hyperinflation.
11. A middle-aged housewife presents with exertion and dyspnoea. She also has a dry cough, and general malaise and is mildly cyanosed. On auscultation of chest you find crepitations. She has a history of arthritis.
12. A middle-aged smoker presents with chronic cough and phlegm. His sputum is tenacious but not yellow or blood stained. His chest is hyperinflated. His arterial carbon dioxide is high and arterial oxygen is low.

THEME: 3
PATHOLOGY OF LUNG DISORDERS

Options

a. Sarcoidosis.
b. Goodpasture's syndrome.
c. Wegener's granulomatosis.
d. Alveolar proteinosis.
e. Alveolar microlithiasis.
f. Rheumatoid arthritis.
g. Fibrosing alveolitis.
h. Cor pulmonale.
i. Cystic fibrosis.

For each of the situations/conditions given below, choose the one most appropriate/discriminatory option from above. The options may be used once, more than once, or not at all.

Questions

13. X-ray shows honeycombed appearance. PFT reveals TLC 65% of normal. FEV1/FVC = 90%. ESR 55 mm but ANA and DS-DNA negative.
14. This progressive disease of the lungs and kidneys can produce intra-alveolar hemorrhage and glomerulonephritis.
15. Granulomatous inflammation and necrosis of the lung and other organs are characteristic of this disease.
16. This disease is characterized by massive accumulations of a phospholipid-rich material in alveoli.
17. This systematic disease is characterized by the presence of non-caseating granulomas in the lung and other organs.
18. Cardiac involvement in this disease may manifest as arrhythmias and conduction disturbances.

THEME: 4
PHYSICAL SIGNS IN LUNG DISEASE

Options

Movement on side of lesion	*Trachea*	*Percussion*	*Breath Sounds Tactile Fremitus and Vocal Resonance*
a. Diminished	Usually central may be deviated away from lesion	Dull (Stony)	Diminished
b. Diminished	Usually central may be deviated away from lesion	Hyper-resonant	Diminished
c. Diminished	Central or deviated towards lesion	Dull	Increased
d. Diminished	Deviated towards affected side	Dull	Increased
e. Diminished	Central	Normal or hyper-resonant	Normal

For each of the situations/conditions given below, choose the one most appropriate/discriminatory option from above. The options may be used once, more than once, or not at all.

Questions

19. COPD.
20. Pneumonia.
21. Pneumothorax.
22. Pleural effusion.
23. Fibrosis of lung.

THEME: 5
TYPICAL X-RAY APPEARANCE IN CHEST DISEASES

Options

a. Bats wing appearance.

b. Air bronchogram.
c. Pop corn calcification.
d. Multiple ring shadows of 1 cm or larger.
e. Thin walled air cysts which are associated with a number of consolidated processes.

For each of the situations/conditions given below, choose the one most appropriate/discriminatory option from above. The options may be used once, more than once, or not at all.

Questions

24. Pulmonary oedema.
25. Bronchiectasis.
26. Hamartoma.
27. Lobar pneumonia.
28. Staphylococcal pneumonia.

THEME: 6
INVESTIGATIONS IN RESPIRATORY DISEASES

Options

a. Full blood count.
b. Chest X-ray.
c. Sputum culture and sputum microscopy.
d. PEFR.
e. Arterial blood gas analysis.
f. Lung function tests.
g. Bronchoscopy.
h. CT scan.

For each of the situations/conditions given below, choose the one most appropriate/discriminatory option from above. The options may be used once, more than once, or not at all.

Choose the next most useful investigation

Questions

29. A 45-year-old male presents with an abrupt onset of lightness in the chest, dry cough, breathlessness since last half an hour. It is increasing in severity. The patient has had

such attacks twice in the past and is known case of asthma on regular medication since last 10 years. Regular medications have failed to help. On examination Respiratory rate 50/minute, Pulse = 120/minute. Wheeze ++.

30. A 50-year-old male chronic smoker presents with chronic and a history of 2 episodes of haemoptysis in the past week. On examination, clubbing present. Chest X-ray shows mediastinal widening a large round opacity in the right hilar region.
31. 46-year-old male executive chronic smoker with a history of cough with whitish expectoration in mornings since last few years, presence of cough and increased amount of sputum, intermittently throughout the day since last few weeks. History of mild chest pain and breathlessness since one week clinical examination is non-conclusive.

THEME: 7
INVESTIGATIONS FOR RESPIRATORY DISEASES

Options

a. CT scan thorax.
b. MRI scan thorax.
c. Chest X-ray.
d. Bronchoscopy.
e. Mediastinoscopy.
f. Mediastinostomy.

For each of the situations/conditions given below, choose the one most appropriate/discriminatory option from above. The options may be used once, more than once, or not at all.

Questions

32. Mid zone mass lesions.
33. Quantification of extent of emphysema.
34. Investigation of choice in patient with suspected COPD.
35. First line of investigation for suspected bronchiectasis.
36. Investigation of choice for structural lesions of cardiovascular system.

37. Examination of right hilum.
38. Examination of left hilum.

THEME: 8
CELLULAR CONSTITUENTS IN BRONCHOALVEOLAR LAVAGE FLUID

Options

	Number of cells	*Lymphocytes*	*Macrophages*	*Neutrophils*	*Eosinophils*
a.	N	N	N	+	N
b.	++	N	D	++	N
c.	++	+	D	+	+
d.	++	++	D	N	N

Key: +—increased; N—normal; D—decreased

For each of the situations/conditions given below, choose the one most appropriate/discriminatory option from above. The options may be used once, more than once, or not at all.

Questions

39. Extrinsic allergic alveolitis.
40. Smoker.
41. Sarcoidosis.
42. Idiopathic pulmonary fibrosis.

THEME: 9
INTERPRETATION OF SPIROMETRY

Options

a. $FEV_1/FVC = 80\%$.
b. $FEV_1/FVC = 90\%$.
c. $FEV_1/FVC = 42\%$.

For each of the situations/conditions given below, choose the one most appropriate/discriminatory option from above. The options may be used once, more than once, or not at all.

Questions

43. Normal.
44. Obstructive.
45. Restrictive.

THEME: 10
PLEURAL FLUID ANALYSIS

Options

a. Neutrophils ++.
b. Lymphocytes ++.
c. Mesothelial cells ++.
d. Abnormal mesothelial cells.
e. Multinucleated giant cells.
f. Lupus erythematous cells.

For each of the situations/conditions given below, choose the one most appropriate/discriminatory option from above. The options may be used once, more than once, or not at all.

Questions

46. Mesothelioma.
47. Bacterial infection.
48. Rheumatoid effusion.
49. Secondary malignancy.
50. Pulmonary infarction.

THEME: 11
CAUSES OF EXTRINSIC ALLERGIC ALVEOLITIS

Options

a. Farmers lung.
b. Malt workers lung.
c. Humidified fever.
d. Maple bark strippers lung.
e. Vineyard sprayers lung.
f. Coffee workers lung.

For each of the situations/conditions given below, choose the one most appropriate/discriminatory option from above. The options may be used once, more than once, or not at all.

Questions

51. Cryptostroma corticale.
52. Chemicals in dust.
53. *Aspergillus clavatus.*
54. Thermophilic actinomycetes.
55. *Naegleria gruberi.*

THEME: 12
DIAGNOSIS OF LUNG DISEASES

Options

a. Bronchiectasis.
b. Cystic fibrosis.
c. Lung abscess.
d. Histiocytosis.
e. Wegener's granulomatosis.
f. Churg-Strauss syndrome.
g. Loffler's syndrome.
h. Goodpasture's syndrome.

For each of the situations/conditions given below, choose the one most appropriate/discriminatory option from above. The options may be used once, more than once, or not at all.

Questions

56. Upper respiratory tract granulomas, fleeting lung shadows and necrotising glomerulonephritis.
57. Most common, fatal inherited disease.
58. Repeated episodes of small amounts of hemoptysis with progressive dyspnea and cough.
59. In chronic cases, may be associated with secondary amyloid, which is further associated with peripheral edema and proteinuria.
60. Occurs on background of chronic uncontrolled asthma.

THEME: 13
DIAGNOSIS OF RESPIRATORY DISEASES

Options

	PO_2 mm Hg.	O_2 Saturation (%)	PCO_2 mm Hg.	$[HCO_3]$ (mEq/L)	pH
a.	120	99	20	19	7.60
b.	104	99	24	12	7.25
c.	81	95	51	45	7.58
d.	62	92	34	23	7.46
e.	38	65	65	26.2	7.22
f.	60	80	30	26	7.34

For each of the situations/conditions given below, choose the one most appropriate/discriminatory option from above. The options may be used once, more than once, or not at all.

Questions

61. Fulminant status asthmaticus.
62. Long-standing pyloric obstruction.
63. Hysterical hyperventilation.
64. Diabetic ketoacidosis.
65. Emphysematous chronic obstructive pulmonary disease (COPD).
66. Pulmonary embolism.

THEME: 14
DIAGNOSIS OF BREATHLESSNESS

Options

a. Cor pulmonale.
b. Left ventricular failure.
c. Type II respiratory failure.
d. Bronchospasm.
e. Psychogenic paralysis.

f. Diaphragmatic paralysis.
g. Increased left atrial pressure.
h. Inflammatory infiltration of the interstitium of the lung.

For each of the situations/conditions given below, choose the one most appropriate/discriminatory option from above. The options may be used once, more than once, or not at all.

Questions

67. Recent headache in a patient with chronic cough. ABG shows CO_2 retention.
68. Paroxysmal nocturnal dyspnoea associated with frothy sputum.
69. History of heart attack.
70. Recent episode of ankle swelling with the acute exacerbation of his bronchitis.
71. Occurs immediately after lying down.
72. Occurs 60-120 minutes after onset of sleep.
73. Occurs five minutes after cessation of exercise.
74. Improves or remains unchanged during exercise.
75. Worsens in the late afternoon or evening and improves over the weekend.

THEME: 15
CAUSES OF BREATHLESSNESS

Options

a. Anaemia
b. Bronchogenic carcinoma
c. Pneumothorax
d. Pneumonia
e. Pleural effusion
f. Inhaled foreign body
g. Pulmonary oedema
h. Extrinsic allergic alveolitis
i. Pulmonary embolism
j. Bronchial asthma
k. Cryptogenic fibrosing alveolitis

For each of the situations/conditions given below, choose the one most appropriate/discriminatory option from above. The options may be used once, more than once, or not at all.

Questions

76. An 80-year-old man has been short of breath for a few weeks. His chest X-ray shows a right basal shadow rising towards his axilla.
77. A 30-year-old farmer presents with fever, malaise, cough and breathlessness which he has had for a few days. His symptoms were worse in the evening. Clinical examination demonstrated coarse inspiratory crackles.
78. A 48-year-old train conductor complains of chronic productive cough. He is also a heavy smoker.
79. A 50-year-old woman on HRT presents with swollen left calf, chest pain and shortness of breath.
80. A 50-year-old woman presents with progressive breathlessness and cyanosis. Clinical examination reveals clubbing and bilateral inspiratory crackles.
81. A 30-year-old tall slim porter presents with the sudden onset of chest pain and breathlessness. He has similar episodes in the past.

THEME: 16
CAUSES OF BREATHLESSNESS

Options

a. Valvular heart disease
b. Atelactasis
c. Bronchial carcinoma
d. Pulmonary embolus
e. Metastatic carcinoma
g. Anaemia
h. Bronchial asthma
i. Atypical pneumonia
j. Acute pulmonary oedema
k. Exacerbation of chronic bronchitis
l. Sinusitis

For each of the situations/conditions given below, choose the one most appropriate/discriminatory option from above. The options may be used once, more than once, or not at all.

Questions

82. A 70-year-old man with a history of chronic productive cough now presents to Accident and Emergency with shortness of breath and is drowsy.
83. A 50-year-old male patient on the ward awakes with dyspnoea and frothy sputum. He had suffered an MI a week earlier. On examination, he is cyanosed and tachypnoeic. Auscultation of the lungs reveal bilateral crepitations.
84. An 18-year-old girl is brought into Accident and Emergency with very difficult and noisy breathing.
85. A 35-year-old airline steward presents with one week history of fever, dry cough and shortness of breath. On examination, he is tachypnoeic. His lungs are clear on auscultation.
86. A 58-year-old woman presents with dyspnoea. On examination, she has a firm mass in the left breast and decreased breath sounds in the right lower lung fields. Chest X-ray reveals a pleural effusion.

THEME: 17
CAUSES OF BREATHLESSNESS

Options

a. Cystic fibrosis
b. Histoplasmosis
c. Pneumothorax
d. Pneumocystis carinii infection
e. Acute MI
f. Bronchiectasis
g. Extrinsic allergic alveolitis
h. Cryptogenic fibrosing alveolitis
i. Churg-Strauss syndrome
j. Allergic bronchopulmonary aspergillosis
k. Goodpasture's syndrome

l. Pulmonary embolism
m. Primary thyrotoxicosis

For each of the situations/conditions given below, choose the one most appropriate/discriminatory option from above. The options may be used once, more than once, or not at all.

Questions

87. A 35-year-old man presented with breathlessness at rest, cough and haemoptysis all of which he has had for a few days. On examination he is cyanosed and there are bilateral inspiratory and expiratory wheezes. His peak flow is normal. Blood investigations show evidence of renal failure.
88. A 10-year-old boy has had measles two-year-ago, and now presents with a productive cough associated with occasional haemoptysis.
89. A 45-year-old man presents with progressive burning pains in the soles of his left foot, bilateral cramps in both calves, and left foot drop. He is known asthmatic and suffers from recurrent sinusitis. Full blood count shows eosinophilia.
90. A 70-year-old man presents with pneumonia which he has had for two weeks and which was resistant to antibiotics. He has had asthmatic bronchitis for more than 50 years. Chest X-ray shows consolidation on the right upper zone and left perihilar consolidation. Blood tests show neutrophilia .
91. A healthy young woman comes to you complaining of a swelling in front of the neck and diarrhoea. She also has palpitations and is short of breath.

THEME: 18
TREATMENT OF DYSPNOEA

Options

a. Chest drainage
b. Intravenous antibiotics in combination with steroids
c. Pain relief

d. Rebreathing or sedation
e. Treatment with anti-malarial drugs
f. Anticoagulation
h. Correction of acidosis with IV bicarbonate
i. IV insulin
J. Rapid rehydration with normal saline
k. Thrombolysis

For each of the situations/conditions given below, choose the one most appropriate/discriminatory option from above. The options may be used once, more than once, or not at all.

Questions

92. A 48-year-old man has developed mild dyspnoea and position of chest pain, mainly lying flat. His ECG shows ST Segment elevations in most leads.
93. A 22-year-old patient with non-insulin dependent diabetes has become progressively breathless over the last 24 hours. His PH is 7.2 and his pCO_2 is 2.2 Kpa. The blood glucose concentration was 24 mmol/l.
94. A 30-year-old drug addict complains of severe shortness of breath for the last 3 days. The symptoms have developed gradually. Physical examination of his chest is normal, but his pulse oximeter readings are low at about 65-70% on air.
95. A 35-year-old man has suddenly developed dyspnoea after a prolonged holiday in Thailand. His pulse oximeter reading is 80 %, but you are not able to detect any abnormalities over the lungs.
96. A 25-year-old woman is admitted with severe shortness of breath. Her respiratory rate is 48 breaths per minute. Her blood gas results are pH 7.5, pO_2 of 14 Kpa, pCO_2 2.0 Kpa.

THEME: 19
MANAGEMENT OF BREATHLESSNESS

Options

a. Oxygen therapy

b. Radiotherapy
c. Antidepressants
d. Iron supplements
e. Change of occupation
f. Lobectomy
g. Edrophonium chloride
h. Chemotherapy
i. Blood transfusion
j. Anticoagulants
k. Thymectomy

For each of the situations/conditions given below, choose the one most appropriate/discriminatory option from above. The options may be used once, more than once, or not at all.

Questions

97. A middle-aged woman complains of dyspnoea over the past year. She had to give up her gardening. An ECG shows right ventricular hypertrophy and strain.
98. A 40-year-old shipyard worker complains of gasping for breath. On physical examination you discover mild cyanosis and restricted chest movements.
99. A 60-year-old man says he cannot get enough air. Over the past few months he has become increasingly breathless. Also, he has noticed he has had difficulty finishing his dinner. His jaw tires.
100. A 40-year-old woman presents with increasing breathlessness over a period of 10 months. She now finds herself unable to climb stairs. Also she has just had her third child in three-year-and complains of feeling depressed.
101. An elderly woman cannot carry on her household chores but has to sit down every few minutes. A chest X-ray shows diffused reticular nodular shadows, especially in her lower lobes.

THEME: 20
DIAGNOSIS OF ABNORMAL CHEST X-RAYS

Options

a. Histiocytosis

b. Idiopathic thrombocytopenia
c. Hyperthyroidism
d. Asthma
e. Lung fibrosis
f. Bronchogenic carcinoma
g. Sarcoidosis
h. Aspergillus fumigatus
i. Polyarteritis nodosa
j. Silent MI
k. Pleurisy
l. Tuberculosis

For each of the situations/conditions given below, choose the one most appropriate/discriminatory option from above. The options may be used once, more than once, or not at all.

Questions

102. A middle-aged pharmaceutical engineer presents with increasing breathlessness and cough. He does not smoke. On chest X-ray you find diffuse bilateral mottling and multiple small cystic lesions. Six months ago he had a pneumothorax.
103. A 35-year-old computer engineer with a long history of asthma and rhinitis presents with wheezing, cough and fever. A chest X-ray shows patchy consolidation. Physical examination shows multiple tender subcutaneous nodules and purpura.
104. A 40-year-old man presents with chest pain and cough. He complains of fullness and pressure in the chest and a sharp pain affecting two or three ribs on the right side. A chest X-ray shows a right-sided hilar enlargement.
105. A young woman complains of sore eyes, dull chest pain, malaise and a low grade fever. She thinks she has had a recurrent low grade fever for four months. Her chest X-ray shows bilateral hilar enlargement.
106. For the last four-year-a young man has complained of recurrent bouts of pneumonia and wheeziness, cough, fever and malaise. His sputum is tenacious. Peripheral blood shows a very high ESR and IgE.

THEME: 21
DIAGNOSIS OF CHRONIC OBSTRUCTIVE PULMONARY DISEASE

Options

a. Cystic fibrosis.
b. Extrinsic asthma.
c. Chronic bronchitis.
d. Immotile cilia syndrome.
e. Alpha antitrypsin deficiency.

For each of the situations/conditions given below, choose the one most appropriate/discriminatory option from above. The options may be used once, more than once, or not at all.

Questions

107. A 22-year-old man with mild diabetes mellitus, who has daily cough productive of one-cup thick sputum.
108. A 25-year-old woman with recurrent episodes of shortness of breath and cough shortly after moving into a new apartment.
109. A 26-year-old man with chronic productive cough for 10 years, recurrent sinusitis and infertility.
110. A 42-year-old male cigarette smoker with dyspnea and nonproductive cough associated with a history of recurrent pneumothorax and chronic hepatitis.
111. A 56-year-old nonsmoking male miner with a daily productive cough during the winter months for the past four years.

THEME: 22
SIDE EFFECTS OF DRUGS ON RESPIRATORY SYSTEM

Options

a. Asthma.
b. Pulmonary infiltration.
c. Pulmonary eosinophilia.
d. SLE like syndrome

e. Respiratory depression.
f. Opportunistic infections.

For each of the situations/conditions given below, choose the one most appropriate/discriminatory option from above. The options may be used once, more than once, or not at all.

Questions

112. Nitrofurantoin.
113. Beta-blockers.
114. Barbiturates.
115. Hydralazine.
116. Bleomycin.

THEME: 23
CAUSES OF PNEUMONIA

Options

a. *Bacteroides fragilis.*
b. *Coxiella burnettii.*
c. *E. coli.*
d. *Haemophilus influenzae.*
e. *Leigonella pneumophila.*
f. Mixed growth of organisms.
g. *Mycobacterium tuberculosis.*
h. *Mycoplasma pneumoniae.*
i. *Pneumocystis carinii.*
j. *Staphylococcus aureus.*
k. *Streptococcus pneumoniae.*

For each of the situations/conditions given below, choose the one most appropriate/discriminatory option from above. The options may be used once, more than once, or not at all.

Questions

117. A 25-year-old man has a three-day history of shivering, general malaise and productive cough. The X-ray shows right lower lobe consolidation.

118. A 26-year-old man presents with severe shortness of breath and dry cough which he has had for 24 hours. He is very distressed. He has been an IV drug abuser. The X-ray shows perihilar fine mottling.
119. A 35-year-old previously healthy man returned from holiday five days ago. He smokes 10 cigarettes a day. He presents with mild confusion, a dry cough and marked pyrexia. His chest examination is normal. The X-ray shows widespread upper zone shadowing.
120. A 20-year-old previously healthy woman presents with general malaise, severe cough and breathlessness which has not improved with a seven-day course of amoxycillin. There is nothing significant to find on examination. The X-ray shows patchy shadowing throughout the lung fields. The blood film shows clumping of red cells with suggestion of cold agglutinins.
121. A 40-year-old smoker with a history of acute exacerbation of obstructive airway disease presents with breathlessness not being controlled with nebuliser at home and fever. Examination reveals cyanosis at the lips with pursing, extensive bilateral wheeze and bronchial breathing at the right lower zones. Investigations reveal Hb 16 g/dl, TLC 11.5 x 10^9/lit. Sputum culture showed gram-negative bacilli.

THEME: 24
CAUSES OF PNEUMONIA

Options

a. Bronchiectasis
b. *H. influenzae*
c. Lung cancer
d. *Pneumocystis carinii*
e. *Streptococcus pneumoniae*
f. Viral
g. Aspiration
h. Fungal infection
i. *Klebsiella pneumoniae*

j. *Mycoplasma pneumoniae*
k. *Staphylococcus aureus*
l. Tuberculosis
m. *Legionella pneumoniae*

For each of the situations/conditions given below, choose the one most appropriate/discriminatory option from above. The options may be used once, more than once, or not at all.

Questions

122. A previously well 20-year-old girl has had influenza for the last two weeks. She is deteriorating and has a swinging fever. She is coughing up copious amounts of purulent sputum. Chest X-ray shows cavitating lesions.
123. A 30-year-old male prostitute has felt generally unwell for two months with some weight loss. Over the last three weeks he has noticed a dry cough with increasing breathlessness. Two courses of antibiotics from the GP have produced no improvement. Chest X-ray shows bilateral interstitial infiltrates.
124. A 60-year-old man with COPD presents with pneumonia. Clinically he improves with antibiotics. In the outpatient clinic four weeks later, the consolidation on his chest X-ray has not resolved.
125. A 20-year-old male patient has just returned from holiday abroad and presents with flu-like illness, headaches, high fever. Prior to this he had complained of abdominal pain, vomiting, diarrhoea which was associated with blood per rectum.
126. A 40-year-old woman presents with four months history of productive cough and recent haemoptysis. She has lost 5 kgs in weight. The chest X-ray shows right upper lobe consolidation.
127. A 70-year-old man currently undergoing chemotherapy for chronic leukaemia has felt unwell with fever and unproductive cough for two weeks despite treatment with broad spectrum IV antibiotics. Chest X-ray shows an enlarged right sided mid zone consolidation.

128. On return to University a 24-year-old student presents with the onset of fever, malaise and a dry cough. The student health service gave him Amoxycillin. After a week he felt no better and his chest X-ray showed a patchy bilateral consolidation.

THEME: 25
CAUSES OF PNEUMONIA

Options

a. *Pneumocystis carinii*
b. Tuberculosis
c. Aspergillosis
d. *Streptococcus pneumoniae*
e. *Psuedomonas aeruginosa*
f. *Streptococcus* infection
g. *Chlamydia* infection
h. *Mycoplasma pneumoniae*
i. *Coxiella burnettii*
j. Actinomycosis
k. *Staphylococcus aureus*
l. *Legionella pneumophila*
m. *Klebsiella*

For each of the situations/conditions given below, choose the one most appropriate/discriminatory option from above. The options may be used once, more than once, or not at all.

Questions

129. A 35-year-old man who works in an abattoir presents with sudden onset of fever, mylagia, headache, dry cough and chest pain. His chest X-ray shows patchy consolidation of the right lower lobe giving ground glass appearance.
130. A 35-year-old man with HIV presents with a productive cough and haemoptysis. Chest X-ray shows a round ball in the right upper lobe surmounted by a dome of air.
131. A 20-year-old man presents with dry cough, skin rash and bone and muscle aches. His chest X-ray shows wide

spread patchy shadows. Blood tests show evidence of haemolysis.

132. A 65-year-old alcoholic man presents with sudden purulent productive cough. His chest X-ray shows consolidations in the left upper lobe.
133. A 40-year-old pet shop owner presents with high fever, excruciating headaches and a dry hacking cough. Chest X-ray shows patchy consolidation.
134. A 50-year-old travelling insurance salesman presents with high fever, mylagia and abdominal pain and haemoptysis. Chest X-ray shows diffused patchy lobular shadowing. A cough progressive from a modest non-productive cough to producing mucopurulent sputum. The fever persists for two weeks.
135. A 65-year-old woman presents with confusion and productive cough. Her chest X-ray shows right lower lobe consolidation.

THEME: 26
CAUSES OF HAEMOPTYSIS

Options

a. Tuberculosis
b. Foreign body inhalation
c. Bronchogenic carcinoma
d. Bronchiectasis
e. Wegener's granulomatosis
f. Pulmonary infarction
g. Mitral stenosis
h. Haemorrhagic telangiectasia
i. Pneumonia
j. SLE
k. Polyarteritis nodosa

For each of the situations/conditions given below, choose the one most appropriate/discriminatory option from above. The options may be used once, more than once, or not at all.

Questions

136. A 70-year-old woman who had a total hip replacement a week ago presents with severe chest pains, shortness of breath and haemoptysis.
137. A 50-year-old bank manager presents with cough, pleuritic chest pain and haemoptysis. This was proceeded by rhinitis, recurrent epistaxis and haematuria. Chest X-ray shows multiple nodular masses.
138. A 70-year-old Asian immigrant presents with cough, haemoptysis, night fever and sweating.
139. A 60-year-old smoker with a long history recurrent chest infection presents with haemoptysis and greenish sputum. On examination he has clubbing and coarse crepitations over the bases of both lungs.
140. A 50-year-old diabetic presents with fever, pleuritic pain and rusty coloured sputum.
141. A 65-year-old smoker presents with cough, haemoptysis and weight loss. On examination, there is clubbing and gynaecomastia.

THEME: 27
INVESTIGATION OF HAEMOPTYSIS

Options

a. Clotting studies
b. Chest X-ray
c. Antinuclear antibodies and free DNA
d. CT of chest
e. Urinalysis
f. Tissue biopsy
g. Full blood count
h. Bronchoscopy
i. 12 lead ECG
j. Anti-GBM antibody
k. Heaf test
l. Pulmonary angiogram
m. Sputum cytology

For each of the situations/conditions given below, choose the one most appropriate/discriminatory option from above. The options may be used once, more than once, or not at all.

Question

142. A 35-year-old man presents with haemoptysis, dyspnoea and haematuria. Chest X-ray reveals bilateral alveolar infiltrates. Urinalysis reveals the presence of protein and red cell casts.
143. A 35-year-old IV drug abuser presents with dyspnoea and haemoptysis. His chest X-ray is unremarkable and ECG shows a sinus tachycardia. Blood gas shows a low PCO_2 and elevated pH.
144. A 48-year-old man presents with occasional haemoptysis and chronic productive cough. He has a history of recurrent pneumonia. Chest X-ray reveals peribronchial fibrosis.
145. A 45-year-old man presents with recurrent epistaxis, haemoptysis and haematuria. On examination, he has a nasal septal perforation and nodules on chest X-ray.
146. A 55-year-old man presents with a chronic cough and mild haemoptysis. On examination, he has digital clubbing with pain and swelling around his wrists. Chest X-ray reveals a single nodule.

THEME: 28
INVESTIGATION OF HYPERVENTILATION

Options

a. Chest X-ray
b. CT brain
c. ABG
d. Blood glucose
e. Blood count and blood film
f. V/Q scan
g. Salicylate levels
h. Spiral CT with contrast.
i. Urea and electrolytes

j. Serum lactose
k. Echocardiogram
l. Non required.

For each of the situations/conditions given below, choose the one most appropriate/discriminatory option from above. The options may be used once, more than once, or not at all.

Questions

147. A 20-year-old motorcycle courier was involved in a head on collision with a van. He had an obvious deformity of his left thigh and knee. X-ray confirmed communted fracture of the shaft of the femur that was reduced and placed in traction. Five days later he suddenly deteriorates and becomes drowsy, confused and febrile. He is hyperventilating and cyanosed. There are crackles at both lung bases and petechia over his chest and neck.
148. A 20-year-old car mechanic is brought to casualty by his girlfriend. She describes a two day history of rigors, sweats and intermittent confusion. On examination he is agitated, sweaty and pyrexial with a temperature of 38.6°C. He is hyperventilating and cyanosed despite receiving oxygen by facemask. There is dullness to percussion and bronchial breathing of the left lung base.
149. A 30-year-old teacher who is seven months pregnant, presents with sudden collapse and breathlessness. On examination, she is afebrile, severely cyanosed and hyperventilating. Her pulse is 140/min and blood pressure 70/30 mm Hg.
150. A 30-year-old nurse is brought to casualty as an emergency. She is hyperventilating but drowsy. She has been complaining of nausea and tinnitus and had an episode of haematemesis.
151. A 13-year-old schoolgirl was out with her friends at a party last night. When she returned home this morning she was drowsy, unwell, and vomiting. She has lost 5 kg over last two months. On arrival at hospital, she is drowsy, confused and hyperventilating but not cyanosed. Her breath smells of pear drops.

152. A 16-year-old boy presents to casualty complaining of severe chest pain and difficulty breathing. He is hyperventilating and pale but not cyanosed. He has had 4 similar admissions in the last-year-and his older brother also attends the hospital frequently.

THEME: 29

INVESTIGATION OF RESPIRATORY DISEASE

Options

a. Serum precipitins and high resolution CT
b. Arterial blood gas
c. Sputum culture
d. Fibre-optic bronchoscopy
e. Immediate expertise help
f. Static lung volumes with reversibility
g. Bronchial lavage
h. Mantoux test
i. Serum calcium, ACE levels and transbronchial biopsy
j. Echocardiogram
k. Flow volume loop
l. ECG, blood gases and perfusion scan

For each of the situations/conditions given below, choose the one most appropriate/discriminatory option from above. The options may be used once, more than once, or not at all.

Questions

153. A 50-year-old farmer with intermittent dry cough, fever, dyspnoea, progressive weight loss and fine crepitations on auscultation.
154. A 40-year-old Nigerian woman develops clubbing, erythema nodosum, iritis and dyspnoea. On her chest X-ray you see lymphadenopathy.
155. A 50-year-old caucasian childminder in Glasgow presents with dry cough, nightsweats and haemoptysis.
156. A 60-year-old life long smoker has had a dry cough, weight loss and haemoptysis. Chest xray and CT show right middle lobe collapse. He is sent to the chest clinic for investigation.

157. A 25-year-old male develops sudden onset of dyspnoea, chest pain on inspiration and haemoptysis whilst straining at stool. He had a cholecystectomy 10 days previously. He rapidly becomes cyanosed and loses consciousness. On examination his blood pressure is 75/50 mmHg. His pulse is thready with a rate of 160/min and his pulmonary component of second heart sound is loud. His JVP is raised by 6 cm.

THEME: 30
CAUSES OF PULMONARY OEDEMA

Options

a. Myocarditis
b. Mitral regurgitation
c. Aortic stenosis
d. Iatrogenic
e. Adult respiratory distress syndrome
f. Acute renal failure
h. Myocardial infarction
i. Cardiomyopathy
j. Mitral stenosis
k. Constrictive pericarditis
l. Hypoalbuminaemia
m. Anaemia

For each of the situations/conditions given below, choose the one most appropriate/discriminatory option from above. The options may be used once, more than once, or not at all.

Questions

158. A 40-year-old woman was admitted to hospital two days ago with abdominal pain and vomiting. She was tender in the epigastrium and it was found to have a very high serum amylase level. She has been treated with large volumes of IV fluid and has maintained a good urine output. None the less she has been persistently hypoxic and is deteriorating rapidly. She now has crackles throughout both lung fields and a pO_2 of 5.1Kpa despite receiv-

ing 60% oxygen by mask. A chest X-ray shows massive bilateral pulmonary oedema. Her serum albumin is 30 mmol/litre.

159. A 70-year-old woman presents to casualty with acute breathlessness. She has had 3 similar admissions in the last few months. She has a past history of rheumatic fever. On examination, she has an irregular pulse of 110 bpm. She has a non-displaced tapping beat with no evidence of left ventricular dysfunction. No murmurs are audible. There are crepitations heard in both lower lung fields.
160. A 25-year-old man has become increasingly breathless over a period of four days. He has also had severe central chest pain and a fever. He was previously fit and well. On examination, he looks unwell, cyanosed and dyspnoeic. Pulse is 120/min regular and his blood pressure is 90/40 mmHg. His JVP is elevated and he has a gallop rhythm with no murmurs. There are crackles in both lung bases. Chest X-ray shows pulmonary oedema and a normal heart. ECG shows extensive ST elevation in the anterior and inferior leads without Q waves.

THEME: 31
MANAGEMENT OF PNEUMOTHORAX

Options

a. Observation only.
b. Simple aspiration.
c. Large bore tube drainage.
d. Indwelling catheter drainage.
e. Thoracoscopy/thoracotomy.

For each of the situations/conditions given below, choose the one most appropriate/discriminatory option from above. The options may be used once, more than once, or not at all.

Questions

161. Failed simple aspiration.
162. Traumatic minor pneumothorax.

163. Recurrent pneumothorax.
164. Pneumothorax with mild dyspnea.
165. Spontaneous pneumothorax.
166. Persistent air leak.

THEME: 32
CAUSES OF PLEURAL EFFUSION

Options

a. Hypoalbuminaemia
b. Emphysema
c. Bronchial carcinoma
d. Meig's syndrome
e. Rheumatoid arthritis
f. Yellow nail syndrome
g. Cardiac failure
h. Pneumonia
i. Tuberculosis
j. Mesothelioma
k. Pleural metastasis
l. SLE

For each of the situations/conditions given below, choose the one most appropriate/discriminatory option from above. The options may be used once, more than once, or not at all.

Questions

167. A 55-year-old woman presents with increasing breathlessness and abdominal swelling. She has a right sided pleural effusion. Examination of abdomen reveals ascites and large pelvic mass.
168. A 60-year-old retired builder has a three month history of cough and left sided chest pain. He has a pleural effusion on the left. On chest X-ray there is evidence of pleural calcification.
169. A 70-year-old woman presents with a two months history of increasing breathlessness and swollen legs. On examination, she has a raised JVP and a left sided pleural effusion.

170. A 35-year-old woman presents with a three day history of pyrexia, rigors and sweats. This was proceeded by a one week history of cough and increasing dyspnoea. She had a swinging fever and dullness to percussion at the left lung base.
171. A 30-year-old IV drug abuser presents with a three week history of cough, fever and general malaise with occasional haemoptysis. He has a right sided pleural effusion.
172. A 60-year-old woman presents with a intermittent breathlessness and cough. On examination, she has a right sided pleural effusion and discoloured nails.

THEME: 33
MANAGEMENT OF PLEURAL EFFUSION

Options

a. Observation only.
b. Simple aspiration.
c. Large bore tube drainage.
d. Indwelling catheter drainage.
e. Thoracoscopy/thoracotomy.

For each of the situations/conditions given below, choose the one most appropriate/discriminatory option from above. The options may be used once, more than once, or not at all.

Questions

173. Emphysema.
174. Failed chemical pleurodesis.
175. Asymptomatic pleural effusion of known cause.
176. Traumatic hemothorax.
177. Tuberculosis effusion.
178. For symptomatic relief.

THEME : 34
MANAGEMENT OF BREATHLESSNESS

Options

a. Intramuscular adrenalin.
b. Intubation and assisted ventilation.

c. Chest drain with under water seal.
d. Intravenous frusemide.
e. Nebulised salbutamol.
f. Nebulised beclomethasone.
g. IV hydrocortisone.

For each of the situations/conditions given below, choose the one most appropriate/discriminatory option from above. The options may be used once, more than once, or not at all.

Questions

179. A 15-year-old female came to casualty with sudden onset breathlessness following a bee sting. On examination, she is cyanosed, has puffy eyelids, pulse 112/min, BP 90/60 mm Hg, RR 30/min and bilateral extensive rhonchi.
180. A tall, 30-year-old female collapsed while playing hockey. On examination she is cyanosed, pulse 120/min, RR – 30/min, BP 90/60 mm Hg, trachea shifted to the left, reduced air entry on the right, tympanic note on percussion on the right side of chest.
181. A 40-year-old patient is admitted into casualty with breathlessness on examination she has an irregular pulse 106/min, BP 108/76 mm Hg, a loud 1st heart sound with a mid-diastolic murmur and no third heart sound.
182. A 60-year-old female patient presents with weakness and breathlessness. On examination pulse 105/min, BP 100/68 mm Hg, RR 26/min, equal air entry with central trachea. She has a bilateral ptosis, grade 2/5 power in all her limbs, and deep tendon reflexes are lost. Chest X-ray is normal and blood gases show PaO_2 7.3 kPa and $PaCO_2$ 9.1 kPa.

THEME: 35
MANAGEMENT OF CHEST COMPLAINTS

Options

a. Chest wall drain
b. Stop smoking
c. Amoxycillin

d. Aspiration
e. Bronchial lavage
f. Ipratropium
g. Salbutamol
h. Postural drainage
i. Pleurectomy
j. CPAP
k. Prednisolone
l. Bronchoscopy
m. Surgical excision
n. Aminophylline

For each of the situations/conditions given below, choose the one most appropriate/discriminatory option from above. The options may be used once, more than once, or not at all.

Questions

183. A 40-year-old man who has had recurrent chest infections since a serious bout of influenza three-year-ago presents with chronic productive cough. His sputum is tenacious and blood stained. On auscultation you find crackles.
184. A middle-aged woman brings her husband into your surgery. She complains of his heavy snoring. Also in the middle of the night he stops breathing, gags and wakes up. His performance at work has been declining and he has been threatened with retirement.
185. A young man with chronic hepatitis develops chest complaints. He has become breathless and coughs. He has lost weight and his joints bother him. On physical examination you note mild cyanosis.
186. A 60-year-old man comes to you and complains of wheeziness and coughing. He has tried to give up smoking but he finds it very difficult. He is thin and healthy looking with a rounded chest. His breathing is noisy. His cough is unproductive.
187. A woman who has been treated for hypothyroidism, cannot breath at night. She must sit propped up and she has a constant dull chest pain. On examination of her chest you find stony dullness and bronchial breathing.

THEME: 36
MANAGEMENT OF AIRWAY OBSTRUCTION

Options

a. IM adrenaline 1:1000
b. Oxygen 60% and salbutamol nebuliser
c. IV dexamethasone
d. Tracheostomy
e. Endotracheal intubation
f. Cricothyroidotomy
g. Heimlich manoeuvre
h. Adrenaline nebuliser
i. Oxygen and IV aminophylline
j. Hyperbaric oxygen
k. Needle thoracocentesis
l. Suction of mucus block

For each of the situations/conditions given below, choose the one most appropriate/discriminatory option from above. The options may be used once, more than once, or not at all.

Questions

188. A 7-year-old girl presents acutely with stridor. She is using her accessory muscles of respiration. She is distressed and tacypnoeic.
189. A 25-year-old woman is brought to casualty by ambulance having sustained gross maxillofacial deformities following a high speed RTA. She is now agitated and hypoxic.
190. A 13-year-old girl presents to casualty after being stung by a wasp. She is acutely distressed and dyspnoeic and develops stridor.
191. A 75-year-old woman with tracheostomy tube presents with difficulty in breathing. She is apyrexial. She complains that her tube feels blocked.
192. A 12-year-old boy presents with a boiled sweet stuck in his throat, he is in respiratory distress and cyanotic.

193. A 15-year-old boy with a history of asthma presents acutely with shortness of breath and expiratory wheezing. His respiratory rate is 30 per minute. On auscultation, he now has a silent chest.
194. A 25-year-old man collapses in the street. His wife states that he has been bothered by a sore throat recently. The paramedics arrive, assess his airway, attempt and fail intubation. He now has laryngeal spasm and is turning blue.
195. A 5-year-old boy presents with high fever and stridor. He is in severe respiratory distress. He is drooling saliva.
196. A 65-year-old man with a history of bronchitis presents with tacypnoea and wheezing throughout the chest.

THEME: 37
TREATMENT OF ASTHMA IN CHILDHOOD

Options

a. Adrenaline
b. Inhaled long acting bronchodilator
c. IV aminophylline
d. Oral steroids
e. Oral theophylline
f. Regular oral bronchodilator
g. As required oral bronchodilator
h. Desensitization
i. Inhaled sodium cromoglycate
j. Inhaled steroid
k. Intermittent inhaled bronchodilators
l. Nebulised bronchodilators

For each of the situations/conditions given below, choose the one most appropriate/discriminatory option from above. The options may be used once, more than once, or not at all.

Questions

197. A 9-year-old boy with a mild cough and wheeze after playing football in the cold weather.
198. A 6-year-old girl with asthma uses her bronchodilator twice a day to relieve her mild wheeze. Her parents refuse to give her any treatment containing corticosteriods.

199. A 9-year-old girl with chronic asthma presents to the accident and emergency Department with rapidly worsening wheeze not relieved with inhaled bronchodilators. Steroids have been given orally.
200. A 4-year-old boy with recurrent wheeze whenever he gets a viral infection has now developed night cough. There has been no improvement in spite of using inhaled bronchodilators twice each night.
201. A 14-year-old boy with well controlled asthma using inhaled steroids and a bronchodilator comes to the Accident and Emergency Department with breathlessness and swollen lips after eating a peanut butter sandwich.

THEME: 38
MODES OF ARTIFICIAL RESPIRATION

Options

a. Controlled mandatory.
b. Intermittent mandatory.
c. Synchronized intermittent mandatory.
d. Pressure support.
e. Pressure controlled.
f. Continuous positive airway pressure.
g. Inverse ratio.
h. Assist/control.
i. High-frequency jet.

For each of the situations/conditions given below, choose the one most appropriate/discriminatory option from above. The options may be used once, more than once, or not at all.

Questions

202. All breaths initiated and delivered via the ventilator.
203. Ventilator provides a minimum minute volume, but not synchronized with patient effort.
204. Ventilator provides a minimum minute volume by augmenting a proportion of patient-initiated breaths.
205. Machine delivers an inspiratory pressure in response to patient effort.

206. Similar to pressure support, but does not require patient effort, breath rate, timing determined by the machine.
207. Pressure is the same in inspiration as in expiration: requires spontaneous respiratory effort.
208. Inspiratory time longer than expiratory (converse of normal).
209. Breaths are machine initiated and delivered (controlled. or patient initiated and augmented (assisted; the proportion of each depends on patient effort and machine back-up rate.
210. Ventilation is achieved using tidal volumes lower than the anatomical dead-space at very high frequencies; gas movement in the airways occurs primarily by convection.

THEME: 39
LUNG CARCINOMA

Options

a. Epidermoid carcinoma.
b. Adenocarcinoma.
c. Large cell carcinoma.
d. Small cell carcinoma.
e. Bronchio-alveolar carcinoma.

For each of the situations/conditions given below, choose the one most appropriate/discriminatory option from above. The options may be used once, more than once, or not at all.

Questions

211. The most common type of lung cancer associated with hypercalcemia.
212. Most responsive to cytotoxic chemotherapy.
213. Overall best survival by natural history or after surgery.
214. Most commonly associated with ectopic endocrine syndromes.
215. This variety of lung cancer is frequently diffuse at presentation and may be associated with profuse sputum production.

216. A 58-year-old man with a heavy smoking history who has hemoptysis, a 4 cm mass in the superior segment of the right lower lobe and ipsilateral hilar lymph adenopathy.
217. A 61-year-old man with a heavy smoking history who has a large right hilar mass, mediastinal widening anemia, and abnormal liver function tests.
218. A 66-year-old woman who has progressive systemic sclerosis, diffuse interstitial fibrosis, and multiple enlarging infiltrates through both lung fields.
219. A 66-year-old woman with recent development of grand mal seizures who has a 2.5 cm nodule in the periphery of the left upper lobe.
220. A 68-year-old man with a heavy smoking history who has a 4 cm wide, bulky mass in the periphery of the left lower lobe.

THEME : 40
DIAGNOSIS OF CHEST INJURIES

Options

a. Tension pneumothorax
b. Cardiac tamponade
c. Pulmonary contusion
d. Open pneumothorax
e. Flail chest
f. Haemothorax
g. Rib fracture
h. Myocardial contusion
i. Diaphragmatic rupture

For each of the situations/conditions given below, choose the one most appropriate/discriminatory option from above. The options may be used once, more than once, or not at all.

Questions

221. A 60-year-old man involved in a road traffic accident complains of chest pains. He was driving the car and rear-ended the front car with some force. A friction rub is elic-

ited. His ECG shows multiple premature ventricular ectopic beats.

222. A 42-year-old man is stabbed in the chest and is brought to Accident and Emergency with shortness of breath. A 4 cm stab wound is noted, and the wound is heard to "suck" with each breath.
223. A 35-year-old man is stabbed in the left side of his chest and is brought to Accident and Emergency. He is short of breath and restless. His chest is clear to auscultation. There is a rise in venous pressure with inspiration. The CXR shows a globular-shaped heart.
224. A 35-year-old man is stabbed in the back and is brought to the Accident and Emergency in respiratory distress. His blood pressure is 90/50 with a pulse rate of 110. He has dull breath sounds over his left chest. You leave the knife *in situ*.
225. A 42-year-old man sustains blunt trauma to his chest and presents with marked dyspnoea. A nasogastric tube is inserted to decompress his stomach. On CXR, the nasogastric tube is seen on left side of the chest.

THEME: 41
INVESTIGATION OF CHEST TRAUMA

Options

a. Chest drain
b. CT of the chest
c. MRI scanning
d. Pericardiocentesis
e. Abdominal ultrasound
f. Chest X-ray
g. Needle thoracocentesis

For each of the situations/conditions given below, choose the one most appropriate/discriminatory option from above. The options may be used once, more than once, or not at all.

Questions

226. A 25-year-old horse rider has sustained a crush injury to the chest when her horse landed on her during a fall. On

examination you find tenderness on the right side of her chest with decreased breath sounds and dullness to percussion. Her vital signs are pulse of 110 bpm and blood pressure is 100/80 mm Hg.

227. A 30-year-old motorcyclist involved in a road traffic accident complains of difficulty in breathing. He has a breathing rate of 40/min, decreased chest movements and air entry on the right, along with hyper-resonance on percussion on the right side. His pulse oximeter readings are around 80% on oxygen.
228. A 40-year-old man was involved in a high speed road traffic accident. He is unconscious with evidence of bruising across his chest. Despite intravenous fluid replacement with 4 litres of Hartmann's solution, he remains hypotensive. His X-ray shows a widened mediastinum.
229. A 32-year-old driver of a car involved in a head-on collision has evidence of blunt chest trauma to the sternum area. His blood pressure is 90/60 mm Hg with a pulse of 120/min. He has prominent neck veins and muffled heart sounds. Chest X-ray is normal.
230. A 40-year-old man has been stabbed in the left lower chest from behind with a 5 cm long blade. His BP is 80/60 mmHg with a pulse of 110/min. He has normal breath sounds and no evidence of pneumothorax on X-ray.

THEME: 42
TREATMENT OF CHEST TRAUMA

Options

a. Obtain portable chest X-ray
b. Needle thoracocentesis
c. Thoracotomy tube insertion at the 9 th intercostal space
d. Perform CPR and defibrillate
e. Pericardiocentesis
f. Exploratory laparotomy
g. Peritoneal lavage
h. Immediate thoracotomy of left chest
i. Immediate thoracotomy and simultaneous laparotomy in theatre

j. CPR adrenaline and intubate
k. Atropine one mg IV and intubate

For each of the situations/conditions given below, choose the one most appropriate/discriminatory option from above. The options may be used once, more than once, or not at all.

Questions

231. A 35-year-old man is shot in the left axillary line at the 7th intercostal space. He has a thoracotomy tube inserted that drains 200 mls per hour of blood. The bleeding persists. Abdominal X-ray shows a bullet in the abdomen.
232. A 30-year-old man is stabbed in the left chest under his nipple. His blood pressure is 80/50 with a pulse rate of 120/min. He has distended neck veins. His BP on repeat measuring drops to 70/50. He has vesicular breath sounds bilaterally.
233. A 28-year-old man is brought to casualty after being stabbed in the left anterior chest. He collapses in casualty. ECG shows electromechanical dissociation.
234. A 25-year-old man is stabbed in the left axillary line at the 6th intercostal space. He has no breath sounds on the left side of his chest. He has distended neck veins. His blood pressure is 80/50.
235. A 30-year-old man is shot in the left axillary line at the 7th intercostal space. He has no breath sounds on the left side. At thoracotomy tube is inserted at the 2nd intercostal space. No blood is drained. The blood pressure drops even further.

Three

Neurology

THEME: 1
CAUSATIVE AGENTS FOR MENINGITIS

Options

a. *E. coli.*
b. *H. influenza.*
c. *Meningococcus.*
d. *Pneumococcus.*
e. *Staphylococcus.*
f. *Pseudomonas.*

For each of the situations/conditions given below, choose the one most appropriate/discriminatory option from above. The options may be used once, more than once, or not at all.

Questions

1. From CSF shunts.
2. Adults.
3. Neonates.
4. From spinal procedure.
5. Children.
6. Elderly and immunocompromised.

THEME: 2
CAUSES OF MENINGITIS

Options

a. Malaria
b. Leptospirosis
c. Paramyxovirus
d. *H. influenzae*

e. *Meningococcus*
f. *Pneumococcus*
g. *Staphylococcus aureus*
h. *Mycobacterium tuberculosis*
i. Syphilis
j. Epstein Barr virus
k. Candidiasis
l. *Cryptococcus neoformans*

For each of the situations/conditionss given below. Choose the one most appropriate/discriminatory options from above. The options may be used once, more than once or not at all.

Questions

7. A sewer worker presents with jaundice, fever, signs of meningism painful calves and bruising.
8. A teenager with photophobia, fever, seizures, positive Kernig's sign and a petechial rash.
9. IV drug abuser with established AIDS presents with suspected meningitis. The organism is confirmed in the CSF by India Ink staining.
10. A18-year-old boy presents with fever, malaise and severe unilateral pain and swelling over the parotid area. He subsequently develops headache, neck stiffness and photophobia.
11. A 45-year-old man returns from holiday and develops a dry cough. His wife complains that he sweats excessively at nights. When he finally coughs up blood, she takes him to GP where he also admits to having chronic vague headache, loss of appetite, intermittent vomiting and an episode of collapse at work during which he was seen to jerk all limbs.

THEME: 3
THE IMMEDIATE MANAGEMENT OF MENINGITIS

Options

a. Acyclovir
b. Antipyretics

c. Cranial computed tomography (CT) scan
d. High dose steroids
e. Intravenous (IV) 20% dextrose
f. Intravenous (IV) plasma expansion
g. Intravenous (IV) sodium bicarbonate
h. Lumbar puncture
i. Naso-gastric tube insertion
j. Thick and thin blood film
k. Treat immediate contacts
l. Urinary catheter

For each of the situations/conditions given below, choose the one most appropriate/discriminatory option from above. The options may be used once, more than once, or not at all.

Questions

12. A 6-year-old girl, who has never been immunised,has been treated with amoxycillin for otitis media. After five days, she is more unwell with fever, headache, photophobia, neck stiffness but no alteration in consciousness. Her fundi and blood pressure are normal.
13. A previously well college student aged 19, is found unconscious by his friend. On arrival at the Accident and Emergency Department, he has a tachycardia, weak pulse and a rapidly spreading purpuric rash.His college doctor has given him intramuscular penicillin.
14. A 32-year-old known AIDS patient has three week history of increasing vomiting, headache and weight loss. On examination, she is confused and has papilloedema and pulse rate of 60 beats/minute.
15. A 7-year-old boy developed fever, neck stiffness and photophobia on morning after a schoolmates birthday party. He has a petechial rash and antibiotics were started for suspected meningococcal infection. He is now stable and receiving all necessary immediate treatment.
16. A 43-year-old journalist visited Sierra Leone in west Africa to cover the on going war for 5 days. A day after returning at home in Islington, he has a sudden fever, rigors and stiff neck and shoulders. On examination he has excoriated urticarial lesions of his ankles and mild jaundice.

THEME: 4
TREATMENT OF MENINGITIS

Options

a. Benzylpenicillin
b. Chloramphenicol
c. Ampicillin
d. Rampicin, isoniazid, ethambutol and pyrazinamide.
e. Amphotericin B and flucytosine
f. Gentamicin
g. Erythromycin
h. Cefotaxime
i. Oral rifampicin
j. Vancomycin
k. Supportive treatment

For Each of the situations/conditions given below, choose the one most appropriate/discriminatory option from above.The options may be used once, more than once, or not at all.

Questions

17. A 3-year-old girl presents with acute onset of pyrexia, nausea and vomiting. Lumbar puncture reveals high protein and polymorph count and low glucose. Gram-negative bacilli present in the smear and culture.
18. A 40-year-old man presents with fever and meningeal signs. His lumbar puncture reveals 20/mm^3 mononuclear cells, 2g/l of protein and a glucose level half the plasma level. There are no organisms in the smear.
19. A 17-year-old girl presents with fever, odd behaviour, purpura and conjunctival petechiae. Her lumbar puncture reveals gram -ve cocci.
20. A 22-year-old man presents with fever, headache and drowsiness. His lumbar puncture reveals 1000 mononuclear cells/mm^3, 0.5 g/l of protein and a glucose greater than two-third of his plasma glucose level. Organisms are absent.
21. A 25-year-old husband of a patient admitted with pyogenic meningitis admits to having oral contact with his wife and is anxious.

THEME: 5
CSF ANALYSIS

Options

	Cell count	*Glucose*	*Protein*
a.	$< 4/mm^3$	> 60% of RBS	0.15 – 0.5 g/lit 2.8 – 4.2 m mol/lit
b.	< 90 – 1000	decreased	1.5 g/lit
c.	10-350	decreased	1 – 5 g/lit
d.	50- 1500	normal	< 1 g/lit
e.	0 – 100	decreased	normal/increased
f.	50 – 500	decreased	increased
g.	$< 4/mm^3$	normal	increased
h.	0 – 50	normal	normal

For each of the situations/conditions given below, choose the one most appropriate/discriminatory option from above. The options may be used once, more than once, or not at all.

Questions

22. Malignancy.
23. Tuberculous meningitis.
24. Multiple sclerosis.
25. Normal CSF.
26. Subarachnoid hemorrhage.
27. Pyogenic meningitis.
28. Viral meningitis.
29. Fungal meningitis.

THEME : 6
LOCALISATION OF CNS LESION

Options

a. Non-dominant parietal lobe.
b. Dominant occipital lobe.
c. Dominant temporal lobe.
d. Dominant frontal lobe.
e. Dominant parietal lobe.

For each of the situations/conditions given below, choose the one most appropriate/discriminatory option from above. The options may be used once, more than once, or not at all.

Questions

30. A 45-year-old male stroke patient, who is a college graduate is unable to add the numbers 5, 2 and 3.
31. A 30-year-old woman with a head injury can follow spoken instructions but is unable to express herself verbally.
32. A 40-year-old man who has been involved in a serious automobile accident, seems to be alert and oriented but does not seem to understand what is being said to him.
33. A 48-year-old stroke patient is unable to copy completely, a simple drawing of a clock face.
34. A 45-year-old man who suffered a stroke can write a sentence that is dictated to him but he is unable to read the sentence aloud.

THEME: 7
LOCALISATION OF PATHOLOGY

Options

a. Subarachnoid bleed due to aneurysm in circle of Willis.
b. Pituitary tumor.
c. Left posterior inferior cerebellar artery.
d. Parasagittal meningioma.
e. Tumor localized to right parietal lobe.
f. Left cerebellar tumor.
g. Right cerebellar tumor.
h. Right temporal lobe tumor.

For each of the situations/conditions given below, choose the one most appropriate/discriminatory option from above. The options may be used once, more than once, or not at all.

Questions

35. A 20-year-old student complains of severe headache of 10 minutes duration and collapses. On examination he is febrile, drowsy but arousable. On examination has neck stiffness and a dilated left pupil.

36. Patient presents with gradually progressing weakness of the left upper limb. On examination there is no wasting, has grade 2/6 power, hypertonia and biceps, triceps and supinator jerks are exaggerated.
37. Has sudden onset of vertigo, dizziness and difficulty in swallowing. Preliminary neurological testing reveals a left side's cerebellar signs, nystagmus, loss of sensation over the left half of face and loss of pain and temperature on the right half of the torso and right upper and lower limbs.
38. A 60-year-old female wakes up with weakness of right side of body. Examination reveals no wasting, grade 2/6 power of right upper and lower limbs, hypotonia and diminished deep tendon reflexes on the right side. The right plantar is however upgoing.

THEME: 8
NEUROLOGICAL DISORDERS

Options

a. Subdural haematoma
b. Guillain Barré syndrome
c. Frontal lobe abscess
d. Brainstem haemorrhage
e. Petit mal epilepsy
f. Multiple sclerosis
g. Benign intracranial hypertension
h. Arnold-Chiari malformation
i. Meningitis
j. Normal pressure hydrocephalus
k. Motor neurone disease

For each of the situations/conditions given below, choose the one most appropriate/discriminatory option from above. The option may be used once, more than once, or not at all.

Questions

39. A 37-year-old engineer was started on diuretics 3 months ago for hypertension. A few weeks later he was admitted to A&E with vomiting, acute vertigo and gross incoordination. On examination there was bilateral nystagmus.

40. A 78-year-old hypertensive woman is referred for fluctuating level of consciousness. On examination her blood pressure is 175/110, fundus examination showed some hypertensive changes, her reflexes are bilaterally brisk and her plantars are upgoing.
41. A 26-year-old presents with weeks history of headache and diplopia. On examination she is obese and fundoscopy shows bilateral papilloedema.
42. A 28-year-old diplomat presented with sudden onset blurring of vision in left eye. A week earlier he noted progressive clumsiness of the right hand. A few months earlier he noted progressive clumsiness of the right hand. A few months earlier he had had an episode of left leg stiffness that resolved spontaneously.
43. A 19-year-old soldier is brought semiconscious into A&E. He has been complaining of severe headache and vomiting of 1 day duration. On examination there is widespread maculopapular rash all over his body.
44. A 36-year-old previously fit man developed a flu like illness which was followed 2 days later by burning pain on both legs. He later developed urinary retention and diplopia. On examination his straight leg raising test was positive bilaterally, ocular mobility was limited bilaterally but sensation was intact.

THEME: 9
DIAGNOSIS OF NEUROLOGICAL DISORDER

Options

a. Multiple sclerosis
b. Lateral medullary syndrome
c. Sagittal sinus thrombosis
d. Guillain-Barré syndrome
e. Motor neurone disease
f. Arnold-Chiari malformation
g. Normal pressure hydrocephalus
h. Myasthenia gravis
i. Herpes simplex encephalitis
j. Peripheral neuritis

k. Benign intracranial hypertension

For each of the situations/conditions given below choose the one most appropriate/discriminatory option from above. The option may be used once, more than once, or not at all.

Questions

45. A 35-year-old clerk presents with diplopia and fatigue. Her symptoms are worse towards the evenings.
46. A 33-year-old carpenter presents with unsteadiness of gait, in coordination of both arms and oscillopsia on down gaze. Clinical examination demonstrates a low hair line, positive Romberg's test and bilateral extensor plantars.
47. A 70-year-old man present with urinary incontinence and poor muscle coordination. On examination he is slightly confused, but apyrexial and there is no papilloedema. 2-year-ago he had meningitis which was successfully treated with antibiotics.
48. A previously fit 60-year-old lawyer is admitted to A&E with a 3 day history of progressively bizarre and aggressive behaviour. On examination she is confused and pyrexial. EEG shows abnormal complexes over the temporal lobe.
49. A 58-year-old man presents with progressive clumsiness and difficulty in performing fine tasks with both hands. On examination there is slight wasting of the intrinsic muscles of both hands but more marked on the left. Reflexes and coordination are normal and there is no sensory deficit.

THEME: 10
DIAGNOSIS OF NEUROLOGICAL DISORDERS

Options

a. Guillain-Barré syndrome
b. Labrynthitis
c. Anterior spinal artery occlusion
d. Alzheimer's disease
e. Shy Drager syndrome
f. Multiple sclerosis

g. Gliobastoma multiforme
h. Vertebral artery occlusion
i. C.I. D.P
j. Cauda equina syndrome
k. Parkinson's disease
l. Meningioma

For each of the situations/conditionss given below, choose the one most appriopriate/discriminatoy option from aboce. The options may be used once, more than once, or not at all.

Questions

50. A 24-year-old diver developed headache, dizziness, right sided hemiparesis and loss of pain and temperature sensation in the right facial and left side of the body following a dive.
51. A healthy 76-year-old woman presented after a fall. On examination there was weakness of both legs with loss of pain and temperature sensation and a-reflexia. Her bladder was distended.
52. A 58-year-old man, presented with a 10 month history of impotence. On examination there was bradykinesia, rigidity, postural hypotension, ataxia and tremors.
53. A 75-year-old woman presented with a 3 week history of headache and progressive confusion. On examination she had right hemianopia. CT showed a large irregularly enhancing mass in the left parietal lobe. There was no evidence of systemic disease.
54. A healthy 72-year-old man presented with a 3 month history of progressive difficulty walking. On examination he had distal weakness in the arms and legs. Muscle stretch reflexes were absent. Motor nerve conduction velocities were slowed.

THEME : 11
SEIZURE DISORDER

Options

a. Simple partial seizure.
b. Complex partial seizures.

c. Tonic–clonic (grand mal) seizures.
d. Absence (petit mal) seizures.
e. Myoclonic seizures.
f. Status epilepticus.

For each of the situations/conditions given below, choose the one most appropriate/discriminatory option from above. The options may be used once, more than once, or not at all.

Questions

55. Seen in Creutzfeldt-Jakob disease.
56. Temporal lobe most common site of origin.
57. A generalised seizure without convulsive muscular activity.
58. Can result in "Jacksonian march".
59. Almost always starts in childhood.

THEME: 12
DIAGNOSIS OF EPILEPSY

Options

a. Partial seizures
b. Generalized epilepsy
c. Myoclonic jerks
d. Infantile spasms
e. Gestault seizures
f. Benign rolandic seizure
g. Petit mal epilepsy
h. Fifth day fits
i. Febrile convulsions
j. Hypocalcemic fits
k. Focal with secondary generalized fits

For each of the situations/conditionss given below. Choose the one most appropriate/discriminatory options from above. The options may be used once, more than once or not at all.

Questions

60. A 14-year-old girl who has been academically brilliant lately has had difficulty with her school work. She has been caught day dreaming in class on a number of occasions.

61. A 6-year-old girl was rushed to the hospital with a fit that involved all her upper and lower limbs. She has an upper respiratory infection a few-year-ago. On examination she does have a red throat and is pyrexial.
62. A 12-year-old girl was found in bed- in the early morning having left sided jerks. She was also salivating from the side of the mouth and seemed unresponsive for a few minutes.
63. A newborn baby is born to mother of Pakistani origin. The baby has a generalized seizure involving her arms and legs.
64. A 6-month-old baby has jerking episodes lasting a few minutes at a time. During these episodes the baby is seen to flex his arm and legs and the head also flexes. The child has 3-4 episodes every hour.

THEME: 13
INVESTIGATION OF EPILEPSY

Options

a. Blood culture
b. Blood glucose
c. Lumbar puncture
d. CT scan head
e. Mantoux test
f. EEG
g. Full blood count
h. Chest X-ray
i. Urea and electrolytes
j. Blood alcohol level
k. Toxicology screen
l. Skull X-ray

For each of the situations/conditions given below, Choose the one most appropriate/discriminatory option from above. The option may be used once, more than once, or not at all.

Questions

65. A 53-year-old obese man presents with sweating, tremor, drowsiness, fits and agitation. His wife denies any history of alcoholism.

66. A 12-year-old girl is brought to A&E by her parents complaining of persistent rash, photophobia and neck pain.
67. A 35-year-old mechanic has recurrent epileptiform attacks. He has no history of trauma.
68. An 18-year-old student is brought to the A&E by ambulance having been flung off his bicycle in a RTA. Upon arrival, he is noted to have deterioration in consciousness.
69. A 32-year-old boxer presents with headache, drowsiness, seizures and a rising blood pressure.

THEME: 14
INVESTIGATION OF SEIZURES

Options

a. Serum calcium
b. Serum glucose
c. Serum electrolytes
d. Serum urea and creatinine
e. Serum LFTs
f. Full blood count
g. CT scan of head
h. Lumbar puncture
i. VDRL
j. Chest X-ray
k. Drug levels
l. EEG
m. ESR
n. Anti-ds DNA

For each of the situations/conditions given below. Choose the one most appropriate/discriminatory option form above. The options may be used once, more than once or not at all.

Questions

70. A 50-year-old alcoholic presents with sweating, tachycardia and convulsions.
71. A 40-year-old diabetic started on tetracycline for severe apthous ulceration now presents with epilepsy and vomiting.

72. A 10-year-old boy presents with fits for the first time. His parents report that he stops talking in mid sentence and then continues were he left off 10 secs later.
73. A 15-year-old female presents with fits and fever. She is noted to have petechial rash that does not blanch on pressure.
74. A 30-year-old woman presents with fits and arthralgia. She is noted to have thinning of her hair and oral ulceration.

THEME: 15
MANAGEMENT OF SEIZURE DISORDER

Options

a. Phenytoin.
b. Sodium valporate.
c. Carbamazepine.
d. Ethosuximide.
e. None of the above.

For each of the situations/conditions given below, choose the one most appropriate/discriminatory option from above. The options may be used once, more than once, or not at all.

Questions

75. A 2-year-old boy with generalised seizures and a temperature of 39.5 degree Celsius.
76. A 5-year-old girl who has been mistakenly considered "inattentive" and "a daydreamer".
77. A 20-year-old woman who jerks involuntarily in response to sensory stimulation or movement.
78. A 24-year-old man who persistently smacks the lips with an arrest of other activities.
79. A 37-year-old man with focal motor seizures that spread up the extremities toward the trunk.

THEME: 16
TYPES OF APHASIAS

Options

	Speech output	*Comprehension*	*Repetition*
a.	Very scant, patient May be mute	impaired	impaired
b.	Non-fluent	intact	impaired
c.	Fluent, even excessive	impaired	impaired
d.	Fluent	intact	impaired
e.	Non-fluent	intact	intact
f.	Fluent	impaired	intact

For each of the situations/conditions given below, choose the one most appropriate/discriminatory option from above. The options may be used once, more than once, or not at all.

Questions

80. Conduction aphasia.
81. Global aphasia.
82. Transcortical sensory aphasia.
83. Motor aphasia.
84. Transcortical motor aphasia.

THEME: 17
TYPES OF NEUROGENIC BLADDER

Options

	Bladder Sensation	*Bladder Emptying*	*Bladder Capacity*	*Bladder Tone*
a.	Preserved	complete but uninhibited	reduced	normal
b.	Lost	gets emptied as soon as it gets filled	reduced	increased
c.	Lost	constant dribbling	decreased	increased
d.	Preserved	distended bladder, severe pain	increased	decreased
e.	Lost	distended, painless	increased	decreased

For each of the situations/conditions given below, choose the one most appropriate/discriminatory option from above. The options may be used once, more than once, or not at all.

Questions

85. Motor denervated.
86. Reflex neurogenic.
87. Neuropathic.
88. Sensory denervated.
89. Autonomous.

THEME: 18
DIAGNOSIS OF MYOPATHIES

Options

a. Duchenne dystrophy.
b. Limb-girdle dystrophy.
c. Myotonia congenita.
d. Myotonic dystrophy.
e. Facioscapulohumeral dystrophy.

For each of the situations/conditions given below, choose the one most appropriate/discriminatory option from above. The options may be used once, more than once, or not at all.

Questions

90. An autosomal dominant inheritance; there is difficulty in relaxing muscles but no weakness.
91. An autosomal dominant inheritance; it is associated with cataracts, testicular atrophy, and baldness in males.
92. An autosomal recessive inheritance; it begins in adolescence with normal or slightly increased muscle enzymes.
93. An autosomal dominant inheritance; it begins in adolescence and occasionally involves the truncal muscles.
94. An X-linked recessive inheritance; it begins in childhood and muscle enlargement is common.

THEME: 19
MANAGEMENT OF MYASTHENIA GRAVIS

Options

a. Corticosteroids
b. Radiotherapy and chemotherapy
c. Partial thymectomy
d. Thymectomy and radiotherapy
e. Total thymectomy
f. Expectant management
g. Anticholinesterases
h. Azathioprine
i. Radiotherapy
j. Chemotherapy

For each of the situations/conditions given below. Choose the one most appropriate/discriminatory option from above. The option may be used once, more than once or not at all.

Questions

95. Malignant thymoma
96. Generalized myasthenia gravis with a benign thymoma.
97. Ocular myasthenia gravis with a normal thymus gland
98. Benign thymoma
99. Generalized myasthenia gravis with a normal thymus gland.

THEME: 20
DIAGNOSIS OF MUSCLE WEAKNESS

Options

a. Syringomyelia
b. Charcot-Marie tooth disease
c. Subacute combined degeneration of cord
d. Multiple sclerosis
e. Bell's palsy
f. Guillain-Barré syndrome
g. Poliomyelitis
h. Motor neurone disease

i. Dermatomyositis
j. Polymyalgia rheumatica
k. SLE

For each of the situations/conditions given below. Choose the one most appropriate/discriminatory option from above. The options may be used once, more than once, or not at all.

Questions

100. A 45-year-old woman presents with a purple rash on her cheeks and eyelids and insidious symmetrical proximal muscle weakness.
101. A 40-year-old woman presents with diplopia on lateral gaze, nystagmus paraesthesiae, and muscle weakness, CSF examination reveals oligoclonal band and an increase in IgG.
102. A 30-year-old man presents with week after upper respiratory tract infection with paraesthesiae which rapidly develop to flaccid paralysis of the lower limbs. The CSF examination shows very high protein but no white cells.
103. A 25-year-old man presents with flaccid paralysis of the legs with loss of reflexes. He reports recovering from a mild upper respiratory tract infection but then developing meningitis. The CSF shows raised protein and increased lymphocytes.
104. A 35-year-old man presents solely with palsy of the left side of his face including his forehead. His otological examination and other cranial nerves are normal.

THEME: 21
DIAGNOSIS OF SMALL MUSCLE WASTING OF HAND

Options

a. Parkinson's disease.
b. Syringomyelia.
c. Motor neuron disease.
d. Duchene's muscular dystrophy.
e. Carpal tunnel syndrome.
f. Myotonic dystrophy.
g. Cervical spondylitis.

h. Guillain-Barré syndrome.
i. Hereditary motor sensory neuropathy.

For each of the situations/conditions given below, choose the one most appropriate/discriminatory option from above. The options may be used once, more than once, or not at all.

Questions

105. Overweight female patient comes to you with aching of hands. She is obese and has pulse of 55/min. On examination there is wasting of thenar eminence and weakness of adductor pollicis brevis bilaterally with loss of sensation over the lateral three and half fingers.
106. A 45-year-old male patient complains of weakness of his left hand and arm. On examination he has wasting of the small muscles of the left hand with fasciculation. Biceps and triceps reflexes on the right side were exaggerated and sensation was normal.
107. A 20-year-old male patient presents with a painless ulcer on his right index and middle fingers. On examination he has wasting of the small muscles of the hand bilaterally with loss of pain and temperature sensation over both hands and arms with preservation of vibration and position sense.
108. A balding middle-aged male patient comes to you with weakness of both hands and arms gradually progressing. On examination there is bilateral ptosis, cataracts and there is wasting of small muscles of both hands with no fasciculation or sensory loss.

THEME: 22
DIAGNOSIS OF STROKE /TRANSIENT ISCHAEMIC ATTACK(TIA)

Options

a. Carotid artery stenosis
b. Cerebellar haemorrhage
c. Cerebral embolus
d. Cerebral haemorrhage
e. Cerebral vasculitis

f. Migraine
g. Subarachnoid haemorrhage
h. Subdural haematoma
i. Temporal arteritis
j. Vertebrobasilar TIA

Questions

109. A 27-year-old woman has a long standing history of headaches associated with nausea and vomiting .On this occasion she presents with sudden loss of vision in the right half of the visual field. By the time you see her it has improved considerably.
110. An 82-year-old woman complains of increasing weakness and muscle pain to the point where she is finding it difficult to brush her hair and get out of a chair. She now presents with a sudden loss of vision in her left eye.
111. A 74-year-old woman had a fall two weeks ago. She is brought into the A&E department with slowly increasing drowsiness. On examination you find mild hemiparesis and unequal pupils.
112. A woman previously in good health presents with sudden onset of severe occipital headache and vomiting. Her only physical sign on examination is a stiff neck.

THEME: 23
CEREBROVASCULAR DISEASE

Options

a. TIA involving the carotids
b. Sagittal sinus thrombosis
c. Extradural haemorrhage
d. Lateral medullary syndrome
e. Subarachnoid haemorrhage
f. Subdural hemorrhage
g. Cerebellar haemorrhage
h. Lacunar infarction
i. Hypertensive encephalopathy
j. Pseudobulbar palsy
k. TIA involving the vertebro-basilar system

For each of the situations/conditions given below, choose the one most appropriate/discriminatory option from above. The options may be used once, more than once or not all.

Questions

113. A 73-year-old man presents with hemianopia, hemisensory loss, hemiparesis and aphasia of 16 hrs duration.
114. A 80-year-old women presents with hemianopia, hemisensory loss, ataxia, choking, dysarthria and vertigo.
115. A 60-year-old hypertensive and diabetic is admitted with acute dizziness, vomiting and difficulty in moving his right arm and leg. On examination there is Horner's syndrome on the right side.
116. A 58-year-old man presented to A&E with severe headache and drowsiness which started suddenly while he was working on the computer. He had vomited once. On examination he was apyrexial,his pulse was 100 and blood pressure was 160/100 mmHg.
117. A 72-year-old man was referred by his GP for recurrent headaches and fluctuating level of consciousness. There was no history of direct head trauma.

THEME: 24
SITE OF NEURO MUSCULAR DISORDERS

Options

a. Anterior horn cell.
b. Peripheral nerve.
c. Neuromuscular junction.
d. Muscle.

For each of the situations/conditions given below, choose the one most appropriate/discriminatory option from above. The options may be used once, more than once, or not at all.

Questions

118. Reflexes are decreased out of proportion to weakness.
119. Diurnal fluctuations are common.

120. Atrophy early and marked.
121. Most likely to cause distal weakness.
122. Characteristic facial features.

THEME : 25
DIAGNOSIS OF LEG WEAKNESS

Options

a. Syringomyelia.
b. Myopathies.
c. Disc prolapse.
d. Motor neuron disease.
e. Friedrich's ataxia.

For each of the situations/conditions given below, choose the one most appropriate/discriminatory option from above. The options may be used once, more than once, or not at all.

Questions

123. Unilateral foot drop.
124. Absent knee jerks and extensor plantars.
125. Chronic spastic paraparesis.
126. Weak legs with no sensory loss.
127. Chronic flaccid paraparesis.

THEME : 26
DIAGNOSIS OF HEADACHE

Options

a. Migraine.
b. Tension.
c. Giant cell arteritis.
d. Acute glaucoma.
e. Cluster headache.
f. Carotid artery stenosis
g. Cerebellar haemorrhage
h. Temporal neuralgia
i. Cerebral vasculitis
j. Subarachnoid haemorrhage

k. Chronic subdural haematoma
l. Polymyalgia rheumatica
m. Vertebro-basilar TIA
n. Paget's disease

For each of the situations/conditions given below, choose the one most appropriate/discriminatory option from above. The options may be used once, more than once, or not at all.

Questions

128. A 60-year-old female patient while watching a movie suddenly developed sudden blindness in right eye and headache. Blood reports showed raised ESR, raised alkaline phosphatase and raised CRP.
129. A 50-year-old male executive, following a meeting, develops a headache and notices a tender scalp on combing his hair.
130. A 40-year-old smoker presents with acute onset headache, which lasts for 40 minutes. The pain is localized around the eye and it is bloodshot.
131. A 62-year-old female patient develops sudden onset headache around the right eye while watching a movie. Headache is associated with reduced vision and circumcorneal redness/nausea/vomiting.
132. A 40-year-old female patient develops unilateral headache which is associated with nausea, vomiting and photophobia.
133. A deaf 56-year-old woman complains of a chronic headache. She is found to have sabre tibiae.
134. A 59-year-old man previously in good health presents with sudden onset of severe occipital headache and vomiting. His only physical sign on examination is a stiff neck.
135. A 38-year-old woman suffers paroxysms of intense stabbing pain lasting only a few seconds in the face. It is precipitated by talking.
136. A 34-year-old chronic alcoholic had a fall two weeks ago. He now presents with slowly increasing drowsiness and headache.

THEME: 27
INVESTIGATION FOR HEADACHE

Options

a. Carotid arteriography
b. Computed tomography (CT) scan
c. Electroencephlogram (EEG)
d. Erythrocyte sedimentation rate (ESR)
e. Fundoscopy
f. Intraocular pressure
g. Lumbar puncture
h. Magnetic resonance imaging (MRI)
i. Mental state examination
j. Nasalendoscopy
k. Skull X-ray
l. Temporal artery biopsy
m. Toxoplasma serology
n. Visual fields
o. Psychiatric history

Questions

137. A 34-year-old woman has a generalised headache, described as a tight band, unrelieved by paracetamol. She has difficulty sleeping and says she has lost weight recently.
138. A 51-year-old woman has a severe headache aggravated by brushing her hair. She says she has been generally unwell for a few months with aching muscles.
139. A 71-year-old woman has severe headache aggravated by brushing her hair. She says she has been generally unwell for a few months with aching muscles.
140. A 14-year-old boy presents with drowsiness and generalised headache. He is recovering from a bilateral parotitis. His CT scan is normal.
141. A 32-year-old man presents with headache, photophobia and sudden reduction in visual acuity. His fundi look pale.
142. A 54-year-old man is brought to the Accident and Emergency with a 6 months history of headache. His wife says

that he has also become progressively more forgetful, tends to lose temper and is emotionally labile. There is no history of loss of weight, infectious disease or trauma.

143. A 55-year-old man with blurred vision complains of headache which he has had for past 5 months. Coughing and sneezing seem to worsen the headache.
144. An obese 31-year-old woman is brought to the Accident and Emergency Department with a severe occipital headache of 2 hours duration. She is unable to move her left hand and leg.
145. A 23-year-old homosexual man complains of a headache of 3 weeks duration. A Computed tomography scan is done and shows multiple "ring "enhancing lesions.
146. A 34-year-old man with blurred vision comlpains of a severe headache of 1 hour duration. He also complains of pain on chewing.

THEME: 28
CAUSES OF HEADACHE

Options

a. Meningitis
b. Migraine
c. Cluster headache
d. Tension headache
e. Subarachnoid hemorrhage
f. Sinusitis
g. Benign intracranial hypertension
h. Cervical spondylosis
i. Giant cell arteritis
j. Otitis media
k. Transient ischaemic attack

For each of the situations/conditions given below. Choose the one most appropriate/discriminatory option form above. The options may be used once, more than once or not at all.

Questions

147. A 25-year-old woman presents with episodes of unilateral throbbing headache, nausea and vomiting. She states

that it is aggravated by light. The episodes seem to occur prior to her menstruation.

148. A 40-year-old man presents with severe pain around his right eye with eyelid swelling lasting 20 min. He has had several attacks during past weeks. The attacks are worse at night.
149. A 10-year-old boy presents with fever, headache, left eye pain and swelling. He described his vision as blurry. He has recently recovered from a cold.
150. A 60-year-old female presents with bitemporal headache, unilateral blurry vision and pain on combing hair. Her ESR is elevated.
151. A 30-year-old obese female presents with headache and diplopia. On examination she has papilloedema. She is alert with no focal symptoms or signs.

THEME: 29
MANAGEMENT OF HEADACHE

Options

a. Carbamazepine.
b. Ergotamine.
c. Lithium.
d. Indomethacin.
e. Biofeedback.

For each of the situations/conditions given below, choose the one most appropriate/discriminatory option from above. The options may be used once, more than once, or not at all.

Questions

152. Migraine.
153. Cluster.
154. Tension.
155. Trigeminal neuralgia.
156. Paroxysmal hemicranial headache.

THEME: 30
MANAGEMENT OF HEADACHE

Options

a. Listen, counsel and reassure
b. ESR, high dose steroids
c. Repeated lumbar puncture,dexamethasone
d. CT scan head and lumbar puncture
e. History and clinical features
f. EEG
g. Skull X-ray
h. Autoantibody screen
i. Sinus X-ray
j. Visual acuity
k. High dose IV antibiotics
l. ECG

For each of the situations/conditionss given below. Choose the one most appropriate/discriminatory options from above. The options may be used once, more than once or not at all.

Questions

157. A 52-year-old man presents with chronic dull band like headache with scalp tenderness worse at night.
158. A 17-year-old girl admitted with headache and seizures. On examination she has papilloedema, bradycardia and petechial rash.
159. An 18-year-old girl presents with premenstrual unilateral headache associated with vomiting and a need to lie in the dark.
160. A 58-year-old woman with pain in her jaw on eating, headache and fleeting visual disturbances.
161. A 21-year-old student describes severe headache followed by vomiting, left sided weakness and loss of consciousness. There are no focal neurological sign. Fundoscopy at this stage is normal.
162. A 32-year-old obese woman complains of headache on waking which is worsened by coughing. She also has blurred vision and occasionally sees double. CT scan, head

has ruled out a space occupying lesion. She feels entirely well otherwise and there is no impairment of consciousness.

163. A teenager describes constant unilateral frontal pain with local tenderness

THEME : 31
VESSELS INVOLVED IN STROKE SYNDROMES

Options

a. Right vertebral.
b. Left anterior cerebral.
c. Left middle cerebral.
d. Left posterior cerebral.
e. Right paramedian branch of the basilar.
f. Posterior inferior cerebellar artery.

For each of the situations/conditions given below, choose the one most appropriate/discriminatory option from above. The options may be used once, more than once, or not at all.

Questions

164. Loss of abduction of the right eye with a left hemiplegia and diminished tactile and proprioceptive sense in the left half of the body.
165. Diplopia with gaze to the right, ptosis and pupillary mydriasis on the left, and a right hemiplegia.
166. Loss of pain and temperature in the right half of the face and left half of the body; ataxia with falling to the right, right ptosis and miosis, dysphagia, hoarseness and diminished gag reflex on the right.
167. Aphasia with paralysis and diminished sensation of the right face and right upper extremity.
168. Paresis and diminished sensation of the right leg along with urinary retention, mild confusion, agitation and dysphasia speech.
169. Vertigo with vomiting with dysphasia, nystagmus on looking to side lesion and ipsilateral cranial nerve palsies.

THEME : 32
DIAGNOSIS OF CEREBRAL VENOUS THROMBOSIS

Options

a. Lateral sinus thrombosis.
b. Carvernous sinus thrombosis.
c. Sagittal sinus thrombosis.
d. Temporal lobe abscess.
e. Subdural empyema.

For each of the situations/conditions given below, choose the one most appropriate/discriminatory option from above. The options may be used once, more than once, or not at all.

Questions

170. A 14-year-old girl with right facial pain, high fever, left hemiparesis, nuchal rigidity, and progressive obtundation.
171. A 30-year-old man with prostration, fever, headache, papilloedema amd edema of the right forehead and anterior scalp, with left focal motor seizures.
172. A 47-year-old man with a one week history of left forehead and temporal headache along with nausea and vomiting. Brief episodes of altered awareness with normal consciousness and an inability to follow commands began two days ago. He now speaks fluently, but the speech is remarkably devoid of meaning with much paraphasia.
173. A 51-year-old man with high fever and a generalized headache with malaise, who has chemosis, edema and cyanosis of the upper face with a right oculomotor palsy and hyperaesthesia of the right forehead.
174. A 69-year-old man with fever, right sided headache felt maximally behind the right ear, tenderness over the right mastoid process, right abducens palsy, and right facial numbness.

THEME: 33
DIAGNOSIS OF NERVE LESIONS

Options

a. Musculocutaneous nerve.
b. Peroneal nerve.
c. Median nerve.
d. Femoral nerve.
e. C6 nerve root.

For each of the situations/conditions given below, choose the one most appropriate/discriminatory option from above. The options may be used once, more than once, or not at all.

Questions

175. Decreased sensation on volar aspect of thumb and index and middle fingers; weakness of wrist flexors, long finger flexors (thumb, index and middle fingers., pronators of forearm, and the abductor pollicis brevis; loss of finger reflexes.
176. Decreased sensation over the lateral forearm excluding the thumb, weakness of biceps and brachialis; absent biceps reflex.
177. Decreased sensation over the dorsum of foot; weakness of foot and toe dorsiflexion; no reflex changes.
178. Decreased sensation on lateral forearm including the thumb; weakness of biceps, brachialis and brachioradialis; absent supinator reflex.
179. Decreased sensation on anterior thigh and medial leg, weakness of extension at the knee reflex.

THEME : 34
CAUSES OF FACIAL PALSY

Options

a. Bell's palsy
b. Parotid tumor
c. Ramsay hunt syndrome

d. Multiple sclerosis
e. Facial nerve schwannoma
f. Sarcoidosis
g. Transverse temporal bone fracture
h. Suppurative otitis media
i. Guillain-Barré syndrome
j. Cerebrovascular accident
k. Longitudinal temporal bone fracture
l. Malignant otitis media

For each of the situations/conditionss given below. Choose the one most appropriate/discriminatory option from above. The options may be used once, more than once or not at all.

Questions

180. A 40-year-old man presents with facial pain, a droop to the side of the face and a preauricular facial swelling.
181. A 30-year-old man who has substained a blow to the back of his head presents with facial nerve palsy and haemotympanum.
182. A 55-year-old woman presents with a right-sided lower motor neurone facial nerve palsy and sensorineural hearing loss. She is noted to have vesicles in her ear.
183. A 50-year-old diabetic man presents with a unilateral facial nerve palsy and severe earache. On examination, he has granulation tissue deep in the external auditory meatus.
184. A 40-year-old woman presents with unilateral optic neuritis and facial nerve palsy.

THEME: 35
CAUSES OF UNILATERAL FACIAL PALSY

Options

a. Stroke
b. Brainstem tumor
c. Multiple sclerosis
d. Acoustic neuroma
e. Otitis media

f. Cholesteatoma
g. Bell's palsy
h. Ramsay-Hunt syndrome
i. Parotid tumor
j. Trauma
k. Post-meningitis
l. Sarcoidosis

For each of the situations/conditionss given below. Choose the one most appropriate/discriminatory options from above. The options may be used once, more than once or not at all.

Questions

185. A 30-year-old woman has developed ear pain and facial weakness. On otoscopy she has an inflamed bulging tympanic membrane.
186. A 35-year-old woman has suddenly developed facial palsy. 6 months before this she had an episode of blurred vision and unsteadiness. On examination she has mild ataxia and an afferent papillary defect.
187. A 70-year-old man suddenly developed facial weakness which was preceded by symptoms of severe left ear pain, vertigo and deafness. On examination he has vesicles around his ear and on his soft palate.
188. A 50-year-old woman has developed complete facial palsy of the left side of the face including the forehead. She also has facial pain and watering of the eye on that side. Her sense of taste is impaired.
189. A 56-year-old woman with a history of atrial fibrillation develops sudden weakness of the right side of her face. She is still able to wrinkle both sides of her forehead and her smile is symmetrical.
190. A 35-year-old man has developed a slowly progressive right sided facial palsy with deafness and tinnitus as well as facial asymmetry. He is unable to adduct his right eye. His father had been similarly affected.

THEME: 36
DIAGNOSIS OF FACIAL PAIN

Options

a. Migraine
b. Abscess
c. Coryza
d. Serous otitis media
e. Glaucoma
f. Iritis
g. Trigeminal neuralgia
h. Sinusitis
i. SLE
j. Head lice
k. Herpes zoster
l. Space occupying lesion
m. Meningitis
n. Temporal arteritis

For each of the situations/conditionss given below. Choose the one most appropriate/discriminatory options from above. The options may be used once, more than once or not at all.

Questions

191. A 31-year-old man complains of facial pain between the eyes and on one side of the face. His nose and the affected eye are congested. He says the pain is severe.
192. A 20-year-old man says his face hurts especially around the eyes and cheeks. When he bends forwards it worsens and makes him cry.
193. A 57-year-old teacher says she has facial pain, especially in the temples at night. On the right side of her face it throbs. For the past 3 weeks she has felt unwell and had to miss classes. Also, combing her hair has become painful.
194. A 43-year-old mechanic complains of left sided facial pain. The pain is stabbing and runs up and down his face, especially at meal times. He has been to the dentist, but the dentist has found his teeth to be in good order.

THEME: 37
TREATMENT OF FACIAL PAIN

Options

a. Prednisolone
b. Tricyclic antidepressants
c. Lithium carbonate
d. Broad spectrum antibiotics
e. Ergotamine
f. Serotinin reuptake inhibitor
g. Propanolol
h. Carbamazepine
i. Refer to dentist
j. Augmentin and nasal decongestant
k. Analgesia

For each of the situations/conditions given below. Choose the one most appropriate/discriminatory option from above. The options may be used once, more than once or not at all.

Questions

195. A 30-year-old woman presents with unilateral headache and facial pain. She describes flashing lights preceding the headache and nausea. She is asthmatic and is on the OC pills. She also suffers from Graves' disease.
196. A 40-year-old man complains of a series of headaches that occur ever year and consist of severe pain around the eye for 3 weeks at a time.
197. A 35-year-old woman complains of frontal headaches and pain over the bridge of her nose with catarrhal symptoms and nasal blockage.
198. A 55-year-old woman complains of pain in her face and jaw worse on eating. She also complains of transient loss of vision in her right eye and scalp pain when combing her hair.
199. A 50-year-old woman complains of an electric shock like pain that starts in her jaw and ascends to her temples. She states the pain is agonizing and is triggered by touching a particular spot on her lips.

THEME: 38
CAUSES OF PERIPHERAL NEUROPATHY

Options

a. Carcinomatous neuropathy
b. Side effect of drug therapy
c. Diabetic neuropathy
d. Vitamin B_{12} deficiency
e. Vitamin B_1 deficiency
f. Polyarteritis nodosa
g. Guillain-Barré syndrome
h. Amyloidosis
i. Sarcoidosis
j. Industrial poisoning
k. Porphyria

For each of the situations/conditions given below. Choose the one most appropriate/ discriminatory option from above. The options may be used once, more than once or not at all.

Questions

200. A 50-year-old man presents with distal sensory neuropathy affecting the lower limbs in a stocking distribution and is noted to have Charcot's joints. The ankle reflex is absent.
201. A 55-year-old man who drinks heavily presents with numbness and paraesthesiae in his feet. He complains of walking on cotton wool.
202. A 40-year-old man who is being treated with chemotherapy for lymphoma presents with peripheral paraesthesiae, loss of deep tendon reflexes and abdominal bloating.
203. A 45-year-old woman presents with peripheral neuropathy. She is noted to have bilateral hilar gland enlargement on chest X-ray and a negative Mantoux test. She also suffers from polyarthralgia and has tender red, raised lesions on her shin.
204. A 25-year-old man presents with paraesthesiae followed by a recent upper respiratory tract infection.

THEME: 39
ETIOLOGY OF PERIPHERAL NEUROPATHIES

Options

a. Lead.
b. Acrylamide.
c. Thallium.
d. Arsenic.
e. Organophosphates.

For each of the situations/conditions given below, choose the one most appropriate/discriminatory option from above. The options may be used once, more than once, or not at all.

Questions

205. Sensory loss, hyperkeratosis, brown skin, Mees' lines, and pitting edema of the feet and ankles.
206. Painful paraesthesias of the feet and hands, alopecia, Mees' lines, ataxia, chorea and cranial neuropathies.
207. Wrist drops, abdominal colic, constipation, fatigue, anorexia and weight loss.
208. Truncal ataxia and skin peeling and excessive sweating of feet and hands.
209. Cholinergic symptoms may occur first with slightly delayed onset of neuropathy that maximizes within two weeks.

THEME: 40
DIAGNOSIS OF PERIPHERAL NERVE INJURIES

Options

a. Erb's palsy
b. Klumpke's palsy
c. long thoracic nerve injury
d. Spinal accessory nerve injury
e. Axillary nerve injury
f. Radial nerve injury
g. Ulnar nerve injury
h. Median nerve injury

i. Suprascapular nerve injury
j. Sciatic nerve injury
k. Femoral nerve injury
l. Tibial nerve injury
m. Common peroneal nerve injury
n. Superficial peroneal nerve injury

For each of the situations/conditions given below. Choose the one most appropriate / discriminatory option from above. The options may be used once, more than once or not at all.

Questions

210. A football player presents with foot drop after injuring his knee. He can neither dorsiflex nor evert the foot. Sensation is lost over the front and outer half of the leg and dorsum of the foot.
211. A 50-year-old man postincision and drainage of a posterior triangle neck abscess now presents with pain and drooping of his shoulder. On examination there is mild winging of the scapula on active abduction of the arm against resistance, this then disappears on forward thrusting of the shoulder.
212. A 20-year-old man who has accidently cut his forearm on the shattered glass now presents with hyperextension of metacarpophalangeal joints of the ring and little fingers.
213. A 30-year-old man presents with an elbow dislocation and a hand held with ulnar fingers flexed and the index straight. He is unable to abduct his thumb.
214. A 60-year-old man post total hip replacement now walks with a drop foot and a high stepping gait. Sensation is lost below the knees except over the medial leg.

THEME: 41
TYPES OF POLYNEUROPATHIES

Options

a. Guillain-Barré syndrome.
b. Diabetes neuropathy.
c. Alcoholic neuropathy.

d. Charcot-Marie tooth disease.
e. Amyloidosis.
f. Freidrich's ataxia.

For each of the situations/conditions given below, choose the one most appropriate/discriminatory option from above. The options may be used once, more than once, or not at all.

Questions

215. Multifocal neuropathy.
216. Inherited neuropathy.
217. Predominantly sensory neuropathy.
218. Neuropathy with nerve thickening.
219. Demyelinating neuropathy.
220. Painful, axonal neuropathy.

THEME: 42
DIAGNOSIS OF CHOREIFORM DISORDERS

Options

a. Huntington's disease.
b. Wilson's disease.
c. Ataxia-telangiectasia.
d. Lesch-Nyhan syndrome.
e. Chorea-acanthocytosis.

For each of the situations/conditions given below, choose the one most appropriate/discriminatory option from above. The options may be used once, more than once, or not at all.

Questions

221. A 27-year-old boy with chorea, athetosis, spasticity, aggression, and compulsive self-multilation of the lips, hyperuricemia is present.
222. A 14-year-old girl with recurrent pulmonary infections and a 10 years history of progressive ataxia and choreoathetoid movements, dysarthria, and myoclonic jerks; she is areflexic with a peripheral neuropathy and spider-like vascular abnormalities on the ears, nose and forearms.

223. A 36-year-old woman with a seven years history of tremor of the arms and head progressing to choreiform movements, with dysarthria, dysphagia, drooling, muscle rigidity and mental dulling; ophthalmologic and hepatic dysfunctions are present.
224. A 42-year-old woman with four years history of progressive chorea, orofacial tics, self-multilation of the lips and tongue, areflexia, elevated serum creatinine phosphokinase. "Burr cells" on peripheral blood smear, and atrophy of the caudate nuclei on CT scan.
225. A 49-year-old woman with a seven years history of progressive clumsiness leading to achorea of arms, legs, and bulbar musculature. The gait is characterized by hesitation, stuttering steps, and frequent falls. Emotional problems in earlier-year-have progressed to delusions, paranoia, impulsiveness and agitation with recent impairement of memory and judgement.

THEME: 43
MANAGEMENT OF PARKINSON'S DISEASE

Options

a. L-dopa.
b. Selegiline.
c. Carbidopa.
d. Nortriptylline.
e. Anticholinergics.
f. Apomorphine.
g. Procyclidine.

For each of the situations/conditions given below, choose the one most appropriate/discriminatory option from above. The options may be used once, more than once, or not at all.

Questions

226. For tremors.
227. Improves mobility.
228. For drug induced parkinsonism.
229. For associated depression.

230. Avert's end of dose deterioration of L-dopa.
231. Helps patients with severe on-off effects.

THEME : 44
NEUROLOGICAL LESIONS CAUSING GAIT DISORDERS

Options

a. Stiff, circumduction gait.
b. Flexed posture, shuffling feet, slow to start with postural instability.
c. Shuffling, difficulty in getting feet off the floor.
d. Wide base, unstable.
e. Wide base, falls worse in poor light.
f. Waddling gait.
g. Wild flinging of legs.
h. Walking on ice.
i. Donald duck gait.
j. High stepping gait.

For each of the situations/conditions given below, choose the one most appropriate/discriminatory option from above. The options may be used once, more than once, or not at all.

Questions

232. Cerebellum.
233. Depression.
234. UMN lesion.
235. Foot drop.
236. Alcohol abuse.
237. Frontal lesion.
238. Myopathy.
239. Extrapyramidal.
240. Astasia abasia (over cautious).
241. Posterior column lesion.

THEME: 45
DIAGNOSIS OF DYSKINESIAS

Options

a. Rest tremor.
b. Intentional tremor.
c. Chorea.
d. Anxiety.
e. Hemiballismus.
f. Athetosis.
g. Tics.
h. Myoclonus.
i. Asterixis.
j. Dystonia.
k. Tardive dyskinesia.

For each of the situations/conditions given below, choose the one most appropriate/discriminatory option from above. The options may be used once, more than once, or not at all.

Questions

242. Sudden involuntary focal or general jerks arising from cord, cortex or brainstem, usually seen in infantile spasms.
243. Slow, sinous, confluent, purposeless movements of hands.
244. Involuntary chewing and grimacing movements due to long-term neuroleptics especially in elderly.
245. Nonrhythmic, jerky, purposeless movements of hands.
246. Prolonged muscle contraction producing abnormal postures.

THEME: 46
SITE OF LESIONS IN DYSKINESIAS

Options

a. Substantia nigra.
b. Caudate nucleus.
c. Putamen.
d. Subthalamic nucleus.
e. Basal ganglia.

For each of the situations/conditions given below, choose the one most appropriate/discriminatory option from above. The options may be used once, more than once, or not at all.

Questions

247. Chorea.
248. Torsion dystonia.
249. Athetosis.
250. Parkinsonism.
251. Hemiballismus.

THEME: 47
INVESTIGATIONS OF NEUROLOGICAL DISORDERS

Options

a. Tensilon test.
b. Muscle biopsy.
c. Nerve conduction tests.
d. MRI cervical spine.
e. CT scan brain.
f. Visual evoked potential.
g. Lumbar puncture.
h. EEG.
i. None of the above.

For each of the situations/conditions given below, choose the one most appropriate/discriminatory option from above. The options may be used once, more than once, or not at all.

Questions

252. A middle-aged lady with a history of right-sided facial palsy 4 months ago. Now presents with generalised bodyache and a left sided foot drop, also complains of polydipsia and polyuria and investigations reveal sugar in early morning urine sample.
253. A 46-year-old electrician complains of difficulty in working with arms over his head and feels progressively tired and weak as the day goes on. Chest X-ray reveals a mediastinal mass.

254. A 28-year-old smoker comes to you with complaints of having burns on his finger tips from cigarettes, which he smokes. He says he can not feel the burning end of the cigarettes although he feels the cigarette and has no difficulty in holding it. On examination he has wasted small muscles of the hand.
255. A 40-year-old lady comes to you with difficulty in walking gradually worsening over 48 hours. He now has some breathing difficulty. On examination he has grade 3/6 power in all limbs and loss of deep tendon. Reflexes a nerve conduction test done reveals demyelination.

THEME: 48
DIAGNOSIS OF INTRACRANIAL LESIONS

Options

a. Subdural haematoma
b. Cerebral abscess
c. Astrocytoma
d. Acoustic neuroma
e. Meningioma
f. Pituitary tumor
g. Secondary tumor
h. Cerebral aneurysm
i. Cerebral angioma
j. Subarachnoid hemorrhage
k. Extradural haemorrhage
l. Medulloblastoma

For each of the situations/conditions given below. Choose the one most appropriate/ discriminatory options from above. The options may be used once, more than once or not at all.

Questions

256. A 50-year-old man presents with unilateral tinnitus and dizziness. He also complains of difficulty swallowing and loss of taste.
257. A 45-year-old women presents with sudden onset of headache, neck stiffness and double vision. She lapses into

coma. She had a similar episode 2 weeks prior that was not as severe and resolved spontaneously. She has a history of hypertension and no history of trauma.

258. A 10-year-old boy presents with headache, blurry vision and vomiting. He is noted to have an ataxic gait, nystagmus and pastpointing. His CT scan of the head shows enlarged cerebral ventricles and a cerebellar mass.
259. A 40-year-old woman postradical mastectomy now presents with sudden onset of severe headache and confusion. She is apyrexial and shows no signs of head trauma. The CT scan of the head shows a space occupying lesion.
260. A 30-year-old cricketer presents in a coma. He had been struck by a cricket ball earlier that day and had been fine until now. On examination he has asymmetrical pupils.

THEME: 49
CAUSES OF CEREBRAL LESIONS

Options

a. Arteriovenous malformation
b. Berry aneurysm
c. Brain abscess
d. Extradural haematoma
e. Subdural haematoma
f. Carotid artery occlusion
g. Pituitary adenoma
h. Medulloblastoma
i. Craniopharyngioma
j. Meningioma
k. Metastatic carcinoma

For each of the situations/conditionss given below. Choose the one most appropriate/discriminatory options from above. The options may be used once, more than once or not at all.

Questions

261. A 60-year-old woman treated with total thyroidectomy for thyroid carcinoma now presents with visual changes. On examination she has bitemporal hemianopia. CT scan

of the head shows a cystic lesion compressing the optic chiasma.

262. A 25-year-old man complains of the worst headache of his life. He denies any history of head trauma. He has no focal neurological deficits.
263. A 65-year-old male alcoholic has fluctuating levels of consciousness. He develops focal neurological deficits. His wife reports that he fell down the staircase 2 months ago.
264. A 45-year-old motorcyclist involved in RTA. On examination he has a dilated left pupil and is unconscious. Skull films show a left temporal-parietal fracture.
265. A 55-year-old woman treated with modified radical mastectomy for breast carcinoma 5 years ago now presents with gradual onset of confusion and visual disturbances. CT scan of the head shows a cerebral mass.

THEME: 50
CAUSES OF NEUROLOGICAL SIGNS

Options

a. Middle cerebral artery infarction
b. Anterior cerebral artery infarction
c. Posterior cerebral artery infarction
d. Vertebro-basilar ischaemia
e. Subacute combined degeneration of cord
f. Syringomyelia
g. Cord compression
h. Tabes dorsalis

For each of the situations/conditionss given below. Choose the one most appropriate/discriminatory options from above. The options may be used once, more than once or not at all.

Questions

266. A 50-year-old man presents with severe stabbing pains in his chest and limbs. He has a wide based gait. On examination he has ptosis and small, irregular pupils that react to accommodation but not to light. He has absent deep tendon reflexes and position sense.

267. A 60-year-old man presents with urinary incontinence and contralateral hemiparesis of the foot, leg and shoulder. He is awake but silent and immobile in a coma-vigil state.
268. A 70-year-old man presents with contralateral hemisensory loss and paresis of conjugate gaze to the opposite side.
269. A 70-year-old man presents with dysarthria and incontractable hiccups. On examination he has nystagmus and is noted to have an ataxic gait.
270. A 40-year-old alcoholic man presents with numbness and tingling sensation in his feet. He is noted to have loss of vibration and position senses in his legs with loss of deep tendon reflexes. Full blood count reveals a macrocytic anemia.

THEME: 51
DIAGNOSIS OF NEUROLOGICAL COMPLAINTS

Options

a. Space occupying lesion
b. Polyarteritis nodosa
c. Autonomic neuropathy
d. Bulbar palsy
e. Polyneuropathy
f. Pernicious anemia
g. Parkinson disease
h. Myasthenia grais
i. Multiple sclerosis
j. Spondylosis
k. Myotonia
l. Motor neurone disease
m. Neurofibromatosis
n. Syringomyelia

For each of the situations/conditionss given below. Choose the one most appropriate/discriminatory options from above. The options may be used once, more than once or not at all.

Questions

271. A young teacher complains of being unable to see properly for 3 days. Afterwards she recovers completely. 3 months later she gets out of her car and stumbles to the ground. Again she recovers, but she still has some difficulty walking.
272. An elderly broker has difficulty speaking and walking. He has an idea but finds it difficult to say what he thinks as quickly as formerly. He also trips on entering and leaving rooms. All of this makes him more unhappy.
273. A 32-year-old bank manager complains that he cannot get to work on his Bicycle anymore. He gets tired and must get down before the end of his trip. Also he has noticed some weakness on swallowing and colleagues remark on his aggressive behaviour.
274. A 58-year-old man presents with leg weakness. He complains of stumbling and falling. On physical examination you find some wasting exaggerated reflexes and normal sensation.
275. A 40-year-old man complains of pain, tenderness and numbness in his legs. Recently he has stumbled a couple of times without reason. He says he does drink but that he was very sober at the time.

THEME: 52
DIAGNOSIS OF NEUROLOGICAL COMPLAINTS

Options

a. Diabetes metllitus
b. Vitamin B deficiency
c. Depression
d. Myasthenia gravis
e. Syringomyelia
f. Botulism
g. Lead poisoning
h. Discoid lupus erythematous
i. SLE
j. Cerebrovascular accident
k. Aortic aneurysm

l. Leprosy
m. Dermatomyositis
n. Pyomyositis

For each of the situations/conditionss given below. Choose the one most appropriate/discriminatory options from above. The options may be used once, more than once or not at all.

Questions

276. An elderly man who tins his own food suffers from blurred vision, photophobia and spasticity. He complains of difficulty speaking and is brought in by his son. His breathing is laboured.
277. A young adult complains about loss of sensation and temperature, especially in the neck and shoulders. Recently, he has injured his arm and hands quite badly without feeling anything.
278. A middle-aged woman presents with recurrent nausea, weight loss and fever. She has pain, stiffness and weakness in her hips and shoulders. She does not have a rash but the skin around the neck and shoulders appear thickened.
279. A 48-year-old man complains of ill health, joint pain and muscle weakness. He has a fever, loss of appetite, nausea and weight loss. The patient points to a circular area of white and thickened skin behind the ear. He says the hair has never grown back.

THEME : 53
DIAGNOSIS OF NEUROLOGICAL ABNORMALITIES

Options

a. Vertebro-basilar infarction.
b. Cerebral infarct.
c. Subarachnoid hemorrhage
d. Cerebral hemorrhage.
e. Hypoglycemia.
f. Cerebello-pontine hemorrhage.
g. Hypercalcemia.
h. Multiple sclerosis.
i. Polymyalgia rheumatica.

For each of the situations/conditionss given below. Choose the one most appropriate/discriminatory options from above. The options may be used once, more than once or not at all.

Questions

280. An elderly man wakes up in the morning with numbness of his right hand, blurring of vision in his right eye. He then suffers a drop attack.
281. A 33-year-old man reports a history of walking while swinging to one side.
282. A 32-year-old known hypertensive presents to you with a right hemiparesis.
283. A 34-year-old woman has a six month histiry of on and off hemiparesis which resolves with no neurological deficits.
284. A 55-year-old woman treated for breast cancer with chemotherapy and radiotherapy presented with a history of confusion, tiredness, weakness and polyuria. On examination no neurulogical deficits were found.

THEME: 54
MANAGEMENT OF NEUROLOGICAL PATHOLOGY

Options

a. Consult neurosurgeon at once
b. IV 5 mL/Kg of a 20% solution of mannitol
c. Emergency burr holes
d. Urgent computed tomography (CT)
e. Discharge after check skull X-rays
f. A period of observation and discharge shortly after
g. 50 mL of a 50 % solution of dextrose bolus
h. Naloxone
i. Pyrimethamine-sulphadiazine

For each of the situations/conditionss given below. Choose the one most appropriate/discriminatory options from above. The options may be used once, more than once or not at all.

Questions

285. A 40-year-old man involved in a road traffic accident is brought to A&E. ON examination Glasgow Coma Scale (GCS) of 11 is found . He is found to have a bruise in the left temporal area.
286. A 25-year-old man is brought to A&E . He smells of alcohol. Blood glucose is 5.0 mmol/l and his left pupil is dilated GCS is 7. The nearest consultant neurosurgeon is 2 hours away.
287. A 30-year-old man is brought to A&E after a drunken brawl, unconscious. After initial resuscitation the patient breathing becomes progressively deeper and then shallower and pupils constrict then later become fixed and dilated. CT scan has been done.
288. A 17-year-old boy is brought to the A&E department following a road traffic accident. He has rhinnorhea and periorbital oedema. His GCS is 5.
289. A 30-year-old IV drug abuser is brought to the A&E department with a severe headache and confusion. A CT scan shows multiple ring enhancing lesions. The pulse rate is 60 beats /min and blood pressure is 150/100 mmHg. He is severely wasted.

THEME: 55
MANAGEMENT OF NEUROLOGICAL DISORDERS

Options

a. Reserpine.
b. Guanidine.
c. Haloperidol.
d. Thiamine.
e. Insulin.
f. Glucose.
g. Symptomatic.

For each of the situations/conditions given below, choose the one most appropriate/discriminatory option from above. The options may be used once, more than once, or not at all.

Questions

290. Eaton-Lambert syndrome.
291. Tourette's syndrome.
292. Reye's syndrome.
293. Tardive dyskinesia syndrome.
294. Korsakoff's syndrome.

THEME : 56
INVESTIGATIONS OF NEUROLOGICAL DISORDERS

Options

a. Serum B_{12} levels.
b. MRI cervical spine.
c. Repetitive stimulation by EMG/NCV.
d. CSF analysis.
e. Toxicology screen.
f. Post lunch blood sugar.
g. Plasma lactate before and after exercise.
h. Urinary porphobilinogen.
i. CT brain.
j. Serum CPK and LDH.
k. Serum electrolytes.
l. Evoked visual potentials.

For each of the situations/conditions given below, choose the one most appropriate/discriminatory option from above. The options may be used once, more than once, or not at all.

Questions

295. A 4-year-old boy with delayed motor milestones. Now he cannot run or climb stairs.
296. A 20-year-old trainee nurse complains of fatiguability, occasionally seeing double and intermittent change in voice quality.
297. A 30-year-old estate agent gets severe muscle cramps on moderate exercise but is all right if he does his movements slowly and steadily.
298. A 40-year-old factory worker developed severe weakness of all four limbs and became breathless rapidly within 6

hours of onset. However, he had improved remarkably overnight in hospital.

299. A 20-year-old girl is admitted with generalised weakness of all four limbs developing over 24 hours, also gives past history repeated episodic abdominal pains.

THEME: 57
DIAGNOSIS OF HEAD INJURY

Options

a. Subarachnoid haemorrhage
b. Subdural haemorrhage
c. Fracture base of skull
d. Concussion
e. Compound skull fracture
f. Cerebral haemorrhage
g. Cephalohaematoma
h. Extradural haemorrhage
i. Granulomatous meningitis

For each of the situations/conditionss given below. Choose the one most appropriate/discriminatory options from above. The options may be used once, more than once or not at all.

Questions

300. A cyclist is involved in an accident and is brought into the Accident and Emergency Department with a GCS of 8 and no physical injuries. On examination of the ear, there is a haemotympanum.
301. Following a motoring accident, a patient is brought into the Accident and Emergency Department with deterioration of consciousness. He regains consciousness and complains of headache and is found to have neck stiffness on examination.
302. A 65-year-old man was kicked in the head a week ago. He is brought to A&E in an unconscious state. He smells of alcohol. On examination, he has a rising BP and unequal pupils. His GCS is 8.
303. A 45-year-old man was struck in the head by a cricket ball. He had an episode of LOC lasting 5 minutes. The

patient now complains of headache. He has no lateralising signs on neurological examination.

304. A 45-year-old man with a history of epilepsy has a fit and strikes the side of his head on the edge of the bathtub. He is dazed and complains of headache. Skull X-ray reveals a linear fracture of the parietal area. His level of consciousness diminishes.
305. A 58-year-old man is struck in his head with a dustbin lid and presents with an open scalp wound. Skull X-ray confirms an underlying skull fracture. The dura is intact.

THEME: 58
CAUSES OF LOWER EXTREMITY PARALYSIS

Options

a. Middle cerebral artery infarction
b. Spinal artery occlusion
c. Guillain-Barré syndrome
d. Poliomyelitis
e. Deep vein thrombosis
f. Acute cord compression
g. Intermittent claudication
h. Critical limb ischaemia
i. Compartment syndrome
j. Medial menisus tear

For each of the situations/conditionss given below. Choose the one most appropriate/discriminatory options from above. The options may be used once, more than once or not at all.

Questions

306. A 67-year-old smoker presents with pain in his left calf on walking and also at rest. His ankle-brachial Doppler pressure index is 0.3.
307. A 30-year-old man develops gradual weakness in his extremoties following flu. On examination, he is unable to drink, to raise his legs and has loss of muscle tone and deep tendon reflexes. The lumbar puncture demonstrates 4 lymphocytes/cc, 2 g/l protein and 3 mmol/l of glucose.

308. A 20-year-old man presents with pain on inner aspect of his right knee after being tackled in rugby. He reports a tearing sensation and is unable to move his leg. On examination the knee is swollen and tender and the joint is locked.
309. A 70-year-old woman with a history of multiple myeloma suddenly develops back pain and is unable to move her legs. On examination she has hypotonia, toss of deep tendon reflexes and sensory loss of her tower extremities. She also goes into urinary retention.
310. A 2-year-old boy presents with pain in the calves and inability to move his lower legs. He is also noted to have pneumonia and splenomegaly. On examination, he has loss of motor power and tone, loss of sensation and decreased deep tendon reflexes in his lower extremities.

THEME : 59
NEUROLOGICAL INJURY

Options

a. Anterior cord syndrome.
b. Central cord syndrome.
c. Brown-Sequard syndrome.
d. Spinal shock.
e. Neurogenic shock.

For each of the situations/conditions given below, choose the one most appropriate/discriminatory option from above. The options may be used once, more than once, or not at all.

Questions

311. Motor paralysis, loss of pain and temperature, preserved posterior column function (position sense, light touch, and vibration) usually seen after cervical flexion injury.
312. Paralysis, loss of gross proprioception and vibration on the same side as the lesion, contra-lateral loss of pain and temperature sensation.
313. Often follows hyperextension injury, consists of neurological deficit of the upper extremities that is more pro-

nounced than in the lower extremities with scattered sensory losses.

THEME: 60
DIAGNOSIS OF CONFUSION

Options

a. Viral encephalitis
b. Brain tumor (primary)
c. Epilepsy
d. Cerebrovascular accident
e. Pancreatic tumor
f. Diabetic ketoacidosis
g. Psychiatric illness
h. Influenza
i. Subarachnoid haemorrhage
j. Nephroma
k. Acute intermittent porphyria
l. Variegate porphyria
m. Liver failure
n. Amyloidosis

For each of the situations/conditionss given below. Choose the one most appropriate/discriminatory options from above. The options may be used once, more than once or not at all.

Questions

314. A young woman complains of sweating, palpitations, abdominal pain and weakness. On bringing herself to A&E she is aggressive and confused. She has a seizure and falls unconscious. Her serum insulin is high.
315. A 27-year-old PhD student presents with abdominal pain, nausea and vomiting. His breathing is rapid and shallow. He is confused. On examination you find the breath sweet smelling, the eyes sunken and the body temperature below normal.
316. A 26-year-old woman presents with abdominal pain, vomiting and constipation. She also complains of numb-

ness and clumsiness in her legs. She has been very depressed and anxious. Her urine is dark.

317. An elderly man with a history of rheumatoid arthritis presents with abdominal pain, a swollen face and swollen eyelids. His JVP is normal and his urine is frothy. Urine examination shows paraproteinemia.
318. A student who has ingested 3 bottles full of paracetamol is brought in with acute abdominal pain. She is very angry and confused. She vomits several times and falls unconscious.

THEME: 61
DIAGNOSIS OF CONFUSION

Options

a. Dementia
b. Psychosis
c. Septicemia
d. Pelvic abscess
e. Acute urinary tract infection
f. Tuberculosis
g. Bronchogenic carcinoma
h. Gout
i. Prostatic hypertrophy
j. Carcinoma colon
k. Crohn's disease
l. Creutzfeldt-Jakob disease
m. Depression
n. Secondaries

For each of the situations/conditionss given below. Choose the one most appropriate/discriminatory options from above. The options may be used once, more than once or not at all.

Questions

319. A 51-year-old sales manager complains of nausea, irritability and confusion. He has oliguria and on physical examination you palpate a large suprapubic mass.

320. A middle-aged woman is treated for severe depression with antidepressants and ECT. The antidepressants had no effect upon her mood however and the ECT treatment aggravated her complaints. Now she stumbles and slurs her speech.
321. A 47-year-old woman is confused and irritable. She does not smoke but is brought in by her husband who does. He says that she has become increasingly difficult and very easily confused. She does not have a cough but CXR shows an opacity.
322. A 48-year-old journalist with joint pain and joint swelling in brought to A&E by his wife. He woke up this morning feeling sick and confused. He has been vomiting all morning.
323. A 58-year-old accountant complains of depression and inability to concentrate. Over the past years his performance at work and his relationships with his colleagues have steadily deteriorated. He has also had difficulty with his speech and swallowing.

THEME : 62
CAUSES OF CONFUSION

Options

a. Dementia
b. Delirium tremens
c. Postictal state
d. Hypoxia
e. Cerebrovascular accident
f. Hypoglycemia
g. Hypothermia
h. Encephalitis
i. Urinary tract infection
j. Intoxication
k. Acute psychosis
l. Hypothyroidism

For each of the situations/conditionss given below. Choose the one most appropriate/discriminatory options from above. The options may be used once, more than once or not at all.

Questions

324. A 30-year-old man has been picked up in the street by police. He was initially drowsy but is now agitated and aggressive. His trousers are wet with urine.
325. A 75-year-old woman has gradually become confused over 4 years. She forgets the names and birthdays of her family. She gets lost when she goes shopping alone. She sometimes leaves her cooker on all night.
326. A 20-year-old man is irritable and confused. He appears disturbed by loud noises. He is also complaining of a headache and has pyrexia and mild neck stiffness.
327. A 30-year-old man had an appendicectomy 2 days ago and is now agitated and confused. He is sweaty and has a marked tremor of his hands. He claims that his sleep was disturbed by insects in his bed.
328. A 75-year-old woman was found on the floor at home having collapsed. She is drowsy and confused and has been incontinent of urine. She is shaking. Her pulse is 50/min and her ECG shows J waves.
329. A 20-year-old man who was picked up by the police is behaving irrationally and is confused and irritable. He is pale and sweaty and smells of alcohol. He keeps asking for biscuits.

THEME: 63
INVESTIGATION OF CONFUSION

Options

a. Blood glucose
b. CT scan
c. Full blood count
d. Stool culture
e. Ultrasound abdomen
f. Blood culture
g. Chest X-ray
h. ECG
i. MSU
j. Thyroid function tests
k. Urea and electrolytes

For each of the situations/conditions given below, choose the one most appropriate/discriminatory option from above. The options may be used once, more than once, or not at all.

Questions

330. A previously fit 80-year-old woman has been noted by daughter to be increasingly slow and forgetful over several months. She has gained weight, intends to stay indoors with heating on even in the warm weather.
331. A frail 80-year-old woman presents with poor mobility and recent history of falls. She has deteriorated generally over the past two weeks with fluctuating confusion. On examination she has a mild hemiparesis.
332. An 80-year-old woman in a nursing home has been constipated for a week. Over the past few days she has become increasingly confused and incontinent.
333. A 65-year-old man has recently been started on tablets by his GP. He is brought to the A&E by his wife with sudden onset of aggressive behaviour, confusion and drowsiness. Prior to starting the tablets he was loosing weight and complained of thirst.
334. An 80-year-old man with known mild Alzheimer's disease became suddenly more confused yesterday. When seen in A&E, his blood pressure was 90/60 mm mercury and his pulse was 40/min and regular.

THEME: 64
DIAGNOSIS OF DIZZINESS

Options

a. Benign postural vertigo
b. Acute vestibular failure
c. Migraine
d. Brainstem tumor
e. Multiple sclerosis
f. Phaeochromocytoma
g. Encephalitis
h. Hypoglycaemia

i. Hyperglycemia
j. Diabetes mellitus
k. Meniere's disease
l. Barbiturates
m. Space occupying lesions

For each of the situations/conditionss given below. Choose the one most appropriate/discriminatory options from above. The options may be used once, more than once or not at all.

Questions

335. A young housewife complains of repeated attacks of dizziness. Over the past 3 months she has repeatedly lost her balance and has had to sit down. She says everything rotates and she feels sick.
336. A 50-year-old man says he goes dizzy and falls over, always to the left side. He says it happens whenever he lowers his head 6 months ago he was assaulted and knocked down unconscious.
337. A 32-year-old hotelier complains of dizziness. Things suddenly start turning around and she falls down. She has no nausea or tinnitus. Over the past year she has had 3 bouts of unexplained dizziness. She has also had numbness in her right leg and has had occasionally stumbled.
338. A young man with a sharp cough looses his balance and takes to his bed. Rising makes him dizzy and makes him want to vomit. He has no auricular signs or symptoms.
339. An elderly man complains of fits of dizziness, palpitations and headache. He is worried about another attack. During his last attack he suddenly became very pale and very weak and he wanted to throw up but could not. He had to sit down for 15 mins.

THEME: 65
IMMEDIATE INVESTIGATIONS OF THE UNCONSCIOUS PATIENT

Options

a. Arterial blood gases
b. Blood carbon monoxide levels

c. Blood culture
d. Blood glucose
e. Blood paracetamol levels
f. Blood salicylate
g. Chest X-ray
h. Computed tomography (CT) scan brain
i. Electrocardiogram (ECG)
j. Lumbar puncture
k. Serum osmolality
l. Temperature

Questions

340. A 43-year-old man is brought to the A&E department unconscious (Glasgow Coma Scale =7). On initial examination his pulse rate is 80 beats /min. He is sweating and has a SaO_2 of 98 % on air.
341. A 45-year-old woman is brought to the Accident and Emergency Department unconscious (GCS=7). On examination her pulse rate is 110 beats/min, temperature normal, BM (glucose) 4.6. She was found with an empty bottle of antidepressant Dothiepin (Prothiaden).
342. A 43-year-old man is brought to Accident and Emergency Department unconscious (GCS=7). On initial examination her pulse rate is 90 beats/min, BM 5.3, SaO_2 97 % on air. He smells of alcohol. There are no external signs of injury.
343. A 44-year-old man is brought to the A&E Department unconscious (GCS=7). On initial examination his pulse rate is 100 beats/min. BM= 4.3. SaO_2 100 % on air. He is accompanied by other members of his family who also report to be feeling unwell.
344. A 41-year-old woman is brought to the Accident and Emergency Department unconscious (GCS=7). On initial examination her pulse rate is 110 beats/min. SaO_2 95 % on air, BM (glucose) 4.5. A purpuric rash is noted on both her arms.
345. A 30-year-old man collapsed at a nightclub. He has GCS of 3. He has evidence of neck stiffness. His pulse is 60/min and his BP is 170/100 mmHg.

346. A 62-year-old man was brought into casualty complaining of chest pain. His ECG at that time was normal and he is awaiting the results of blood tests. After 2 hours, he suddenly complains of feeling very faint and collapses. His BP is barely recordable and his pulse is very weak.
347. A 20-year-old woman collapsed at a party. Her friends say that she had drunk several bottles of beer before acting strangely for about half an hour prior to collapsing. She has been incontinent of urine. On examination she is clammy, sweaty and tachycardic.

THEME: 66
INVESTIGATION OF COLLAPSE

Options

a. Full blood count
b. ECG
c. Lumbar puncture
d. Pelvic ultrasound
e. Ultrasound abdomen
f. Serum calcium
g. Urine pregnancy test
h. Thyroid function test
i. Urea and electrolytes
j. Chest X-ray
k. CT scan of the head
l. Blood glucose

For each of the situations/conditions given below, choose the one most appropriate/discriminatory option from above. The options may be used once, more than once, or not at all.

Questions

348. A 16-year-old girl is brought to her GP after collapsing. She is noted to be febrile with a purpuric rash that does not blanch on pressure.
349. A 65-year-old female is brought into the A&E department after collapsing at home. Her thighs show evidence of lipoatrophy and her shins of necrobiosis lipoidica.

350. A 35-year-old man presents to A&E after collapsing on a cricket pitch. He takes carbamazepine. There is a haematoma over his right temple.
351. A 24-year-old presents to her GP after collapsing at home. She reports nausea worse in the morning. Her last menstrual period was five weeks ago.
352. An 18-year-old college student presents to the A&E department after collapsing at school. Her last menstrual period was three weeks ago and lasted three days. She is anxious. Her pulse is irregular and rapid.
353. A 70-year-old woman with a history of chronic renal failure presents with fits and fainting. She complains of cramps in her limbs and circumoral numbness.
354. A 55-year-old woman complains of dizziness and blackouts. On examination, her pulse rate is 50.

THEME: 67
INVESTIGATION OF LOSS OF CONSCIOUSNESS

Options

a. Electroencephalography
b. Ambulatory ECG
c. Exercise ECG
d. Carotid arteriography.
e. Computer tomography
f. Echocardiography.
g. Do nothing.

Questions

355. A 12-year-old girl loses consciousness after a period of prolonged standing. She becomes pale but regains consciousness within a few seconds.
356. An elderly woman reports history of loss of consciousness on five occasions. Each time she regains consciousness in few minutes.
357. A 34-year-old man has a history of falling with jerky movements of the hands and the feet associated with urinary incontinence.

358. A 12-year-old girl has a history of falling with jerky movements of the body on several occasions. She bites her tongue during the falls.

THEME 68
CAUSES OF BLACK OUTS

Options

a. Vasovagal reflex.
b. Carotid sinus hypersensitivity.
c. Strokes-Adams syndrome.
d. Transient ischemic syndrome.
e. Hypoglycemic episode.
f. Hysteria.
g. Orthostatic hypotension.
h. Micturition blackout.
i. Drop attacks.
j. Epilepsy.

For each of the situations/conditions given below, choose the one most appropriate/discriminatory option from above. The options may be used once, more than once, or not at all.

Questions

359. A 50-year-old presents with history of episode of blackouts for last one week when he gets up to micturate at night.
360. A 50-year-old female presents with episodes of sudden weakness of legs with no warning and says she has never lost consciousness.
361. A 50-year-old female presents with history of multiple episodes of blackouts yesterday evening and each episode was preceded by nausea and sweating and lasted about 2 minutes during which she lost her consciousness. It was later found that yesterday was her husband's death anniversary.
362. A 50-year-old patient with part history of MI now complains that for last 10 days he has been having episodes of unconsciousness, which start without warning. Wife says she also noticed few clonic jerks during attacks, which were prolonged.

THEME: 69
THE MANAGEMENT OF PATIENTS IN COMA

Options

a. Alcohol levels
b. Angiography
c. Arterial blood gases
d. Blood cultures
e. Blood sugar
f. Computed tomography
g. Naloxone
h. Paracetamol screen
i. Plasma osmolality
j. Toxocology
k. Urea and electrolytes

Questions

363. A 25-year-old found deeply unconscious is brought to the Accident and Emergency Department. He has an abrasion over his left temple and puncture marks on his left forearm.
364. A 37-year-old alcoholic is found wandering in a park. His partner says he has had a number of falls recently and in the Accident and Emergency the patient is confused. The blood sugar level is normal.
365. A 19-year-old university student went home from class because of a headache. The next morning she is found unconscious at home. She has purpuric rash and a fever.
366. A 23-year-old known diabetic arrives in the A&E Department. She is pale, sweaty and unconscious. Her companion says she was well 30 min ago but suddenly became confused and then cold not be roused.
367. A 45-year-old is brought to the Accident and Emergency by her husband who reports that she collapsed in the bathroom. Upon examination she is unconscious with bilateral upgoing plantar responses. Her blood sugar level is normal.

THEME: 70
TREATMENT OF COMA

Options

a. Cefotaxime IV
b. Phentolamine IV
c. Triiodothyronine IV
d. Propanolol IV
e. Insulin infusion
f. 50% Dextrose IV
g. Neurosurgical decompression dependant on CT scan findings
h. Naloxone IV
i. Hydrocortisone sodium succinate IV
j. Benzylpenicillin IV
k. Acyclovir IV

For each of the situations/conditions given below. Choose the one most appropriate/discriminatory option from above. The options may be used once, more than once or not at all.

Questions

368. A 22-year-old man involved in a RTA presents to A&E comatose with pinpoint pupils.
369. A 30-year-old man with a history of epilepsy is brought to A&E in a comatose state. He is pyrexial and noted to have a purpuric rash. His family state that he is allergic to penicillin.
370. A 55-year-old man undergoing an IV urogram suddenly complains of severe headache and palpitations. His BP is noted to be 189/120 and rising.
371. A 50-year-old man is brought into A&E in a comatose state. He smells of alcohol. He is pyrexial with a BP of 180/110 and a pulse of 50. His pupils are unequal.
372. A 70-year-old man is brought to A&E in a coma. His temperature is 35C, pulse is 50 and he has a goitre on examination.

THEME : 71
CAUSES OF DELIRIUM

Options

a. Hepatic failure
b. Renal failure
c. Hypoxia
d. Pellagra
e. Wernicke-Korsakoff syndrome
f. Beriberi disease
g. Hypoglycemia instructions
h. Alcohol withdrawal
i. Drug withdrawal
j. Brain tumor
k. Subarachnoid hemorrhage
l. Drug intoxication
m. Brain abscess

For each of the situations/conditions given below. Choose the one most appropriate/discriminatory option from above. The options may be used once, more than once or not at all.

Questions

373. A 60-year-old man presents with confusion, restlessness and walks with a broad based gait. On examination, he has nystagmus and bilateral lateral rectus palsies and smells of alcohol.
374. A 40-year-old man taking isoniazid for tuberculosis now presents with dermatitis, diarrhoea and dementia.
375. A 30-year-old man presents with pinpoint pupils and delirium. He is noted to have nasal septal perforation.
376. A 35-year-old man presents with fever, delirium and fits. He has a history of chronic sinusitis. On examination, he has asymmetrical pupils and a rising blood pressure. There are no external signs of head trauma.
377. A 55-year-old man presents with seizures and hallucinations. He is tachycardic with a low blood pressure. He insists there are insects crawling over his body. He has a history of alcoholism.

THEME: 72
DIAGNOSIS OF DEMENTIA

Options

a. Alcoholic dementia
b. Alzheimer's dementia
c. Creutzfeldt-Jacob's disease
d. Head trauma
e. Human immunodeficiency virus
f. Huntington's chorea
g. Parkinsonism
h. Pick's disease
i. Repeated trauma
j. Space occupying lesions
k. Substance induced dementia
l. Toxin induced dementia
m. Vascular dementia

Question

378. A 56-year-old man with no previous history is brought to the A&E Department by his wife who says he has become progressively more forgetful, tends to lose his temper and is emotionally labile. There is no history of infectious diseases or trauma.
379. A 74-year-old man presents with weakness in his arm and leg (from which he recovered within a few days) and short term memory loss. He has an extensor plantar response. He had a similar episode two year ago and became unable to identify objects and to make proper judgements.
380. A 38-year-old haemophliliac who received several blood transfusions a few year ago presents with irritability and increasing memory deficiet. He is unable to speak properly. He is on antitubercular treatment.
381. A 34-year-old woman presents with memory loss, poor concentration and inability to recognise household objects. On examination she has a right handed involuntary writhing movement. There is a strong family history of similar complaints.

382. A 62-year-old patient with chronic schizophrenia presents with mask-like face and involuntary movement in both hands. He complains of chronic cough and forgetfullness.

THEME: 73
INVESTIGATION OF DEMENTIA

Options

a. Chest X-ray
b. Serum calcium level
c. TSH and T4 levels
d. FBC and blood film
e. EEG
f. Lumbar puncture
g. Serum urea
h. Liver function tests
i. CT scan
j. Serum glucose
k. VDRL
l. HIV serology
m. Serum copper and ceruloplasmin
n. Dietary history
o. Drug levels

For each of the situations/conditions given below. Choose the one most appropriate / discriminatory option from above. The options may be used once, more than once or not at all.

Questions

383. A 50-year-old woman who underwent hysterectomy a week prior now presents with dementia, she also complains of perioral tingling.
384. A 70-year-old man presents with progressive dementia and tremor. On examination he has extensor plantar reflexes and Argyl Robertson pupils.
385. A 40-year-old man with a history of epilepsy presents with progressive dementia with fluctuating levels of consciousness. On examination he has unequal pupils.

386. A 30-year-old homosexual man presents with weight loss chronic diarrhoea and progressive dementia. On examination he has purple papules on the legs.
387. A 30-year-old man presents with sweating, agitation, tremors and dementia. He admits to binge drinking.

THEME: 74
PROGNOSIS OF DEMENTIA

Options

a. Alzheimer's disease
b. Cardiovascular accident
c. Lewy body dementia
d. Cataract
e. Parkinsonism
f. Huntington's chorea
g. Pick's disease
h. Creutzfeldt Jakob's disease

Questions

388. A 57-year-old woman whose son mentioned that she was becoming progressively forgetful with names of things and chores was diagnosed 5-7 year ago with dementia now dies.
389. An elderly woman has a history of episodic weakness of her right arm,all the episodes lasting about 12 hours is brought by her daughter who says the former has become progressively forgetful.
390. A 45-year-old man presents with difficulty in initiating movement and general slowness in doing anything. He is put on dopaminergic drugs by his GP but shows no response.

THEME: 75
MANAGEMENT OF HEAD INJURIES

Options

a. Discharge home with head injury advice
b. Urgent CT head

c. Immediate left sided burr hole
d. Immediate right sided burr hole
e. Admit for 24 hour observation
f. Intravenous dexamethasone
g. Perform skull X-ray examination
h. Intubate the patient
i. Airway assessment with cervical spine control
j. Transfer to neurosurgical colleagues
k. Pronounce the patient dead

For each of the situations/conditions given below, choose the one most appropriate/discriminatory option from above. The options may be used once, more than once, or not at all.

Questions

391. A 30-year-old woman tripped in the street and hit her head on the sharp doorway. She thinks she briefly lost consciousness at the time. She had amnesia for about half an hour after treatment but clearly remembers hitting her head. She lives with her husband.
392. A five-year-old boy has a large fresh bruise on the side of his head. His father thinks that he fell off his swing in the garden. There are a number of bruises on both arms and legs. The boy refuses to talk and is uncooperative with examination. Skull X-rays show an old occipital fracture but no new fractures.
393. A 55-year-old man is brought into A&E department following an assault and battery to the head. He has a face mask and reservoir bag delivering 15 litres per minute of oxygen, a stiff cervical collar and is attached to intravenous drip. He has no spontaneous eye opening except to pain, makes incomprehensive sounds, and does not obey commands. He demonstrates flexion with control to painful stimuli. On suction, he has no gag reflex.
394. A 28-year-old man hit his head on a plank in his garden. He did not loose consciousness and is alert and orientated with no focal neurological signs. He is complaining of a headache but has no other symptoms. He lives alone.

395. A 50-year-old man slipped at an ice rink. He lost consciousness for five minutes. He does not recall falling but does remember skating with his children. He has a severe headache and some bruising around both eyes. There is clear liquid running from his left nostril which tests positive for glucose on the stick.
396. A 35-year-old cyclist has been struck by a car on a head on collision and arrives incubated in A&E. On arrival his classical coma scale is 3. He has fixed and dilated pupils.
397. A 35-year-old man involved in an RTA presents to A&E with a large open scalp wound, multiple facial injuries and a deformed right.

Four

Hematology

THEME: 1
DIAGNOSIS OF ANEMIA

Options

a. Sideroblastic anemia.
b. Lead poisoning.
c. Pernicious anemia.
d. Folate deficiency.
e. Aplastic anemia.
f. Hereditary spherocytosis.
g. Beta-thalassemia.
h. Sickle cell anemia.
i. Iron deficiency anemia.
j. Hodgkin's disease.

For each of the situations/conditions given below, choose the one most appropriate/discriminatory option from above. The options may be used once, more than once, or not at all.

Questions

1. A 35-year-old male presents with fatigue of insidious onset, tachycardia, c/o tingling and numbness of extremities, serum bilirubin is slightly raised and the MCV is 104.
2. Anemia with petechiae after sulfonamide therapy.
3. A 29-year-old radiology technician presents with bleeding gums, epistaxis, sore throat and has breathlessness and tachycardia.
4. A 15-year-old boy presents with ulcers of the leg and splenomegaly. On examination he has pallor and reports that his elder brother also had a similar problem.
5. A 30-year-old female, a native of central Africa presents with intense pain in the flanks, reports that she had similar episodes earlier. On examination, she has low grade fever and blood investigations reveal anemia

6. A 50-year-old male who works with scrape metals presents with constipation, tingling and numbness of extremities, weakness of muscles, anorexia. On examination, he has pallor.
7. A 40-year-old male presents with neck nodes, weight loss and fever.

THEME: 2
DIAGNOSIS OF ANEMIA

Options

a. Iron deficiency anemia.
b. Anemia of chronic disease.
c. Thalassemia.
d. Sideroblastic anemia.
e. Aplastic anemia.
f. Pernicious anemia.

For each of the situations/conditions given below, choose the one most appropriate/discriminatory option from above. The options may be used once, more than once, or not at all.

Questions

	Serum Iron	*TIBC*	*Ferritin*	*Iron in Marrow*	*Iron in erythroblasts*
8.	Reduced	Reduced	Increased	Absent	Absent
9.	Reduced/normal	Reduced	Reduced	N/Increased	A/reduced
10.	Normal	Normal	Normal	Present	Present
11.	Increased	Normal	Increased	Present	Ring form.

THEME : 3
DIAGNOSIS OF ANEMIA

Options

a. Microcytic anemia.
b. Normocytic anemia.
c. Macrocytic anemia.

d. None of the above

For each of the situations/conditions given below, choose the one most appropriate/discriminatory option from above. The options may be used once, more than once, or not at all.

Questions

12. Renal failure.
13. Liver disease.
14. Sideroblastic anemia.
15. Pregnancy.
16. Thalassemia.

THEME : 4
INVESTIGATIONS OF ANEMIA

Options

a. Serum ferritin.
b. Total iron-binding capacity.
c. Serum iron.
d. Whole body RBC counting with radioactive vitamin B_{12}.
e. Schilling test.
f. Serum folate.
g. Folate in RBC.
h. Hemoglobin electrophoresis.
i. Sickling test.
j. Bone marrow aspiration.
k. LAP score.

For each of the situations/conditions given below, choose the one most appropriate/discriminatory option from above. The options may be used once, more than once, or not at all.

Questions

17. Iron deficiency anemia.
18. Pernicious deficiency anemia.
19. Folate deficiency anemia.
20. Thalassemia.
21. A 16-year-old male with icterus but no splenomegaly and history of leg ulcers.

22. A 55-year-old male with pancytopenia.
23. A 50-year-old male with leucocytosis with myelocytes and metamyelocytes in the peripheral blood.

THEME : 5
INVESTIGATIONS OF HEMOLYTIC ANEMIA

Options

a. Full blood count.
b. Monospot test.
c. Urine microscopy.
d. Ham's test.
e. Reticulocyte count.
f. Thick and thin blood film.
g. Coomb's test.
h. Hemoglobin electrophoresis.
i. Red cell fragility test.

For each of the situations/conditions given below, choose the one most appropriate/discriminatory option from above. The options may be used once, more than once, or not at all.

Questions

24. A 25-year-old man returns from holiday in Africa. He is pale on admission and pyrexial.
25. A 15-year-old girl presents with tiredness, splenomegaly and a sore throat with white exudates.
26. A 25-year-old has pancytopenia, abdominal pain and has had thrombotic events 5 years ago.
27. A rhesus positive baby (group A) is born to rhesus negative mother.
28. A 30-year-old man has mild anaemia, splenomegaly and has had gallstones. He is of Caucasian origin.

THEME :6
ANEMIAS WHICH ARE MORE THAN ANEMIAS

Options

a. Pernicious anemia.

b. Aplastic anemia.
c. Myelodysplastic syndrome.
d. Felty's syndrome.
e. Pure red cell aplasia.
f. Paroxysmal nocturnal hemoglobinuria.
g. Evan's syndrome.
h. Hypersplenism.
i. Thrombotic thrombocytopenic purpura.

For each of the situations/conditions given below, choose the one most appropriate/discriminatory option from above. The options may be used once, more than once, or not at all.

Questions

29. Stem cell failure.
30. Non-immune destruction of platelets and erythrocytes.
31. Impaired thymidine synthesis.
32. Complement mediated lysis of all cells.
33. Immune destruction of platelets and erythrocytes.

THEME: 7
BLOOD INVESTIGATIONS

Options

	RBC mass	*Plasma volume*	*Oxygen saturation*	*Erythropoietin*
a.	Normal	Reduced	Normal	Normal
b.	Increased	Normal	Normal	Reduced
c.	Increased	Normal	Normal	Increased
d.	Increased	Normal	Normal	Increased

For each of the situations/conditions given below, choose the one most appropriate/discriminatory option from above. The options may be used once, more than once, or not at all.

Questions

34. A 60-year-old male with a plethoric face, neutrophilic leukocytosis, thrombocytosis, splenomegaly and an ESR of zero.

35. A 72-year-old woman with a 4 cm cystic renal mass, cannot ball metastases in the lung, and polycythemia.
36. A 4-year-old boy with uncorrected tetralogy of Fallot.
37. A 20-year-old female marathon runner who is dehydrated from lack of water supplementation during the race.

THEME: 8
INTERPRETATION OF HAEMATOLOGY RESULTS

Options

a. Alcoholism
b. Beta thalassaemia major
c. Chronic blood loss
d. Cytotoxic drugs
e. Dietary deficiency
f. Haemolysis
g. Hypothyroidism
h. Perinicious anaemia
i. Rheumatoid arthritis
j. Untreated hyperthyroidism

For each of the situations/conditions given below, choose the one most appropriate/discriminatory option from above. The options may be used once, more than once, or not at all.

Questions

38. Hb 7.9g/dl
 MCV 57fl
 MCHC 21g/dl
 WBC 9.0 *1.000,000,000/L
 Platelets 523* 1,000,000,000/L
 Retics 6%
 ESR 14 min/hr
39. Hb 10.9g/dl
 MCV 106 fl
 HCH 37g/dl
 WBC 8.0*1,000,000,000/L
 Platelets 223*1,000,000,000/L

	Retics	< 1%
	ESR	8 min/hr
	Blood film	target cells
40.	Hb	5.6g/l
	MCV	83fl
	MCHC	37 g/dl
	WBC	1.3*1,000,000,000/L
	Platelets	62*1,000,000,000/L
	Retics	<1%
	ESR	6 min/hr
	Blood film	Normal
41.	Hb	9.8g/dl
	MCV	84fl
	MCHC	32g/dl
	WBC	7.1*1,000,000,000/L
	Platelets	194*1,000,000,000/L
	Retics	<1%
	ESR	90 min/hr
	Blood film	normal
42.	Hb	10.1g/dL
	MCV	73fl
	MCHC	31g.dL
	WBC	6.1 * 1,000,000,000?L
	Platelets	283 * 1,000,000,000/L
	Retics	9%
	ESR	15min/hr
	Blood film	small irregular shaped RBC, anisocytosis

THEME: 9
INTERPRETATION OF PERIPHERAL BLOOD SMEAR

Options

a. Infectious mononucleosis
b. Megaloblastic anaemia
c. Multiple myeloma
d. Iron deficiency anaemia
e. Beta thalassemia major
f. Malaria
g. Myelofibrosis

h. AML
i. Thrombotic thrombocytopenia.
j. CLL
k. Sickle cell anaemia

For each of the situations/conditions given below, choose the one most appropriate/discriminatory option from above. The options may be used once, more than once, or not at all.

Questions

43. Microcytosis, anisocytosis, poikilocytosis, hypochromia, target cells and tear drop cells.
44. Stacking of red cells into rouleaux and abnormal plasma cells.
45. Hypochromic, microcytic red cells and cigar-shaped cells.
46. Sickle cells, target cells and nucleated red cells.
47. Poikilocytosis, anisocytosis, macrocytosis, tear drop cells and hypersegmented polymorphs.
48. Leucoerythroblastic blood film with immature white cells and nucleated red cells, anisocytosis, poikilocytosis and tear drop cells.

THEME: 10
COMPLICATIONS OF BLOOD DYSCRASIA

Options

a. Generalised lymphadenopathy
b. Meningitis
c. Massive splenomegaly
d. Purpura
e. Bone pain
f. Gum hyperplasia
g. Thrombophilia

For each of the situations/conditions given below, choose the one most appropriate/discriminatory option from above. The options may be used once, more than once, or not at all.

Questions

49. A 34-year-old woman with increased granulocyte series and a raised platelet count.

50. A young boy with cervical lymphadenopathy and a raised white cell blood count.
51. A 3-year-old boy presents with neck stiffness, photophobia and headache. Blood film shows a marked lymphocytosis.
52. A 38-year-old woman with cervical lymphadenopathy, Mature lymphoblasts are seen on the blood film. Examination reveals a mild splenomegaly. He is on phenytoin for epilepsy.

THEME: 11
CAUSES OF BRUISING

Options

a. Haemophilia A
b. Scurvy
c. Anticoagulant therapy
d. Leukemia
e. Side effects of steroids
f. DIC
g. HSP
h. ITP
i. TTP
j. Christmas disease
k. VWD
l. Hereditary hemorrhagic telangiectasia

For each of the situations/conditions given below, choose the one most appropriate/discriminatory option from above. The options may be used once, more than once, or not at all.

Questions

53. A 15-year-old male presents with fever, abdominal pains, purpura and focal neurological deficits.
54. A 45-year-old female is noted to have capillary angiectases on the buccal mucosa and tongue. She has suffered from intermittent gastrointestinal bleeding.
55. A 15-year-old girl has history of arthralgia and abdominal pain. She now presents with purpura around the but-

tocks and upper thighs after an upper respiratory infection.

56. A 65-year-old man presents with epistaxis and bruising. She has a recent history of a deep vein thrombosis.
57. A 65-year-old female who lives alone presents with ecchymoses of the lower limbs. She has a poor diet lacking fruit and vegetables and suffers from rheumatoid arthritis.

THEME: 12
DIAGNOSIS OF CLOTTING ABNORMALITIES

Options

a. Idiopathic thrombocytopenic purpura.
b. DIC.
c. Factor VIII deficiency.
d. Factor XI deficiency.
e. Anticoagulant therapy.
f. Factor VII deficiency.
g. Bernard-Soulier syndrome.
h. I.T.P.

Key: TTP—Thrombotic thrombocytopenic purpura
TT—Thrombin time
PT—Prothrombin time
APTT—Activated partial thromboplastin time

For each of the situations/conditions given below, choose the one most appropriate/discriminatory option from above. The options may be used once, more than once, or not at all.

Questions

58. A 20-year-old male with prolonged PTT but a normal PT, TT and platelet count.
59. A 30-year-old female with intrauterine fetal death and prolonged PT, APTT and TT with thrombocytopenia.
60. A 20-year-old female with thrombocytopenia with normal PT, APTT and TT and a normal LDH.
61. A 60-year-old female on treatment for unilateral foot edema with prolonged PT and APTT.
62. A 25-year-old woman with thrombocytopenia and anemia with normal prothrombin time PTT and TT and an elevated LDH.

THEME: 13
INVESTIGATIONS OF BLEEDING DISORDERS

Options

	INR	KCCT	Thrombin	Platelet Count	Bleeding Time
a.	Normal	Raised	Raised	Normal	Normal
b.	Raised	raised	raised	low	raised
c.	Raised	raised	normal	normal/low	normal/raised
d.	Normal	normal	normal	normal	raised
e.	Raised	raised	normal	normal	normal
f.	Normal	raised	normal	normal	normal
g.	Normal	raised	normal	normal	raised
h.	Normal	normal	normal	low	raised

For each of the situations/conditions given below, choose the one most appropriate/discriminatory option from above. The options may be used once, more than once, or not at all.

Questions

63. Platelet defect.
64. ITP.
65. Heparin.
66. Hemophilia.
67. V.W.D.
68. DIC.
69. Vitamin K deficiency.
70. Liver disease.

THEME: 14
TREATMENT OF CLOTTING DISORDERS.

Options

a. Warfarin.
b. Factor 8 concentrate.
c. Fresh frozen plasma.
d. Oral ferrous sulphate.
e. IM Iron formulation.
f. Heparin.

g. Vitamin K.
h. Desmopressin.
i. Factor 10.
j. Blood transfusion.
k. No treatment required.

For each of the situations/conditions given below, choose the one most appropriate/discriminatory option from above. The options may be used once, more than once, or not at all.

Questions

71. A 70-year-old man has liver failure and bleeding varices, the surgeon has decided to take her to theatre to try and stop the bleeding.
72. A 10-year-old boy with thalassemia disease is breathless with a hemoglobin of 8.0.
73. A lady who has a prosthetic heart valve is now pregnant. She needs advice on anticoagulation.
74. A 12-year-old girl is found to have a prolonged bleeding time, serum factor 8 levels are found to be normal.

THEME: 15
PREVENTION AND TREATMENT OF THROMBOTIC DISEASE

Options

a. Early mobilisation
b. Aspirin
c. Thrombolysis
d. Compression stockings
e. Foot pump
f. Intravenous heparin
g. Phenindione
h. Warfarin (INR 2-3)
i. Warfarin (INR 3-4.5)
j. Subcutaneous unfractionated heparin
k. Subcutaneous low molecular weight heparin
l. Nothing

For each of the situations/conditions given below, choose the one most appropriate/discriminatory option from above. The options may be used once, more than once, or not at all.

Questions

75. A 25-year-old man is admitted for an elective haemorrhoidectomy. He has no other medical problems.
76. A 55-year-old woman is admitted for an elective total hip replacement. She has a history of peptic ulcer disease and takes lansoprazole. She is otherwise well. What prophylaxis against thrombosis is indicated.
77. A 30-year-old woman has had four spontaneous abortions, two deep vein thrombosis and suffers from migraine. Blood test confirms the presence of anti-cardiolipin antibodies.
78. A 25-year-old woman is 16 weeks pregnant and develops a painful, swollen leg. A femoral vein thrombosis is diagnosed with doppler ultarsound. She has already been started on intravenous heparin.
79. A 65-year-old man is in atrial fibrillation secondary to rheumatic mitral valve disease. Echocardiogram shows a dilated left atrium and mild mitral stenosis only. He has developed a severe rash with warfarin in the past.

THEME: 16
TARGET LEVELS OF INR ON WARFARIN TREATMENT

Options

a. 3 – 4.0
b. 4 – 4.9
c. 2.5 – 3.5
d. 2 – 3.0
e. 3.5 – 4.5

For each of the situations/conditions given below, choose the one most appropriate/discriminatory option from above. The options may be used once, more than once, or not at all.

Questions

80. Pulmonary embolism.
81. Caged ball prosthetic heart valve.
82. Atrial fibrillation.
83. Above knee deep vein thrombosis.

THEME: 17
DIAGNOSIS OF HEMATOLOGICAL DISORDERS

Options

a. Sickle cell anemia.
b. Paroxysmal nocturnal hemoglobinuria.
c. Acute myeloid leukemia.
d. Hodgkin's lymphoma.
e. Myelofibrosis.
f. Primary polycythemia.
g. Gaisbock's syndrome.
h. Middle cerebral artery hemorrhage.
i. Multiple myeloma.
j. Fe deficiency anemia.

For each of the situations/conditions given below, choose the one most appropriate/discriminatory option from above. The options may be used once, more than once, or not at all.

Questions

84. A 28-year-old man recovering from surgery, presents with recurrent abdominal pain and his urine which he had voided at night was dark in colour.
85. A 63-year-old female presents with tinnitus, vertigo, feeling depressed. On examinations she has hypertension, intermittent claudication and also complains of severe itching after a hot bath.
86. A 50-year obese male, who is a hypertensive and has been smoking since the last 15 years, presents with a history suggestive of transient ischemic attacks.
87. A 45-year-old female presents with insidious onset of weight loss, weakness and lethargy. She c/o fullness bone pain. On examination, spleen is enlarged. Philadelphia chromosome is absent.
88. A 25-year-old female presents with an enlarged painless lymph node in the neck. She also reports of fever and weight loss. Her peripheral blood smear shows Reed-Sternberg cells with a bilobed mirror-imaged nucleolus.

89. A 65-year-old man presents with bone pain, anemia and renal failure. His bone marrow reveals abundance of malignant plasma cells.
90. A 12-year-old boy presents with swelling of the hands and feet and anemia. His peripheral blood smear reveals target cells and elongated crescent-shaped red blood cells.
91. A 70-year-old woman presents with anemia. She is noted to have koilonychias and atrophic glossitis. Her blood smear reveals microcytic, hypochromic blood cells.

THEME: 18
DIAGNOSIS OF HEMATOLOGICAL DISORDERS

Options

a. ALL.
b. Multiple myeloma.
c. Acute myeloid leukemia.
d. Acute promyelocytic leukemia.
e. ITP.
f. CLL.
g. TTP.
h. CML.
i. Polycythemia rubra vera
j. Amyloidosis.
k. Aplastic anemia.
l. Non-hodgkin's lymphoma.
m. Hodgkin's lymphoma.

For each of the situations/conditions given below, choose the one most appropriate/discriminatory option from above. The options may be used once, more than once, or not at all.

Questions

92. A 70-year-old retired farmer presents to his GP with weakness and bone pain. He is noted to be anemic with increased calcium and uric acid levels. X-ray reveals osteolytic lesions.
93. A 4-year-old boy presents with recurrent infections, bone pains and weakness. Investigations reveal a pancytopenia and blasts.

94. A 65-year-old woman presents with malaise. She is noted to have gum hypertrophy and skin nodules. Investigations reveal a pancytopenia and blasts.
95. A 60-year-old farmer presents with epistaxis. His peripheral blood shows lymphocytosis.
96. An HIV- positive man on effective antiretroviral therapy presents with painless lymphadenopathy and fevers, drenching night sweats and weight loss.
97. A 40-year-old bank manager presents with tiredness, weight loss, fever and sweating. Examination reveals an enlarged spleen. Blood tests show lymphocytosis and anemia. The patient is tested positive for Philadelphia chromosome.

THEME: 19
DIAGNOSIS OF HEMATOLOGICAL DISORDERS

Options

a. Protein C deficiency.
b. Paroxysmal nocturnal hemoglobinuria (PNH).
c. Lupus inhibitor syndrome.
d. Trousseau's syndrome.

For each of the situations/conditions given below,, choose the one most appropriate/discriminatory option from above. The options may be used once, more than once, or not at all.

Questions

98. A 30-year-old woman with a history of rash and arthritis has deep vein thrombosis. She has had a problem with recurrent abortions.
99. A 45-year-old man, who has been followed up by his physician for 4 years for chronic iron deficiency anemia with unknown source of blood loss, has portal vein thrombosis.
100. A 60-year-old man had deep vein thrombosis of his left leg last month and is being appropriately managed with warfarin. He has symptoms of new clot formation in the right leg as well as a clot in his left forearm.

101. A 67-year-old woman with mitral stenosis is started on warfarin by her cardiologist. On the third day, painful red areas appear on her thigh and breast.

THEME: 20
PATHOGENESIS OF HEMATOLOGICAL DISORDERS

Options

a. Hereditary spherocytosis.
b. Haemophilia.
c. Iron deficiency anemia.
d. Vitamin B_{12} deficiency anemia.
e. G6PD deficiency.
f. ITP.
g. Sickle cell anemia.
h. Hypersplenism.
i. Chronic renal failure.
j. Myelofibrosis.
k. None of the above.

For each of the situations/conditions given below, choose the one most appropriate/discriminatory option from above. The options may be used once, more than once, or not at all.

Questions

102. Autoimmune disease.
103. Crystallization of haemoglobin.
104. Membrane oxidation.
105. Membrane loss.
106. Impaired generation of factor IX.

THEME: 21
TREATMENT OF HEMATOLOGICAL DISEASES

Options

a. Oral iron therapy.
b. Parenteral iron therapy.
c. Corticosteroids.

d. Bone marrow transplant.
e. Intravenous immunoglobulin.
f. Anti-thymocyte globulin.
g. Cobalamine and folate.
h. Blood transfusion.
i. Warfarin therapy.

For each of the situations/conditions given below, choose the one most appropriate/discriminatory option from above. The options may be used once, more than once, or not at all.

Questions

107. A 10-year-old boy with a hemoglobin of 6 gm/dl and microcytic anemia.
108. A 63-year-old male with lymphadenopathy, leucocytosis count 60000 with 80 lymphocytes, anemia amd spherocytosis.
109. A 6-year-old boy with thrombocytopenia, increased megakaryocytes in the bone marrow and antiplatelet antibodies.
110. A 40-year-old male with tropical sprue and macrocytic anemia.
111. A 50-year-old male with pancytopenia and replacement of bone marrow and fat.

THEME: 22
DIAGNOSIS OF HEMATOLOGICAL MALIGNANCIES

Options

a. A.M.L.
b. A.L.L.
c. C.M.L.
d. C.L.L.
e. N.H.L.
f. Hodgkin's lymphoma.
g. Myeloma.
h. Hairy cell leukemia.
i. Burkitt's lymphoma.

For each of the situations/conditions given below, choose the one most appropriate/discriminatory option from above. The options may be used once, more than once, or not at all.

Questions

112. A 50-year-old male presents with an insidious onset of anemia weight loss, low grade fever and abdominal discomfort. Bone marrow aspirate shows an increase in the myeloid precursors.
113. A 48-year-old male presents with breathlessness, tachycardia, recurrent infections, he has a palpable spleen and the blood film shows a low WBC count and cells with a filament like cytoplasm.
114. An elderly female presents with an insidious onset of breathlessness, feeling tired easily, palpitations. On examination there is fracture of L_4 and L_5. On investigations the level of urea is also increased.
115. A 4-year-old patient with pancytopenia and circulating blasts.
116. A 24-year-old male with blasts in the peripheral smear but no lymphadenopathy.
117. A 72-year-old male with lymphocytosis and decreased platelets.

THEME: 23
CLASSIFICATION OF NON-HODGKIN'S LYMPHOMA

Options

a. Nodular lymphocytic, poorly differentiated type.
b. Histiocytic type.
c. Undifferentiated, Burkitt's type.
d. Lymphoblastic type.

For each of the situations/conditions given below, choose the one most appropriate/discriminatory option from above. The options may be used once, more than once, or not at all.

Questions

118. Infiltrate of large, irregular, cleaved or noncleaved cells derived from lymphoid elements, usually occurring in a

diffuse pattern and frequently appearing in an extranodal site.

119. Diffuse pattern of aggressively disseminating t cells with round or convoluted nuclei and scanty cytoplasm, often presenting as a localized mediastinal mass.
120. Infiltrates of small, cleaved, and variably sized cells of B cell origin, usually presenting in adult life as asymptomatic lymphadenopathy.
121. Radio sensitive, slowly progressive lymphoma associated with prolonged survival despite early dissemination to liver, bone marrow, and peripheral blood.
122. Occurring in children and young adults; when untreated, there is rapid dissemination to peripheral blood and meninges, with a median survival time of less than one year.
123. Rapidly growing, diffuse infiltrate of large, uniform and noncleaved B cells; often presenting as an abdominal mass in children.
124. Occurring predominantly in later adult years; potentially curable when drug combinations that include doxorubicin are used.
125. Surgery and chemotherapy with cyclophosphamide containing drug combination are used for effective primary treatment.

THEME: 24
CHROMOSOMAL ANOMALIES IN HEMATOLOGY

Options

a. Deletions of chromosome 5 and/or 7.
b. Hyperdiploidy with more than 50 chromosomes.
c. Translocation of the *abl* oncogene from chromosome 9 to chromosome 22.
d. Translocation of the *myc* oncogene from chromosome 8 to the heavy chain immunoglobulin locus on chromosome 14.

For each of the situations/conditions given below, choose the one most appropriate/discriminatory option from above. The options may be used once, more than once, or not at all.

Questions

126. Burkitt's lymphoma.
127. Acute myeloid leukemia (AML) following chemotherapy.
128. Chronic myeloid leukemia (CML).

THEME: 25
CAUSES OF HIGH ESR

Options

a. Disseminated malignancy.
b. Uraemia.
c. Anaemia.
d. Tuberculosis.
e. Giant cell arteritis.
f. Sarcoidosis.
g. Bacterial infection.
h. Amyloidosis.
i. Multiple myeloma.
j. Rheumatoid arthritis
k. Waldenstorm's macroglobulinemia
l. SLE

For each of the situations/conditions given below, choose the one most appropriate/discriminatory option from above. The options may be used once, more than once, or not at all.

Questions

129. A 70-year-old woman develops severe hip pain while gardening. Hip joint X-ray shows fracture of neck of femur. She gives a history of lower back pain and malaise. She is tender over the lumbar spine. ESR is 110 mm/hr.
130. An 18-year-old woman from Trinidad presents with pleuritic chest pain, breathlessness, arthralgia, myalgia and facial rash. She has a small left pleural effusion. ESR is 80 mm/hr. C-reactive protein is within normal limits.
131. A 70-year-old woman presents with bitemporal headache and visual loss in the left eye. ESR is 90 mm/hr.

132. A 60-year-old woman has blurred vision, headaches and lethargy. On examination she has tortuous retinal vessels with evidence of recent retinal hemorrhages. ESR is 80 mm/hr and she has a marked increase in IgM levels.
133. A 55-year-old man has had bronchiectasis for 30 years. His chest is stable and there is no infection. He complains of malaise and arthralgia and has proteinuria and an enlarged liver and spleen. ESR is 110 mm/hr.

THEME: 26
IMMUNODEFICIENCY DISORDERS

Options

a. Ataxia-telangiectasia.
b. Di-George syndrome.
c. X-linked hypogammaglobulinemia.
d. Thymic aplasia.
e. Severe combined immunodeficiency disease.
f. Wiskott-Aldrich syndrome.
g. Graft versus host reaction.
h. Febrile transfusion reaction.
i. None of the above.

For each of the situations/conditions given below, choose the one most appropriate/discriminatory option from above. The options may be used once, more than once, or not at all.

Questions

134. A 9-months-old infant has a small fish like mouth, low set notched ears, cardiac insufficiency, hypocalcemia and lymphopenia. The patient has had several episodes of viral pneumonia, a fungal infection of the oral mucosa and fever, blisters caused by herpes simplex virus. The infant is diagnosed as having an immunodeficiency disease.
135. A 8-months-old infant has a history of chronic diarrhea, several episodes of pneumonia, and otitis media. He also has had oral candidiases and infections with herpes simplex virus. He has no detectable thymus upon radiography and B lymphocytes are absent. A rash was evident at birth.

136. A newborn boy with Di-George syndrome in adverently received crossmatch compatible blood that was not irrigated. The infant developed fever, diarrhea, liver abnormalities, skin rash and lost weight.
137. A newborn boy with truncus arteriosus has carpopedal spasm and absence of the mediastinal shadow on a chest X-ray.

THEME: 27
IMMUNODEFICIENCY AND INFECTION

Options

a. Neutrophil.
b. T lymphocyte.
c. Eosinophils.
d. Antibody.
e. Complement.

For each of the situations/conditions given below, choose the one most appropriate/discriminatory option from above. The options may be used once, more than once, or not at all.

Questions

138. Mycobacterium.
139. Neisseria species.
140. Candidiasis.
141. Nocardia species.
142. *Pseudomonas aeruginosa.*
143. Pyogenic bacteria.

Five

Endocrinology

THEME: 1
MULTIPLE ENDOCRINE ADENOMATOSIS

Options

a. Elevated serum calcium level.
b. Elevated serum thyrocalcitonin level.
c. Severe watery diarrhea.
d. Abdominal pain secondary to peptic ulceration.
e. Distorted body habitus

For each of the situations/conditions given below,, choose the one most appropriate/discriminatory option from above. The options may be used once, more than once, or not at all.

Questions

1. MEA type I (Wermer's syndrome).
2. MEA type II (Sipple's syndrome).
3. MEA type III (mucosal neuroma syndrome).
4. Pancreatic gastrinoma (Zollinger – Ellison syndrome).
5. Pancreatic cholera.

THEME: 2
DIAGNOSIS OF ENDOCRINE EMERGENCIES

Options

a. Myxoedema coma.
b. Thyrotoxic storm.
c. Addisonian crises.
d. Hypopituitary coma.
e. Phaeochromocytoma.

For each of the situations/conditions given below,, choose the one most appropriate/discriminatory option from above. The options may be used once, more than once, or not at all.

Questions

6. A 40-year-old male presents with headache and is in a state of lowered consciousness. On examination he has ophthalmoplegia, is hypotensive and hypothermic but deep tendon reflexes are normal.
7. A 40-year-old male presents in a state of lowered consciousness. On examination he has ophthalmoplegia, is hypotensive and hypothermic and deep tendon reflexes are depressed.
8. A 40-year-old agitated and febrile patient comes with severe abdominal pain.
9. A 40-year-old male presents with sudden onset headache and is formed to be hypertensive.

THEME: 3
INVESTIGATION OF ENDOCRINE DISORDERS

Options

a. ACTH stimulation test
b. Serum aldosterone levels
c. T3, T4 and TSH levels
d. Examination of old X-rays
e. Water deprivation test
f. C- peptide levels
g. Dexamethasone suppression test
h. Fasting blood glucose
i. Urinary ketone levels
j. Glycosylated haemoglobin levels
k. Basal plasma protein levels
l. Liver function tests

For each of the situations/conditions given below, choose the one most appropriate/discriminatory option from above. The options may be used once, more than once, or not at all.

Questions

10. A 40-year-old woman presents with tachycardia, atrial fibrillation, double vision and swelling above her ankles. She has lidlag on examination.

11. A 35-year-old man presents with insidious onset weakness and weight loss. On examination, he has hyperpigmentation of the palmar creases and postural hypotension.
12. A 50-year-old man is admitted for investigation of his glycosuria. His wife comments that his appearance has changed over the last few years and everything seems to have got bigger. He also complains of tingling in his left hand and excessive sweating.
13. A 15-year-old boy presents with four weeks history of weight loss, polyuria and polydipsia.
14. A 40-year-old man has hypotension, hyperglycaemia, myopathy, thinning of the skin, buffalo hump and truncal obesity.

THEME: 4
TREATMENT OF ENDOCRINE CONDITIONS

Options

a. Calciferol
b. Phenoxybenzamine and propranolol
c. Long-term replacement with glucocorticoid steroids and mineralocorticoids
d. Carbimazole
e. Thyroxine
f. Ocreotide
g. Propylthiouracil
h. Propranolol
i. IV calcium gluconate
j. Desmopressin
k. Metyrapone

For each of the situations/conditions given below, choose the one most appropriate/discriminatory option from above. The options may be used once, more than once, or not at all.

Questions

15. A 48-year-old woman presents to her GP with fatigue, depression and weight gain. She also complains of constipation and poor memory. On examination she has a

smooth "peaches and cream" complexion, thin eyebrows and a large tongue.

16. A 45-year-old obese woman presents to casualty with rib fractures and bruising following a fall in the bathroom. She is noted to be hypertensive and has glycosuria.
17. A 72-year-old woman presents to her GP with weight loss and depression. On examination she is noted to have buccal pigmentation and pigmented scars. She appears dehydrated. Her blood pressure in 100/60 mmHg .
18. A 32-year-old pregnant woman presents to her GP with anxiety. On examination she is a nervous woman with exophthalmos, warm peripheries and atrial fibrillation.
19. A 42-year-old man presents to his GP complaining of change in appearance and headaches. His eyebrow is more prominent and his nose has broadened. He states that his shoes are too small and he has tingling in certain fingers, worse at night.

THEME: 5
CAUSES OF CUSHING'S SYNDROME

Options

a. Cushing's disease due to pituitary adrenocorticotrophic hormone (ATCH) excess.
b. Cushing's syndrome due to an adrenal tumor.
c. Ectopic ACTH syndrome.
d. Adrenal insufficiency.
e. No adrenal disease.

A patient is suspected of having Cushing's disease. For diagnostic purposes, dexamethasone is given in a low dose (2 mg daily) for 2 days and high dose (8 mg daily) for 2 days. For each change in urinary free cortisol levels, select the diagnosis it indicates.

For each of the situations/conditions given below,, choose the one most appropriate/discriminatory option from above. The options may be used once, more than once, or not at all.

Questions

20. They fall distinctly with low-dose dexame
high-dose dexamethasone.
21. They do not change with low-dose dexamethasone but fall distinctly with high-dose dexamethasone.
22. They do not fall with either low-dose or high-dose dexamethasone; the plasma ACTH level is elevated.
23. They do not with either low-dose or high-dose dexamethasone; the plasma ACTH level is low.

THEME: 6
PHYSICAL FACIES

Options

a. Toad face.
b. Round face.
c. Monkey face.
d. Moon face.
e. Coarse face.
f. Hippocratic face.
g. Sallow face.
h. Haggered face.

For each of the situations/conditions given below,, choose the one most appropriate/discriminatory option from above. The options may be used once, more than once, or not at all.

Questions

24. Acromegaly.
25. Uraemia.
26. Hypothyroidism.
27. Peritonitis.
28. Hypopituitarism.
29. Myotonia.
30. Pseudohypoparathyroidism.
31. Cushing's syndrome.

THEME: 7
DIAGNOSIS OF THYROID DISEASE

Options

a. De Quervain's thyroiditis
b. MEN -I
c. Hashimoto's disease
d. MEN -II
e. Thyroid carcinoma
f. Thyroid storm
g. Graves disease
h. Simple goitre
i. Hypothyroidism
j. Thyroglossal cyst

For each of the situations/conditions given below, choose the one most appropriate/discriminatory option from above. The options may be used once, more than once, or not at all.

Questions

32. A 40-year-old man presents with weight loss despite a good appetite, constipation, frontal headaches and menorrhagia. She also complains of recurrent dyspepsia and peptic ulcer symptoms. Her abdominal X-ray shows renal stones.
33. A 40-year-old woman presents with weight loss, muscular weakness, oligomenorrhoea, diarrhoea and blurring of vision. On examination there is exophthalmos and proximal myopathy.
34. A 50-year-old woman presents with goitre. On examination the thyroid is firm and rubbery. Thyroid microsomal antibodies are positive in high titre.
35. A 30-year-old man presents with a hard nodular midline neck mass that moves upward on swallowing. Thyroid radio-nucleotide scan shows cold spots.
36. A 45-year-old woman presents with fever, tachycardia, restlessness, hypertension and vomiting. On examination she has a diffused swelling of the thyroid gland and strabismus with diplopia.

37. A 20-year-old student presents with a neck swelling. On examination the swelling moves up with swallowing and profusion of the tongue.
38. A 28-year-old woman presents with weight gain, constipation, lethargy and flaky rash.
39. A 30-year-old woman presents with fever, sore throat and dysphagia. On examination she has a fine tremor and a diffusely tender thyroid. Radioisotopes scan shows no uptake.

THEME: 8
DIAGNOSIS OF NECK SWELLING

Options

a. Toxic adenoma
b. Toxic multinodular goitre
c. Hyperthyroidism
d. Hypothyroidism
e. Parathyroid carcinoma
f. Secondary hyperparathyroidism
g. Hypoparathyroidism
h. Adrenal hyperplasic
i. Hyperprolactinoma
j. Acromegaly
k. Follicular carcinoma
l. Anaplastic carcinoma
m. Papillary carcinoma
n. Chromophobe adenoma

For each of the situations/conditions given below, choose the one most appropriate/discriminatory option from above. The option may be used once, more than once, or not at all

Questions

40. A 52-year-old man presents with painless lump in the neck and chronic cough. Physical examination finds tachycardia and pallor. He feels that he has lost weight, but he is not certain. He does not smoke or drink.

41. On a routine blood examination a 43-year-old woman is found to have high serum calcium levels. She has complained recently of bouts of abdominal pain and recurrent UTI. On physical examination you find an enlarged thyroid gland.
42. A young woman is warm, even when resting. She turns the central heating off, opens the windows and annoys her family. Her pulse rate is high and her skin is moist.
43. A middle-aged woman complains of irritability and weight loss. She says she has palpitations. On physical examination you find mild tachycardia and goitre. There are no eye changes. A thyroid scan determines a single hot nodule.
44. A young man presents with a neck lump. It is painless and had been bothering him for the past 4 months. He has no other symptoms or signs. On palpitation you find the lump to be single discrete not particular hard and confined to the thyroid gland itself. His cervical lymph nodes are enlarged.

THEME : 9
THYROID FUNCTION TESTS

Options

a. Graves disease.
b. Hypothyroidism.
c. Subacute thyroiditis.
d. Nontoxic goiter.

For each of the situations/conditions given below, choose the one most appropriate/discriminatory option from above. The options may be used once, more than once, or not at all.

Questions

45. Elevated serum thyroxine (T_4), low radioactive iodine uptake.
46. Elevated serum T_4, low triiodothyronine (T_3) resin uptake.
47. Elevated serum T_4, elevated radioactive iodine uptake.

THEME: 10
PATHOLOGY OF THYROID DISORDERS

Options

a. Graves' disease.
b. Testicular feminization syndrome.
c. Addison's disease.
d. Hypopituitarism.
e. Acromegaly.

For each of the situations/conditions given below, choose the one most appropriate/discriminatory option from above. The options may be used once, more than once, or not at all.

Questions

48. Excessive production of hormone by an endocrine tumor.
49. Destruction of an endocrine gland by tumor, trauma or infarction.
50. Stimulation of an endocrine gland by autoimmune mechanisms.
51. Destruction of an endocrine gland by autoimmune mechanisms.
52. Impaired sensitivity of peripheral tissues to normal circulating levels of a hormone.

THEME: 11
TREATMENT OF THYROID DISORDER

Options

a. Subtotal thyroidectomy
b. Carbimazole
c. Thyroxine
d. Beta blockers
e. Total thyroidectomy
f. Thyroid lobectomy
g. Radiotherapy
h. Corticosteroids
i. Potassium iodide
j. Propranolol
k. Radioactive iodine

For each of the situations/conditions given below, choose the one most appropriate/discriminatory option from above. The options may be used once, more than once, or not at all.

Questions

53. A 12-year-old girl presents with thyrotoxicosis. A radio-isotope scan shows an enlarged thyroid with uniform uptake throughout.
54. A 55-year-old woman is found to have an enlarged toxic nodular goitre.
55. A 48-year-old woman presents with thyroid enlargement. Thyroid function tests are normal. Needle biopsy confirms the diagnosis of Hashimoto's thyroiditis.
56. A 28-year-old woman is found to have Graves' disease. She remains thyrotoxic after treatment with carbimazole for one year.
57. A 30-year-old pregnant woman is found to have thyro-toxicosis due to Graves' disease during second trimester of pregnancy.

THEME: 12
DIABETES

Options

a. True of diabetes mellitus (DM) but not diabetes insipidus (DI).
b. True of DI but not DM.
c. True of both DM and DI.
d. True of neither DM nor DI.

For each of the situations/conditions given below, choose the one most appropriate/discriminatory option from above. The options may be used once, more than once, or not at all.

Questions

58. Polyuria and polydipsia.
59. Does not cause renal disease in adults.
60. Does not occur as a result of tumors.
61. Related in some manner to obesity.

THEME: 13
DIAGNOSIS OF INSULIN ABNORMALITIES

Options

a. Insulinoma.
b. Factitious hypoglycemia.
c. Gestastional diabetes.
d. Type II diabetes.
e. Type I diabetes.

For each of the situations/conditions given below, choose the one most appropriate/discriminatory option from above. The options may be used once, more than once, or not at all.

Questions

62. Patient with raised plasma insulin and serum C-peptide concentration and reduced blood glucose.
63. An obese 52-year-old man with polyuria, polydipsia and glycosuria but negative for ketone bodies.
64. A patient with reduced blood glucose and serum C-peptide and raised plasma insulin.
65. A 17-year-old woman with a 2 weeks history of increased thirst, increased frequency of urination, weight loss of 6 Kgs, nausea, vomiting and difficulty in breathing.

THEME: 14
INTERPRETATION OF HYPOGLYCEMIA

Options

	Insulin	*Ketones*	*C - Peptide*
a.	Raised/normal	No	Present
b.	Low/undetectable	No	Absent
c.	Low/undetectable	Raised	Absent
d.	Raised/normal	No	Absent

For each of the situations/conditions given below, choose the one most appropriate/discriminatory option from above. The options may be used once, more than once, or not at all.

Questions

66. Non-pancreatic neoplasm.
67. Alcohol.
68. Insulinoma.
69. Adrenal failure.
70. Exogenous insulin administration.
71. Anti-insulin receptor antibody.

THEME: 15
INVESTIGATION OF HYPOGLYCAEMIA

Options

a. Liver function tests
b. Thick blood films
c. Oral hypoglycaemic drug levels
d. Anti-insulin receptor antibodies
e. Gamma glutaryl transpeptidase
f. Prolonged GTT
g. Insulin and C-peptide levels
h. Synacthen test
i. Abdominal ultrasound

For each of the situations/conditions given below, choose the one most appropriate/discriminatory option from above. The options may be used once, more than once, or not at all.

Questions

72. A 50-year-old alcoholic presents with a collapse. He is sweaty, slightly confused and has a fine tremor. He is hypoglycaemic.
73. A 38-year-old man returns from holiday. He becomes febrile, confused and drowsy and complains of a headache. His blood glucose is low.
74. A 50-year-old Asian woman with a history of pulmonary tuberculosis presents with episodes of faintness, particularly on standing. She is found to have postural hypotension and a blood glucose of 2.3 mmol per litre. She is also hyponatraemic with a sodium of 127 mmol per litre.

75. A 22-year-old patient presents with a witnessed seizure and is found to have a blood glucose of less than 1mmol per litre. There is no family history of epilepsy but mother has had diabetes for 30 years.
76. A 48-year-old man complains of nausea and light headedness after meals and is found to have low blood sugar at the time of these symptoms. He has had a subtotal gastrectomy for carcinoma.

THEME: 16
ORAL HYPOGLYCAEMIC AGENTS

Options

a. Phenformin.
b. Metformin.
c. Gliclazide.
d. Chlorpropamide.
e. Tolbutamide.
f. Glibenclamide.
g. Troglitazone.

For each of the situations/conditions given below, choose the one most appropriate/discriminatory option from above. The options may be used once, more than once, or not at all.

Questions

77. Most widely used OHA.
78. Shortest acting OHA, best suited for elderly patients because the risk of hypoglycemia is low.
79. Major complication is lactic acidosis.
80. Longest acting OHA, its side effect include development of photosensitivity.

THEME : 17
MODE OF ACTION OF ORAL HYPOGLYCEMIA AGENTS

Options

a. Raises the insulin sensitivity.
b. Increases insulin secretion from pancreas.

c. Decreases insulin resistance.
d. Decreases breakdown of starch to sugar.
e. None of the above.

For each of the situations/conditions given below, choose the one most appropriate/discriminatory option from above. The options may be used once, more than once, or not at all.

Questions

81. Troglitazone.
82. Metformin.
83. Starch carbohydrates in diet.
84. Glibenclamide.
85. Acarbose.
86. Regular exercise.

THEME : 18
MANAGEMENT OF DIABETIC AUTONOMIC NEUROPATHY

Options

a. Tetracycline.
b. Fludrocortisone.
c. Cisapride.
d. Poldine methylsulphate.
e. Ephedrine hydrochloride.

For each of the situations/conditions given below, choose the one most appropriate/discriminatory option from above. The options may be used once, more than once, or not at all.

Questions

87. Gustatory sweating.
88. Nocturnal diarrhoea.
89. Neuropathic edema.
90. Vomiting due to gastroparesis.
91. Postural hypotension.

THEME: 19
MANAGEMENT OF DIABETIC PATIENT DURING INTER CURRENT ILLNESS

Options

a. Pneumonia in a patient on insulin.
b. Trauma in a patient on insulin.
c. Gastroenteritis in a patient on insulin.
d. Pneumonia in a patient on insulin.

For each of the situations/conditions given below, choose the one most appropriate/discriminatory option from above. The options may be used once, more than once, or not at all.

Questions

92. Maintain calorie intake, and continue normal insulin. Increase it only if blood glucose levels are consistently > 10 mmol/lit.
93. Start the patient on IV soluble insulin by pump.
94. Stop the initial treatment. Start on insulin using the sliding scale.
95. Continue initial treatment. Start on supplementary insulin using the sliding scale.

THEME: 20
COMPLICATIONS OF DIABETES MELLITUS

Options

a. Cerebrovascular disease
b. Nephropathy
c. Retinopathy
d. Polyneuropathy
e. Amyotrophy
f. Coronary artery disease
g. Peripheral vascular disease
h. Cataracts
i. Rubeosis iridis
j. Mononeuritis multiplex
k. Autonomic neuropathy

For each of the situations/conditions given below, choose the one most appropriate/discriminatory option from above. The options may be used once, more than once, or not at all.

Questions

96. A 60-year-old patient is becoming increasingly confused. She has periods where her confusions seems to be stable and then seems to rapidly deteriorate in stepwise progression. On examination there are extensor plantars but leg reflexes are diminished.
97. A 52-year-old patient complains of burning pain in the feet, worse at night or walking. He describes the sensation as like "walking on hot coals".
98. A 40-year-old patient complains of giddiness and falls. She also suffers with intermittent vomiting and sweating and occasional faecal incontinence at night.
99. A 22-year-old patient complains of worsening vision over several months. The fundoscopy is difficult in this patient even through dilated pupils. There appears to be opacity of the lens.
100. A 38-year-old patient complains of sudden loss of vision in his left eye. On examination there is complete ptosis of the left eye, the pupil is dilated and the eye is abducted and deviated inferiorly.

THEME: 21
TREATMENT OF DIABETIC COMPLICATIONS

Options

a. Insulin sliding scale, heparin and half strength normal saline
b. Insulin sliding scale, half strength normal saline and potassium replacement
c. Insulin sliding scale, normal saline and potassium replacement
d. Insulin sliding scale, heparin and half strength normal saline
e. 50 ml of 50 % dextrose given intravenously

f. Sugary drink
g. Measure C-peptide levels
h. Chest X-ray

For each of the situations/conditions given below, choose the one most appropriate/discriminatory option from above. The options may be used once, more than once, or not at all.

Questions

101. A 55-year-old man is brought to A&E in an unconscious state. His glucose is 35 mmol per litre. His arterial blood gas shows a pH of 7.2 and $PaCO_2$ of 2.0. His serum sodium is 140, potassium is 3, chloride is 100 and bicarbonate is 5 mmol per litre.
102. A 55-year-old diabetic presents in a state of coma. He is febrile with diminished breath sounds on auscultation. He has warm extremities. His glucose is 20 mmol per litre and his white cell count is 22 *10^9 with increased neutrophils.
103. A 48-year-old woman presents with tachycardia, sweating and agitation. Her husband is a diabetic. She has a history of Munchausen's syndrome.
104. A 70-year-old man is noted to have a glucose level of 37 mmol per litre and sodium of 163 mmol per litre. He has no prior history of diabetes and has been on IV fluids for a week. His other medications include IV Cefuroxime, Metronidazole and Dexamethasone.
105. A 38-year-old diabetic who is an actor by profession is started on Propranolol for stage fright. He collapses after a day shooting. He has not changed his insulin regime.

THEME: 22
MANAGEMENT OF DIABETES MELLITUS

Options

a. Acarbose
b. Gliclizide
c. Dietary adjustment

d. Twice daily mixed insulin
e. IV Insulin sliding scale
f. Subcutaneous insulin sliding scale
g. One long acting and three short acting insulin injections
h. Once daily long acting insulin
i. Repaglinide
j. Glibenclamide
k. Metformin
l. No change in treatment required

For each of the situations/conditions given below, choose the one most appropriate/discriminatory option from above. The options may be used once, more than once, or not at all.

Questions

106. A 30-year-old woman was found to have glycosuria at a routine antenatal clinic visit. A glucose tolerance test confirmed diagnosis of gestational diabetes.
107. A 60-year-old man was diagnosed with diabetes at routine medical examination three months ago. His BMI is 32 despite losing 5 kgs by following the dietician's advice. His home blood glucose readings range from 7 to 11 and his glycolated haemoglobin is 10 %.
108. A 30-year-old woman has had type one diabetes for 15 years. She injects Isophane insulin twice a day and rarely tests her blood sugars at home. She attends the diabetic clinic for the first time in over a-year-and informs you that she is twelve weeks pregnant.
109. A 65-year-old man has had type 2 diabetes for 4 years, for which he was taking Chlorpropamide. He presents with an acute MI and his laboratory blood glucose is 11 mmol per litre.
110. An 80-year-old woman was diagnosed with diabetes after she was found to have a high blood glucose during an admission to hospital with a fall. Despite following appropriate dietary advice her glycolated haemoglobin remains elevated at 11 %. She is visually impaired and finds it impossible to test her blood glucose at home. She is not obese.

THEME: 23
MANAGEMENT OF HYPERALDOSTRERONISM

Options

a. Surgery followed by spironolactone.
b. Only spironolactone.
c. Dexamethasone followed by spironolactone
d. K^+ and Cl^- replacement followed by amiloride.

For each of the situations/conditions given below, choose the one most appropriate/discriminatory option from above. The options may be used once, more than once, or not at all.

Questions

111. Glucocorticoid responsive aldosteronism.
112. Conn's disease.
113. Primary hyperreninemia.
114. Adrenal hyperplasia.

THEME: 24
CIRCADIAN RHYTHM

Options

a. Maximum levels at 8 a.m.
b. Maximum levels at 12 noon.
c. Maximum at night.
d. Maximum 1 hour after sleep.
e. Maximum at 4 p.m.

For each of the situations/conditions given below, choose the one most appropriate/discriminatory option from above. The options may be used once, more than once, or not at all.

Questions

115. Body temperature.
116. Cortisol.
117. Growth hormone.
118. Prolactin.
119. Intellectual performance.

THEME: 25
DIAGNOSIS OF CAUSES OF OBESITY

Options

a. Bulimia nervosa.
b. Hypothyroidism.
c. Cushing's syndrome.
d. Laurence-Moon-Biedl syndrome.
e. Anorexia nervosa.
f. None of the above

For each of the situations/conditions given below, choose the one most appropriate/discriminatory option from above. The options may be used once, more than once, or not at all.

Questions

120. A 20-year-old female comes with 2 years history of eating in binges, slightly overweight and forcibly vomiting along with use of laxatives.
121. A 38-year-old female patient, a known diabetic presents with increased weight of 5 kgs, c/o lethargy, menorrhagia. She also gives history of change of voice.
122. A 40-year-old female presents with 1 year history of increased weight, easy bruising, oligomenorrhea. On examination hypertension is present.
123. A boy of 6 years comes with history of difficulty of seeing at night, his parents complain that he feels very dull. On examination he is obese, has cataract and polydactyly.

THEME: 26
CAUSES OF HIRSUTISM

Options

a. Exogenous androgen administration.
b. Adrenal tumor.
c. Polycystic ovarian disease.
d. Congenital adrenal hyperplasia.
e. Ovarian tumor.

For each of the situations/conditions given below, choose the one most appropriate/discriminatory option from above. The options may be used once, more than once, or not at all.

Questions

124. Slight elevation of plasma testosterone and androstenedione.
125. Can be associated with anovulation, obesity, amenorrhea.
126. An obese woman with secondary infertility and hirsutism. Lab value shows LH: FSH=3:1.
127. Often associated with elevated 17 – hydroxyprogesterone levels.

THEME: 27
ENZYME DEFICIENCIES

Options

a. Complete androgen resistance.
b. 5-alpha reductase deficiency.
c. Testicular dysgenesis.
d. 17- alpha hydroxylase deficiency.
e. 3-beta hydroxy steroid dehydrogenase deficiency.

For each of the situations/conditions given below, choose the one most appropriate/discriminatory option from above. The options may be used once, more than once, or not at all.

Questions

128. A genotypic male (XY) infant with male phenotypic internal reproductive tract but ambigous external genitalia.
129. A genotypic male (XY) infant with female phenotypic external genitalia characterized by a vagina that ends as a blind sac (i.e. no internal reproductive tract).
130. A genotypic male (XY) infant with female phenotypic internal and external reproductive system.
131. A genotypic female (XX) born with female phenotypic internal and external reproductive system but fails to mature at puberty.

Six

Gastroenterology

THEME: 1
INTERPRETATION OF LFT'S

Options

a. Serum bilirubin.
b. Serum aminotransferases.
c. S. alkaline phosphatase.
d. S. gamma glutaryl transferase.
e. Serum albumin and prothrombin time.

For each of the statements/situations given below, choose the one most appropriate/discriminatory option. The options can be used once, more than once or not at all.

Questions

1. Biliary obstructions.
2. Hepatic enzyme induction.
3. Transport.
4. Hepatic synthesis.
5. Hepato cellular damage.

THEME: 2
DIAGNOSIS OF HEPATIC CONDITIONS

Options

a. Chronic persistent hepatitis.
b. Chronic active hepatitis.
c. Autoimmune hepatitis.
d. Primary sclerosing cholangitis.
e. Primary biliary cirrhosis.
f. Primary hematochromatosis.
g. Wilson's disease.

For each of the statements/situations given below, choose the one most appropriate/discriminatory option.The options can be used once ,more than once or not at all.

Questions

6. Chronic hepatitis B infection.
7. Chronic hepatitis C infection.
8. A 40-year-old male comes with 3 months history of jaundice and pale stools. He also gives history of altered bowel habits and bloody stools.
9. A 45-year-old female comes with 3 months history of jaundice and pale stools. She also complains of joint pains and dysphagia, on examination clubbing and xanthelesmata are noticed.
10. A 35-year-old attends infertility clinic. His skin is of grey complexion and mild jaundice is noticed.

THEME : 3
CAUSES OF ASCITES

Options

a. Carcinomatosis peritonei
b. Budd-Chiari syndrome
c. Liver cirrhosis
d. Nephrotic syndrome
e. Primary hepatoma
f. Hepatocellular carcinoma
g. Bacterial peritonitis
h. TB peritonitis
i. Congestive cardiac failure

For each of the statements/situations given below, choose the one most appropriate/discriminatory option. The options can be used once, more than once or not at all.

Questions

11. A 54-year-old man with metastatic liver disease develops exudative ascitis.

12. A 57-year-old man has a history of recurrent ascitis which is exudative in nature. On abdominal paracentesis numerous neutrophils are found in the ascitic fluid.
13. An immigrant from India has been in the UK for 10 years ,but regularly goes back to her country for summer holidays. She frequently develops exudative ascitis, and has lost considerable.
14. A middle-aged man presents with bilateral pitting pedal oedema.

THEME: 4
DIAGNOSIS OF ABDOMINAL DISTENSION

Options

a. Portal vein thrombosis
b. Cirrhosis
c. Malabsorption
d. Secondaries
e. Peptic ulcer
f. Tuberculosis
g. Fibrosing alveolitis
h. Alcoholism
i. Pancreatitis
j. Hepatoma
k. Bronchogenic carcinoma
l. Gallstones
m. Portal hypertension
n. Epulis

For each of the situation/condition given below, choose the one most appropriate/discriminatory option from above. The options may be used once, more than once, or not at all.

Questions

15. A 52-year-old man is admitted with abdominal swelling and pain in the right hypochondrium. His symptoms and signs developed rapidly over the last 12 days and a liver scan shows a filling detect in the left lobe of the liver.

16. A 48-year-old secretary is brought to you with jaundice, malaise and tender hepatomegaly. She has been drinking heavily for the past 2 weeks.
17. A middle-aged alcoholic and heavy smoker is brought to A and E with a chronic cough and a distended abdomen. Examination of the ascitic fluid shows atypical cells.
18. A middle-aged public complains of steadily losing weight over a period of 3 months. She is weak and pale with a protuberant abdomen and her gums bleed easily. Her stools have a high fat content.
19. A agricultural worker complains of a chronic cough, purulent sputum and abdominal distension. He has just arrived in England from Spain where he was picking grapes.

THEME: 5
CONDITIONS OF THE BOWEL

Options

a. Haemochromatosis.
b. Ulcerative colitis.
c. Crohn's disease.
d. Coeliac disease.
e. Carcinoid tumors.
f. Liver failure.
g. Hepatocellular carcinoma.
h. Carcinoma esophagus.

For each of the statements/situations given below, choose the one most appropriate/discriminatory option. The options can be used once, more than once or not at all.

Questions

20. Increased serum iron, decreased TIBC.
21. Increased alpha-fetoprotein.
22. Squamous cell carcinoma.
23. Granulomas and strictures.
24. Antiendomyseal/alpha gliadin antibodies.

THEME: 6
COLONIC DISORDERS

Options

a. Carcinoma of the caecum
b. Carcinoma of the sigmoid colon
c. Colonic polyp
d. Diverticulitis
e. Haemorrhoids
f. Irritable bowel syndrome
g. Sigmoid volvulus
h. Ulcerative colitis

For each of the situation/condition given below, choose the one most appropriate/discriminatory option from above. The options may be used once, more than once, or not at all.

Questions

25. A 72-year-old man presents with increasing tiredness over a 2-year-period. He has a microcytic anaemia and a mass in the right iliac fossa.
26. A 33-year-old woman consults you regarding symptoms of alternating diarrhoea and constipation associated with cramp-like abdominal pain.
27. A 76-year-old man presents with weight loss, pain on eating and abdominal distension. Plain abdominal X-ray films show the so called 'coffee bean' sign.
28. An 82-year-old woman presents to A and E with a distended abdomen. A plain abdominal X-ray film shows gross faecal loading in the colon and gas in the small bowel. The rectum is empty.
29. A 39-year-old woman presents with passage of bloodstained motions and mucus 5 times a day. Symptoms have persisted for over 1 month and are associated with weight loss. Barium enema shows no evidence of Colonic neoplasm, but a granular mucosa.

THEME: 7
DIAGNOSIS OF ORAL ULCERS

Options

a. SLE.
b. Tolbutamide.
c. Herpes simplex I.
d. Squamous cell carcinoma.
e. Vitamin B_{12} deficiency.
f. Syphilis.
g. Dentures.

For each of the statements/situations given below, choose the one most appropriate/discriminatory option.The options can be used once ,more than once or not at all.

Questions

30. A 27-year-old female presents with history of depression, pallor and edema and muscle weakness since last 4 months. Her husband died 6 months back. She also developed oral ulcers since 2 months.
31. A 48-year-old female, mother of 4 children developed oral ulceration since 3 months. She comes from a poor socio-economic status.
32. A 32-year-old male complains of painful oral ulceration and vesicles for the last 4 days. Last week he just returned back from a local sea resort where he had vacationed.
33. A 58-year-old male executive, chain smoker and alcoholic develops an indurated ulcer over lateral border of tongue.

THEME: 8
CAUSES OF ORAL ULCERATION

Options

a. Behcet's disease
b. Crohn's disease
c. Erythema multiforme
d. Lichen planus
e. Oral mucositis
f. Recurrent oral ulceration

g. Reiter's syndrome
h. Shingles
i. Squamous cell carcinoma
j. Syphilis
k. Systemic lupus erythematosus
l. Ulcerative colitis

For each of the situation/condition given below, choose the one most appropriate/discriminatory option from above. The options may be used once, more than once, or not at all.

Questions

34. A 40-year-old HIV positive patients presents with a 2 day history of pain affecting the right side of his face, followed by a vesicular rash affecting both his midface and the right side of his palate.
35. A 15-year-old schoolgirl presents with a 2 years history of up to five painful oral ulcers occurring at intervals of 1-2 months. She is otherwise well.
36. A 25-year-old Turkish man has been suffering from recurrent orogenital ulceration. He is now complaining of floaters affecting his vision, increasing acne-like lesions and joint pains.
37. A 30-year-old woman given oral Trimethoprim for a urinary tract infection develops discrete target-like lesions on her skin with severe oral ulceration and crusting of the lips.
38. A 35-year-old man returns from an extended period of overseas travel and develops a small papule on his upper lip which rapidly breaks down into a large painless indurated ulcer.

THEME: 9
PREVENTION /HEALTH PROMOTION OF JAUNDICE /HEPATITIS

Options

a. Cirrhosis
b. Hepatitis A

c. Hepatitis B
d. Hepatitis C
e. Hepatocellular carcinoma
f. Leptospirosis
g. Lyme's disease
h. Sclerosing cholangitis

For each of the statements/situations given below, choose the one most appropriate/discriminatory option.The options can be used once ,more than once or not at all.

Questions

39. Care in preparation of shellfish.
40. Immunisation of sewage workers.
41. Immunisation of paramedics who come into contact with body fluids.
42. Counselling for intravenous (IV) drug users to use needle exchange facilities.
43. Avoidance of swimming in rivers and reservoirs.
44. Avoidance of alcohol for six months after hepatitis A.
45. Mass immunisation against Hepatitis B, other than for the prevention of hepatitis B.

THEME: 10
ABDOMINAL SWELLINGS

Options

a. Ca caecum.
b. Ileocolic intussusception.
c. Aortic aneurysm.
d. Appendicular abscess.
e. Inguinal hernia.
f. Pyosalpinx.

For each of the statements/situations given below, choose the one most appropriate/discriminatory option. The options can be used once, more than once or not at all.

Questions

46. A 45-year-old male patient presents with history of irregular bowel motions since 2 months and occult blood stool test positive/lump in RIF.

47. A 45-year-old male patient presents with history of pain abdomen 3 months back which was associated with constipation. Presently there is a lump in RIF and occult blood test in stools is negative.
48. A 32-year-old male patient presents with complaints of back pain since last 4 months. Examination reveals mass in umbilical region.
49. A 6-year-old female child c/o intermittent pain abdomen associated with vomiting for the last one month. On examination a mass felt in right lumbar/RIF region.

THEME: 11
CAUSES OF ASCITES

Options

a. Tuberculous peritonitis
b. Meig's syndrome
c. Budd-Chiari syndrome
d. Constrictive pericarditis
e. Portal vein thrombosis
f. Compression of portal vein by LN
g. Cirrhosis
h. Right heart failure due to MS
i. Pseudomyxoma peritonei
j. Protein losing enteropathy

For each of the situation/condition given below, choose the one most appropriate/discriminatory option from above. The options may be used once, more than once, or not at all.

Questions

50. A 40-year-old woman presents with ovarian fibroma, right hydrothorax and ascites.
51. A 25-year-old woman develops nausea, vomiting and abdominal pain. On examination she has tender hepatomegaly and ascites. She has recently started on OC pills.
52. A 30-year-old man develops ascites and right lower quadrant colicky pain. The ascitic fluid is viscous and mucinoid in nature.

53. A 40-year-old woman presents with ascites. On examination she has a dominant 'a' wave in the JVP, a loud P2 and low volume peripheral artery pulse volume. She has a history of rheumatic fever.
54. A 50-year-old woman presents with fatigue and ascites. She is noted to have a rapid, irregular pulse rate with small volume. The CXR reveals a small heart with calcification seen on the lateral view. The 12 lead ECG demonstrates low QRS voltage and T wave inversion.

THEME: 12
DIAGNOSIS OF CONSTIPATION

Options

a. Carcinoma of the colon
b. Parkinsonism
c. Anorexia nervosa
d. Myxoedema
e. Bulimia
f. Diverticulosis
g. Chronic pseudo-obstruction
h. Systemic sclerosis
i. Hypercalcemia
j. Diabetic neuropathy
k. Irritable bowel syndrome
l. Multiple sclerosis

For each of the statements/situations given below, choose the one most appropriate/discriminatory option. The options can be used once ,more than once or not at all.

Questions

55. A 42-year-old woman complains of excessive thirst, polyuria, polydipsia and constipation. She admits to losing weight. Her fasting blood glucose is 5.4 mmol/l.
56. A 23-year-old man being treated for myeloma is brought to the A and E department, confused. This followed a hour history of severe abdominal pain, vomiting. Prior to this, the patient had complained of polyuria, polydipsia and constipation.

57. A 16-year-old frail girl complains of constipation. Her Body Mass Index (BMI) is found to be 17. She is extremely afraid of eating and admits to sticking a finger down her throat to indulge vomiting after meals. She is unsually sensitive to cold.
58. A 60-year-old man with a history of weight loss,presents with bleeding per rectum. He also reports a history of diarrhoeawhich seems alternate with constipation. His haemoglobin is 10 g/dl.
59. A 65-year-old woman presents with constipation and reports difficulty in starting or stopping to walk. She has dysarthria and dribbling.

THEME: 13
VOMITING

Options

a. Gastric erosions.
b. Henoch-Schonlein purpura.
c. Pyloric stenosis.
d. Acute pancreatitis.
e. Viral gastroenteritis.
f. Renal colic.
g. Hysterical vomiting.
h. Meniere's syndrome.

For each of the statements/situations given below, choose the one most appropriate/discriminatory option.The options can be used once ,more than once or not at all.

Questions

60. A 45-year-old female, known patient of rheumatoid arthritis complains of upper abdomen pain associated with vomiting since last 2 days. She has recently returned back from a vacation.
61. A 3 months old male child following a breastfeed develops projectile vomiting.
62. A 5-year-old child c/o pain abdomen associated with vomiting since last 3 days. He also has hematuria and arthralgia.

63. A 38-year-old male patient known alcoholic and smoker develops pain abdomen with vomiting since 2 days. He also develops a greyish skin discoloration over abdominal wall.

THEME: 14
INVESTIGATIONS OF WEIGHT PROBLEMS

Options

a. Ultrasound abdomen
b. Thyroid function tests
c. Short ACTH stimulation test
d. Chest X-ray
e. Upper GI endoscopy
f. Blood glucose
g. 24 hour urine collection for vanillyl-mandelic acid
h. Proctosigmoidoscopy
i. 24 hour collection for urine-free cortisol

For each of the situation/condition given below, choose the one most appropriate/discriminatory option from above. The options may be used once, more than once, or not at all.

Questions

64. A 20-year-old man presents with intermittent abdominal pain with diarrhoea, and weight loss. He is noted to have anal lesions, clubbing, arthritis and erythema nodosum.
65. A 40-year-old woman presents with weight gain and truncal obesity. She suffers from amenorrhoea, hirsutism, hypertension and is noted to have glycosuria.
66. A 30-year-old insulin dependent diabetic presents with weight loss, weakness, vitiligo, and hyperpigmentation of the palmar creases. His serum electrolytes are abnormal.
67. A 20-year-old female presents with an insidious onset of weight gain, hoarseness, and menorrhagia. Her mother states that she is depressed of late.
68. A 15-year-old girl presents with a few weeks history of weight loss, polyuria and polydipsia.

THEME: 15
INVESTIGATION OF WEIGHT LOSS

Options

a. Stool for cysts, ova and parasites
b. Urea and electrolytes
c. Chest X-ray
d. Full blood count
e. Serum glucose
f. Urinalysis
g. Thyroid function tests
h. Ultrasound of abdomen
i. Barium swallow
j. Blood cultures
k. Plasma ACTH and cortisol

For each of the situation/condition given below, choose the one most appropriate/discriminatory option from above. The options may be used once, more than once, or not at all.

Questions

69. A 60-year-old man recently treated for renal tuberculosis presents with weight loss, diarrhoea, anorexia, hypotension, and is noted to have hyperpigmented buccal mucosa and hand creases.
70. A 50-year-old woman presents with weight loss, increased appetite, sweating, palpitations, preference for cold weather, hot moist palms and tremors.
71. A 25-year-old man presents with steatorrhoea, diarrhoea and weight loss after eating contaminated food.
72. A 65-year-old man presents with a sudden onset of diabetes, anorexia, weight loss, epigastric and back pain.
73. A 70-year-old woman presents with progressive dysphagia, weight loss and a sensation of food sticking in her throat.

THEME: 16
DYSPHAGIA

Options

a. Pseudobulbar palsy.
b. Squamous cell carcinoma of the oesophagus.
c. Pharyngeal carcinoma.
d. Oesophageal candidiasis.
e. Achalasia.
f. Bronchial carcinoma.

For each of the statements/situations given below, choose the one most appropriate/discriminatory option. The options can be used once ,more than once or not at all.

Questions

74. A 55-year-old male patient known hypertensive and is on irregular medications, is brought to the casualty and is found to have suffered a CVA. On examination slurred speech and spastic tongue. Two days later patient developed aspiration pneumonitis.
75. A 28-year-old female drug addict complains of painful swallowing since 3 days.
76. A 49-year-old promiscuous male patient known smoker and alcoholic complains of difficulty in swallowing solids since last 3 weeks.
77. A 58-year-old male patient smoker c/o difficulty in swallowing since one month. He also casually mentioned hoarseness of voice since last 3 months, which he attributes to smoking.

THEME: 17
CAUSES OF DYSPHAGIA

Options

a. Benign stricture.
b. Malignant stricture.
c. Achalasia cardia.
d. Peptic stricture.

For each of the statements/situations given below, choose the one most appropriate/discriminatory option. The options can be used once, more than once or not at all.

Questions

78. A young patient c/o difficulty in swallowing, it is not associated with pain. She also gives history of accidental ingestion of caustic soda 6 weeks back-for which she had taken treatment.
79. A 34-year-old male, bank manager, chronic smoker and alcoholic gives history of difficulty in swallowing, also gives history of pain epigastrium relieved with food. He also gives history of water brash often.
80. A 75-year-old male presents with difficulty in swallowing which has progressively increased over last 2 months. Patient has lost dysphagia for solids as well as liquids.
81. A 38-year-old female c/o difficulty in swallowing which has progressively in creased over last 3 months. Patient also gives history of chest infection for which she had taken treatment. She has difficulty in swallowing fluids more than solids.

THEME: 18
CASUES OF DYSPHAGI A

Options

a. Achalasia
b. Pharyngeal pouch
c. Diffuse oesophageal spasm
d. Globus pharyngeus
e. Plummer-Vinson syndrome
f. Carcinoma of oesophagus
g. Peptic stricture
h. Myasthenia gravis
i. Swallowed foreign body
j. Caustic stricture
k. Retrosternal goitre

For each of the situation/condition given below, choose the one most appropriate/discriminatory option from above. The options may be used once, more than once, or not at all.

Questions

82. A 32-year-old female presents with progressive dysphagia with regurgitation of fluids. She denies weight loss.
83. A 27-year-old man with a history of depression presents with acute dysphagia. He has a prior history of repeated suicide attempts. These are associated with burns in the oropharynx.
84. A 60-year-old woman presents with progressive dysphagia. On examination she has a smooth tongue, koilonychias and suffers from iron deficiency anaemia.
85. A 65-year-old woman presents with regurgitation of food, dysphagia, halitosis and a sensation of a lump in her throat.
86. A 70-year-old man presents with a short history of dysphagia, weight loss and has palpable neck nodes on examination.

THEME: 19
THE TREATMENT OF DYSPHAGIA

Options

a. Antifungal therapy
b. Incision and drainage
c. Endoscopic diverticulotomy
d. External excision of pharyngeal pouch
e. Reassurance
f. Nasogastric intubation
g. Intravenous antibiotics and analgesia
h. Antispasmodics
i. Dilation of the lower oesophageal sphincter

For each of the situation/condition given below, choose the one most appropriate/discriminatory option from above. The options may be used once, more than once, or not at all.

Questions

87. A 50-year-old man complains of dysphagia after eating bread. Barium swallow reveals a lower oesophageal ring.
88. A 40-year-old woman on chemotherapy for metastatic breast carcinoma now presents with painful swallowing. On examination, she has white plaques on top of friable mucosa in her mouth and more seen on oesophagoscopy.
89. A 20-year-old man presents with painful swallowing. On examination, he has trismus and unilateral enlargement of his tonsil. The peritonsillar region is red, inflamed and swollen.
90. A 40-year-old woman presents with dysphagia. On examination, she is afebrile with neck erythema and a midline neck swelling.
91. A 40-year-old woman complains of dysphagia for both solids and liquids. She sometimes suffers from severe retrosternal chest pain. Barium swallow reveals a dilated oesophagus which tapers to a fine distal end.

THEME: 20
TREATMENT OF OESOPHAGEAL PATHOLOGY

Options

a. Endoscopic dilatation
b. Ketoconazole systemically administered.
c. Topical nystatin
d. IV ganclovir (High dose)
e. IV acyclovir (low dose)
f. Surgical resection.
g. Endoscopic insertion of Atkinson's tube.
h. Heller's myotomy.
i. Triple therapy
j. Surgical repair
k. Sclerotherapy.

For each of the statements/situations given below, choose the one most appropriate/discriminatory option.The options can be used once ,more than once or not at all.

Questions

92. A 32-year-old man has been receiving cyclosporin for the treatment of her rheumatoid arthritis presents with odynophagia (painful swallowing) and mild dysphagia. Oesophageal endoscopy reveals multiple small white plaques on background of an abnormally reddened mucosa.
93. A 31-year-old woman with AIDS presents with odynophagia. Oesophageal endoscopy reveals multiple shallow ulcers in the lower oesophagus. The mucosa contains multiple vesicles.
94. A 29-year-obese man presents with dysphagia. Barium swallow demonstrates a smooth "rat tail " appearance. He has complained of heartburn for the last 6 months.
95. A 62-year-old woman presents with dysphagia. She has been progressively started with initial difficulty for swallowing solids but now also has involved liquids. She looks wasted.

THEME: 21
INVESTIGATIONS OF LIVER DISEASES

Options

a. Anti-mitochondrial antibody.
b. Alpha–Fetoprotein.
c. Viral markers.
d. Antinuclear cytoplasmic antibodies.
e. Antinuclear/smooth muscle antibody.
f. Urinary copper.
g. Alpha, antitrypsin deficiency.

For each of the statements/situations given below, choose the one most appropriate/discriminatory option. The options can be used once, more than once or not at all.

Questions

96. Primary biliary cirrhosis.
97. Wilson's disease.

98. Hepatitis B.
99. Sclerosing cholangitis.
100. Autoimmune hepatitis.

THEME: 22
PRECRIBING AND LIVER FAILURE

Options

a. Spirolactone 100 mg/24 hr PO
b. Frusemide 100 mg/24hr PO
c. Paracentesis
d. Paracentesis with albumin infusion
e. Ciprofloxacin 250 mg PO
f. Flucloxacillin 500 mg/24hr PO
g. Chlorpheniramine 75 mg PO
h. Cholestyramine 4 g/8hr PO
i. Tetracycline 250 mg/8hr PO
j. Stop Warfarin
k. Warfarin-increased dosage
l. Warfarin reduced dosage
m. Bedrest, salt and fluid restriction.

For each of the statements/situations given below, choose the one most appropriate/discriminatory option.The options can be used once ,more than once or not at all.

Questions

101. A 32-year-old chronic alcoholic is in liver failure. He has severe pruritis.
102. A 30-year-old chronic alcoholic is on warfarin following an acute myocardial infarction he suffered 3 months ago. He now develops liver cirrhosis.
103. A 32-year-old man has had hepatitis B for the last one year and now presents with a grossly distended abdomen and other stigmata of liver disease. You are worried he may develop spontaneous bacterial peritonitis.
104. A 30-year-old woman presents with a mildly distended abdomen, yellowing of the mucous membranes. She is found to have spider naevi on her chest.

THEME: 23
HEPATO-BILIARY DISORDERS

Options

a. Budd-Chiari syndrome.
b. Secondary biliary cirrhosis.
c. Neonatal hepatitis.
d. Amoebiasis.
e. Extrahepatic biliary atresia.
f. Intrahepatic biliary atresia.
g. Ascending cholangitis.

For each of the statements/situations given below, choose the one most appropriate/discriminatory option. The options can be used once, more than once or not at all.

Questions

105. Most common cause of neonatal cholestasis in the first week of life.
106. A patient with polycythemia vera presents with painful hepatosplenomegaly, jaundice, ascites and portal hypertension.
107. Immigrant from Mexico with a space occupying mass in the right lobe of the liver and bloody diarrhea with mucus.
108. Neonatal jaundice, bile duct proliferation in the portal triads and normal uptake of radio nuclide but absence of radio nuclide in the small intestine 24 hours later.
109. Triad of fever, right upper quadrant pain and jaundice.

THEME: 24
INVESTIGATION OF BILIARY SYSTEM

Options

a. ERCP
b. Percutaneous transhepatic cholangiography
c. HIDA scan
d. CT scan
e. Oral cholecystogram

f. Serum CA 19-9
g. Barium follow through
h. Plain abdominal X-ray
i. MRI scan
j. Oesophagogastroduodenoscopy
k. Laparoscopy

For each of the situation/condition given below, choose the one most appropriate/discriminatory option from above. The options may be used once, more than once, or not at all.

Questions

110. A 59-year-old man presents with obstructive jaundice. USG shows no gallstones. The liver appears normal and the common bile duct measures 12 mm in diameter. His past medical history includes partial gastrectomy 15 years ago for peptic ulcer.
111. A 45-year-old woman presents with upper abdominal pain and obstructive jaundice. The gallbladder is not palpable clinically. USG shows gallstones and a dilated common bile duct.
112. A 50-year-old obese woman presents with acute upper abdominal pain. Examination demonstrates pyrexia, tachycardia and tenderness in the right upper abdomen. An erect chest radiograph reveals no free intraperitoneal gas. USG fails to confirm diagnosis.
113. A 70-year-old woman presents with obstructive jaundice and a palpable gallbladder. USG shows a dilated common bile duct and enlargement of pancreatic head. Her past medical history includes partial gastrectomy for a bleeding peptic ulcer.

THEME: 25
CAUSES OF GASTROENTERITIS

Options

a. Giardiasis.
b. Rotavirus.
c. Ulcerative colitis.

d. *Staphylococcus aureus.*
e. Scormbotoxin.
f. Salmonella.
g. Appendicitis.
h. Cryptosporidium.
i. *Entamoeba histolytica.*
j. *Clostridium botulinum*

For each of the statements/situations given below, choose the one most appropriate/discriminatory option. The options can be used once, more than once or not at all.

Questions

114. A 35 years hemophilic with AIDS with loss of weight pain abdomen, diarrhea for 4 weeks. On examination febrile, not dehydrated, abdomen is non-tender. Investigations reveal Hb 12 gm/dl, TLC 4000 X 10 I/lit, Na 12 g mmol/lit k 3.6 mmol/lit. Stool is positive for blood. Modified acid fast staining shows 1-3 micrometer in diameter.
115. A 56-year-old female and her daughter came from a wedding and develop pain abdomen diarrhoea vomiting 2 hours after returning home. On examination Pulse 110/min BP 96/68 mmHg. Abdominal examination revealed generalised tenderness. Stool is watery and is negative for blood.
116. A 23-year-old returns from overnight camping trip and c/o feeling weak and has difficulty in swallowing. On examination pulse 74/min. BP 112/78 mmHg. Not dehydrated. On examination neurological status reveals bilateral ptosis, loss of ankle and knee jerks.
117. A 44-year-old presents with pain abdomen, bloody diarrhea, vomiting history of attended party 24 hours ago. On examination Temperature up, P 98/min BP 100/70 mmHg dehydrated. Bloody and foul smelling stools.

THEME: 26
DIAGNOSIS OF ABDOMINAL PAIN

Options

a. Peritonitis
b. Gallstones

c. Crohn's disease
d. Duodenal ulcer
e. Hiatus hernia
f. Reflux oesophagitis
g. Carcinoma head of pancreas
h. Carcinoma tail of pancreas
i. Acute pancreatitis
j. Chronic pancreatitis
k. Gastric ulcer
l. Oesophageal tear
m. Helicobacter pylori

For each of the situation/condition given below, choose the one most appropriate/discriminatory option from above. The options may be used once, more than once, or not at all.

Questions

118. An elderly man presents with abdominal pain, anorexia and weight loss. The pain is dull and penetrating through to the back. It helps him with the pain to stoop forwards. His right leg is inflamed and tender.
119. A middle-aged man complains of persistent abdominal pain. He says antacids and food help him with the pain but it will not go away. Sometimes he feels sick and vomits and that helps. Recently he has lost weight and appetite.
120. An elderly woman presents with painless jaundice and weight loss. On physical examination you find the gall-bladder to be enlarged. She enjoys smoking and drinking.
121. A middle-aged man presents with acute abdominal pain in the epigastrium. The pain radiates to the back between the scapulae. It is excruciating. The patient is nauseous and vomits repeatedly.
122. A 38-year-old man complains of recurrent bouts of abdominal pain. The pain begins below the sternum and moves through to the back. Sometimes the pain is disabling and the patient cannot leave his bed. When he has the pain he looses his appetite and has lost as much as a stone in weight.

THEME: 27
DIAGNOSIS OF ABDOMINAL PAIN

Options

a. Gastric ulcer
b. Gastric atrophy
c. Non-ulcer dyspepsia
d. Basal pneumonia
e. Retrocaecal appendicitis
f. Helicobacter pylori
g. Duodenitis
h. Carcinoma stomach
i. Oesophagitis
j. Hepatitis
k. Acute pancreatitis
l. Duodenal peptic ulcer
m. Acute cholecystitis
n. MI

For each of the situation/condition given below, choose the one most appropriate/discriminatory option from above. The options may be used once, more than once, or not at all.

Questions

123. A 32-year-old man points to an area of acute epigastric pain with his right index finger. The pain is worse at night and taking food relieves him. Taking antacids also relieves it. His serum amylase is slightly elevated.
124. A 48-year-old short order cook presents with nausea and acute abdominal pain boring through to the back. The epigastrium is very tender. He has had 3 similar bouts in the past 18 months. A barium meal is normal.
125. A 51-year-old woman complains of chronic abdominal pain around the umbilicus. She often suffers from indigestion, abdominal pain and vomiting. She had a thyroidectomy 12 years ago and is on replacement regime. A barium meal shows an absence of mucosal folds.
126. A 39-year-old marketing executive presents with acute epigastric pain. The pain is continuous and it has been

increasing in intensity over the past day. It radiates to the right hypochondrium.

127. A middle aged man presents with acute abdominal pain that radiates through to the back. The pain is severe and causes him to feel sick and vomit repeatedly. On physical examination you find the abdomen to be tender. His serum amylase is 5 times greater than normal.

THEME: 28
DIAGNOSIS OF ABDOMINAL PAIN

Options

a. Perforated appendix.
b. Pancreatitis.
c. Pelvic inflammatory disease.
d. Biliary colic.
e. Intestinal obstruction.
f. Sickle cell anemia.
g. Lead poisoning.
h. Ruptured aortic aneurysm.
i. Porphyria.
j. Hysteria.
k. Lead poisoning.
l. Ketoacidosis.

For each of the statements/situations given below, choose the one most appropriate/discriminatory option. The options can be used once, more than once or not at all.

Questions

128. A 15-year-old west Indian boy with severe pain abdomen, with ulcers on skin and looks pale.
129. A 48-year-old house wife having pain right hypochondrium, recurrent with a tinge of icterus.
130. A 39-year-old with taking alternative medicine for chronic rheumatoid arthritis, with pain abdomen 2 weeks, gums have dark bluish pigment in a linear distribution.
131. A 18-year-old boy with insulin dependent DM presents with breathlessness, dizziness, vomiting with pain abdomen.

132. A 30-year-old house wife has pain in abdomen (lower) and tenderness in it. Illiac fossa since 2 weeks.

THEME: 29
DIAGNOSIS OF ABDOMINAL PAIN

Options

a. Faecal impaction
b. Carcinoma colon
c. Chronic pancreatitis
d. Acute pancreatitis
e. Gastric carcinoma
f. Angina
g. MI
h. Oesophagitis
i. Hiatus hernia
j. Acute constipation
k. Acute appendicitis
l. Peptic ulcer
m. Chronic cholecystitis
n. Basal pneumonia

For each of the situation/condition given below, choose the one most appropriate/discriminatory option from above. The options may be used once, more than once, or not at all.

Questions

133. A 38-year-old stock broker comes in to A and E with sever upper abdominal pain. His breath smells of alcohol. He is pale and sweaty. On physical examination you find board like rigidity.
134. A 50-year-old woman complains of flatulence and chest pains after meals. She is overweight and enjoys looking after many grandchildren.
135. A young lawyer presents with stomach pains. Over the past years he has gained weight because eating relieves his hunger pangs, but now the pangs are almost constant. He does not have a fever or jaundice and a physical examination shows nothing abnormal.

136. A healthy young woman complains of abdominal pain. She says she has had 3 episodes in the last month. On examination you find she has a low grade fever and tenderness in the right flank.
137. A hospital doctor complains of abdominal pain and vomiting after meals. He has no previous history of indigestion. Over the past six months the incidents have increased in number and severity.

THEME: 30
DIAGNOSIS OF ABDOMINAL PAIN

Options

a. Familial polyposis
b. Food poisoning
c. Anorexia – bulimia
d. Irritable bowel syndrome
e. Crohn's disease
f. Ulcerative colitis
g. Diverticular disease
h. Gallstone ileus
i. Adhesions
j. Faecal impaction
k. Pelvic abscess
l. Rectal carcinoma
m. Colonic cancer
n. Blood dyscrasia

For each of the situation/condition given below, choose the one most appropriate/discriminatory option from above. The options may be used once, more than once, or not at all.

Questions

138. For the past 2 weeks a middle-aged railway engineer has complained of acute constipation. His stools are dark but not apparently bloodstained. Abdominal palpation detects a mass with moderate tenderness.
139. A 43-year-old man says he cannot finish passing his stool and that what he does pass is streaked with blood. He

says he has always been regular. He wants to know if a laxative will help.

140. A 50-year-old lawyer complains of blood and diarrhoea. Recently she has suffered abdominal pain, fever and general ill health. On examination you find tenderness in the lower abdomen.
141. A young woman presents with recurrent abdominal pain, episodic diarrhoea, malaise and fever. Over the past few years she has felt her health to be declining. At presentation she complains of severe abdominal pain and constipation.
142. A young woman complains of cramp like abdominal pain and difficulties with bowel movements. Acute abdominal pain is relieved by embarrassing flatulence. Barium studies and sigmoidoscopy have proved inconclusive.

THEME: 31
MANAGEMENT OF ABDOMINAL PAIN

Options

a. Mannitol
b. Dexamethasone
c. Craniotomy
d. Eye drops
e. Regular follow-up
f. Interferon
g. Aciclovir
h. Primary closure
i. Laparotomy
j. Oesophageal stapling
k. Sclerotherapy
l. Tinidazole
m. Metronidazole
n. Penicillin

For each of the situation/condition given below, choose the one most appropriate/discriminatory option from above. The options may be used once, more than once, or not at all.

Questions

143. A young woman who has ingested 3 bottles of paracetamol earlier in the day presents with fever, sweating, jaundice and confusion. Examination of her eyes demonstrates increasing papilloedema.
144. A middle-aged man presents with enlarged liver and feeling of unwell. On physical examination you find no signs of liver disease. Investigations are normal. Liver biopsy demonstrates enlarged portal tracts and a chronic inflammatory cell infiltrate.
145. A 52-year-old man complains of ill health. He presents with malaise, low grade fever and jaundice. His liver is large and tender and is jaundiced. Biopsy of the live demonstrates piecemeal necrosis. His HbsAG is positive and HbE antigen is negative.
146. A 38-year-old man presents with blood-stained vomitus. After a heavy meal in a restaurant he collapsed in the street and was brought by the ambulance team. His condition has been stabilised but he continues to cough up blood. He is jaundiced and you palpate a mass in the right upper quadrant of the abdomen.
147. A middle-aged man who presents in A and E with acute abdominal pain. He has spent an evening celebrating. Over the past year he has presented to A and E 3 times with a similar complaint. Barium studies have demonstrated some smoothness in the stomach lining.

THEME: 32
INVESTIGATIONS

Options

a. X-ray cholecystography.
b. FBC.
c. Liver biopsy.
d. USG.
e. EEG.
f. Endoscopy.
g. CXR.

h. Laparoscopy.
i. LFT.
j. Cholangiography.
k. Blood glucose.
l. ECG.
m. Ba enema.

For each of the statements/situations given below, choose the one most appropriate/discriminatory option. The options can be used once, more than once or not at all.

Questions

148. A 40-year-old overweight female patient c/o right upper abdomen pain, feels sick and vomits. Had celebrated her birthday in a restaurant where she had taken rich food.
149. A 23-year-old c/o lower right side pain. Was perfectly well then developed central abdomen pain which disappeared and was replaced by a sharp pain in lower abdomen on one side.
150. A 45-year-old vegetarian c/o chronic breathlessness, fatigue. Had been fit earlier. Recently had a child and feels under pressure at work.
151. Middle-aged male patient c/o loss of body hair, mild confusion. On examination mild hepatosplenomegaly. He is a moderate drinker.
152. A 60-year-old collapses while working at his market stall. He is brought in with soiled trousers and blood at mouth.

THEME: 33
CAUSES OF CONSTIPATION

Options

a. Colorectal carcinoma
b. Diverticular disease
c. Hypothyroidism
d. Hypercalcemia
e. Parkinson's disease
f. Hirschsprung's disease
g. Chronic laxative abuse

h. Pelvic trauma
i. Adverse effect of drug
j. Irritable bowel syndrome

For each of the situation/condition given below, choose the one most appropriate/discriminatory option from above. The options may be used once, more than once, or not at all.

Questions

153. A 20-year-old man has been constipated since childhood. He opens his bowels once or twice a week and has noticed faecal soiling.
154. A 40-year-old woman has constipated weight gain and menorrhagia. She opens her bowels only twice a week. Pulse is 50/min and she has dry skin.
155. A 35-year-old woman has long-standing constipation with weight loss. She passes hard pellet like stools, often with straining and feeling of incomplete evacuation. Examination is normal.
156. A 50-year-old man fell from a ladder and injured his back. He requires regular painkillers for his back. Since the accident he has had difficulty opening his bowels and has noticed reduced bowel frequency.
157. A 52-year-old woman has recently developed constipation and feels that she does not completely empty her rectum on defecation. She has passed blood per rectum on 2 occasions.
158. A 70-year-old woman has seen her GP for depression on several occasions. She now complains of abdominal pain, constipation and thirst. She has also recently noticed a breast lump.

THEME: 34
DIAGNOSIS OF ANAL COMPLAINTS

Options

a. Venereal warts
b. Condyloma
c. Pelvic abscess
d. Anaemia

e. Anal carcinoma
f. Rectal carcinoma
g. Colonic carcinoma
h. Prolapse
i. Haemorrhoids
j. Diverticular disease
k. Ulcerative colitis
l. Crohn's disease
m. Syphilis
n. Gonorrhoea

For each of the situation/condition given below, choose the one most appropriate/discriminatory option from above. The options may be used once, more than once, or not at all.

Questions

159. A 61-year-old woman presents with pallor and tiredness. Her stools are heavily streaked with blood. Recently she has passed fewer and fewer motions. She does not complain of pain and abdominal palpation reveals no abdominal masses, although the liver is slightly enlarged.
160. A healthy young woman presents with ulcer near her anus. It is painless, macular and hard.
161. A 29-year-old woman presents with abdominal pain and bleeding per rectum. She has had a swinging fever for the past few days and passed mucus.
162. A 62-year-old man complains of dripping blood on to his stool after defaecation. He looks pale. He has no other complaints.
163. A young man with a history of sexually transmitted disease presents with acute anal pain and bleeding. Over the past few months he has suffered from increasing constipation.

THEME: 35
INVESTIGATION OF GASTROINTESTINAL DISORDERS

Options

a. Sigmoidoscopy and biopsy

b. Barium enema
c. Abdominal X-ray
d. Upright chest X-ray
e. Abdominal USG
f. Abdominal CT scan
g. Liver biopsy
h. Endocervical smear and culture
i. Paracentesis
j. FBC
k. LFTs

For each of the situation/condition given below, choose the one most appropriate/discriminatory option from above. The options may be used once, more than once, or not at all.

Questions

164. A 30-year-old female taking OC pills presents to her GP complaining of right upper quadrant abdominal discomfort.
165. A 22-year-old female presents with fever and right upper quadrant pain. On examination she has adnexal tenderness and purulent cervical discharge.
166. A 35-year-old obese female presents with fever, vomiting and right upper quadrant abdominal pain. The pain is worse on inspiration.
167. A 50-year-old heavy drinker presents with fever, jaundice, ascites and right upper quadrant abdominal pain. Blood tests reveal a leukocytosis, increased LFTs and a raised serum bilirubin. SGOT was higher than SGPT.
168. A 20-year-old female presents with recurrent episodes of colicky abdominal pain and diarrhoea. On examination, she is also noted to have perianal fistulae.

THEME: 36
TREATMENT OF INTESTINAL OBSTRUCTION

Options

a. Right hemicolectomy
b. Urgent herniorrhaphy

c. Sigmoid colectomy
d. Nasogastric aspiration with fluid and electrolyte replacement
e. Subtotal colectomy and ileorectal anastomosis
f. Anterior resection
g. Exploratory laparotomy and Hartmann's procedure
h. Abdominoperineal resection with end colostomy
i. Transverse colectomy
j. Proximal loop colostomy

For each of the situation/condition given below, choose the one most appropriate/discriminatory option from above. The options may be used once, more than once, or not at all.

Questions

169. A 60-year-old man presents with abdominal pain in the right iliac fossa and distension. X-ray shows a single dilated loop of bowel of 12 cm in diameter with the convexity under the left hemidiaphragm.
170. A 70-year-old man presents with bowel obstruction and pain in the rectum. Rectal examination and biopsy confirms an obstructing carcinoma of the rectum.
171. A 50-year-old man complains of constant groin pain, associated with nausea and vomiting. On examination, he has a positive cough impulse. A tender, tense lump is palpated and is not reducible.
172. A 60-year-old man presents with fever, vomiting and intense left iliac fossa pain. On examination, he has a rigid, distended abdomen with rebound tenderness on the left. Erect chest X-ray reveals free air under the diaphragm.
173. An 80-year-old man presents with abdominal distension and pain. Sigmoidoscopy and barium enema confirm an obstructing carcinoma of the rectosigmoid.

THEME: 37
DIAGNOSIS OF DIARRHOEA

Options

a. Viral gastroenteritis
b. Ulcerative colitis

c. Coeliac disease
d. Laxative abuse
e. Thyrotoxicosis
f. Campylobacter infection
g. Pseudomembranous colitis
h. Giardiasis
i. Collagenous colitis
j. Irritable bowel syndrome
k. Chronic pancreatitis

For each of the situation/condition given below, choose the one most appropriate/discriminatory option from above. The options may be used once, more than once, or not at all.

Questions

174. A 52-year-old woman presented with a 4 years history of recurrent non bloody diarrhoea. All investigations were normal apart from a raised ESR and colonic biopsy which showed an eosinophilic band in the subepithelial layer.
175. A previously fit 22-year-old man presented with acute bloody diarrhoea, crampy abdominal pain and low grade fever. His symptoms resolved spontaneously in 6 days and never recurred.
176. A 28-year-old woman presented with chronic watery diarrhoea. The stools showed a positive osmotic gap. Her diarrhoea stopped within 3 days after admission and fasting.
177. A previously healthy 21-year-old man presented with a six weeks history of bloody diarrhoea, crampy abdominal pain and fever. Proctosigmoidoscopy showed bleeding and friable Colonic mucosa.
178. A 27-year-old woman developed severe watery diarrhoea 12 days after starting antibiotics for pelvic inflammatory disease. Proctosigmoidoscopy showed plaque like lesions.
179. An anxious 28-year-old sales assistant presented with a 45 months history of diarrhoea alternating with constipation. The stools were usually soft and there was not history of bleeding. No abnormality was found on examination. All investigations including flexible fibre optic Sigmoidoscopy and radiography were normal.

THEME: 38
CAUSES OF DIARRHOEA

Options

a. Campylobacter infection
b. Viral gastroenteritis
c. Ulcerative colitis
d. Crohn's disease
e. Laxative abuse
f. Pseudomembranous cells
g. Shigella infection
h. Cryptosporidiosis
i. Salmonellosis
j. Irritable bowel syndrome
k. *Clostridium perferingens*
l. *E. coli* infection

For each of the situation/condition given below, choose the one most appropriate/discriminatory option from above. The options may be used once, more than once, or not at all.

Questions

180. A 30-year-old man with AIDS presents with profuse watery diarrhoea. Oocysts are detected in stool.
181. A 25-year-old man presents with fever, bloody diarrhoea and cramping for several weeks that does not resolve with antibiotic therapy. Proctosigmoidoscopy reveals red raw mucosa and pseudopolyps.
182. A 60-year-old man presents with fever, watery diarrhoea, and crampy abdominal pain. He had completed antibiotic therapy for osteomyelitis a month ago. Proctosigmoidoscopy reveals yellowish white plaques on the mucosa.
183. A 20-year-old man recently back from holiday in the far east presents with abrupt onset of severe diarrhoea. The diarrhoea is self-limiting and lasts only for 3 days.
184. A 20-year-old female presents with chronic watery diarrhoea. She is emaciated. Stool electrolyte studies show an osmotic gap. Blood tests reveal hypokalemia.

THEME: 39
NONINFECTIOUS CAUSES OF DIARRHOEA

Options

a. Gluganoma
b. Coeliac disease
c. Adenocarcinoma of pancreas
d. Colorectal carcinoma
e. Crohn's disease
f. Ulcerative colitis
g. Thyrotoxicosis
h. Diabetic neuropathy
i. Faecal impaction
j. Metastatic carcinoid syndrome
k. Zollinger-Ellison syndrome

For each of the situation/condition given below, choose the one most appropriate/discriminatory option from above. The options may be used once, more than once, or not at all.

Questions

185. A 40-year-old man presents with epigastric pain and diarrhoea. The basal gastric acid output is quite high.
186. A 50-year-old diabetic woman presents with weight loss, anaemia and diarrhoea. She is noted to have migratory necrolytic erythema.
187. A 40-year-old woman presents with weight loss and diarrhoea. Small bowel biopsy reveals villous atrophy.
188. A 40-year-old man presents with weight loss and chronic diarrhoea. He is noted to have osteomas and colonic polyps.
189. A 20-year-old female presents with fever, weight loss and diarrhoea. She is noted to have perianal fistulae. X-ray reveals a string sign.

THEME: 40
DIAGNOSIS OF CHRONIC DIARRHOEA

Options

a. Anxiety
b. Pancreatic adenoma

c. Carcinoid syndrome
d. Bowel cancer
e. Diverticular disease
f. Malnutrition
g. Gastroenteritis
h. Addison's disease
i. Conn's syndrome
j. Ulcerative colitis
k. Crohn's disease
l. Idiopathic steatorrhoea
m. Peptic ulcer
n. Gastric carcinoma

For each of the situation/condition given below, choose the one most appropriate/discriminatory option from above. The options may be used once, more than once, or not at all.

Questions

190. A 52-year-old woman presents with recurrent peptic ulceration intractable to medical treatment. He complains of recurrent abdominal pain, diarrhoea and steatorrhoea. His serum gastrin level is high.
191. A young woman complains of recurrent abdominal pain and diarrhoea. She is subject to fevers and has lost weight over the past year. On sigmoidoscopy you find the bowel wall to be inflamed and granular.
192. A 23-year-old woman with a history of grumbling appendix presents with persisting diarrhoea. On physical examination you find the liver to be slightly enlarged. She also complains of flushing and difficulty in breathing.
193. A 28-year-old lecturer complains of diarrhoea. His stools are pale, frothy and copious. His mouth and tongue are very painful on swallowing.
194. A middle-aged man complains of frequent stools. Examination of the stools shows mucus and blood. Sigmoidoscopy shows the bowel wall to be friable.

THEME: 41
DIAGNOSIS OF GASTROINTESTINAL CONDITIONS.

Options

a. Hepatoma
b. Oesophageal varices
c. Mallory Weiss tear
d. Perforated peptic ulcer
e. Fractured rib
f. Haematoma of rectus sheath
g. Umbilical hernia
h. Sigmoid volvulus
i. Splenic rupture
j. Pancreatic pseudocyst
k. Divarication of recti
l. Acute pancreatitis

For each of the situation/condition given below, choose the one most appropriate/discriminatory option from above. The options may be used once, more than once, or not at all.

Questions

195. A 50-year-old man presents with nausea, vomiting and epigastric pain. On examination he has a palpable epigastric mass and a raised amylase. CT scan of the abdomen shows a round well circumscribed mass in the epigastrium.
196. A 40-year-old multiparous woman presents with midline abdominal mass. The mass is non-tender and appears when she is straining. On examination the midline mass is visible when she raised her head off the examining bed.
197. A 19-year-old man presents with sudden severe upper abdominal pain after being tackled during a rugby practice. He was recently diagnosed with glandular fever.
198. A 7-year-old girl presents with spontaneous massive haematemesis.
199. A 55-year-old male alcoholic presents with vomiting 800 ml of blood. His blood pressure is 80/50 mmHg with a pulse rate of 120. He also has ascites.

THEME: 42
DIAGNOSIS OF MALABSORPTION

Options

a. Chronic pancreatitis
b. Crohn's disease
c. Cystic fibrosis
d. Intestinal lymphangiectasis
e. Immunodeficiency
f. Pancreatic carcinoma
g. Coeliac disease
h. Whipple's disease
i. Thyrotoxicosis
j. Postinfectious malabsorption
k. Obstructive jaundice

For each of the situation/condition given below, choose the one most appropriate/discriminatory option from above. The options may be used once, more than once, or not at all.

Questions

200. A 38-year-old man presented with recurrent arthritis, diarrhoea and steatorrhoea. On examination there was bilateral small knee effusions. Small bowel biopsy showed PAS +ve material in the lamina propria.
201. A 50-year-old architect presented with a 1 year history of lethargy, weight loss, diarrhoea and low back pain. On examination there was evidence of proximal myopathy and mild pitting oedema. Faecal fat excretion was increased.
202. A 65-year-old man presents with severe epigastric pain and weight loss. The pain is severe and radiating to his back. On examination there is a palpable epigastric mass and hepatomegaly.
203. A 38-year-old man presents with bloody diarrhoea, abdominal discomfort and weight loss. On examination there is a tender palpable mass in the right iliac fossa.
204. A 19-year-old student presents with abdominal pain and diarrhoea. She has had recurrent chest infections for most of her life.

205. A 58-year-old alcoholic complains of epigastric pain for 5 months duration. The pain gets worse after heavy alcoholic consumption. He also complains of diarrhoea and weight loss. Abdominal X-rays show multiple calcifications.

THEME: 43
CAUSES OF CONSTIPATION

Options

a. Poor fibre intake
b. Hypothyroidism
c. Irritable bowel syndrome
d. Hypocalcaemia
e. Iatrogenic
f. Anal fissure
g. Carcinoma rectum
h. Carcinoma colon
i. Bowel obstruction
j. Pregnancy
k. Depression
l. Bedrest

For each of the situation/condition given below, choose the one most appropriate/discriminatory option from above. The options may be used once, more than once, or not at all.

Questions

206. A 40-year-old woman presents with a 3 days history of constipation, colicky abdominal pain, distension and vomiting. She has not even passed wind. Bowel sounds are active and high pitched.
207. A 30-year-old man complains of constipation and pain on defaecation. He also notices small amounts of fresh blood on the paper afterwards. He is unable to tolerate rectal examination.
208. A 21-year-old woman with learning difficulties complains of recent onset of abdominal distension, constipation, indigestion and amenorrhoea.

209. A 65-year-old man complains of constipation, low mood, low back pain that prevents him sleeping, fatigue and thirst He has bony tenderness over his lumbar spine.
210. A 52-year-old woman complains of constipation and nausea four days after abdominal hysterectomy for fibroids. On examination she has active bowel sounds of normal pitch and pinpoint pupils.
211. A 60-year-old man presents with a 2 months history of increasing constipation with occasional diarrhoea. He also describes anorexia, weight loss and a feeling of tenesmus.

THEME: 44
DIAGNOSIS OF LOWER GI BLEED

Options

a. Ulcerative colitis
b. Amoebic dysentery
c. Crohn's disease
d. Carcinoma rectum
e. Carcinoma sigmoid
f. Diverticular disease
g. Diverticulosis
h. Ulcerative pancolitis
i. Trauma
j. Tuberculous adenitis
k. HIV enteropathy

For each of the situation/condition given below, choose the one most appropriate/discriminatory option from above. The options may be used once, more than once, or not at all.

Questions

212. A young man presents with abdominal pain, bleeding per rectum. Barium enema reveals an ulcerated stricture of the sigmoid colon.
213. A young man presents with per rectal bleeding. Investigation shows granular inflammation in the distal 12 cm of the sigmoid colon. The proximal area is normal.

214. A young woman with per rectal bleeding is found to have ulcers in the anal area and vulva. Colonoscopy revealed ulcers in the transverse colon.
215. A 45-year-old man presents with abdominal pain, frequent stools. He denied they were blood stained and barium studies show a filling defect in the ascending colon. His HB was 8 gm/dl, MCV 67 fl.

THEME: 45
DIAGNOSIS OF MAELENA

Options

a. Alcoholism.
b. Duodenal ulcer.
c. Stomal ulcer.
d. Acute anxiety.
e. Gastric erosion.
f. Gallstones.
g. Portal hypertention.
h. Hodgkin's disease.
i. Transfusion reactions.
j. Ca stomach.
k. Gastric ulcer.
l. Hiatus hernia.
m. Esophageal varices.

For each of the statements/situations given below, choose the one most appropriate/discriminatory option. The options can be used once, more than once or not at all.

Questions

216. A 50-year-old c/o epigastric pain. Pain before meals or wakes him at night. Relieved by milk.
217. A 60-year-old c/o pain abdomen putting her off food. Cannot bear the idea of eating and has lost weight over few months. She forces herself to vomit after eating. This makes her feel better.
218. Elderly female with rheumatoid arthritis c/o malaise, pallor, takes aspirin for joint pains. Recently had acute stomach pain.

219. A 40-year-old c/o weakeness and pain abdomen. 6 weeks ago pyloroplasty was done for duodenal ulcer.
220. Chronic alcoholic with ascites, large spleen and jaundice. Past history of hematemesis for which sclerotherapy was done.

THEME: 47
CAUSES OF HAEMATEMESIS

Options

a. Duodenal ulcer
b. Vascular malformation
c. Mallory-Weiss tear
d. Oesophageal varices
e. Gastric carcinoma
f. Crohn's disease
g. Oesophageal carcinoma
h. Haemophilia
i. Gastric ulcer
j. Oesophagitis
k. Meckel's diverticulum

For each of the situation/condition given below, choose the one most appropriate/discriminatory option from above. The options may be used once, more than once, or not at all.

Questions

221. A 53-year-old unemployed alcoholic presents with haematemesis, history of alcoholic liver disease and ascites.
222. A 77-year-old man with a history of dysphagia mainly to solid food and weight loss for three months.
223. A 34-year-old bank manager with a long history of indigestion presents with haematemesis, severe constant epigastric pain and weight loss.
224. A 42-year-old secretary presents with haematemesis. She also complained of epigastric pain which usually occurs at night. The pain is relieved by antacids and is worse when she is hungry.

THEME: 48
INVESTIGATION OF VOMITING

Options

a. FBC
b. Erect chest X-ray
c. Plasma cortisol levels
d. CT head
e. Serum calcium
f. Urea and electrolytes
g. USG abdomen
h. Urinary porphobilinogen and ALA synthetase
i. Thyroid function tests
j. Blood glucose
k. Midstream urine specimen

For each of the situation/condition given below, choose the one most appropriate/discriminatory option from above. The options may be used once, more than once, or not at all.

Questions

225. A 60-year-old man on insulin presents with itching, nausea and vomiting. He is noted to have peripheral oedema and normocytic anaemia.
226. A 50-year-old woman with a known breast carcinoma presents acutely with nausea, vomiting, polydipsia, confusion and drowsiness.
227. A 30-year-old woman with Hodgkin's lymphoma presents with an insidious onset of weakness, weight loss, nausea and vomiting. She is noted to have hyperpigmented hand creases.
228. A 30-year-old woman started on OC pills presents acutely with abdominal pain, vomiting, tachycardia, hypertension and peripheral neuropathy.
229. A 30-year-old man involved in an RTA present acutely with severe epigastric pain, left shoulder pain and vomiting. He has no bowel sounds.

THEME: 49
CAUSES OF HAEMATEMESIS

Options

a. Chronic peptic ulceration
b. Gastritis
c. Oesophageal varices
d. Mallory-Weiss tear
e. Carcinoma oesophagus
f. Carcinoma stomach
g. Oesophagitis
h. Haemophilia
i. Epistaxis
j. Angiodysplasia
k. Peutz-Jegher syndrome
l. Ehlers-Danlos syndrome

For each of the situation/condition given below, choose the one most appropriate/discriminatory option from above. The options may be used once, more than once, or not at all.

Questions

230. A 40-year-old obese man presents with projectile haematemesis after ingestion of a 5 course meal and wine.
231. A 50-year-old man presents with massive haematemesis. He is noted to have freckles on his lower lip.
232. A 60-year-old alcoholic man presents with massive haematemesis and shock. He is noted to have finger clubbing and ascites.
233. A 70-year-old man with chronic hoarseness presents with retrosternal chest pain and haematemesis. He has a history of Achalasia and has lost one stone in weight.
234. A 65-year-old man presents with haematemesis. He is noted to have an enlarged left supraclavicular node, ascites and anaemia.

THEME: 50
CAUSES OF HAEMATEMESIS AND MELENA

Options

a. Peptic ulcer
b. Gastric erosions
c. Oesophagitis
d. Oesophageal carcinoma
e. Oesophageal varices
f. Carcinoma stomach
g. Bleeding diathesis
h. Osler-Weber-Rendu syndrome
i. Mallory-Weiss syndrome
j. Peutz-Jegher's syndrome

For each of the situation/condition given below, choose the one most appropriate/discriminatory option from above. The options may be used once, more than once, or not at all.

Questions

235. A 21-year-old student has been on a drinking binge to celebrate the end of his exams. He has a 6 hours history of profuse vomiting with small amounts of fresh blood mixed in his vomit. His vital signs are stable.
236. A 24-year-old woman has had 24 hours of diarrhoea and vomiting which she thinks followed eating reheated take away food. There was fresh blood in the last 3 vomits. Vital signs are stable.
237. A 55-year-old man has chronic back pain for which he takes Diclofenac. He has epigastric pain after meals and recently has developed black tarry stools and has had an episode of coffee ground vomiting.
238. A 35-year-old man with a long history of excess drinking of alcohol presents with massive haematemesis. He is also noted to be jaundiced, hypotensive and tachycardic.
239. A 40-year-old woman describes intermittent haemoptysis as well as small amounts of haematemesis. She has Telangiectasia on her face.

THEME: 51
DIAGNOSIS OF FEELING UNWELL

Options

a. Hepatitis A
b. Hepatitis B
c. Hepatitis C
d. Gallstones
e. Pancreatitis
f. Cholangiosclerosis
g. HIV infection
h. Cirrhosis
i. Chronic persistent hepatitis
j. Chronic active hepatitis
k. Secondaries
l. Hepatocellular carcinoma
m. Leukaemia
n. Lymphoma

For each of the situation/condition given below, choose the one most appropriate/discriminatory option from above. The options may be used once, more than once, or not at all.

Questions

240. An elderly man presents with severe epigastric pain radiating to the right hypochondrium. The pain has been worsening over the past day and a half and goes through to his back and shoulders. The patient feels sick and has vomited several times. He is jaundiced.
241. A middle-aged man complains of his appearance. His wife says his eyes are yellow. On physical examination you find mild hepatomegaly. His alkaline phosphatase, albumin and globulin are normal. He says he is a teetotaler.
242. A healthy young waiter complains of feeling unwell with nausea, vomiting and diarrhoea. He has a headache, fever and abdominal pain. On palpation you find the liver to be tender and enlarged.

243. A 34-year-old stockbroker presents with jaundice and physical exhaustion. His liver and spleen are enlarged and you notice he has spider naevi on both cheeks. He says he is a moderate drinker and that he has been unwell for more than a-year-now.
244. A middle-aged social worker presents with abdominal pain and fever. She has been unwell for 2 weeks and feels she is getting worse rather than better. Her urine is dark and her stools are pale. She has tender lymph nodes and joint pain.

THEME: 52
INVESTIGATION OF GASTROINTESTINAL DISORDERS

Options

a. Jejunal biopsy
b. Antireticulin and antigliadin antibodies
c. Serum TNF levels
d. ESR
e. Anti DNA antibodies
f. Barium meal and follow through
g. Barium enema and colonic biopsy
h. Stool for reducing substances
i. Serum electrolytes
j. Serum amylase
k. Arterial blood gases
l. Lateral and AP abdominal X-ray

For each of the situation/condition given below, choose the one most appropriate/discriminatory option from above. The options may be used once, more than once, or not at all.

Questions

245. A 15-year-old girl has tiredness for the last 4 years. She has delayed puberty and does not like eating gluten-containing foods.
246. A 25-year-old man with on and off diarrhoea. On examination he has finger clubbing.

247. A 4-year-old girl has had gastroenteritis recently. Mother complains that her diarrhoea continues now 2 weeks after the illness began.
248. A 25-year-old man who was driving was involved with a high speed collision. He was wearing his seat belt and now complains of upper abdominal pain. His CXR is normal.
249. An 80-year-old lady with bilious vomiting and abdominal pain. On examination tenderness is noted.

THEME: 53
INVESTIGATIONS OF GASTROINTESTINAL DISORDERS

Options

a. CT abdomen
b. Oesophageal manometry
c. Motility studies
d. Mesenteric angiography
e. PTC
f. Barium enema
g. Upper GI endoscopy
h. Barium meal
i. Ultrasound scan
j. Erect and supine abdominal X-ray

For each of the situation/condition given below, choose the one most appropriate/discriminatory option from above. The options may be used once, more than once, or not at all.

Questions

250. A 49-year-old alcoholic presents with haematemesis and melaena. He is stable and being transfused.
251. A 56-year-old man presents with massive persistent fresh rectal bleeding. A recent barium enema showed no evidence of diverticulosis or tumours. Nasogastric suction showed yellow bile and no evidence of bleeding.
252. A 59-year-old man presents with a 2 days history of worsening crampy abdominal pain, constipation and

recurrent vomiting. On examination his abdomen is distended with high pitched bowel sounds. There is no localised tenderness or rectal mass.

253. A 65-year-old woman presents with a 1 year history of pain in the right upper quadrant exacerbated by eating rich foods.

254. A 68-year-old man presents with obstructive jaundice and severe weight loss of a 2 months duration. Abdominal USG shows a 5 cm mass with dilated bile ducts in the heads of the pancreas.

THEME: 54
LIVER DISEASE

Options

a. Gilbert's syndrome
b. Chronic active hepatitis
c. Gaucher's disease
d. Galactosaemia
e. Primary biliary cirrhosis
f. Alcoholic liver disease
g. Wilson's disease
h. Haemochromatosis
i. Cholecystitis
j. Hepatic adenoma
k. Hepatic amoebiasis

For each of the situation/condition given below, choose the one most appropriate/discriminatory option from above. The options may be used once, more than once, or not at all.

Questions

255. A 37-year-old woman presented with generalised pruritus for 5 months. On examination she was tanned and there were spider naevi on her chest. The liver was palpable one finger breadth below the costal margin as well as the tip of the spleen.

256. A 30-year-old woman presented with anorexia, weight loss, lethargy and arthralgia for 3 weeks. On examination,

she was pale and jaundiced. The liver was palpable 2 finger breadths below the costal margin as well as the tip of the spleen. Test results were: ALP 150, U, AST 875, Bilirubin 39 umol, albumin 21 g/l, globulin 52 g/l.

257. A 29-year-old woman presented with acute abdominal pain. Her bowels were regular with normal stools. She was taking OC pills. On examination there was no features of chronic liver disease. Pulse 120, BP 90/50 and temperature was 37.2°C. Her abdomen was tender and guarding present. The right lobe was palpable.
258. A 40-year-old man presents with worsening limb twitches and facial tics. He has been an inpatient in a psychiatric hospital for the last 5 years. His father had a similar history and died in a psychiatric hospital.
259. A 32-year-old man presented with haematemesis and shock. On examination there were multiple surgical scars over both knees, the right hip and the right hypochondrium. His liver was palpable four finger breadths below the costal margin.
260. A fit 17-year-old developed flu like illness followed 3 days later by abdominal pain, nausea, vomiting and jaundice. All his blood tests were normal apart from increased, unconjugated bilirubin.

THEME: 55
DIAGNOSIS OF JAUNDICE

Options

a. Hemolytic anaemia
b. Leptospirosis
c. Halothane
d. Gallstones
e. Hepatitis B associated with primary hepatocellular carcinoma
f. Pancreatic carcinoma
g. Primary biliary cirrhosis
h. Chronic active hepatitis
i. Gilbert's syndrome

j. Alcoholic hepatitis
k. Paracetamol overdosage
l. Sclerosing cholangitis

For each of the situation/condition given below, choose the one most appropriate/discriminatory option from above. The options may be used once, more than once, or not at all.

Questions

261. A 45-year-old woman has melanotic skin pigmentation, pruritus, hepatosplenomegaly and dark urine. She develops jaundice 5 years after onset.
262. A 60-year-old man presents with jaundice, hepatomegaly, nocturnal abdominal pain radiating through to the back and weight loss.
263. A 50-year-old Asian man develops jaundice, right upper quadrant pain, weakness, proximal myopathy and depression.
264. A 45-year-old man develops deep jaundice, abdominal pain, hypoglycaemia, fever and increased PT. Liver biopsy shows Mallory's hyaline and collagen deposition.
265. A 32-year-old man presents with jaundice, fever, mouth ulceration, blood and mucus per rectum and pyoderma gangrenosum.

THEME: 56
DIFFERENTIAL DIAGNOSIS OF JAUNDICE

Options

a. Hepatoma
b. Hepatitis
c. Carcinoma of bile duct
d. Alcoholism
e. Phenelzine induced jaundice
f. Spherocytosis
g. Secondaries
h. Carcinoma pancreas
i. Hemolytic anaemia
j. Primary biliary cirrhosis

k. Gallstones
l. CLL
m. Thalassemia

For each of the situation/condition given below, choose the one most appropriate/discriminatory option from above. The options may be used once, more than once, or not at all.

Questions

266. A 60-year-old man presents with jaundice. On physical examination you notice his liver is enlarged, irregular and tender. You also notice that his index finger and forefinger are also dark.
267. A 55-year-old divorced office worker was admitted to hospital with a history of increasing jaundice and weight loss for 2 months. She noticed that her urine has become much darker and that her stools had become pale.
268. A 40-year-old mother of five, complained of yellow skin and abdominal pain, especially after meals. She was overweight and she said that she did not like going out to restaurants because of embarrassing flatulence.
269. A 30-year-old woman complains of jaundice. She is unemployed and depressed and undergoing psychotherapy. For the past 5 months she has been under treatment at the Tavistock Clinic in London.
270. A middle-aged women complains of intense pruritus and yellowing of her skin. On physical examination you notice xanthomata and skin pigmentation.

THEME: 57
INVESTIGATION OF MALABSORPTION

Options

a. Sweat test
b. ERCP
c. Abdominal USG
d. Abdominal X-ray
e. Jejunal biopsy
f. Barium follow through

g. Endomysial antibodies
h. Thyroid function tests
i. Faecal fat content
j. Immunoglobulins
k. Hydrogen breath test
l. HIV test

For each of the situation/condition given below, choose the one most appropriate/discriminatory option from above. The options may be used once, more than once, or not at all.

Questions

271. A 50-year-old woman has developed weight loss and passes loose pale stools. She has mouth ulcers and is anaemic. She takes thyroxine for myxoedema.
272. A 35-year-old man presents with weight loss, diarrhoea and pain on swallowing. On examination he has oral candidiasis and molluscum contagiosum.
273. A 10-year-old girl with a history of recurrent chest infection has developed pale floating stools and weight loss.
274. A 45-year-old man has recurrent abdominal pain, weight loss and diarrhoea. He has a previous history of alcoholism.
275. A 40-year-old man has a small bowel resection. He now has symptoms of malabsorption and barium investigation is inconclusive.

THEME: 58
DIAGNOSIS OF VITAMIN DEFICIENCY

Options

a. Vitamin A deficiency
b. Vitamin D deficiency
c. Vitamin K deficiency
d. Vitamin E deficiency
e. Thiamine deficiency
f. Riboflavin deficiency
g. Niacin deficiency

h. Pyridoxine deficiency
i. Biotin deficiency
j. Folic acid deficiency
k. Cobalamin deficiency
l. Ascorbic acid deficiency

For each of the situation/condition given below, choose the one most appropriate/discriminatory option from above. The options may be used once, more than once, or not at all.

Questions

276. A 9-year-old boy is noted to have a bitot spot on his conjunctiva.
277. A 40-year-old female with a history of coeliac disease presents with epistaxis. Her Prothrombin time is elevated.
278. A 30-year-old man presents with fissuring of the angles of his mouth and seborrheic dermatitis around his nose.
279. A 40-year-old man complains of flushing after coffee and alcohol and diarrhoea. On examination, he has angular stomatitis, a Casal's collar rash and oedema.
280. A 30-year-old woman presents to her dentist with bleeding gums. She does not like to eat vegetables.

THEME: 59
CHOOSE THE CORRECT DIAGNOSIS

Options

a. Ulcerative colitis
b. Crohn's disease.
c. Amoebic dysentry.
d. Diverticulitis.
e. Food poisoning and acute gastroenteritis.

For each of the statements/situations given below, choose the one most appropriate/discriminatory option. The options can be used once, more than once or not at all.

Questions

281. A 30-year-old patient c/o diarrhea, blood +, mucus + pus +, taking treatment on and off, crampy pain abdomen +, fever +.

282. A lady 40-year-old history of has going to marriage reception at night and next day she had diarrhea, she has been vomiting since midnight.
283. Young patient c/o diarrhea, blood +, abdomen pain+, relevant microscopy stool.
284. A 30 years old patient with diarrhoea , mucous +, blood +, pain abdomen +, loss of weight ++. On examination patient has anal fistula too.

THEME: 60
CASUES OF ACUTE PANCREATITIS

Options

a. Gallstones
b. Hypertriglyceridemia
c. Mumps
d. Alcohol
e. Polyarteritis nodosa
f. Hypothermia
g. Cystic fibrosis
h. Pancreatic carcinoma
i. Iatrogenic
j. Thiazide diuretics
k. Hypercalcemia

For each of the situation/condition given below, choose the one most appropriate/discriminatory option from above. The options may be used once, more than once, or not at all.

Questions

285. A 10-year-old girl with a history of recurrent chest infections and sinusitis with acute abdominal pain.
286. A 45-year-old obese woman with a history of recurrent pain in the right hypochondrium.
287. A 38-year-old driver presenting with recurrent central abdominal pain, diarrhoea and bleeding per rectum. 3 weeks earlier he had a flu like illness with productive cough and myalgia. Chest examination shows inspiratory bilateral wheezes.

288. A 49-year-old woman presenting with polyuria, haematuria, abdominal pain and bone aches. On examination her blood pressure is 170/100 mmHg.
289. A 12-year-old student presenting with fever, anorexia, headache, malaise and trismus.

THEME: 61
INVESTIGATING GASTROINTESTINAL DISORDERS

Options

a. Oesophageal manometry
b. Barium swallow
c. Chest radiography
d. Upper GI endoscopy and biopsy
e. CT chest
f. Motility studies
g. MRI abdomen and pelvis
h. CT abdomen and pelvis
i. Colonoscopy
j. Barium enema
k. Oesophageal PH testing

For each of the situation/condition given below, choose the one most appropriate/discriminatory option from above. The options may be used once, more than once, or not at all.

Questions

290. A 70-year-old alcoholic and heavy smoker presents with a 3 month history of progressive dysphagia and weight loss.
291. A 53-year-old man underwent upper GI endoscopy for assessment of dysphagia. 3 hours later he complained of severe chest pain. On examination there was crepitus in his neck.
292. A 69-year-old man has been on medications for gastric ulcer for 12 weeks. A repeat upper gastrogaffin series shows moderate shrinkage of the ulcer.

293. A 57-year-old with an 8 weeks history of dysphagia undergoes a barium swallow. It shows bird peak deformity of the distal oesophagus with proximal dilatation.
294. A 60-year-old presents with a 2 days history of worsening left lower quadrant abdominal pain. On examination he is pyrexial and there is tenderness in the left lower quadrant. FBC shows leukocytosis.

THEME: 62
INVESTIGATION OF LIVER DISEASE

Options

a. Mitochondrial antibodies
b. Serum, Iron and TIBC
c. Serum copper and ceruloplasmin
d. Serum bilirubin and LFTs
e. HbsAg
f. Antibodies to HCV
g. Antibodies against nuclei and actin
h. Antibodies to HAV
i. Gamma glutamyl transferase levels
j. Alpha 1 antitrypsin

For each of the situation/condition given below, choose the one most appropriate/discriminatory option from above. The options may be used once, more than once, or not at all.

Questions

295. A 60-year-old man with emphysema presents with liver disease. His sputum is purulent and found to contain elastases and proteases.
296. A 50-year-old woman presents with pruritus and jaundice. She complains of dry eyes and mouth. On examination she has xanthelasma and hepatosplenomegaly.
297. A 50-year-old bronzed man presents with a loss of libido. He is noted to have hepatomegaly. He take humulin and actrapid insulin.

298. A 22-year-old man presents with tremor and dysarthria. On examination he is noted to have a greenish brown pigment at the corneoscleral junction.
299. A 30-year-old woman presents with acute hepatitis. She is pyrexial, jaundiced with hepatosplenomegaly, bruising and migratory polyarthritis. She is noted to have a goitre.

THEME: 63
DIAGNOSIS OF LIVER DISEASE

Options

a. Budd-Chiari syndrome
b. Cholestasis
c. Hemolytic jaundice
d. Hepatocellular failure
e. Acute hepatitis C
f. Acute hepatitis B
g. Acute hepatitis A
h. Primary biliary cirrhosis
i. Alcoholic hepatitis
j. Haemochromatosis
k. Wilson's disease
l. Hepato cellular carcinoma

For each of the situation/condition given below, choose the one most appropriate/discriminatory option from above. The options may be used once, more than once, or not at all.

Questions

300. A 22-year-old woman presents with right upper quadrant pain and ascites. On examination she has hepatomegaly. Diagnostic liver scintiscan shows maximal take-up in the caudate lobe alone. Her regular medication includes OC pills and Prozac.
301. A 50-year-old woman presents with hepatomegaly and dark skin pigmentation. She admits to drinking heavily. She is noted to have glycosuria. .
302. A 40-year-old man presents with jaundice. He was started on chlorpromazine for intractable hiccups 3 weeks ago.

303. A 50-year-old man presents with hepatomegaly and fever. His blood test reveal an elevated MCV and an elevated gamma glutamyl transpeptidase.
304. A 40-year-old woman presents with hepatomegaly and weight loss. She takes OC pills and Atenolol. She is noted to have a raised alpha-fetoprotein.

THEME: 64
DIAGNOSIS OF JAUNDICE

Options

a. Primary biliary cirrhosis
b. Chronic active hepatitis
c. Carcinoma head of pancreas
d. Sclerosing cholangitis
e. Hepatocellular carcinoma
f. Cholangiocarcinoma
g. Gilbert's syndrome
h. Dubin-Johnson syndrome
i. Common bile ducts
j. Rotor's syndrome
k. Hepatitis A

For each of the situation/condition given below, choose the one most appropriate/discriminatory option from above. The options may be used once, more than once, or not at all.

Questions

305. A 12-year-old boy presents with jaundice after recent episode of tonsillitis. Serum bilirubin rises further on fasting. USG and liver biopsy reveal no abnormality.
306. A 27-year-old man presents with jaundice. He also describes a 6 month history of bloody diarrhoea. HB is 10, bilirubin 75 umol and AST, ALT and ALP are all raised. LFTs improve with ursodeoxycholic acid administration.
307. A 45-year-old woman presents with a painless jaundice 4 weeks after laparoscopic cholecystectomy. Bilirubin 105, AST 150 and ALP 750.

308. A 69-year-old woman presents with jaundice and backache. Clinical examination shows a mass in the right upper quadrant, acanthosis, nigrans and superficial thrombophlebitis.
309. A 49-year-old woman with Sjögren's syndrome presents with jaundice and hepatosplenomegaly. Her urine is dark and serum contains antimitochondrial antibody. Liver biopsy shows ductal destruction, proliferation and granulomas.

THEME: 65
INVESTIGATING CHANGE IN BOWEL HABIT

Options

a. ESR
b. Stool culture
c. Per rectal examination
d. FBC
e. Haemoglobuin
f. Plain abdominal X-ray
g. Procotoscopy
h. Sigmoidoscopy
i. Abdominal palpation
j. Barium enema
k. Laparotomy
l. Double enema test
m. WBC count
n. Stool examination

For each of the situation/condition given below, choose the one most appropriate/discriminatory option from above. The options may be used once, more than once, or not at all.

Questions

310. A teenager complains of acute abdominal pain. He has felt unwell and unable to pass stools since a game of football yesterday afternoon. On physical examination you find a tense smooth tender lower abdominal swelling.

311. A 55-year-old man complains of constipation and colicky abdominal pain. On physical examination you find a palpable and mobile abdominal mass. The patient appears very pale.
312. A young adult complains of recurrent attacks of diarrhoea. She says her stools contain blood and mucus. Sometimes she has a low grade fever.
313. A 42-year-old train driver complains of diarrhoea. He says he has always been regular. He says his stools contain blood and that he passes mucus first thing in the morning.
314. An elderly woman cannot pass stools. She is bedridden and incontinent. She has taken laxatives and they did give her some relief, but she still feels very constipated.

THEME: 66
DIAGNOSIS OF MEDICAL SYNDROMES

Options

a. Pendred's syndrome
b. Patterson-Brown Kelly syndrome
c. Plummer-Vinson syndrome
d. Reiter's syndrome
e. Waterhouse-Friedrichsen syndrome
f. Shieie's syndrome
g. Peutz-Jegher syndrome
h. Fanconi's syndrome
i. Zollinger-Ellison syndrome
j. Reye's syndrome
k. Mallory-Weiss syndrome
l. Sjögren's syndrome
m. Felty's syndrome

For each of the situation/condition given below, choose the one most appropriate/discriminatory option from above. The options may be used once, more than once, or not at all.

Questions

315. A 50-year-old man presents with a low white count and anaemia. He is noted to have splenomegaly. He is taking Diclofenac for arthritis.

316. A 55-year-old man is noted to have freckles on his lips and occasional rectal bleeding.
317. A 20-year-old man presents with bone pain, polyuria, and polydipsia. He is noted to have glycosuria and aminoaciduritis.
318. A 25-year-old man presents with arthritis, urethritis, conjunctivitis and keratoderma blenorrhagicum.
319. A 50-year-old woman presents with rheumatoid arthritis and complains of diminished lacrimation and salivation.

THEME: 67
DIAGNOSIS OF MASS IN R.U.Q.

Options

a. Hepatoma.
b. Hydatid cyst.
c. Secondaries in liver.
d. Amoebic liver abscess.

For each of the statements/situations given below, choose the one most appropriate/discriminatory option. The options can be used once, more than once or not at all.

Questions

320. A young Chinese patient c/o right upper quadrant fullness, pain abdomen but it is not related to food. Patient has lost weight significantly over last 4 months. Patient gives history of jaundice in past.
321. A 30-year-old lady gives history of right upper quadrant, also gives history of fever, gives history of travel abroad and had diarrhea for which she had been treated.
322. A 60-year-old female comes with mass in right upper quadrant and ascitis. On examination mass is hard. She gives history of radical mastectomy done for Ca breast 2 years back.
323. A young patient (who was fond of dogs), has a mass in the right upper quadrant, not painful. X-ray shows a clear zone with fleeks of calcification in the wall.

THEME: 68
CAUSES OF SPLENOMEGALY

Options

a. CML
b. Myelofibrosis
c. Malaria
d. Schistosomiasis
e. Visceral leishmaniasis
f. Glandular fever
g. Portal hypertension
h. Lymphoma
i. Felty's syndrome
j. Gaucher's syndrome
k. Infective endocarditis

For each of the situation/condition given below, choose the one most appropriate/discriminatory option from above. The options may be used once, more than once, or not at all.

Questions

324. A 50-year-old man presents with malaise, recurrent chest infections and intermittent low grade fever. He has massive splenomegaly. HB 9, WBC 3 x 10, platelets 90 x 10. Bone marrow aspirate is dry.
325. A 40-year-old woman has a long history of pruritus, arthralgia and mild jaundice. She presents with haematemesis and is found to have splenomegaly. Endoscopy shows oesophageal varices.
326. A 60-year-old woman has had rheumatoid arthritis for 30 years. She presents with recurrent infections and easy bruising and is found to have a grossly enlarged spleen. Liver is not enlarged.
327. A 50-year-old refugee from Iraq presents with weight loss, cough, diarrhoea, recurrent fevers and epistaxis. He is pale and has massive splenomegaly. HB 8, WBC 2.0 x $10^{9,}$ albumin 22g/l.

328. A 52-year-old woman from Russia presents with malaise and low grade fever for 1 month. She has splinter haemorrhages in her finger nailbeds and macroscopic haematuria. Her spleen is just palpable.

THEME: 69
CAUSES OF SPLENOMEGALY

Options

a. Typhoid
b. Gaucher's disease
c. Malaria
d. Schistosomiasis
e. Lymphoma
f. Leishmaniasis
g. Idiopathic thrombocytopenic purpura
h. Polycythaemia rubra vera
i. Felty's syndrome
j. Leptospirosis
k. Chronic myeloid leukaemia

For each of the situation/condition given below, choose the one most appropriate/discriminatory option from above. The options may be used once, more than once, or not at all.

Questions

329. A 20-year-old man presents acutely with fever, jaundice, Purpura, injected conjunctiva and painful calves after swimming outdoors.
330. A 26-year-old man recently returned from a trip to India presents with intermittent fevers, cough, diarrhoea, epistaxis and massive splenomegaly.
331. A 22-year-old female presents with epistaxis and easy bruising and massive splenomegaly.
332. A 30-year-old Jewish man presents with incidental splenomegaly on a routine physical exam at his GP's clinic. His serum acid phosphatase is elevated. He admits to having episodes of bone pain. His uncle also has an enlarged spleen.

333. A 60-year-old female with rheumatoid arthritis presents with splenomegaly. Her full blood count shows a white count of 1500/mm^3.

THEME: 70
INVESTIGATION OF SPLENOMEGALY

Options

a. Lumbar puncture
b. Liver biopsy
c. Bone marrow biopsy
d. Blood culture
e. Heterophil antibody agglutination
f. White cell count
g. Serology
h. Packed cell volume
i. Blood film
j. Full blood count
k. Rheumatoid factor
l. Liver function test
m. Abdominal USG
n. Serial blood pressure

For each of the situation/condition given below, choose the one most appropriate/discriminatory option from above. The options may be used once, more than once, or not at all.

Questions

334. An adolescent girl presents with fever, lymphadenopathy and splenic enlargement. She has a very sore throat.
335. A 27-year-old abattoir worker has an undiagnosed fever for 2 weeks. He complains of headache, cough and sweating. A CXR shows consolidation. Physical examination shows dehydration and splenomegaly.
336. A young woman complains of lacking energy. On physical examination you find the spleen and lymph nodes to be enlarged. You also detect a mild cyanosis.
337. A middle-aged man complains of joint pain, chest pain and weight loss. He is pale and breathless and anaemic.

On physical examination you find a large spleen and enlarged lymph nodes.

338. A 52-year-old man who enjoys drinking presents with pallor, epistaxis and bleeding. On physical examination you find the spleen to be enlarged and the liver to be slightly enlarged.

THEME: 71
CAUSES OF HEPATOMEGALY

Options

a. Congestive cardiac failure
b. Tricuspid regurgitation
c. Malaria
d. Infections mononucleosis
e. Hepatocellular carcinoma
f. Liver metastases
g. CML
h. CLL
i. AML
j. Lymphoma
k. Myelofibrosis
l. Amyloidosis

For each of the situation/condition given below, choose the one most appropriate/discriminatory option from above. The options may be used once, more than once, or not at all.

Questions

339. A 20-year-old student presented to her GP with a 1 week history of fever and sore throat. On examination, she has tender cervical lymphadenopathy and an enlarged tender liver.
340. A 62-year-old man presents with a 3 months history of intermittent constipation and diarrhoea and progressive weight loss. On examination he is cachetic and has knobbly hepatomegaly. He is not jaundiced. His LFTs are normal.

341. An 81-year-old woman presents to her GP with a 6 months history of abdominal swelling, hepatomegaly and leg oedema. She has a past history of rheumatic fever as a child and hypertension for the last few years. She takes Atenolol for her hypertension.
342. A 56-year-old woman has a 20 years history of rheumatoid arthritis. Despite numerous drugs, her arthritis has only recently come under control. Recently she has noticed that she bruises easily. On examination she has a large beefy tongue, lymphadenopathy and hepatomegaly.
343. A 31-year-old man presents to casualty with a 2 weeks history of night sweats, weight loss and pruritus. He has noticed some enlarged glands in his groin that are painful if he drinks alcohol. On examination he has no other evidence of lymphadenopathy and a smooth enlarged liver.

THEME: 72
DIAGNOSIS OF JAUNDICE

Options

a. Gallstones
b. Alcoholic cirrhosis
c. Hepatitis
d. Well's disease
e. Hemolysis
f. Gilbert's syndrome
g. Carcinoma of head of pancreas
h. Cholangiocarcinoma
i. Dubin-Johnson syndrome
j. Drug induced cholestasis
k. Hepatocellular carcinoma
l. Acute pancreatitis

For each of the situation/condition given below, choose the one most appropriate/discriminatory option from above. The options may be used once, more than once, or not at all.

Questions

344. A 50-year-old man: Bilibrubin 50 umol/l, Alkaline phosphate 200 IU, Alanine aminotransferase 120, gamma glutamyl transpeptidase 600 IU.

345. A 50-year-old man: Bilirubin 110/umol/l, ALT 110 IU, alpha fetoprotein 260 IU/l
346. A 35-year-old woman: Bilirubin 80 umol/l alkaline phosphatase 300 IU, ALT 30 IU, gamma glutamyl transpeptidase 30 IU, amylase 35 IU/l.
347. A 20-year-old man: Bilirubin 45 umol/l – conjugated 7, unconjugated 38, alkaline phosphatase 40 IU, ALT 12 IU, HB 15gm/dl, blood film reported as normal.

THEME: 73
DIAGNOSIS OF LIVER DISEASE

Options

a. Wilson's disease
b. Sclerosing cholangitis
c. Primary biliary cirrhosis
d. Haemochromatosis
e. Galactosemia
f. Gaucher's disease
g. Dubin-Johnson syndrome
h. Gilbert's syndrome
i. Hepatocellular carcinoma
j. Pancreatic carcinoma
k. Chronic active hepatitis

For each of the situation/condition given below, choose the one most appropriate/discriminatory option from above. The options may be used once, more than once, or not at all.

Questions

348. A 48-year-old man presents with dull aching pain in the right hypochondrium, which he has had for 3 weeks. Other complaints include impotence, arthritis, lethargy and weight loss.
349. A 47-year-old alcoholic presents with weight loss, fever, ascites and pain in the right hypochondrium. Abdominal USG shows a focal lesion in a cirrhotic liver. Serum AFP is grossly elevated.

350. A 41-year-old man with known ulcerative colitis presented with progressive abdominal pain and itching. On examination he was jaundiced.
351. A 35-year-old woman presented with jaundice and painless depigmented patches on her hands, neck and face. On examination multiple naevi were found.
352. A 4 weeks old baby was seen with vomiting, diarrhoea and failure to thrive. On examination there was hepatosplenomegaly.

THEME: 74
HEPATITIS

Options

a. Chronic acute hepatitis.
b. Acute hepatitis B.
c. Chronic hepatitis C.
d. Acute hepatitis A.
e. Immunised to hepatitis B.
f. Acute hepatitis D.
g. Acute hepatitis E.
h. Past infection with hepatitis A.

For each of the statements/situations given below, choose the one most appropriate/discriminatory option. The options can be used once, more than once or not at all.

Questions

353. A 30-year-old drug addict known to be Hbs Ag positive, comes to you with weight loss, nausea and lethargy of 3 weeks duration. On examination he is icteric, febrile and has spider nevi. Examination of the abdomen revealed ascitis and 8 cm hepatosplenomegaly. Tests done reveal bilirubin of 44 mmol/l, ALT 420 IU/l, AST 400 IU/l, abdomen 28 gm/l, INR 2.1, Viral marker revealed Hbs Ag positive, IgG anti HBc Ag positive, HBc Ag negative and IgM anti HDV positive.
354. A 30-year-old male salesman returns from a holiday in Thailand and complains of myalgia, headache and dark

colored urine. On examination he was icteric and had a 4 cm tender hepatomegaly. Blood tests done showed a bilirubin of 40 m mol/l , ACT 845 IU/l, AST 455 IU/l. Viral markers showed HBs Ag negative, IgM anti HBs Ag negative, HBe Ag negative, IgM anti HAV positive, anti HBc negative.

355. During screening health care workers in a inner city nursing home, a male nurse was found to have the following blood tests. S.bilirubin 10 mmol/l AST 33 IU/l, ACT 24 Iu/l, albumin 44 gm/l. viral titres revealed Hbs Ag negative, IgG anti HBC negative, IgM anti Hbc negative, IgG anti Hbs Ag positive, anti HCU negative, IgG anti HAv negative.
356. A 30-year-old hemophilic patient had routine screening done which revealed a bilirubin of 33 mmol/l, AST 89 IU/l, ALT 66 IU/l, albumin 34 gm/l. viral markers revealed HBs Ag negative, IgG anti HBc negative, IgM anti HBc negative, anti HCU positive, IgG anti HAv negative.

THEME: 75
CHOOSE THE BEST DIAGNOSIS.

Options

a. Hepatitis E.
b. Paracetamol poisoning.
c. Hepatitis G.
d. Carcinoma pancreas.
e. Wilson's disease.
f. Gibert's disease.
g. Hemolytic jaundice.
h. Drug induced cholestasis.
i. Alcoholic hepatitis.
j. Primary biliary cirrhosis.
k. Primary sclerosing cholangitis.
l. Cholangio carcinoma.

For each of the statements/situations given below, choose the one most appropriate/discriminatory option. The options can be used once, more than once or not at all.

Questions

357. A 65-year-old lady has pain in the upper abdomen and back, severe weight loss, anorexia and now develops typical obstructive jaundice.
358. A 20-year-old boy has severe episodes of jaundice in the last 3 years. He has now developed tremors and choreo athetosis.
359. A 20-year-old student undergoing treatment for depression is found unconscious in his room. The next day in hospital, he develops jaundice and bleeding tendency.
360. A 40-year-old female teacher had pruritis and joint aches since six months. Now she has icterus, mild diarrhea, direct bilirubin and alkaline phosphatase increased, AMA positive.
361. A 30-year-old executive has history of recurrent transient episodes of mild jaundice four times in last five years. Indirect bilirubin increased, enzymes normal, HBs Ag negative.

THEME: 76
DIAGNOSIS OF JAUNDICE

Options

a. Cholestatic jaundice
b. Hepatitis A
c. Hemolytic anaemia
d. Criggler – Najjar syndrome
e. Gilbert's syndrome
f. Chronic active hepatitis
g. Hepatitis B
h. Alcoholic hepatitis
i. Leptospirosis
j. Primary biliary cirrhosis

For each of the situation/condition given below, choose the one most appropriate/discriminatory option from above. The options may be used once, more than once, or not at all.

Questions

362. A 35-year-old IV drug abuser on penicillin and flucloxacillin for cellulitis now presents with jaundice, pale stools and dark urine.
363. A 20-year-old man presents with mild jaundice following an upper respiratory tract infection. On fasting, his bilirubin level is high.
364. A 20-year-old woman presents with abdominal pain, increasing jaundice and arthralgia. She is noted to have hepatosplenomegaly. She recently donated her blood. She is found to have an increase in both unconjugated and conjugated Bilirubin.
365. A 45-year-old woman presents with pruritus, jaundice and pigmentation. Both the liver and spleen are palpable. Investigations reveal a high alkaline phosphatase and a high Bilirubin.
366. A 55-year-old man presents with pale stools and jaundice. 3 days earlier he had fever, malaise, vomiting and upper abdominal discomfort associated with tender enlargement of the liver. He takes methyldopa for hypertension.

THEME: 77
INVESTIGATIONS FOR JAUNDICE

Options

a. Anti HCV antibody.
b. Serum iron.
c. IVC venogram.
d. Antimitochondrial antibody.
e. ANA.
f. HBc Ag.
g. Plasma ceruloplasmin.

For each of the statements/situations given below, choose the one most appropriate/discriminatory option. The options can be used once, more than once or not at all.

Questions

367. A 30-year-old female patient with recurrent abortions comes with a history of myalgia, arthralgia and PUO. In

course of investigations she was found to have deranged liver functions like bilirubin 44 mmol/l, ALT 110 IU/l, AST 99 IU/l. HBs Ag negative and anti HCU negative.

368. A 25-year-old drug addict complains of weight loss and fatigue. On examination, he has signs of liver failure like icterus and ascites and spider nevi. Investigations reveal a bilirubin of 56 m mol/l , AST 56 IU/L, ALT 98IU/L, alkaline phosphatase 220 IU/L, HBs Ag positive anti Hcu negative.
369. A 50-year-old female patient presented with myalgia and fatigue. On examination she has generalized pigmentation, 5 cm hepatomegaly, no splenomegaly and a few spider nevi. Investigations reveal she has a bilirubin of 34 m mmol/L, AST 114 IU/L, ALT 89 IU/L, HBs Ag negative, anti HCV negative and an impaired glucose tolerance test.
370. A 60-year-old female patient presents with generalized pruritis, dark coloured urine, diarrhea. On examination she is icteric, has xanthalesma, multiple scratch marks over her torso, liver just palpable and no ascites. Tests reveal bilirubin of 78 mmol/L, AST 50 IU/L, ALT 65 IU/L, alkaline phospahtase 1200 IU/L, HBs Ag negative, anti HCV negative.

THEME: 78
DIAGNOSIS OF ABDOMINAL PAIN

Options

a. Perforated appendix
b. Pelvic inflammatory disease
c. Pancreatitis
d. Mittleschmers
e. Biliary colic
f. Intestinal obstruction
g. Sickle cell anemia
h. Lead poisoning
i. Ruptured aneurysm of aorta
j. Ketoacidosis

k. Prophyria
l. Hysterical

Questions

371. A 15-year-old west Indian boy is admitted with severe abdominal pain. He was ulcers on his skin and looks pale.
372. A 50-year-old house wife has been having recurrent pain in right hypochondrium and a ginge of icterus.
373. A 40-year-old woman taking 'alternative medicines' for chronic rheumatoid arthritis has abdominal pain since two weeks. Her gums show dark, bluish pigmentation in a linear distribution.
374. A 20-year-old diabetic boy is admitted with breathlessness, dizziness and vomiting will abdominal pain.
375. A 35-year-old house wife has pain in lower abdomen and tenderness in the left iliac fossa, since two weeks.

THEME: 79
INVESTIGATION OF ABDOMINAL PAIN

Options

a. USG abdomen
b. Rectal examination
c. Upper GI endoscopy
d. Barium meal
e. Sigmoidoscopy
f. Colonoscopy
g. CT abdomen
h. KUB X-ray
i. Pelvic ultrasound
j. Laparoscopy
k. Erect chest X-ray

For each of the situation/condition given below, choose the one most appropriate/discriminatory option from above. The options may be used once, more than once, or not at all.

Questions

376. A 60-year-old man complains of severe colicky pain from his right flank radiating to his groin. His urinalysis reveals trace red blood cells.
377. A 25-year-old woman complains of severe lower abdominal pain and increasing abdominal girth. Her urine HCG is negative.
378. A 60-year-old obese man complains of severe epigastric pain radiating to his back. The pain is relieved by eating and is worse at night.
379. A 65-year-old hypertensive man presents with lower abdominal pain and back pain. An expansive abdominal mass is palpated lateral and superior to the umbilicus
380. An 80-year-old woman suffering from rheumatoid arthritis presents with severe epigastric pain and vomiting. She also complains of shoulder tip pain.

THEME: 80
ALCOHOL AND DRUG ABUSE

Options

a. Alcohol
b. Ecstacy
c. LSD
d. Amphetamines
e. Cocaine
f. Caffeine

For each of the statements/situations given below, choose the one most appropriate/discriminatory option.The options can be used once ,more than once or not at all.

Questions

381. An 18-year-old girl is found collapsed outside angenoir (a local discotheque). She has a marked tachycardia and is found to have water intoxication.

382. A medical student who is about to sit for her exams is complaining of insomnia,tremor and excessive sweating.
383. A divorced middle-aged aged woman who is a chief executive in a bank is found to have deranged liver enzymes.

Seven

Rheumatology

THEME: 1
DIAGNOSIS OF JOINT PAIN

Options

a. Ankylosing spondylitis.
b. Erythema nodosum.
c. Gout.
d. Hemochromatosis.
e. Hyperparathyroidism.
f. Joint sepsis.
g. Medial cartilage tear.
h. Osteoarthritis.
i. Psoriatic arthropathy.
j. Pseudogout.
k. Reactive arthritis.
l. Lyme disease.
m. Rheumatoid arthritis.
n. Gonococcal arthritis.
o. SLE.
p. Sjögren's syndrome.
q. Prolapsed intervertebral disc
r. Stills disease
s. Felty's syndrome

For each of the situation/condition given below, choose the one most appropriate/discriminatory option from above. The options may be used once, more than once, or not at all.

Questions

1. A 20-year-old woman complains of 2 weeks of fever, pleuritic chest pain, stiffness and swelling in wrists and

MCP and PIP joints, an erythematous rash over both cheeks and bilateral pretibial edema.

2. A 70-year-old fit farmer presents with pain on weight bearing and restricted movements of the right hip.
3. A 73-year-old woman with rheumatoid arthritis on immunosuppressive drugs presents with systemic malaise and fever and has redness, heat and swelling of the wrist.
4. An elderly woman started frusemide two weeks ago and now presents with a red, hot, swollen metatarsal phalangeal joint.
5. A 22-year-old male soldier presents with a two-week history of a swollen right knee, conjunctivitis and arthritis.
6. A 30-year-old man presents with a 10-year history of back pain, worse in the morning and one episode of iritis.
7. A 50-year-old man complains of a gritty sensation in his eyes and dry mouth, which he has experienced for several months. He has vague arthralgia in his hands and knees but only bulge signs in the knees on examination. He has scattered purpuric lesions over both calves and ankles.
8. A condition which affects males more than females, which starts with inflammatory symptoms in late teens or early twenties. There is a gradual worsening of symptoms in later life.
9. An acute presentation of back pain radiating down the leg with resolution in the majority of cases over a six weeks period. It may recover even without treatment.
10. Intermittent acute attacks of a severe asymmetrical monoarthritis over a period of several years with symptom free intervals.
11. A 15-year-old boy complains of pain in the temporo-mandibular joint for three months. On examination, there is micrognathia, loss of neck extension and unequal lengths of the boys lower limbs. Tests for Rh factor were negative.
12. A 36-year-old lady presented with swollen tender knee joints. She says they feel stiff especially in the morning. On examination she was found to have a temperature of 39°C and ulcerated lower limbs with evidence of hyperpigmentation.

13. A 40-year-old obese man presented with a painful and swollen ankle. The symptoms had started gradually in the previous month. Joint fluid aspiration was done and positively birefringent crystals were found. The patient gave a history of consuming alcohol but was a non-smoker.

THEME: 2
DIAGNOSIS OF JOINT PAIN

Options

a. Rheumatoid arthritis.
b. Osteoarthritis.
c. Gout.

For each of the situation/condition given below, choose the one most appropriate/discriminatory option from above. The options may be used once, more than once, or not at all.

Questions

14. Episodic.
15. Remitting and relapsing.
16. Persistent and may be insiduously progressive.

THEME: 3
DEFORMITIES IN RHEUMATOID ARTHRITIS

Options

a. Proximal interphalangeal joints.
b. Wrist.
c. Metacarpophalangeal joints.
d. Distal interphalangeal joints.

For each of the situation/condition given below, choose the one most appropriate/discriminatory option from above. The options may be used once, more than once, or not at all.

Questions

17. Fusiform swelling.
18. Ulnar deviation.

19. Boutennaire's deformity.
20. Swan neck deformity.
21. Dorsal deviation.

THEME: 4
DISEASES AND THEIR SYSTEMIC INVOLVEMENT

Options

a. Felty's syndrome.
b. Rheumatoid vasculitis.
c. Episcleritis.
d. Sjögren's syndrome.
e. Rheumatoid nodules.
f. Rheumatoid pleural involvement.
g. Caplan syndrome.
h. Pericardial disease.
i. Rheumatoid nodules.
j. SLE.
k. Dermatomyositis.
l. Juvenile rheumatoid arthritis.
m. Rheumatic fever.
n. Lyme disease.

For each of the situation/condition given below, choose the one most appropriate/discriminatory option from above. The options may be used once, more than once, or not at all.

Questions

22. May present as small brown spots in the nail folds.
23. Most common form of eye involvement.
24. Associated with increased frequency of infections.
25. Found in association with occupational lung disease.
26. Commonly involves Achilles tendon.
27. Chronic renal involvement.
28. Cholera.
29. Subcutaneous calcification.
30. Iridocyclitis.

THEME: 5
DISEASES WITH HLA ASSOCIATION

Options

a. HLA B27.
b. HLA DR4.
c. HLA DR3.
d. HLA B17.
e. HLA B8.

For each of the situation/condition given below, choose the one most appropriate/discriminatory option from above. The options may be used once, more than once, or not at all.

Questions

31. Ankylosing spondylitis.
32. Lupus erythematosus (SLE).
33. Juvenile rheumatoid arthritis.
34. Insulin-dependent diabetes mellitus.
35. Reiter's syndrome.
36. Rheumatoid arthritis.
37. Reactive arthritis (Yersinia).

THEME: 6
DIAGNOSIS OF RHEUMATOID DISEASE

Options

a. Rheumatoid arthritis
b. Scleroderma
c. Reiter's syndrome
d. Sjögren's syndrome
e. Dermatomyositis
f. SLE
g. Polymyalgia rheumatica
h. Polymyositis
i. Giant cell arteritis
j. Takayasu's arteritis
k. Churg-Strauss syndrome
l. Antiphospholipid antibody syndrome

For each of the situation/condition given below, choose the one most appropriate/discriminatory option from above. The option may be used once, more than once, or not at all

Questions

38. A 52-year-old woman complains of 4-month history of Raynaud's phenomenon, progressive skin tightness, thickening of fingers and hands, dyspnoea on exertion and dysphagia.
39. A 22-year-old woman complains of loss of appetite, low grade fever, shoulder and buttock pains and severe cramps in her arms and hands during exercise. On examination her pulse is weak in both arms her BP is 75/55 in the left arm, 60/40 in the right arm and 125/75 in both legs.
40. A 73-year-old man presents with persistent malaise, anorexia, pain in the shoulder and hips and loss of 10 kg over the last 10 weeks. On examination there is mild painful limitation of hip and shoulder motion and muscle tenderness but no weakness.
41. A 25-year-old woman presents with deep venous thrombosis in the right leg. Her past history includes 3 miscarriages. Her blood test show mild thrombocytopenia and a positive serology test for syphilis.

THEME: 7
DIAGNOSIS OF ARTHRITIS

Options

a. SLE
b. Antiphospholipid syndrome
c. Reiter's disease
d. Rheumatoid arthritis
e. Felty's syndrome
f. Giant cell syndrome
g. Sjögren's syndrome
h. Scleroderma
i. Polyarteritis nodosa

j. Osteoarthritis
k. Pseudogout

For each of the situation/condition given below, choose the one most appropriate/discriminatory option from above. The option may be used once, more than once, or not at all.

Questions

42. A 60-year-old previously fit man presents with a 2-month history of fatigue, dyspnoea on exertion, abdominal pain and progressive numbness in his feet. He recently developed mild polyarthritis in his hands. On examination there was evidence of left medial nerve mononeuritis. Chest radiography showed cardiomegaly.
43. A 79-year-old man complains of pain and swelling of the right knee. He has bilaterally swollen wrists, metacarpophalangeal, and proximal interphalangeal and distal phalangeal joints. His knee is also swollen with limitation of the range of motion by pain. Radiography shows calcification of the meniscal cartilage of the knee.
44. A 22-year-old woman presents with a 3 weeks history of fever, pleuritic chest pain, stiffness and swelling in the wrists. MCP joints and PIP joints. On examination, there is bilateral periorbital oedema.
45. A 27-year-old man presented with low back pain, pain in the right knee and sore eyes. His past history included an episode of diarrhoea 3 weeks earlier and he has a positive history of back pain. Pelvic radiography sclerosis and erosions of lower joint margins.
46. A 77-year-old woman with long-standing rheumatoid arthritis presented with fever and dysuria. Her past history included recurrent chest and urinary infections. On examination she was hyperpigmented and emaciated. Her hands and feet were severely deformed. Abdominal examination revealed splenomegaly but no hepatomegaly or lymhadenopathy.

THEME: 8
DIAGNOSIS OF RHEUMATOID CONDITIONS

Options

a. Scleroderma
b. Giant cell arteritis
c. Ankylosing spondylitis
d. Polymyositis
e. CREST syndrome
f. SLE
g. Polyarteritis nodosa
h. Rheumatoid arthritis
i. Reiter's syndrome
j. Antiphospholipid syndrome
k. Sjögren's syndrome

For each of the situation/condition given below, choose the one most appropriate/discriminatory option from above. The option may be used once, more than once, or not at all.

Questions

47. A 38-year-old man presented with progressive breathlessness, dry cough and difficulty in swallowing. He also noted that his hands become painful and pale in cold weather. Chest radiographs show patchy shadows in both mid-zones and bases. Radiography of hands showed calcification.
48. A 78-year-old woman presented with headache, anorexia and fever, which she had had for a few weeks. ESR, CRP and platelets were elevated. HB was low.
49. A 36-year-old woman complains of recurrent chest pain, which is worse on inspiration and progressive breathlessness. She also suffers from Raynaud's phenomenon. On examination she has a butterfly rash and a pericardial rub is audible.
50. A 45-year-old woman presented with 4-month history of multiple joint pains and progressive difficulty in climbing stairs. Muscle biopsy was normal. EMG showed

spontaneous fibrillation, high frequency repetitive potentials and polyphasic potentials on voluntary movements.

51. A 46-year-old woman complains of dryness of the mouth and eyes, joint pain and difficulty in swallowing. Schirmer tear test and Rose Bengal staining are both positive.

THEME: 9
DIAGNOSIS OF ARTHRITIS

Options

a. Rheumatoid arthritis
b. Psoriatic arthropathy
c. SLE
d. Septic arthritis
e. Seronegative arthritis
f. Pyrophosphate arthropathy
g. Haemarthrosis
h. Osteoarthritis
i. Gout
j. Hyperparathyroidism
k. Erythema nodosum

For each of the situation/condition given below, choose the one most appropriate/discriminatory option from above. The option may be used once, more than once, or not at all.

Questions

52. A 77-year-old woman presents with pain and various deformities of both knees. She also complains of pain in both hips and hands.
53. A 72-year-old woman presents with pain in both knees. Knee radiography shows a rim of calcification of the lateral meniscus.
54. A 30-year-old woman presents with pain and morning stiffness of the small joints of both hands.
55. A 30-year-old flight attendant presents with gritty eyes and painful knees especially during standing. He has just returned from Thailand.

56. A 78-year-old man presented with pain and swelling of the left first metatarsal joint. He started on thiazide diuretics 3 weeks earlier.
57. A 22-year-old soldier previously fit presents with a red-hot tender swollen knee. Leg muscles show marked spasm.

THEME: 10
INVESTIGATION OF RHEUMATIC DISEASE

Options

a. HLA B27 antigen
b. Bone scan
c. Antibody to DS DNA
d. Anti-nucleolus antibody
e. Rheumatoid factor
f. HLA-DR4 antigen
g. Synovial fluid analysis with polarised-light microscopy
h. X-ray
i. Anti-centromere antibody
j. Anti-jo antibody
k. Serum uric acid
l. Anti-RO antibody

For each of the situation/condition given below, choose the one most appropriate/discriminatory option from above. The option may be used once, more than once, or not at all.

Questions

58. A 60-year-old alcoholic man presents with a hot swollen first metatarsophalangeal joint and a lesion on the rim of his left pinna.
59. A 65-year-old woman with a history of hypothyroidism presents with a warm, painful swollen knee with effusion. The serum calcium is normal. X-ray reveals chondrocalcinosis.
60. A 40-year-old woman presents with flexion deformities of her fingers. She has soft tissue swelling of her digits. She also complains of difficulty swallowing and is noted to have a beaked nose and facial telangiectasia.

61. A 30-year-old woman presents with painful digits worse in the cold and difficulty swallowing. She is noted to have tapered fingers and a fixed facial expression with facial telangiectasia. X-ray reveals calcium around her fingers.
62. A 20-year-old woman presents with dry eyes, arthralgia, dysphagia and Raynaud's phenomenon.

THEME: 11
INVESTIGATION OF SWOLLEN JOINTS

Options

a. Urate crystals on joint aspirate
b. High serum urate
c. Pus cells on joint aspirate
d. Positive rheumatoid factor
e. Positive antinuclear antibody
f. Pyrophosphate crystals on joint aspirate
g. High ESR
h. Erosions on X-ray
i. Positive blood culture
j. High WBC count

For each of the situation/condition given below, choose the one most appropriate/discriminatory option from above. The option may be used once, more than once, or not at all.

Questions

63. A 35-year-old woman has pain and stiffness in her hands, wrists, elbows, knees and ankles. There is swelling of her MCP joints bilaterally. There is a nodule on her left elbow.
64. A 65-year-old man has started chemotherapy for lymphoma. He has developed a painful swollen hot right knee. He is apyrexial.
65. A 75-year-old man has had painful knees for many years, his left knee has become acutely hot and swollen with no history of trauma.
66. A 70-year-old woman has pain and stiffness of her shoulders and hips. She finds it difficult to comb her hair in the morning but is less stiff by the end of the day.

67. A 25-year-old man with severe Crohn's disease suddenly develops a painful swollen knee and cannot put weight through it. He is febrile.

THEME: 12
INVESTIGATION OF JOINT DISEASE

Options

a. Microscopy and culture of urethral discharge, ESR and joint X-ray.
b. Rheumatoid factor and joint X-ray
c. Joint aspiration, swab and blood cultures.
d. Clinical history and joint X-ray
e. Joint aspiration and microscopy
f. Sigmoidoscopy, biopsy and enema
g. Pelvic spring test
h. Thomas's test
i. Anti-sdDNA and complement
j. MRI scan
k. Bone scan
l. Spinal X-ray and HLA profile

For each of the situation/condition given below, choose the one most appropriate/discriminatory option from above. The option may be used once, more than once, or not at all.

Questions

68. A man presents with a single swollen red-hot knee joint. A small laceration is noted on the foot.
69. A 38-year-old woman presents with bilateral tender swellings of the MCP joints of both hands, ulnar deviation and dry eyes. Her joint symptoms are worse in the morning and eased by movement.
70. A 52-year-old lady presents with symmetrical DIP joint swelling and stiffness, worse in the night and exacerbated by movement.
71. A man presents with excruciating pain and swelling of the first metatarsophalangeal joint of his left foot.

72. A 25-year-old male returns from a holiday in Thailand. He present one month later with dysuria, conjunctivitis and a swollen painful knee.

THEME: 13
INVESTIGATIONS OF JOINT DISEASES

Options

a. X-ray of sacroiliac joints.
b. Joint fluid Gram stain and culture.
c. Serum rheumatoid factor determination.
d. Antibody titer to *Borrelia burgdorferi*.
e. Erythrocyte sedimentation rate.
f. X-ray of lumbar spine.
g. Paired blood cultures.
h. Abdominal arteriogram.

For each of the situation/condition given below, choose the one most appropriate/discriminatory option from above. The options may be used once, more than once, or not at all.

Questions

73. A 28-year-old man complains of a 3-months history of morning low back pain, lasting 2 hours each day. He has also noticed a "sausage-like" swelling of his left second toe for 2 months, and has had pain in the bottoms of both heels when he walks. He reports that he had "pink eye" 1-year-ago, around the time of an episode of bloody diarrhea that was treated by his family doctor with an antibiotic.
74. A 24-year-old woman has experienced extreme fatigue and polyarticular joint pain for 6 months. She has taken aspirin irregularly over that time with some relief, but she still complains of prolonged morning stiffness as well as bilateral pain and swelling in her wrists and metacarpophalangeal (MCP) and proximal interphalangeal (PIP) joints. She has no history of fever or other complaints. The only remarkable findings upon physical examination are swelling of the joints and mild limitation of motion of the involved joints due to pain.

75. A 60-year-old man, who had a red, target-shaped rash on his leg during the summer, experiences fatigue, radicular left arm pain and numbness, and difficulty using his left hand for gripping in September. Two months later, he notices pain and swelling of the left wrist and right knee.

THEME: 14
DIAGNOSIS OF VASCULITIC SYNDROMES

Options

a. Henoch Schonlein purpura.
b. Polyarteritis nodosa.
c. Churg-Strauss disease.
d. Wegener's granulomatosis.
e. Temporal arteritis.
f. Takayasu's arteritis.
g. Behcet syndrome.
h. Kawasaki disease.

For each of the situation/condition given below, choose the one most appropriate/discriminatory option from above. The options may be used once, more than once, or not at all.

Questions

76. Pulseless arteritis.
77. Prominent allergic, asthmatic history with lung involvement. Vessel wall shows granulomatous infitrates with eosinophils.
78. Major arterial ischemic lesions that spare lungs and spleen vessel wall show necrotising arteritis at vessel branch points. Aneurysms and renal involvement are characteristic.
79. A 60-year-old male with symptoms of polymyalgia rheumatica. Vessel wall shows giant cell and chronic mononuclear infiltrates in vessel walls.
80. Skin involvement predominant. Visceral involvement typically minimal and self-limiting. Pathologically there is leukocytoclastic vasculitis.
81. Characterized by oral and genital ulceration.

THEME: 15
DIAGNOSIS OF VASCULITIS

Options

a. Microscopic polyangitis
b. Takayasu's arteritis
c. Wegener's granulamotosis
d. Kawasaki's disease
e. Henoch-Schonlein purpura
f. Churg-Stauss syndrome
g. Polyarteritis nodosa
h. Giant cell arteritis
i. Cryoglobulinemia
j. Goodpasture's syndrome
k. Behcet's disease

For each of the situation/condition given below, choose the one most appropriate/discriminatory option from above. The option may be used once, more than once, or not at all

Questions

82. A 22-year-old woman presented with worsening headache, nausea, painful neck and fever. A year ago she had developed pain in her legs on running. On examination her BP was 190/105, femoral pulses were weak with a radio-femoral delay and an abdominal bruit is heard.
83. A 16-year-old student presented with severe chest pain. On examination his temperature was 38.8°C BP was 100/60 and pulse was 120. There was also conjuctival congestion, polymorphous rash and palpable lymphedenopathy.
84. A 79-year-old man presented with acute loss of vision in his left eye, which he had had for 24 hours. He had had severe temporal headaches for about 6 months. On examination the left optic disc was swollen with flame-shaped haemorrhages at 7'O clock position. Eye movements were full and painless.
85. A 28-year-old man presented with fever, mylagia and abdominal pain. On examination his temperature was

38.8°C bp was 190/110 and pulse was 120. His abdomen was tender with guarding and absent bowel sounds.

86. A 42-year-old man presented with shortness of breath and sinusitis. He also complained of numbness and weakness of the left leg, which he had had for 3 months. On examination, his temperature was 38.1°C and there was evidence of left sensory motor neuropathy. FBC showed eosinophilia. CXR showed pulmonary infiltrates.
87. A 13-year-old boy was admitted with a tender swollen left knee and a tender right elbow. His past history included recurrent sore throats and dull abdominal pain for a few days. On examination his temperature was 37.9°C and there was some periumbilical tenderness. Both urine and stools were positive for blood.

THEME: 16
DIAGNOSIS OF CONNECTIVE TISSUE DISORDERS

Options

a. Primary Sjögren's syndrome.
b. Antiphospholipid antibody syndrome.
c. SLE.
d. Primary systemic sclerosis.
e. Secondary Sjögren's syndrome.
f. Polymyositis.
g. Duchene's muscular dystrophy.
h. Sickle cell anemia.
i. Measles.
j. Kawasaki disease.
k. Henoch-Schonlien purpura.
l. Dermatomyositis
m. Osteoarthritis.

For each of the situation/condition given below, choose the one most appropriate/discriminatory option from above. The options may be used once, more than once, or not at all.

Questions

88. A 7-year-old boy had a URI, which was followed by an acute arthritis and abdominal pain. Raised, dark coloured

skin lesions were palpable over the buttocks and lower limbs. He also had hematuria with history of rectal bleeding during a previous episode.

89. A 4-year-old boy with history of fever of one week duration, bilateral conjunctival congestion, erythema of lips and oral mucosa, exanthematous lesions over the body, with cervical lymphadenopathy. Angiography demonstrated coronary dilatation.
90. A 35-year-old woman presents with history of dusky discolouration of fingers and toes in winter, along with restriction of finger movements and difficulty in opening the mouth. She also c/o intermittent abdominal pain and constipation.
91. A 39-year-old female presenting with difficulty in climbing stairs and rising from a low chair, has swelling around her eyes and violet discolouration of upper eyelids. Weight loss has also been noticed.
92. A 40-year-old female with butterfly-rash and joint pain presents with c/o dry mouth and frequent eye problems.
93. A 22-year-old pregnant lady presents with pain of multiple joints. She also gives history of chest pain, which is sharp and which is influenced by movement, associated with tachycardia in the past as well as history of swelling of lower limbs and around the eyes in the past. She has had 2 abortions earlier. On examination, skin lesions are found.

THEME: 17
INVESTIGATION OF AUTOIMMUNE DISORDERS

Options

a. Antinuclear antibody
b. Gastric parietal cell antibody
c. Smooth muscle antibody
d. Antibody to mitochondria
e. Throglobulin antibodies
f. Antiacetylcholine receptor antibodies
g. Antineutrophil cytoplasmic antibody
h. Antibody to reticulin
i. Antibody to platelets
j. Rheumatoid factor

For each of the situation/condition given below, choose the one most appropriate/discriminatory option from above. The option may be used once, more than once, or not at all.

Questions

94. A 44-year-old woman presents with stiff sausage-shaped fingers and MCP joint swelling worse in the morning.
95. A 23-year-old woman presents with diplopia, ptosis and is unable to count to 50 without her voice tiring. She complains of muscle fatigue.
96. A 20-year-old woman presents with a plethora of signs and symptoms. She complains of arthralgia, depression, alopecia, fits, oral ulceration and facial rash. She is found to have proteinuria and a normocytic anaemia.
97. A 40-year-old man presents with a septal perforation, proteinuria and hypertension.
98. A 50-year-old man presents with vitamin B_{12} deficiency and peripheral neuritis.

THEME: 18
AUTOANTIBODIES

Options

a. Antismooth muscle antibody
b. Anti-DS DNA
c. Anti-jo 1
d. Anti-La
e. Anti RNP
f. Anti-Ro
g. Anti-Scl 70
h. Centromere staining pattern of antinuclear antibodies
i. Homogeneous staining pattern of antinuclear antibodies
j. Rheumatoid factor

For each of the situation/condition given below, choose the one most appropriate/discriminatory option from above. The option may be used once, more than once, or not at all.

Questions

99. A neonate born with congenital heart block.
100. A patient who has been receiving isoniazid for tuberculosis develops a photosensitive rash, oral ulcers and pleurisy.
101. A 50-year-old jaundiced woman with xanthelesma, hepatosplenomegaly and a raised alkaline phosphatase on liver function tests. Liver biopsy shows granulomas around the bile ducts.
102. A patient with dysphagia, thin tapering fingers with calcified subcutaneous nodules and Raynaud's phenomenon.
103. An elderly woman with severe symmetrical metacarpophalangeal joint and wrist arthritis and subcutaneous nodules affecting the extensor surfaces of her elbows.

THEME: 19
INVESTIGATIONS OF CONNECTIVE TISSUE DISORDERS

Options

a. Anti Ds–DNA.
b. Anti Ro and Anti La.
c. Anti Jo–1.
d. Anti topoisomerase 1.
e. Antineutrophil cytoplasmic antibody and anti–endothelial cell antibodies.
f. Mesangial IgA deposition.
g. Anticentromere.
h. ANA.

For each of the situation/condition given below, choose the one most appropriate/discriminatory option from above. The options may be used once, more than once, or not at all.

Questions

104. A 7-year-old boy had a URI, which was followed by an acute arthritis and abdominal pain. Raised, dark coloured skin lesions were palpable over the buttocks and lower limbs. He also had hematuria with history of rectal bleeding during a previous episode.

105. A 4-year-old boy with history of fever of one week duration, bilateral conjunctival congestion, erythema of lips and oral mucosa, exanthematous lesions over the body, with cervical lymphadenopathy. Angiography demonstrated coronary dilatation.
106. A 35-year-old woman presents with history of dusky discolouration of fingers and toes in winter, along with restriction of finger movements and difficulty in opening the mouth. She also c/o intermittent abdominal pain and constipation.
107. A 39-year-old female presenting with difficulty in climbing stairs and rising from a low chair, has swelling around her eyes and violet discolouration of upper eyelids. Weight loss has also been noticed.
108. A 40-year-old female with butterfly-rash and joint pain presents with c/o dry mouth and frequent eye problems.
109. A 22-year-old pregnant lady presents with pain of multiple joints. She also gives history of chest pain, which is sharp and which is influenced by movement, associated with tachycardia in the past as well as history of swelling of lower limbs and around the eyes in the past. She has had 2 abortions earlier. On examination skin lesions are found.

THEME : 20
MANAGEMENT OF CONNECTIVE TISSUE DISORDERS

Options

a. Regular monitoring of renal function.
b. Prednisolone 40-60 mg/day.
c. Prednisolone, hypermellose drops, soft contact lenses.
d. Supportive care, e.g. analgesic fluids.
e. Nifedipine and prostaglandin infusions.
f. Aspirin and high dose IV gamma globulin.
g. Low dose steroids.

For each of the situation/condition given below, choose the one most appropriate/discriminatory option from above. The options may be used once, more than once, or not at all.

Questions

110. A 7-year-old boy had a URI, which was followed by an acute arthritis and abdominal pain. Raised, dark coloured skin lesions were palpable over the buttocks and lower limbs. He also had hematuria with history of rectal bleeding during a previous episode.
111. A 4-year-old boy with history of fever of one week duration, bilateral conjunctival congestion, erythema of lips and oral mucosa, exanthematous lesions over the body, with cervical lymphadenopathy. Angiography demonstrated coronary dilatation.
112. A 35-year-old woman presents with history of dusky discolouration of fingers and toes in winter, along with restriction of finger movements and difficulty in opening the mouth. She also c/o intermittent abdominal pain and constipation.
113. A 39-year-old female presenting with difficulty in climbing stairs and rising from a low chair, has swelling around her eyes and violet discolouration of upper eyelids. Weight loss has also been noticed.
114. A 40-year-old female with butterfly-rash and joint pain presents with c/o dry mouth and frequent eye problems.
115. A 22-year-old pregnant lady presents with pain of multiple joints. She also gives history of chest pain, which is sharp and which is influenced by movement, associated with tachycardia in the past as well as history of swelling of lower limbs and around the eyes in the past. She has had 2 abortions earlier. On examination skin lesions are found.

THEME: 21
DIAGNOSIS OF CONDITIONS OF THE HAND

Options

a. Volkmann's ischaemic contracture
b. Dupuytren's contracture
c. Carpal tunnel syndrome
d. Claw hand
e. Raynaud's phenomenon

f. Scleroderma
g. Rheumatoid arthritis
h. Paronychia
i. Psoriasis
j. Koilonychia
k. Glomus tumour
l. Subungual haematoma

For each of the situation/condition given below, choose the one most appropriate/discriminatory option from above. The option may be used once, more than once, or not at all.

Questions

116. A 20-year-old female presents with a painful fingertip that throbs and has kept the patient up all night. The skin at the base and side of the nail is red, tender and bulging.
117. A 30-year-old female presents with a painful fingernail. On examination, there is a small purple, red spot beneath the nail. She denies trauma to the finger.
118. A 60-year-old man with acromegaly presents with pins and needles in the index and middle fingers of his right hand, worse at night.
119. A 20-year-old man presents with fingers that are permanently flexed in his right hand. However, the deformity is abolished by flexion of the wrist. He admits to trauma to his elbow recently. He also complains of pins and needles.
120. A 20-year-old female complains of intermittent pain in her fingertips. She describes the fingers undergoing colour changes from white to blue then red. The symptoms are worse in the winter.

THEME: 22
CAUSES OF A PAINFUL FOOT

Options

a. Morton's neuroma
b. Stress fracture
c. Avulsion fracture

d. Jones fracture
e. Hallux fracture
f. Plantar fascitis
g. Osteochondritis- Freiberg's disease
h. Metatarsalgia
i. Osteochondritis Kohler's disease
j. Bunion
k. Gout

For each of the situation/condition given below, choose the one most appropriate/discriminatory option from above. The option may be used once, more than once, or not at all.

Questions

121. A 50-year-old man presents with pain over the medial calcaneum and pain on doriflexion and eversion of the forefoot.
122. A 60-year-man complains of continual pain in his forefoot worse on walking. X-ray shows widening and flattening of the second metatarsal head and degenerative changes in the metatarsophalangeal joint.
123. A 50-year-old woman complains of painful shooting pains in her right foot when walking. She is tender in the third/forth toe interspace.
124. A 30-year-old soldier complains of pain in his foot when weight bearing. X-ray shows no facture. He is tender around the proximal fifth metatarsal bone.
125. A 20-year-old man complains of pain over the lateral aspect of his right foot. X-ray shows a transverse fracture of the basal shaft of the 5th metatarsal bone.

THEME : 23
RADIOLOGICAL INVESTIGATIONS

Options

a. Rheumatoid arthritis.
b. Osteoarthritis.
c. Psoriatic arthritis.
d. Gout.
e. Ankylosing spondylitis.

f. Pyrophosphate arthropathy.
g. Chondrocalcinosis.
h. Calcific periarthritis.

For each of the situation/condition given below, choose the one most appropriate/discriminatory option from above. The options may be used once, more than once, or not at all.

Questions

126. Ossification of anterior longitudinal ligament of lumbar spine, syndesmophyte formation, erosion and sclerosis of anterior corners of vertebrae, facetal joint changes.
127. Asymmetrical disease with involvement of terminal IP joints and little periarticular osteoporosis.
128. Terminal IP joint involvement, subchondral erosions, loss of joint space, formation of marginal osteophytes.
129. Punched out erosions with soft tissue swelling.
130. Periarticular osteoporosis, loss of articular cartilage, erosions, subluxation and ankylosis.

THEME: 24
RADIOLOGICAL INVESTIGATIONS

Options

a. Pepper pot skull.
b. Onion peel appearance.
c. Sunray appearance.
d. Soap bubble appearance.
e. Pencil in cup appearance.
f. Champagne glass appearance.
g. Rugger jersey spine.

For each of the situation/condition given below, choose the one most appropriate/discriminatory option from above. The options may be used once, more than once, or not at all.

Questions

131. Psoriatic arthropathy.
132. Hyperparathyroidism.
133. Multiple myeloma.
134. Ewings.

135. Osteomalacia.
136. Osteoclastoma.

THEME: 25
MANAGEMENT OF CHRONIC JOINT PAIN

Options

a. Allopurinol
b. Antidepressants
c. Cognitive behavioural therapy
d. Cochicine
e. Gold
f. Joint replacement
g. Methotrexate
h. NSAID
i. Joint aspiration and blood culture
j. Paracetamol
k. Sulphasalazine

Questions

137. A 45-year-old obese asthmatic businessman who drinks 40 units of alcohol a week, presents with 5th episode of a red hot ankle. Aspiration of the joint has revealed uric acid crystals.
138. A healthy 68-year-old woman complains of increasing pain in her left knee and episodes of the joint "giving way". She is no longer able to climb her stairs. On examination, she is found to have a marked valgus deformity with obvious instability.
139. A 45-year-old woman with long-standing rheumatoid arthritis, presents with a red, swollen, inflamed right knee. She has a swinging temperature.
140. A 25-year-old brick layer with ankylosing spondylitis has increasing early morning back pain and stiffness. He is on no medication.
141. A 70-year-old man with severe ischaemic heart disease complains of stiff, painful hands, neck, knees and feet. Examination of the hands reveals Heberden's nodes.

Eight

Infectious Disease

THEME: 1
STAINS USED IN DIAGNOSTICS

Options

a. Leishman's stain.
b. Field's stain.
c. Zeihl-Neelson stain.
d. Congo red stain.
e. Gram's stain.
f. Congo-O stain.
g. Auramine stain.

For each of the situation/condition given below, choose the one most appropriate/discriminatory option from above. The options may be used once, more than once, or not at all.

Questions

1. Bacteria.
2. Fat.
3. Malarial parasite.
4. Blood cells.
5. Mycobacterium.
6. Tuberculosis specific.
7. Amyloidosis.

THEME: 2
DIAGNOSIS OF INFECTIONS

Options

a. *Pseudomonas aeruginosa*
b. *Escherichia coli*

c. *Staphylococcus aureus*
d. *Proteus mirabilis*
e. *Streptococcus viridans*
f. *Chlamydia trachomatis*
g. *Chlamydia psittaci*
h. *Trichomonas vaginalis*
i. *Neisseria gonorrhoea*
j. *Neisseria meningitis*
k. *Haemophilus influenzae*

Questions

8. A 20-year-old woman presents with a subacute onset of lower abdominal pain associated with frequency and dysuria.
9. A 10-year-old Nigerian boy presents with a 3-month history of a purulent eye discharge and increased lacrymation. His 16-year brother has a similar condition.
10. A 4-year-old boy who has just started schoolsents with a high fever, vomiting, headache and a stiff neck.
11. A 30-year-old man presents with a fever, dyspnoea and palpitations. ON auscultation a pan-systolic murmur is heard in the tricuspid area. He was previously healthy.
12. A 24-year-old man presents with a swelling in his right axilla. Aspiration yeilds yellowish-green pus.

THEME: 3
DIAGNOSIS OF COMMON INFECTIOUS DISEASES

Options

a. Measles
b. Tuberculosis
c. Meningitis
d. Sickle cell trait
e. Hepatitis
f. Hepatitis B
g. Malaria
h. Acquired immune deficiency syndrome
i. Influenzae

j. Glandular fever
k. Chickenpox
l. Scarlet fever
m. Mumps
n. Rubella

Questions

13. A 34-year-old man has lost 4 Kg over the past 3 months, and complains of a 4 months history of a productive cough.
14. A 30-year-old man who has just returned from Africa complains of joint pains and fever associated with chills and rigors. A blood smear shows numerous "ring" trophozoites.
15. A 23-year-old male homosexual complains of joint pains associated with malaise and mild icterus.
16. A mother brings her 2-year-old son to the A&E Deptt., who is drowsy and vomiting. On examination, koplik spots were found with a generalised maculo-papular rash.
17. A 5-year-old girl was given antibiotics for an ear infection 6 hours ago but is now afraid to look at bright light and refused to eat.

THEME: 4
CAUSES OF INFECTION

Options

a. *E. coli*
b. *Staphylococcus aureus*
c. Group A Streptococcus
d. *Staphylococcus epidermidis*
e. Group B Streptococcus
f. *Clostridium perfringens*
g. *Klebsiella pneumoniae*
h. *Proteus mirabilis*
i. *Mycobacterium tuberculosis*
j. *Enterobacter aerogenes*

For each of the situation/condition given below, choose the one most appropriate/discriminatory option from above. The option may be used once, more than once, or not at all.

Questions

18. A 20-year-old woman presents with dysuria. She has no prior history of UTI. Urinanlysis demonstrates white cells and pus.
19. A 30-year-old multiparous woman presents with spiking fever and a foul smelling vaginal discharge 24 hours after delivery of her baby.
20. A 55-year-old woman presents with back pain. Investigations reveal a pyogenic vertebral osteomyelitis.
21. A 40-year-old woman presents with dysuria and urinary incontinence. Her urine is noted to be alkaline.
22. A 50-year-old diabetic woman presents with fever, redness, swelling and pain over the right side of her face.

THEME: 5
CAUSES OF INFECTIONS

Options

a. *Pseudomonas aeruginosa*
b. *E. coli*
c. *Staphyococcus aureus*
d. *Clostridium aureus*
e. *Clostridium difficile*
f. *Yersinia enterocolitica*
g. *Neisseria gonorrhoeae*
h. *Chlamydia trachomatis*
i. *Camylobacter*
j. *Streptococcus pneumoniae*
k. *Mycobacterium*
l. *Mycoplasma*

For each of the situation/condition given below, choose the one most appropriate/discriminatory option from above. The option may be used once, more than once, or not at all.

Questions

23. A 50-year-old man in ITU had remained intubated for 10 days. He is now pyrexial. He has diminished breath sounds. Swabs from the ventilator tubing show gram-negative rods.
24. A 30-year-old woman complains of severe right lower quadrant pain and watery diarrhoea. She is pyrrexial. She had visited her parents in the country a week ago.
25. A 20-year-old man presents with right knee pain and swelling not associated with trauma. Synovial fluid is aspirated and reveals may diplococci. He also admits to a creamy yellow penile discharge.
26. A 50-year-old diabetic man presents with a painful and swollen right leg. X-ray demonstrates air in the soft tissues.
27. A 40-year-old man complains of profuse watery diarrhoea after 2 weeks of antibiotics therapy. Sigmoidoscopy reveals yellow necrotic regions.

THEME: 6
CAUSES OF BACTERIAL INFECTIONS

Options

a. *Bacillus anthracis*
b. *Pseudomonas pyocaneus*
c. *Streptococcus pyogenes*
d. *Staphylococcus aureus*
e. *Corynebacterium diphtheriae*
f. *Listeria monocytogenes*
g. *Clostridium perfringens*
h. *Borrelia burgdoferi*
i. *Pseudomonas aerunginosa*
j. *E. coli*
k. *Bordetella pertussis*
l. *Yersinia enterocolitica*
m. *Moraxella catarrhalis*
n. *Myobacterium tubercolusis*

For each of the situation/condition given below, choose the one most appropriate/discriminatory option from above. The option may be used once, more than once, or not at all.

Questions

28. A 50-year-old diabetic complains of sever otalgia. On examination there is granulation tissue present in the ear canal.
29. A 20-year-old man presents with fever, rash and is unable to close his left eye. On examination he is noted to have a skin rash with a central clearing spreading from a tick bite and a left sided facial palsy.
30. A 50-year-old alcoholic with known liver disease present with fever, abdominal pain and distension. Paracentesis of the peritoneal fluid with gram staining reveals Gram-negative rods.
31. A 55-year-old abattoir worker presents with fever, oedema and a cutaneous papule. Scraping of the skin lesion reveals gram-positive rods.
32. A 60-year-old IDDM male presents with a painful and swollen leg. X-ray of the leg reveals air in the soft tissues.
33. A 25-year-old man has had problems with a recent middle ear infection he is found unconscious.
34. An IV drug abuser who regularly injects has a temprature of 40°C.
35. A 35-year-old Asian lady with a 5-month history of persistent headache.

THEME: 7
DIAGNOSIS OF SEXUALLY TRANSMITTED DISEASES

Options

a. Syphilis
b. Gonorrhoea
c. AIDS
d. Lymphogranuloma venereum
e. Granuloma inguinale
f. Molloscum contagiosum
g. Herpes simplex hominis type 2 virus
h. Gardenella vaginalis
i. *Chlamydia trachomatis*

j. Trichomoniasis
k. Candidiasis

For each of the situation/condition given below, choose the one most appropriate/discriminatory option from above. The option may be used once, more than once, or not at all.

Questions

36. A 23-year-old man presents with dysuria, urethral discharge and joint paint. Gram staining shows gram-negative intracellular diplococci.
37. A 27-year-old African immigrant presents with painful fixed inguinal lymphadenopathy, 3 week earlier he had had a painless papule on his genitalia which ulcerated, then healed.
38. A 31-year-old woman presents with fever, myalgia, headache and multiple painful shallow ulcers in the vulva. On examination there are also ulcers in the cervix and tender inguinal lymphedenopathy. 4 weeks after treatment and recovery her symptoms recur but are less severe.
39. A 37-year-old multipara presented with vaginal discharge. 10 days earlier she had used a medication for yeast infection. She also complains of strong odour after intercourse.
40. A 20-year-old married woman presents with a 2-week history of sporadic lower abdominal pain, accompanied by a low-grade fever. She also reports and increasing amount of cloudy, non-irritating discharge and dysuria.
41. A 25-year-old sexually active woman presents with mucopurulent vaginal discharge, pelvic pain and fever. The symptoms begin towards the end of her menstrual period.

THEME: 8
DIAGNOSIS OF INFECTIONS

Options

a. Tuberculosis
b. Lyme disease

c. Toxic shock syndrome
d. Salmonellosis
e. Trichinosis
f. Bacillary dysentery
g. Leptospirosis
h. Toxoplasmosis
i. Amoebic hepatitis
j. Visceral leishmaniasis
k. Actinomycosis

For each of the situation/condition given below, choose the one most appropriate/discriminatory option from above. The option may be used once, more than once, or not at all.

Questions

42. A 30-year-old HIV positive man developed fits. On examination there were generalized lymphadenopathy, tender nodules on his legs, right homonymous heminopia and mild right pyramidal weakness. CT showed a right fronto-parietal space-occupying lesion.
43. A 29-year-old photographer presented with diplopia. He has a past history of facial palsy and recurrent knee swelling. On examination there was mild meningism and partial left 3rd palsy. There was no evidence of residual 7th nerve palsy. Both knees were swollen and tender. There were increased protein and white cells in the CSF.
44. A 19-year-old student presented with acute diplopia, fever and tongue pain. He had had an episode of gastroenteritis during the trip to Alaska 2 weeks earlier. On examination the conjunctivae were swollen and there was bilateral opthalmoplegia. Tongue movements were weak bilaterally. The rest of the examination was normal.
45. A 42-year-old Asian immigrant presented with a 2-month history of fever and weight loss. On examination there was generalized lymphedenopathy, hepatomegaly and huge splenomegaly. His ankles are swollen but there was no evidence of chronic liver disease.

THEME: 9
INVESTIGATION OF INFECTIOUS DISEASE

Options

a. Paul-Bunnell test
b. VDRL
c. Ziehl-Neilsen stain for AFB
d. ASO titre
e. Widal test
f. Weil-Felix
g. ELISA
h. Gram stain
i. Schuffner agglutination test

For each of the situation/condition given below, choose the one most appropriate/discriminatory option from above. The option may be used once, more than once, or not at all.

Questions

46. A 25-year-old man presents unwell with a 2-day history of fever, headache and vomiting. He is noted to have a eschar. You suspect Typhus.
47. A 30-year-old man presents with fever, headache and diarrhoea. He is noted to have rose spots on his trunk.
48. A 23-year-old man presents with a red maculopapular rash on his soles and anal papules.
49. A 30-year-old man presents with fever, Jaundice and painful calves. He is an avid swimmer.
50. A 20-year-old female presents with sore throat and is noted to have petechae on the palate.

THEME: 10
TREATMENT OF INFECTIONS

Options

a. Vancomycin
b. Flucloxacillin
c. Trimethoprim

d. Gentamicin
e. Penicillin
f. Cefotaxime
g. Erythromycin
h. Tetracycline
i. Rifampicin, isoniazid and pyrazinamide
j. Amoxycillin
k. Pentamidine

For each of the situation/condition given below, choose the one most appropriate/discriminatory option from above. The option may be used once, more than once, or not at all

Questions

51. A 4-year-old child present to A&E with fever and stridous breathing. He is sitting forward and drooling saliva. He requires intubation for respiratory distress.
52. A 60-year-old man presents with urinary retention on the ward. He had undergone elective abdominal aortic aneurysm repair in the morning. Foley's catheterisation is suggested.
53. A 60-year-old woman presents with dysuria and increased frequency of micturition. She has white cells and pus in her urine.
54. A 20-year-old man presents with a neck mass in the posterior triangle. FNAC demonstrates acid-fast bacilli.
55. A 60-year-old male patient presents with diarrhoea on the ward. He has been on broad spectrum antibiotics for several weeks for a discharging fistula post hip replacement.

THEME: 11
SEXUALLY TRANSMITTED DISEASES

Options

a. Gonococcal urethritis.
b. Non-gonococcal urethritis.
c. AIDS.
d. Syphilis.

e. *Chlamydiae trachomatis*.
f. Chancroid.
g. *Trichomonas vaginalis*.
h. *Candida albicans*.
i. Hepatitis B.
j. Sarcoptes scabeii.
k. Human papilloma virus.
l. Herpes simplex.
m. Herpes zoster.
n. Molluscum contagiosum.
o. Gardrenella.

For each of the situation/condition given below, choose the one most appropriate/discriminatory option from above. The options may be used once, more than once, or not at all.

Questions

56. A 22-year-old promiscous male gives history of painful micturition and early morning discharge.
57. Causes condyloma acuminata and may cause cervical smear abnormalities.
58. A 14-year-old boy with thalassemia presents with nausea, tender hepatomegaly, and anorexia and also has pain in joints.
59. Causes small umbilicated white papules.
60. A 27-year-old pregnant female presents with history of discharge per vaginum. On examination, she has few white patches on vaginal mucosa which bleed on scrapping.
61. A 28-year-old female presents with two-month history of thick bubbly discharge and intense itching.
62. Commonly causes dysuria in both sexes and pelvic inflammatory disease in females. It is the most common cause of ophthalmia neonatorum.
63. A 22-year-old male from Acrid region presents with complaints of burning micturition for past 3 months. He also complains of discharge from eyes. On examination he was found to have clear discharge per urethra and urine examination showed IRBC/HPF and 2 5 WBC's/ HPF.

THEME : 12
HUMAN IMMUNODEFICIENCY VIRUS

Options

a. Prophylactic AZT
b. Needle exchange
c. Refer to your consultant
d. Methadone
e. Counselling
f. Condoms
g. Combination therapy
h. Pentamidine
i. Pyridoxine and sulphadiazine
j. Cotrimoxazole

Questions

64. A 23-year-old woman has been using heroin (iv) for last 4 years. She is not willing to stop using heroin.
65. A third year medical student was drawing blood from an unknown HIV positive patient gets a needle stick injury.
66. A healthy 20-year-old pregnant woman whose partner is a haemophiliac.
67. A 28-year-old haemophiliac with history of 20 previous blood transfusion, gets a needle stick injury from a known HIV positive patient.
68. A 20-year-old sexually active woman who is going to Thailand for a holiday.
69. A known HIV positive patient presents with increasing dyspnoea.The chest X-ray looks normal.

THEME: 13
CLINICAL FEATURES IN HIV INFECTED PATIENTS

Options

a. *Cryptosporidium parvum.*
b. *Toxoplasma gondii* infection.
c. CNS lymphoma.
d. *Pneumocystis carinii* infection.

e. Non-bacterial thrombotic endocarditis.
f. Cytomegalovirus.
g. Persistent generalised lymphadenopathy.
h. Dementia.
i. Chronic inflammatory demyelinating polyneuropathy.
j. Seroconversion illness.
k. Cryptococcal menigitis.
l. Kaposi's sarcoma.
m. Chronic sensory polyneuropathy.
n. Salmonellosis.
o. Isospora belli infection.
p. Candidiasis.
q. *Mycobacterium avium* complex.

For each of the situation/condition given below, choose the one most appropriate/discriminatory option from above. The options may be used once, more than once, or not at all.

Questions

70. Chronic diarrhea responded to cotrimoxazole therapy.
71. Painful test.
72. Progressively increasing cough and breathlessness over 3 weeks.
73. Acute delirium.
74. Convulsions and headache. CT shows ring enhancing lesion.
75. Progressive hemiparesis.
76. Fleshy pink enlarging skin lesions on legs.
77. Acute hemiparesis.
78. Insidious visual loss.
79. Progressive leg weakness.

THEME: 14
LATE COMPLICATIONS OF AIDS

Options

a. Kaposi's sarcoma
b. Molluscum contagiosum
c. Hairy leukoplakia

d. Tuberculosis
e. Cryptosporidum
f. CMV infection
g. Candida infection
h. Pneumocystis carinii infection
i. Cryptococcal infection
j. Toxoplasma abscess
k. AIDS dementia
l. Lymphoma

For each of the situation/condition given below, choose the one most appropriate/discriminatory option from above. The option may be used once, more than once, or not at all

Questions

80. A patient presents with progressive visual deterioration. On examination there are large cotton wool spots in both eyes.
81. A patient presents with gradual onset of headache, neck stiffness, photophobia and fluctuating level of consciousness. CSF shows a lymphocytosis but no organisims on Gram stain. CT brain is normal.
82. A patient presents with purple popular lesions on his face and upper trunk measuring one to two centimetres across. They are not painful or itchy.
83. A patient presents with dysphagia and pain on swallowing. He has ulcers in his mouth covered in a whitish discharge and soreness in the corners of the mouth.
84. A patient presents with fever, dry cough and breathlessness. He is tachypnoeic but chest is clear on auscultation. Oxygen saturation is normal at rest but drops on exercise.
85. A patient presents with profuse water diarrhoea for several months without rectal bleeding and minimal abdominal pain.

THEME: 15
MANAGEMENT OF HIV RELATED CONDITIONS

Options

a. IV ganciclovir
b. Emergency oesophageal surgery
c. HAART (Highly Active Antiretroviral)
d. Adjust the treatment
e. Oral acyclovir
f. Omeprazole-Amoxycillin-Metronidazole
g. Nystatin
h. Vitamin supplements

For each of the situation/condition given below, choose the one most appropriate/discriminatory option from above. The options may be used once, more than once, or not at all.

Questions

86. A 25-year-old gay male presents to his GP with bruises which he says are brought on by the slightest of trauma. On examination he is found to have oral candidiasis. His WBC count is 2.9 *1,000,000/L.
87. A male patient with HIV presents to the STD clinic. The following investigations are done:

Hb	8.9g/dl
WBC	1.4 *1,000,000,000/L
Platelets	90 *1,000,000,000/L
Packed cell volume	96fl
Urea and electrolytes	not done
Alkaline phosphate	98 iu/L
Alanine aminotransferase	45 iu/l

88. A 36-year-old journalist had AIDS for 2 years. He presented with a 3 weeks history of dysphagia, which has failed to fluconazole. He was on Zidovudine 200 mg tds and Dapsone. Pyrimethamine for *Pneumocysttis Carinii pnemonia* prophylaxis. Endoscopy revealed a singe deep ulcer in the lower third of the oesophagus

THEME: 16
ZOONOSES

Options

a. Butchers.
b. Agricultural and forestry workers.
c. Rice farmers.
d. Cave explorers.
e. Granary and ware house workers.
f. Fishermen.
g. Pet shop workers.
h. Sewer workers.
i. Domestic cats.

For each of the situation/condition given below, choose the one most appropriate/discriminatory option from above. The options may be used once, more than once, or not at all.

Questions

89. Brucellosis.
90. Leptospirosis.
91. Anthrax.
92. Rabies.
93. Murine (epidemic) typhus.
94. California encephalitis.
95. Psittacosis.
96. Pasteurella.

THEME: 17
CAUSATIVE ORGANISMS

Options

a. Coagulase positive *Staphylococcus aureus.*
b. *Erysipelothrix.*
c. Group A *Streptococcus.*
d. *Hemophilus influenzae.*
e. *Helicobacter pylori.*
f. *E. coli.*
g. *Pneumocystis carinii.*

h. *Rickettsia prowazekii.*
i. *Mycoplasma pneumoniae.*
j. *Clostridium perfringens.*
k. *Klebsiella pneumoniae.*
l. Group B *Streptococcus.*
m. *Neisseria meningitidis.*
n. *Neisseria gonococcus.*
o. *Staphylococcus epidermidis.*
p. *Pseudomonas aeruginosa.*
q. *Nocardia.*
r. *Listeria monocytogenes.*
s. *Giardia lamblia.*

For each of the situation/condition given below, choose the one most appropriate/discriminatory option from above. The options may be used once, more than once, or not at all.

Questions

97. Erysipelas.
98. Neonatal sepsis.
99. Intravenous drug user with inflammation of the sacroiliac joint.
100. Bilateral adrenal hemorrhage, DIC and hemorrhagic vasculitis in a 6-year-old girl.
101. Gastric ulcer.
102. Chronic diarrhea in a homosexual male.
103. Cervical adenitis.
104. Acute epiglottitis.
105. Patient with rheumatoid arthritis and a bacterial infection of the left wrist.
106. A pruritic creeping violaceous rash on the hands of a fish packing plant employee.
107. Chronic cough and low grade fever in a young patient.
108. Occult bacteremia.
109. Bacterial meningitis in children beyond the newborn period.
110. Young adult with hot, swollen knee and skin lesions.
111. A neonate develops septicemia, maculopapular rash on the legs and trunk, pneumonia, diarrhea and seizures with in a few hours of birth and dies a short while later.

112. Nursery epidemics of watery diarrhea.
113. Elderly patient with symptomatic prosthetic knee joint.
114. Acute otitis media.
115. Bilateral ophthalmia neonatorum in a 4 day old infant.
116. Food poisoning at a banquet.
117. Epidemic typhus.
118. Large red areas of denuded skin and generalised bullae in an infant.
119. Ankylosing spondylitis.
120. Elderly, immunocompromised patient with sepsis and purulent joint fluid.
121. Furuncolosis.

THEME: 18
CLINICAL DIAGNOSIS OF COMMON INFECTIONS

Options

a. Influenza
b. Hepatitis
c. Meningitis
d. Coryza
e. Diptheria
f. Rubella
g. Infectious mononucleosis
h. Candidiasis
i. Poliomyelitis
j. Tuberculosis
k. Brucellosis
l. Staphylococcus
m. Stretococcus
n. Herpes virus

For each of the situation/condition given below, choose the one most appropriate/discriminatory option from above. The option may be used once, more than once, or not at all

Questions

122. An elderly man presents with a sore throat and complains of loosing his voice. Examination of the throat finds the

oral cavity erythematous and sporadically covered with white and yellow patches. He is apparently healthy otherwise.

123. A young farmer complains of high fever and drenching sweats lasting 2 to 3 days. He has had a severe headache, backache and felt very depressed. He says he has had 3 similar episodes in the past month.
124. A 23-year-old student presents with weakness, malaise, fever and yellow sclera. Her upper right abdomen is very tender and her joints ache.
125. A teenager has a terrible headache and a skin rash on the face. His cervical lymph nodes are enlarged. After admission the rash involves the chest and upper arms. He says his joints are very painful, especially his knees.
126. An immigrant child is brought to you with a sore throat and feet. His breathing is laboured and his voice is deep. The trachea is covered with a thin membrane. His cervical lymph nodes are enlarged.

THEME: 19
FEVER AND RASHES

Options

a. Erythema toxicum
b. Impetigo
c. Roseala infantum
d. Epstein-Barr virus
e. Herpes simplex virus
f. Kawasaki's disease
g. Measles
h. Meningitis
i. Psoriasis
j. Ptyiasis rosea
k. Scabies
l. Varicella

For each of the situation/condition given below, choose the one most appropriate/discriminatory option from above. The options may be used once, more than once, or not at all.

Questions

127. A 16-year-old girl ,with a sore throat and fever is found to have cervical lymphadenopathy. She is given ampicillin and gets a generalized erythematous rash.
128. A young boy with fever, a headache, neck stiffness and photophobia,is found to have a generalised non-blanching skin rash.
129. A 1-year-old child with oedematous lips, a red and desquamating rash of the finger tips, is found to be febrile.
130. A 15-month-old girl with a fever for 48 hours, is admitted to hospital. Her fever subsides but on discharge develops a generalised erythematous rash.

THEME: 20
CHEMOPROPHYLAXIS

Options

a. Group A Streptococci.
b. Pneumococci.
c. Meningococci.
d. Plague.
e. Traveller's diarrhea.
f. Recurrent urinary infections.
g. Chronic bronchitis.

For each of the situation/condition given below, choose the one most appropriate/discriminatory option from above. The options may be used once, more than once, or not at all.

Questions

131. Rifampicin.
132. Doxycycline.
133. Ampicillin.
134. Benzathine penicillin.
135. Procaine penicillin.
136. Co-trimoxazole.
137. Tetracycline.

THEME: 21
INVESTIGATION AND MANAGEMENT OF PERSISTENT FEVER

Options

a. Aspirin
b. Cotrimoxazole
c. Chest X-ray
d. CT scan skull
e. Amoxycillin
f. Quinine
g. Benzylpenicillin
h. IV pyelogram
i. Midstream urine collection
j. Lumbar puncture
k. Hospital admission
l. Sputum for culture
m. Chloroquine

For each of the situation/condition given below, choose the one most appropriate/discriminatory option from above. The option may be used once, more than once, or not at all.

Questions

138. A 50-year-old clothes buyer complains of a very high fever and pains in the small area of her back. She complains of increased frequency and dysuria.
139. An elderly man living alone presents with a chesty cough and complains of a very high fever. He says that his temperature has been more than 38 degrees for 3 days. As he is talking to you he clears his throat and blows thick brown phlegm into his hanky.
140. An engineer returned for Malaysia 2 months ago. There he worked for a large hydroelectric project. He complains of high fever and drenching sweats.

THEME: 21
DISEASE PREVENTION

Options

a. Immunoglobulin indicated.
b. Immunoglobulin not proven effective.
c. Immunoglobulin not indicated.
d. Immunoglobulin contraindicated.

For each of the situation/condition given below, choose the one most appropriate/discriminatory option from above. The options may be used once, more than once, or not at all.

Questions

141. Hepatitis A prophylaxis.
142. Hepatitis B prophylaxis.
143. Hepatitis C prophylaxis.
144. Measles prophylaxis.
145. Rubella prophylaxis.
146. Thrombocytopenia.
147. Asthma.

THEME: 22
ARTHROPOD-BORNE DISEASES

Options

a. Aedes
b. Sandfly.
c. Dermacentor andersoni.
d. Black fly.
e. Pediculus humanus corporis.
f. Trombiculid mite.
g. Xenopsylla cheopis.
h. Soft tick.
i. Sarcoptes scabei.
j. House fly.

For each of the situation/condition given below, choose the one most appropriate/discriminatory option from above. The options may be used once, more than once, or not at all.

Questions

148. Epidemic typhus.
149. Relapsing fever.
150. Murine typhus.
151. Trachoma.
152. Dengue fever.
153. Onchocerciasis.
154. Colorado tick fever.
155. Yellow fever.
156. Scrub typhus.

THEME: 23
VIRUSES ASSOCIATED WITH SYSTEMIC DISEASES

Options

a. Bronchiolitis.
b. Erythema infectiosum.
c. Myocarditis.
d. Hemorrhagic cystitis.
e. Vesicular eruption.

For each of the situation/condition given below, choose the one most appropriate/discriminatory option from above. The options may be used once, more than once, or not at all.

Questions

157. Parvovirus.
158. Coxsackie virus.
159. Respiratory syncytial virus.
160. Herpes simplex virus.
161. Adenovirus.

THEME: 24
MANAGEMENT OF VIRAL INFECTIONS

Options

a. Acylovir.
b. Stavudine.

c. Interferon-alpha.
d. Ganciclovir.
e. 5 – Fluorouracil.
f. Amantadine.
g. Zinc gluconate trihydrate.

For each of the situation/condition given below, choose the one most appropriate/discriminatory option from above. The options may be used once, more than once, or not at all.

Questions

162. Life-threatening cytomegalovirus infection.
163. Mild cytomegalovirus infection.
164. HIV.
165. Coryza.
166. Herpes simplex encephalitis.
167. Influenza.
168. Varicella.

THEME: 25
COMPLICATIONS OF PARASITIC INFECTIONS

Options

a. Gastrointestinal obstruction.
b. Pruritis ani.
c. Growth stunting.
d. Cutaneous larva migrans.
e. Rectal prolapse.
f. Pernicious anemia.
g. Periorbital edema.

For each of the situation/condition given below, choose the one most appropriate/discriminatory option from above. The options may be used once, more than once, or not at all.

Questions

169. Threadworm infection.
170. Trichuriasis.
171. Pinworm infection.

172. Ascariasis.
173. Hookworm infections.
174. Trichinellosis.
175. Fish tapeworm.

THEME: 26
INVESTIGATION OF TROPICAL DISEASE

Options

a. Thick and thin blood films
b. Other blood films
c. Blood cultures
d. Stool cultures
e. Stool examination
f. Serology
g. Urine microscopy
h. Urine culture
i. Abdominal USG
j. Skin biopsy
k. Nerve biopsy
l. Clinical diagnosis

For each of the situation/condition given below, choose the one most appropriate/discriminatory option from above. The option may be used once, more than once, or not at all.

Questions

176. A 30-year-old man returns from Pakistan with a 1-week history of headache, fever, constipation and drowsiness. On examination he has a pulse of 60/min, a palpable spleen and rose spots on his trunk.
177. A 35-year-old woman returns from South Africa with diarrhoea and high swinging fever. She has tenderness in the right upper quadrant.
178. A 45-year-old man returns from Vietnam. 2 weeks later he developed headache, malaise, sweats, fever and rigors. Examination is normal.
179. A 60-year-old man returned 1 month ago from a trip to France. He complains of headache, fever and agitation.

He becomes fearful when offered water and develops muscular spasms of face and arms.

180. A 20-year-old student returns from America with acute onset of headache, vomiting, photophobia and deafness. There is a pink macular rash on his palms and soles.
181. A 25-year-old man returned from holiday in Malawi last month. He now complains of haematuria, dysuria and urinary frequency. He had mildly impaired renal function.

THEME: 27
MANAGEMENT OF PROTOZOAL INFECTIONS

Options

a. Praziquantel.
b. Triclabendazole.
c. Albendazole.
d. Niclosamide.
e. Pyrantel Pamoate.
f. Thiabendazole.
g. Ivermectin.

For each of the situation/condition given below, choose the one most appropriate/discriminatory option from above. The options may be used once, more than once, or not at all.

Questions

182. *Toxocara canis.*
183. *Diphyllobothruim latum.*
184. *Fasciola hepatica.*
185. *Fasciolopsis buski.*
186. Schistosomasis.
187. Filariasis.
188. Dog tapeworm.
189. Threadworms.

THEME: 28
ADVICE FOR TRAVELLERS

Options

a. No precautions required

b. Hepatitis A vaccine only
c. Typhoid vaccine only
d. Typhoid vaccine + polio vaccine
e. Rabies vaccine only
f. Hepatitis A, typhoid and polio vaccine
g. Hepatitis A and B, typhoid, polio diphtheria and rabies vaccine.
h. All of G and yellow fever vaccine also
i. All of H and meningitis also

For each of the situation/condition given below, choose the one most appropriate/discriminatory option from above. The option may be used once, more than once, or not at all.

Questions

190. A doctor is travelling to Somalia to work for International Red Cross.
191. A businessman is going to a conference to Thailand.
192. A 40-year-old intends to travel to Barbados for a holiday. He had hepatitis A 4 years ago and received polio vaccine as a child.
193. A 12-year-old girl is travelling to rural France with her parents.

THEME: 29
ADVICE FOR TRAVELLERS- MALARIA PROPHYLAXIS

Options

a. No precautions required
b. Chloroquine only
c. Mefloquine only
d. Proguanil only
e. Doxycycline only
f. Proguanil and chloroquine
g. Maloprim and chloroquine

For each of the situation/condition given below, choose the one most appropriate/discriminatory option from above. The option may be used once, more than once, or not at all

Questions

194. A sports fan is travelling to Jamaica for a 3-week cricket holiday.
195. A young backpacker is planning to travel through Thailand and Western Cambodia.
196. A Ghanaian who is now resident in London is returning to Guana for a month's holiday. He had had malaria in the past.
197. A student is travelling to Kenya for a 2-week holiday. He has a history of manic depression but is currently taking no medication.

THEME: 30
MANAGEMENT OF INFECTIONS

Options

a. Acyclovir.
b. Sulphonamide.
c. Benzylpenicillin + flucoxacillin.
d. Benzylpenicillin + chloramphenicol.
e. Ketoconazole.
f. Ticarcillin + gentamicin.
g. Azithromycin.
h. Ganciclovir
i. Clindamycin.
j. Vancomycin + gentamicin.
k. Doxycycline + penicillin.
l. Cefadroxil netilmicin

For each of the situation/condition given below, choose the one most appropriate/discriminatory option from above. The options may be used once, more than once, or not at all.

Questions

198. A 30-year-old male with fever since 12 days and splenomegaly. A mitral valve replacement with prosthetic valve implantation was done 3-year-ago.
199. A 30-year-old male, hospitalized for the chemotherapy of acute leukemia, develops pneumonia in hospital.

200. A 10-year-old child is admitted with atypical pyogenic meningitis. CSF culture report is awaited.
201. A promiscuous 20-year-old male has recurrent penile vesicles and pain.

THEME: 31
MALARIAL PARASITE

Options

a. *Plasmodium falciparum.*
b. *Plasmodium vivax.*
c. *Plasmodium ovale.*
d. *Plasmodium malariae.*

For each of the situation/condition given below, choose the one most appropriate/discriminatory option from above. The options may be used once, more than once, or not at all.

Questions

202. Incubation period 12-17 days.
203. Incubation period 18-40 days.
204. Incubation period 7-14 days.
205. Incubation period 15-18 days.
206. Reservoir stage in RBC's.
207. No reservoir stage.

THEME: 32
SIDE EFFECTS OF ANTIMALARIAL DRUGS

Options

a. Chloroquine.
b. Fansidar.
c. Primaquine.
d. Mefloquine.
e. Quinine.

For each of the situation/condition given below, choose the one most appropriate/discriminatory option from above. The options may be used once, more than once, or not at all.

Questions

208. Hemolysis.
209. Arrhythmias.
210. Retinopathy.
211. Neuropsychiatric signs.
212. Steven-Johnsons syndrome.
213. Decreased hemopoiesis.

THEME: 33
ANTITUBERCULOSIS DRUGS

Options

a. Isoniazid.
b. Ethambutol.
c. Pyrazinamide.
d. Ethionamide.
e. Rifampicin.

For each of the situation/condition given below, choose the one most appropriate/discriminatory option from above. The options may be used once, more than once, or not at all.

Questions

214. Best anti TB agent.
215. Can cause hepatitis.
216 Can cause optic neuritis.
217. Can cause neuropathy.
218. Is 2nd line agent.
219. Can cause arthralgias.

THEME: 34
AGENTS CAUSING GASTROENTERITIS

Options

a. *Giardia lambba.*
b. *Staphylococcus aureus.*
c. *Salmonella sp.*
d. *Shigella sp.*
e. *Clostridium botulinum.*

For each of the situation/condition given below, choose the one most appropriate/discriminatory option from above. The options may be used once, more than once, or not at all.

Questions

220. Diarrhea, vomiting, hypotension.
221. Diarrhea, vomiting, fever, septicemia.
222. Vomiting, paralysis.
223. Bloody diarrhea.
224. Bloating, flatulance, explosive diarrhea.

THEME: 35
TREATMENT OF INFECTIOUS DISEASE

Options

a. Ganciclovir
b. Pyrimethamine-sulphadiazine
c. No treatment required
d. Bed-rest and avoid alcohol
e. Interferon alpha
f. Co-trimoxazole
g. Zidovudine (AZT) Didanosine (DDI)- Ritonavir
h. Lamivudine Stavudine
i. Fluconazole
j. Flucloxacillin
k. Ribavirin
l. Antihistamines ans careful observation for one week

For each of the situation/condition given below, choose the one most appropriate/discriminatory option from above. The options may be used once, more than once, or not at all.

Questions

225. A 23-year-old male homosexual presents with tachycardia, tachypnoea and a dry cough associated with exertional dyspnoea. Chest X-ray shows a granular appearance. Echocardiography is normal.
226. A 20-year-old feamle air hostess presents to the dermatology clinic where she is found to have seborrheic

dermatitis. On examination she is found to have oral candidiasis and dusky red lesions on the buccal mucosa. Further examination reveals axillary and supraclavicular lymphadenopathy. She has lost weight in recent months.

227. A 23-year-old woman presents with a mild dry cough and a running nose. She is found to have enlarged axillary nodes and a maculo-papular rash all over the body which she says developed after taking ampicillin at home.
228. A 32-year-old known HIV patient presents with headache, photophobia. He is found to have a CD4 count of 99 cells/ml. A computerized tomograph shows ring lesion.

THEME: 36
DIAGNOSIS OF A RASH

Options

a. Pulmonary tuberculosis
b. Sarcoidosis
c. Reiter's syndrome
d. Urticaria
e. Lyme's disease
f. Dystonia mtotonica
g. Herpes simplex
h. Behcet's syndrome
i. Myasthenia
j. Dermatomyositis

For each of the situation/condition given below, choose the one most appropriate/discriminatory option from above. The options may be used once, more than once, or not at all.

Questions

229. A 29-year-old man with known arthritis presented with a painful red eye and a brownish rash on his feet. He has recently been treated for dysentry.
230. A 30-year-old woman presented to the family GP complaining of difficulty in lifting her arms up. She also reported having difficulty getting up and down stairs. A scaly, erythematous rash was noticed on the dorsum of

the hand, and knucles. She had earlier compared dysphagia.

231. A mother brought her 10-year-old son to the GP, with a history of joint pains and recurrent oral ulcers. On examination the boy had hypopyon and mild conjuctivitis.
232. A 40-year-old sheep farmer from Kent presented to her GP complaining of muscle and joint pain with an associated chronic headache, which has been present for 3 weeks. On examination, she had an erythematous annular rash with a central clear, on her abdomen.
233. A 30-year-old woman presented with tender, red nodular on both lower limbs and forearms. She had painful joints and was febrile. She had a month's history of a productive cough and investigation revealed raised angiotensin converting enzyme levels.

THEME: 37
MANAGEMENT OF RASH

Options

a. Isolation/Quarantine
b. Reassure
c. Acyclovir
d. Hydrocortisone cream
e. PUVA
f. A half day course of Rifampicin
g. Immunize against measles
h. Check anticardiolipin antibodies

For each of the situation/condition given below, choose the one most appropriate/discriminatory option from above. The options may be used once, more than once, or not at all.

Questions

234. A distressed mother rings you. She is found out that one of the children at her daughters school has maningitis.
235. A pregnant woman gets a transient rash which disappears. The young woman is otherwise well.

236. A boy with a vesicular rash and fever goes to his GP. His sister has just been discharged following a renal transplant

THEME: 38
MANAGEMENT OF SEPTICEMIA

Options

a. Intravenous catecholamines
b. Intravenous dopamine
c. Intravenous corticosteroids
d. Intravenous dobutamine
e. Oxygen by mask
f. Oral cefuroxime
g. Stenting
h. Laprotomy and removal of dead tissue
i. Wide excision of soft tissues
j. Percutaneous drainage

For each of the situation/condition given below, choose the one most appropriate/discriminatory option from above. The options may be used once, more than once, or not at all.

Questions

237. A 28-year-old woman after cholecystectomy following a perforated gall bladder has a raised right diaphragm with a temperature of 38°C and a pulse of 120 beats.
238. A febrile 39-year-old woman with hypertension, has a history of recurrent urinary tract infection. Abdominal ultrasound showed a dilated calyx.
239. A 32-year-old woman has chikenpox. She scratches herself excessively and develops a blue discoloration on the abdomen. She has a history of not passing urine in the last 24 hours. She continues to scratch herself and the discoloration increases in size.

THEME: 39
DIAGNOSIS OF HIGH FEVER AND COUGH

Options

a. Listeriosis

b. Strychnine poisoning
c. Mushroom poisoning
d. Rabies
e. Enteric fever
f. Shigella
g. Dental abscess
h. Erysipelas
i. Bordetella pertussis
j. Tetanus
k. Coryza
l. Bronchiectasis
m. Influenza
n. Meningitis

For each of the situation/condition given below, choose the one most appropriate/discriminatory option from above. The option may be used once, more than once, or not at all

Questions

240. A child has a cough and a fever. During the day and especially at night he has fits of coughing and cannot help himself. His inspirations are harsh. At first his mother thought he had a cold but he has not got better.
241. A healthy young woman who likes growing vegetables, raising animals and preparing food, complains of fever and aches. She also has a sore throat, conjunctivitis and diarrhoea.
242. A young woman recently returned from holiday in Kenya presents with a severe headache and fever. She also complains of anorexia, abdominal pain and constipation. On physical examination you find multiple small raised pink spots on his chest.
243. A child with abdominal pain and bloody diarrhoea is brought in by her parents. The child has a fever, headache and some neck stiffness. The CSF is sterile. The mother say's a number of children at her daughter's school are similarly affected.
244. A young farmer presents with facial spasms and difficulty closing his mouth. For the past week he has had fever,

malaise and headache. A month earlier he had been involved in a tractor accident.

THEME: 40
DIAGNOSIS OF PUO

Options

a. Abscess
b. Malaria
c. Tuberculosis
d. Infective endocarditis
e. Brucellosis
f. Q fever
g. Lymphoma
h. Renal cell carcinoma
i. Rheumatoid arthritis
j. Adults Still's disease
k. SLE
l. Familial mediterannean fever

For each of the situation/condition given below, choose the one most appropriate/discriminatory option from above. The option may be used once, more than once, or not at all

Questions

245. A 30-year-old woman complains of relapsing high fever every day or 2. She has painful small joints and a faint rash, most notable during fever. Her serum ferritin levels are very high.
246. A 40-year-old man returned from Kenya 2 months ago. He has a 1-month history of low-grade fever and malaise. The fever occurs about twice a week. Examination is unremarkable.
247. A 25-year-old woman complains of malaise, weight loss, intermittent fever and nigh sweats and pruritis, She has a large mass in right axilla and smaller masses in both iliac fossae.
248. A 60-year-old man had rheumatic fever as a child but has been otherwise well. He presents with a 3-week history

of fever and malaise. He has a loud PSM and has microscopic haematuria on dipstick.

249. A 35-year-old man from Turkey present with recurrent fevers, pleuritic chest pain, abdominal pain and joint pain.
250. A 50-year-old man went on a pilgramage to Mecca 6 months ago. Since his return, he has had fever, sweats, painful joints and muscles. Clinically he has sacroilitis and hepatosplenomegaly.

THEME: 41
INVESTIGATION OF PYREXIA OF UNKNOWN ORIGIN

Options

a. Haemoglobin
b. Full blood count
c. Erythrocyte sedimentation rate
d. Lymph node biopsy
e. Computerised tomography of the chest
f. Stool cultures
g. Mantoux test
h. Monospot
i. Echocardiography for vegetations
j. Kveim test
k. HIV antibody titres

For each of the situation/condition given below, choose the one most appropriate/discriminatory option from above. The option may be used once, more than once, or not at all

Questions

251. A 17-year-old boy presents with a 2-week history of fever, malaise and cervical lymphadenopathy. On examination, he has tenderness in the right upper quadrant of his abdomen and has yellow sclerae.
252. A 25-year-old male drug addict presents with a low grade fever, malaise, a change in heart murmur, splinter haemorrhages in the nailbeds, and Osler's nodes in the finger pulp.

253. A 54-year-old man presents with a 2-month history of unilateral enlargement of his right tonsil, fluctuating pyrexia, and multiple neck nodes.
254. A 25-year-old woman presents with fever, malaise, erythema, nodosum and polyarthralgia. Chest X-ray reveals mediastinal hilar lymphadenopathy.
255. A 29-year-old intravenous drug abuser presents with fever and a neck node discharging a cheese, foul smelling substance.

Nine

Oncology

THEME: 1
RISK FACTORS FOR COMMON CANCERS

Options

a. Aflatoxin.
b. Alcoholic beverages.
c. Alkylating agents.
d. Anabolic steroids.
e. Arsenic.
f. Asbestos.
g. Benzene.
h. Chewing tobacco.
i. Tobacco smoke.
j. Ultraviolet radiations.
k. Virus, Epstein-Barr.
l. Virus, Hepatitis B.
m. Virus, human papilloma virus.
n. Vinyl chloride.
o. Pernicious anemia.

For each of the situation/condition given below, choose the one most appropriate/discriminatory option from above. The options may be used once, more than once, or not at all.

Questions

1. Associated with cancer of the mouth and liver.
2. Increases risk of lung cancer two-fold and cancer of peritoneum 100-fold.
3. Can cause different cancers, some secondary to intermittent severe exposure, others due to cumulative dose.

4. Is linked to cancer of the cervix, vulva, and penis.
5. Is linked to cancer even with indirect exposure.
6. Is linked to nasopharyngeal carcinoma.
7. Most common cause of oral cancer.
8. Gastric carcinoma.

THEME: 2
RISK FACTORS OF MALIGNANCIES

Options

a. Nasopharyngeal carcinoma
b. Colorectal carcinoma
c. Non-Hodgkin's lymphoma
d. Sinonasal tumors
e. Gastric carcinoma
f. Lung carcinoma
g. Salivary gland carcinoma
h. Carcinoma of pancreas
i. Thyroid carcinoma
j. Hodgkin's disease
k. Oesophageal carcinoma

For each of the situation/condition given below, choose the one most appropriate/discriminatory option from above. The option may be used once, more than once, or not at all

Questions

9. A 50-year-old man of southern Chinese origin presents with unilateral conductive hearing loss. He is noted to have Epstein-Barr virus.
10. A 40-year-old woman with Sjögrens syndrome now presents with painless neck nodes.
11. A 40-year-old woman with blood group A and a history of pernicious anaemia now presents with weight loss and epigastric discomfort.
12. A 40-year-old man of Nerthern Chinese origin presents with hoarseness and dysphasia. He has a prior history of suicidal attempt with lye ingestion.
13. A 70-year-old woman presents with stridor and a neck mass. She has a prior history of radiation to the neck as a child.

THEME: 3
RISK FACTORS FOR CARCINOMA

Options

a. Basal cell carcinoma
b. Oesophageal carcinoma
c. Cancer of the stomach
d. Bladder carcinoma
e. Lare-bowel carcinoma
f. Bronchial carcinoma
g. Nasopharyngeal carcinoma
h. Oral carcinoma
i. Small-bowel carcinoma
j. Breast cancer
k. Squamous cell carcinoma of the skin

For each of the situation/condition given below, choose the one most appropriate/discriminatory option from above. The option may be used once, more than once, or not at all.

Questions

14. A 40-year-old New Zealander presents with an ulcer on the side of his nose.
15. A 55-year-old male smoker has worked in the rubber industry for a decade.
16. 45-year-old woman with folic acid and iron deficiencies presents with weight loss and bowel habit changes
17. A 75-year-old Indian notes a chronic ulcer on his lower lip. He admits to heavy drinking and betel nut chewing.
18. A 70-year-old man admits to asbestos exposure 20 year ago and has attempted to quit smoking. He has noted weight loss and hoarseness of voice.

THEME: 4
RISK FACTORS FOR ONCOLOGICAL DISEASE

Options

a. Nasopharyngeal carcinoma
b. Colorectal carcinoma

c. Non-Hodgkins lymphoma
d. Sinonasal tumours
e. Garstric carcinoma
f. Lung carcinoma
g. Salivary gland carcinoma
h. Carcinoma of the pancreas
i. Thyroid carcinoma
j. Hodgkin's disease
k. Oesophageal carcinoma
l. Basal cell carcinoma
m. Bladder carcinoma
n. Bronchial carcinoma
o. Oral carcinoma
p. Small bowel tumour

For each of the situation/condition given below, choose the one most appropriate/discriminatory option from above. The option may be used once, more than once, or not at all

Questions

19. A 50-year-old man of Southern Chinese origin presents with unilateral conductive hearing loss. He is noted to have Epstein-Barr virus.
20. A 40-year-old woman with Sjögrens disease now presents with painless neck nodes.
21. A 50-year-old woman with blood group A and a history of pernicious anaemia now presents with weight loss and epigastric discomfort.
22. A 40-year-old man on Northern Chinese origin presents with hoarseness and dysphasia. He has a prior history of suicidal attempt with lye ingestion.
23. A 70-year-old woman presents with stridor and a neck mass. She has a prior history of radiation to the neck as a child.

THEME: 5
RISK FACTORS FOR CARCINOMA

Options

a. Basal cell carcinoma

b. Oesophageal carcinoma
c. Gastric cancer
d. Bladder carcinoma
e. Large bowel carcinoma
f. Bronchial carcinoma
g. Nasopharyngeal carcinoma
h. Oral cancer
i. Small bowel cancer
j. Breast cancer
k. Squamous cell carcinoma of the skin

For each of the situation/condition given below, choose the one most appropriate/discriminatory option from above. The option may be used once, more than once, or not at all

Questions

24. A 40-year-old New Zealander presents with an ulcer on the side of the nose.
25. A 55-year-old male smoker has worked in the rubber industry for a decade.
26. A 45-year-old woman with folic acid and iron deficiencies presents with weight loss and bowel habit changes.
27. A 65-year-old Indian notes a chronic ulcer on his lower lip. He admits to heavy drinking and betel nut chewing.
28. A 70-year-old man admits to asbestos exposure 20 years ago and has attempted to quit smoking. He has noted weight loss and hoarseness of voice.

THEME: 6
DECISION MAKING IN TERMINAL CARE

Options

a. Add amitriptyline or similar drugs
b. Add midazolam methotrimeprazine
c. Antibiotics
d. Administer enema
e. Gastric intubation
f. High fibre diet
g. Increase opiate analgesia

h. Intravenous fluids
i. Nutritional supplements
j. Palliative deep X-ray therapy
k. Prescribe bisphosphate
l. Prescribe laxative
m. Reduce opiate analgesia
n. Set up syringe driver
o. Start steroids
p. Pleurodesis
q. Intercostal nerve block
r. Betadine gel
s. High dose frusemide

For each of the situation/condition given below, choose the one most appropriate/discriminatory option from above. The option may be used once, more than once, or not at all

Questions

29. A 70-year-old woman with terminal endometrial carcinoma is distressed by a foul vaginal discharge.
30. A 70-year-old woman with terminal breast carcinoma gets recurrent pleural effusions.
31. A 70-year-old woman with metastatic bowel carcinoma is distressed by severe pleural pain. She is already on 80 mg 12 h PO of diamorphine.
32. An 80-year-old man with metastatic carcinoma becomes confused with abdominal distension and faecal incontinence. He is on high doses of opiates.
33. A 55-year-old woman with known spinal metastases from breast cancer becomes nauseated and confused. Creatinine is 120 mmol. Blood sugar is 5.4 mmol calcium 3.2 mmol she is receiving intravenous fluids.
34. A 45-year-old man is dying of pain of AIDS. Acquired immunodeficiency syndrome. He is in considerable pain. Despite the morphine sulphate slow release 20 mg daily. Amitriptyline 100 mg at night and naproven 500 mg twice daily.
35. A 65-year-old man with prostate cancer has extensive pelvic spread of disease with pain not adequately controlled by full analgesic cover.

36. An 82-year-old man with bronchial carcinoma is distressed by breathlessness. He is depressed and anorexic but in no pain.

THEME: 7
TUMOUR MARKERS

Options

a. CA 153
b. CA12.9
c. CEA
d. Alpha FP
e. BHCG
f. NSE
g. PSA
h. Serum acid phosphatase
i. S. Calcitonin
j. Thyroglobulin
k. CA 125
l. PLAP (placental alkaline phosphate)
m. PAP

For each of the situation/condition given below, choose the one most appropriate/discriminatory option from above. The options may be used once, more than once, or not at all.

Questions

37. Carcinoma ovary.
38. Choriocarcinoma.
39. Hepatocellular carcinoma.
40. Open neural tube defects.
41. Carcinoma breast and benign breast disease.
42. Colorectal carcinoma.
43. Pancreatic carcinoma.
44. Small cell carcinoma lung.
45. Prostatic carcinoma.
46. Medullary carcinoma thyroid.
47. Seminoma.
48. Extracapsular spread of prostate carcinoma.

THEME: 8
INVESTIGATION OF MALIGNANT DISEASE

Options

a. Prostate-specific antigen (PSA)
b. Alpha-fetoprotein (AFP)
c. Carcino-embryonic antigen (CEA)
d. CA 19-9
e. Chest X-ray
f. Cytology
g. Incision biopsy
h. Excision biopsy
i. Ultrasound
j. CT scan
k. Mammogram
l. Endoscopic examination

For each of the situation/condition given below, choose the one most appropriate/discriminatory option from above. The option may be used once, more than once, or not at all

Questions

49. A 42-year-old woman has noticed a lump in her left breast. There is a strong family history of breast cancer, which affected her mother and sister. There has been no pain in the breast or discharge from the nipple. On examination, she has generally lumpy breast, but says that one particular lump is new and increasing in size.
50. A 23-year-old man has developed a swelling in his scrotum over a three-month period. It is firm and painless and arises from the left testicle. He has a history of asthma and orchidopexy.
51. A 68-year-old man presents with a one year history of urinary frequency and postmicturition dribble. He has a medical history of atrial fibrillation and takes warfarin. On examination, he has an enlarged prostate with an irregular surface and loss of the medial sulcus.
52. A 55-year-old woman had a left hemicolectomy two years ago for carcinoma of the sigmoid colon. Histology was reported as showing tumour invasion through the

muscularis mucosa. She has recently developed a change in bowel habit with no weight loss or rectal bleeding. Abdominal examination is normal.

53. A 72-year-old woman has a six month history of abdominal swelling and malaise. On examination there is generalised abdominal distension with shifting dullness and the suggestion of a pelvic mass. She is on warfarin fro a pulmonary embolism.

THEME: 9
INVESTIGATION OF TUMOURS

Options

a. Alpha-fetoprotein
b. Terminal de-oxyribonuclear transferase (tdt)
c. Carcino-embyonic antigen
d. Placental alkaline phosphatase
e. Human chorionic gonadotrophin
f. Oestrogen receptors (ER)
g. Squamous cell carcinoma antigen (SCC)
h. Cancer antigen radio-immuno-assay (CA 19.9)
i. Calcitonin
j. Acid phosphatase
k. Cancer antigen (CA-125)

For each of the situation/condition given below, choose the one most appropriate/discriminatory option from above. The option may be used once, more than once, or not at all.

Questions

54. A 60-year-old man presents with a firm prostate nodule. He is confirmed to have prostate carcinoma on biopsy.
55. A 40-year-old man presents with a thyroid swelling. Fine needle aspirate reveals medullary carcinoma.
56. A 65-year-old man presents with hepatomegaly, weight loss, and jaundice. Abdominal ultrasound reveals hepatic carcinoma.
57. A 23-year-old woman presents with back pain and increasing abdominal girth. She is found to have an epithelial tumour of one ovary.

58. A 35-year-old man presents with an enlarged smooth firm testes. He is found to have had a seminoma following orchidectomy.

THEME : 10
ONCOLOGICAL EMERGENCIES

Options

a. Hypercalcemia.
b. Superior vena cava obstruction.
c. Cord compression.
d. Increased ICT.
e. Tumor lysis syndrome.

For each of the situation/condition given below, choose the one most appropriate/discriminatory option from above. The options may be used once, more than once, or not at all.

Questions

59. Lung carcinoma.
60. Tumor which cause secondaries very rarely.
61. Prostatic cancer.
62. Leukemia.
63. Neurofibromatosis.

THEME: 11
MANAGEMENT OF PAIN RELIEF

Options

a. A bolus of iv opiate
b. A subcutaneous opiate infusion
c. Acupuncture
d. Carbamazepine
e. Corticosteroids
f. Hypnotherapy
g. Intramuscular NSAIDS
h. Oral NSAIDS
i. Oral opiates
j. Proton pump inhibitors

k. Selective serotonin re-uptake inhibitor, e.g. Fluoxetine
l. Simple analgesics
m. Transcutaneous electrical nerve stimulation

Questions

64. A 70-year-old man presents with severe retrosternal chest pain and sweating. An ECG shows an acute MI.
65. A 65-year-old man with inoperable gastric cancer causing obstruction, and mutiple liver metastasis, is taking a large dose of oral analgesia. Despite this his pain is currently unrelieved.
66. A 50-year-old obese man with a known hiatus hernia presents with recurrent, severe, burning retrosternal chest pain associated with acid regurgitation and increased oral flatulence.
67. A 70-year-old woman reports severe paroxysms of knife –like or electric shock like pain, lasting seconds in the lower part of the right side of her face.
68. A 30-year-old man presents with an 10-year history of back pain, worse in the morning and one episode of uveitis.

THEME: 12
SIDE EFFECTS OF CHEMOTHERAPY DRUGS

Options

a. Hemorrhagic cystitis.
b. Seizures.
c. Pancreatitis.
d. Pulmonary fibrosis.
e. Visceral fibrosis.
f. Gastrointestinal ulceration.
g. Peripheral neuropathy.
h. Bone marrow suppression.
i. Cardiotoxicity.
j. Hepatotoxicity.
k. Vomiting.

For each of the situation/condition given below, choose the one most appropriate/discriminatory option from above. The options may be used once, more than once, or not at all.

Questions

69. Vinblastine.
70. Cisplatin.
71. Methotrexate.
72. Vincristine.
73. Busulfan.
74. Nitrosourea.
75. Chorambucail.
76. Cyclophosphamide.
77. Actinomycin D.
78. L Asparaginase.
79. Melphalan.

THEME: 13
REGIONAL VARIATION IN PREVALENCE OF CANCER

Options

a. White (Caucasians).
b. Black (Africans).
c. Chinese.
d. Japanese.

For each of the situation/condition given below, choose the one most appropriate/discriminatory option from above. The options may be used once, more than once, or not at all.

Questions

80. High rates of melanomas.
81. Highest rates for breast, corpus and ovarian cancers.
82. Have elevated rates for nasopharyngeal and liver carcinomas.

83. High rates for stomach cancer.
84. High cancer rates, attest partially due to socioeconomic factors.

THEME: 14
DIAGNOSIS OF LYMPHOMAS

Options

a. Lymphocyte predominant Hodgkin's disease.
b. Nodular sclerosing Hodgkin's disease.
c. Mixed cellularity Hodgkin's disease.
d. Lymphocyte depleted Hodgkin's disease, reticular type.
e. Lymphocyte depleted Hodgkin's disease, diffuse type.
f. All variants of Hodgkin's disease.

For each of the situation/condition given below, choose the one most appropriate/discriminatory option from above. The options may be used once, more than once, or not at all.

Questions

85. The only form of Hodgkin's disease more common in women.
86. Reed-Sternberg cells can be difficult to locate in this variant.
87. This variant has a particularly good outcome.
88. Can be accompanied by a non-necrotizing epithelioid granulomatous reaction.
89. This variant has particularly a bad outcome.

Ten

Emergencies

THEME:1
MANAGEMENT OF CARDIAC ARREST

Options

a. Defibrillate.
b. CPR for 1 minute.
c. CPR for 3 minutes.
d. Lignocaine.
e. External pacing.

For each of the situation/condition given below, choose the one most appropriate/discriminatory option from above. The options may be used once, more than once, or not at all.

Questions

1. Resistant ventricular fibrillation.
2. Ventricular fibrillation.
3. Cardiac arrest with no ventricular fibrillation.
4. Asystole with P waves.

THEME: 2
BASIC DIFFERENTIAL DIAGNOSIS AND TREATMENT OF EMERGENCIES

Options

a. Acute myocardial infarction
b. Acute pulmonary oedema
c. Cardiogenic shock
d. Epileptic fit
e. Occult internal haemorrhage
f. Pneumonia
g. Pneumothorax

h. Pulmonary embolism
i. Septic shock

For each of the situation/condition given below, choose the one most appropriate/discriminatory option from above. The option may be used once, more than once, or not at all.

Questions

5. A 30-year-old woman has been unwell for six hours. Her vital signs are: pulse 130/min. BP 100/60 mmHg, temperature 30°C, respiratory rate 44 breaths/min
6. A 76-year-old man has collapsed in the street. His vital signs are: pulse 180/min, BP 60/40 mmHg, temperature 36°C, respiratory rate 29 breaths/min.
7. A 50-year-old builder develops severe dyspnoea and chest pain. His vital signs are pulse 100/min BP 240/160 mmHg, temperature 36°C respiratory rate 32 breaths/min.
8. An 18-year-old nanny has become increasingly drowsy and in delirium. She was well the day before her admission. Her vital signs are: Pulse 100/min BP 80/50 mmHg Temperature 39.5°C. Respiratory rate 26 breaths/min. There is a rash over her lower legs.
9. A 63-year-old heavy smoker has suddenly collapsed at home. His vital signs are pulse 130/min BP 60/40 mmHg temperature 36°C. Respiratory rate 30 breaths/min. There are no neurological deficits; electrocardiogram and chest X-ray is normal.

THEME: 3
THE TREATMENT OF MEDICAL EMERGENCIES

Options

a. Cardioversion
b. Cricothyroidotomy
c. Needle thoracocentesis
d. Needle pericardiocentesis
e. Insertion of chest drain
f. Endotracheal intubation
g. Defibrillation

h. Needle aspiration
i. Intravenous heparin
j. Intramuscular adrenaline
k. Intravenous aminophylline

For each of the situation/condition given below, choose the one most appropriate/discriminatory option from above. The option may be used once, more than once, or not at all.

Questions

10. A 45-year-old woman presents with acute dyspnoea and stridor. Her tongue is swollen.
11. A 20-year-old student presents with respiratory distress and pleuritic pain. On examination, he has distended neck veins and no breath sounds over the right lung field.
12. A 30-year-old man presents with chest pain. He has distended neck veins and muffled heart sound. His blood pressure is 80/50.
13. A 55-year-old woman presents with stridor and difficulty swallowing following thyroidectomy. On examination, she has a tense swelling over the surgical site.
14. 30-year-old female presents with acute dyspnoea and pleuritic pain. Her regular medication includes salbutamol inhaler and an oral contraceptive. Her respiratory rate is 30, with a small volume rapid pulse rate or 110 and a blood pressure of 80/50. She has a raised jugular venous pressure. The chest X-ray is normal. Her ECG shows sinus tachycardia.

THEME: 4
THE TREATMENT OF MEDICAL EMERGENCIES

Options

a. Intramuscular adrenaline
b. Emergency tracheostomy
c. Urgent endotracheal intubation
d. Type and crossmatch blood
e. Transfuse "O" negative blood and apply external fixer
f. Transfer to burns unit

g. Tetanus prophylaxis
h. Intravenous antibiotics
i. Intravenous dexamethasone
j. Oxygen and nebulised salbutamol
k. Take patient straight to theatre

For each of the situation/condition given below, choose the one most appropriate/discriminatory option from above. The option may be used once, more than once, or not at all.

Questions

15. A 40-year-old pedestrian has been struck by a speeding car. She is brought into Accident and Emergency wearing a pneumatic antishock garment for an extensive open avulsion injury to her pelvis. She is resuscitated with fluids running via two large bore intravenous cannulas. Her blood pressure is 120/60. The pelvis is grossly distorted.
16. A 10-year-old boy burn victim is brought into casualty with worsening stridor. A facemask with 100% oxygen is covering his face, but his oxygen saturation continues to fall. His midface and mouth have been severely burned.
17. A 4-year-old girl presents with fever, stridor and dyspnoea. She is sitting forward, drooling saliva. She has no history of asthma. She is becoming more distressed.
18. An 18-year-old man presents with fever, trismus and stridor. His breathing becomes laboured with use of accessory muscles. He becomes cyanotic. He initially presented to his GP with a sore throat a few days ago.
19. A 13-year-old known asthmatic presents with severe wheezing and a respiratory rate of 30. Her pulse rate is 120.

THEME : 5
MANAGEMENT OF HYPOTHERMIA

Options

a. Rewarming/space blanket.
b. Ventilate with oxygen.
c. IV access.

d. Cardiac monitor.
e. Antibiotics.
f. All of the above.

For each of the situation/condition given below, choose the one most appropriate/discriminatory option from above. The options may be used once, more than once, or not at all.

Questions

20. An 80-year-old man was brought to A and E with history of loss of consciousness. He had no history of fall nor he is a diabetic. His rectal temperature is 30 degree Celsius.
21. An alcoholic after a bout of alcohol intake was admitted in A and E department, on a winter night with disorientation. Rectal temperature was 34°C. Blood alcohol level was found to be within normal limit.

THEME: 6
MANAGEMENT OF PULMONARY EDEMA

Options

a. Frusemide.
b. Dimorphine.
c. Nitrates.
d. Digoxin.
e. Nifedipine.

For each of the situation/condition given below, choose the one most appropriate/discriminatory option from above. The options may be used once, more than once, or not at all.

Questions

22. Decrease the dose in-patient with COPD.
23. Increase the dose in-patient with renal failure.
24. To be used in-patient with fast AF.
25. To be given for hypertensive LVF.

THEME: 7
IMMEDIATE MANAGEMENT OF A TRAUMA PATIENT

Options

a. Plain abdominal X-ray
b. Asses airway and stablilize spine
c. CT scan of abdomen
d. Transfer to operating theatre
e. Call ambulance only after full recovery
f. Chest drain after needle thoracocentesis
g. Electrocardiogram
h. Immediate blood transfusion
i. Cervical spine immobilisation
j. Bolus of 50% dextrose followed by a saline infusion
k. Computed tomography(CT) brain scan
l. Normal saline infusion
m. Burr hole(s) should be drilled
n. Lumbar puncture
o. Call neurosurgeon immediately
p. Splint limb

Questions

26. A 43-year-old man is brought to the Accident and Emergency Department delirious, following an injury at a rugby match. His Glasgow Coma Scale (GCS) at the scene of injury is 13. On examination his right pupil is fixed and dilated and GCS is now 7. Initial resuscitation has been done. The neurosurgeon is 30 minutes away.
27. A 22-year-old motorist arrives in the Accident & Emergency Department after an accident. His airway is patent. He is noted to have a splinted right leg.
28. A 30-year-old man is involved in a fight. He has a bruise on the cheek. He complains of an acute abdominal pain and is vomiting. He had a herniorrhaphy two weeks ago. He is conscious and fundoscopy has not been done.
29. A 29-year-old motorist, in the A&E Department resuscitation room, appears to be stable after an accident.

While standing up, he becomes progressively dyspoenic. There is reduced air entry on the left side of chest.

30. An 18-year-old girl is being resuscitated after an accident. Her airway is secure. She complains of neck pain. Her pulse rate is 100 beats/min and blood pressure is 110/70 mmHg. Glasgow Coma Scale is 13. She has a deformed left thigh.
31. A 22-year-old motorist is being resuscitated after an accident .He is noted to have external injuries on the right side and a deformed right hand.

THEME: 8
CALCULATE GLASGOW COMA SCALE

Options

a. 6
b. 10
c. 8
d. 5
e. 11
f. 7
g. 12
h. 9

For each of the situation/condition given below, choose the one most appropriate/discriminatory option from above. The options may be used once, more than once, or not at all.

Questions

	Best motor response	*Best verbal response*	*Eye opening*
32.	Flexor response to pain	confused conversation	No opening
33.	Extensor response to pain	incomprehensible	Response to speech
34.	Withdrawal to pain	inappropriate	Response to pain

THEME: 9
HEAD TRAUMA

Options

a. Epidural hematoma.
b. Subarachnoid hemorrhage.

c. Subdural hematoma.
d. Diffuse axonal injury.
e. Concussion.
f. Cerebro-vascular accident

For each of the situation/condition given below, choose the one most appropriate/discriminatory option from above. The options may be used once, more than once, or not at all.

Questions

35. A patient presents to the emergency department (ED) after blunt head trauma with unknown loss of consciousness. His family reports that he was initially confused, become alert, but again appears less awake. He has bruising over the left temporal area.
36. A patient with a known history of alcohol abuse is brought to the emergency department (ED) after a fall in which he struck his head. A head computed tomography (CT) scan reveals a cresent-shaped hyperdense lesion.
37. A 50-year-old man presents to the emergency department (ED) after a high speed motor vehicle collision. He has burise on his head and is comatose. The head computed tomography (CT) scan reveals no focal lesion
38. A 74 years male known hypertensive, fell on his feet and develops lacerated scalp lost consciousness for few minutes but subsequently normal, 3 days later drowsy, confused later aggressive, restless, deficient breathing, unconscious.
39. A 48 years bus driver was finishing his work when getting out of his bus pitched head long onto the garage floor—unconscious but no obvious injury, small skull fracture. Regained consciousness 2 days later but was unable to move his left side.

THEME: 10
FACIAL TRAUMA

Options

a. Simple alveolar fracture.
b. Le Fort's fracture type I.

c. Le Fort's fracture type II.
d. Le Fort's fracture type III.

For each of the situation/condition given below, choose the one most appropriate/discriminatory option from above. The options may be used once, more than once, or not at all.

Questions

40. A fracture that runs through the lateral nose obliquely downward through the maxillary sinus and orbit, separating the zygoma and orbit from the nose.
41. A fracture across the base of the upper incisors.
42. A fracture that extends from the nose through the orbit and zygoma, separating facial bones from the cranium (craniofacial disjunction).
43. A horizontal fracture that runs through the nose and above the heart palate, separating the heart palate from the rest of the face.

THEME: 11
CHEST TRAUMA

Options

a. Tension pneumothorax.
b. Flail chest.
c. Esophageal rupture.
d. Pericardial tamponade.
e. Pulmonary contusion.

For each of the situation/condition given below, choose the one most appropriate/discriminatory option from above. The options may be used once, more than once, or not at all.

Questions

44. A restrained passenger was in a car that was driven at a high speed before colliding into a wall. The passenger had recently eaten a heavy meal and complained of severe pain in the epigastric area. Examination revealed tenderness in the upper abdominal area. A chest radiograph reveals pneumomediastinum.

45. A patient presents after being struck in the chest by a heavy piece of equipment at work. He appears in marked respiratory distress. Examination reveals distended neck veins, hypotension, decreased breath sounds over the right side of the chest, and tracheal deviation to the left side.
46. An unrestrained driver is involved in a motor vehicle collision, striking his chest against the steering wheel, which is deformed. He complains of severe pain over his chest and difficulty breathing. Physical examination reveals crepitus, chest wall tenderness and abnormal chest wall motion.

THEME: 12
THE MANAGEMENT OF TRAUMATIC INJURIES

Options

a. Peritoneal lavage
b. Observation alone
c. Closed thoracotomy tube drainage
d. Pressure dressing
e. Cricothyroidotomy
f. Nasogastric tube suction and observation
g. Surgical repair of the flexor digitorum superficialis tendon
h. Surgical repair of the flexor digitorum profundus tendon
i. Urgent surgical exploration
j. Debridement and repair
k. Endotracheal intubation
l. Needle pericardiocentesis
m. Fasciotomy

For each of the situation/condition given below, choose the one most appropriate/discriminatory option from above. The option may be used once, more than once, or not at all

Questions

47. A 23-year-old man present to Accident and Emergency having been stabbed in the neck. He complains of difficulty swallowing and talking. He has no stridor. On examination, there is a small penetrating wound with diffuse neck swelling.

48. A 12-year-old boy presents with a hand injury sustained while playing rugby and attempting to catch the ball. On examination, he is unable to bend the tip of his right middle finger.
49. A 35-year-old woman is brought into Accident and Emergency acutely short of breath. Her respiratory rate is 50/min. She was involved in a traffic accident. She has no breath sounds on the left. Her trachea is deviated to the right.
50. An 18-year-old man sustains a stab wound to the right thigh. On examination, he has a large haematoma over the thigh and weak distal pulses. He is unable to move his foot and complains of pins and needles in his foot.
51. A 30-year-old woman involved in a head on car collision presents with diffuse abdominal pain. Upright chest X-ray shows elevation of the diaphragm with a stomach gas bubble in the left lower field.

THEME: 13
CAUSES OF SHOCK

Options

a. Pulmonary embolism
b. Myocardial ischaemia
c. Cardiac tamponade
d. Trauma
e. Burns
f. Sepsis
g. Anaphylaxis
h. Major surgery
i. Ruptured aortic aneurysm
j. Ectopic pregnancy
k. Addisonian crisis
l. Hypothyroidism
m. Acute pancreatitis

For each of the situation/condition given below, choose the one most appropriate/discriminatory option from above. The option may be used once, more than once, or not at all.

Questions

52. A 50-year-old man arrives in casualty in shock. His BP is 80/50. His heart sounds are muffled. His jugular venous pressure is noted to increase with inspiration.
53. A 30-year-old woman presents to casualty in respiratory distress and shock. She is noted to have stidor. Her lips are swollen and blue.
54. A 55-year-old man present to casualty with severe abdominal pain, vomiting and shock. The pain is in the upper abdomen and radiates to the back. He takes diuretics. The abdomen is rigid, and the X-ray shows absent psoas shadow.
55. A 40-year-old woman presents to casualty in shock with continuous abdominal pain radiating to her back. The abdomen is rigid with an expansile abdominal mass.
56. A 35-year-old woman presents to casualty in shock with a BP of 80/50 and tachycardia. She is confused and weak. Her husband states that she forgot to take her prednisolone tables with her on holiday and has missed several doses.

THEME: 14
DIAGNOSIS OF PAIN DISORDERS

Options

a. S1 radiculopathy.
b. Midline herniated disk.
c. Spinal stenosis.
d. Posterolateral herniated disk.
e. Vertebral compression fracture secondary to osteoporosis.

For each of the situation/condition given below, choose the one most appropriate/discriminatory option from above. The options may be used once, more than once, or not at all.

Questions

57. An 80-year-old woman with severe midthoracic pain without a history of trauma.

58. A 45-year-old man with lumbosacral pain associated with bilateral leg pain radiation and loss of bladder control.
59. A 60-year-old man with lumbar and gluteal pain when ambulating, relieved with rest.
60. A 56-year-old man with muscular pain in the calf and paresthesias in the little toe.
61. A 36-year-old woman with lumbosacral pain radiating down the right leg and a positive crossed straight-leg raising test.

THEME: 15
CAUSES OF POISONING

Options

a. Lead
b. Paracetamol
c. Salicylate
d. Arsenic
e. Ethanol
f. Mercury
g. Cyanide
h. Carbon manoxide
i. Organphosphate insecticides
j. Paraquat
k. Ethylene glycol
l. Methanol

For each of the situation/condition given below, choose the one most appropriate/discriminatory option from above. The option may be used once, more than once, or not at all.

Questions

62. A 4-year-old child presents with anorexia, nausea and vomiting. On examination, he has a blue line on the gums and is noted to have a foot drop. Blood tests reveals anaemia.
63. A 16-year-old girl presents with weakness, excessive salivation, vomiting, abdominal pain and diarrhoea. There is 'raindrop' pigmentation of the skin. Diagnosis is made from nail clippings.

64. A 40-year-old farmer presents with acute shortness of breath and headache. His skin is red in colour, and he smells of bitter almonds.
65. A 40 -year-old woman complains of headache and memory impairment following the installation of a gas fireplace. Her skin colour is pink.
66. A 50--year-old agricultural farmer presents with nausea, vomiting, hypersalivation, and bronchospasm.

THEME: 16
MANAGEMENT OF POISONING

Options

a. IV n-acetylcysteine
b. Oral methionine
c. Hemodialysis
d. Forced alkaline diuresis
e. IV glucagon
f. IV desferroxamine
g. IV ethanol
h. Activated charcoal
i. Gastric lavage
j. Forces emesis
k. Hyperbaric oxygen
l. iv naloxone

For each of the situation/condition given below, choose the one most appropriate/discriminatory option from above. The option may be used once, more than once, or not at all.

Questions

67. A 50-year-old man with epilepsy took an overdose of his medication 1 hr ago. He has a dry mouth and dilated pupils.
68. A 30-year-old woman with toothache has taken 50 paracetamol tablets 6 hrs back. She feels nauseated and still has toothache, but is otherwise well.
69. A 20-year-old heroin addict arrives in casualty unconscious and cyanosed. His respiratory rate is 6/min and he has pinpoint pupils.

70. A 40-year-old woman with a history of hypertension arrived in casualty 2 hrs ago having taken a whole bottle of her medication in an attempt to commit suicide. She suddenly collapses with a pulse of 30 and BP of 70/30.
71. A 45-year-old homeless man complains of headache, abdominal pain, nausea and dizziness. He admits to having drunk anti-freeze the previous night. He is hyperventilating and slightly drowsy.
72. A 3-year-old boy was found unconscious at home by his mother with an empty medicine bottle next to him. The bottle had contained ferrous sulphate tablets.

THEME: 17
MANAGEMENT OF ACUTE POISONING

Options

a. Dimercapol
b. Atropine
c. Flumazenil
d. Dicobalt edetate
e. Specific antibody fragments
f. Antitoxin
g. Desferroxamine
h. Naloxone
i. Vitamin K
j. Fresh frozen plasma and vitamin K
k. N acetylcysteine
l. Protamine sulphate

For each of the situation/condition given below, choose the one most appropriate/discriminatory option from above. The option may be used once, more than once, or not at all.

Questions

73. A 35-year-old lady who has taken the whole bottle of beta-blocker tablets.
74. A 15-year-old boy who has taken oral benzodiazephines and now has difficulty breathing.

75. A 40-year-old woman who has taken warfarin. She is not normally on anticoagulants and currently she is not actively bleeding.
76. A 35-year-old man has taken Digoxin overdose.
77. A 24-year-old man has taken Opiate analgesic overdose
78. A 6-year-old girl has taken her mother's iron tablets.
79. A 19-year-old girl is rushed to A&E after having taken 30 paracetamol tablets after splitting from her boyfriend.
80. A 20-year-old lady is rushed to A&E after being found moribund. She had old timed meat soup.
81. A 35-year-old lady had ingested cyanide.
82. A 15-year-old girl takes warfarin tablets. She is actively bleeding.

THEME: 18
HEAVY METAL INTOXICATION

Options

a. Muscle spasm.
b. Wrist drops.
c. Cardiovascular collapse.
d. Monday morning fever.

For each of the situation/condition given below, choose the one most appropriate/discriminatory option from above. The options may be used once, more than once, or not at all.

Questions

83. Mercury.
84. Zinc.
85. Arsenic.
86. Lead.

THEME: 19
PHYSIOLOGICAL ANTIDOTES

Options

a. Flumazenil.
b. Atropine.

c. Naltrexone.
d. Pralidoxime.

For each of the situation/condition given below, choose the one most appropriate/discriminatory option from above. The options may be used once, more than once, or not at all.

Questions

87. Beta-blockers.
88. Organo phosphorus compounds.
89. Benzodiazepines.
90. Opioids.

THEME: 20
TELL TALE SIGNS OF SUBSTANCE ABUSE

Options

a. Agitation.
b. Dyspnea.
c. Tachyarrhythmias.
d. Running nose.
e. Neuropathies.

For each of the situation/condition given below, choose the one most appropriate/discriminatory option from above. The options may be used once, more than once, or not at all.

Questions

91. Cocaine.
92. Benzodiazepines.
93. Solvent abuse.
94. Heroin.

THEME: 21
MANAGEMENT OF POISONING

Options

a. Intubation and ventilation.
b. Hydration and hemodialysis.

c. Administration of naloxone.
d. Administration of chloropromazine.
e. Administration of physostigmine.

For each of the situation/condition given below, choose the one most appropriate/discriminatory option from above. The options may be used once, more than once, or not at all.

Questions

95. A hyperactive, agitated patient with dilated pupils, hyperthermia and tachycardia.
96. A drowsy patient with small pupils, shallow respirations, hypothermia and hypotension.
97. A restless, drowsy patient with tachyarrhythmias, hyperpyrexia and convulsions.
98. A confused patient with progressive drowsiness and slightly constricted but reactive pupils.
99. A lethargic patient who is mute and has multifocal seizures.

THEME: 22
DECISION MAKING IN THE INJURED PATIENT

Options

a. 10 units of soluble insulin(IV)
b. Secure airway and stabilize cervical spine
c. IV dexamethasone
d. 2 mg Glucagon (im)
e. Discharge patient after a period of counselling
f. 0.9% Saline (IV)
g. Splint limb
h. Assess airway
i. Asprin
j. Morphine
k. Naproxen
l. 50 ml of 50 % dextrose (IV)
m. Finger prick glucose measurement
n. Cut down should be performed.

Questions

100. An obese 56-year-old man is involved in a road traffic accident and sustains multiple bruises. He now coplains of severe excruciating pain in his right big toe. He had complained of a similar pain last year.
101. You arrive at the scene of major accident and find a 32-year-old man unconsious. He smells of alcohol.
102. A 34-year-old known diabetic is brought to the A& E Department unconscious following a road traffic accident. Initial resuscitation has been done by the paramedics.
103. As part of the ambulance team you arrive at the scane of a major accident. You find a 19-year-old man unconscious smelling of alcohol. His airway and cervical spine are secured by your team.
104. After a heavy bout of drinking a 17-year-old is brought to the A&E Department unconscious. The airway and cervical spine are secure. Several attempts at getting intravenous (IV) access have failed.

THEME: 23
THE MANAGEMENT OF DRUG OVERDOSE AND POISONING

Options

a. Empty stomach with N-G tube
b. IV N-acetylcysteine
c. Dicobalt edetate 300 mg (IV)
d. Specific antibody fragments
e. Nevaripin- Lamuvidine
f. Nevaripin antidote immediately
g. Desferrioxamine-100 % oxygen
h. Charcoal haemoperfusion in ITU
i. Increase urine output by alkaline diuresis
j. ITU
k. ITU-propanolol-muscle relaxation
l. Flumanezil

Questions

105. A mother brings her 5-year-old son who has reportedly swallowed an unknown quantity of 'white' tablets. On examination the child is breathing deeply and biochemical results show an increased anion-gap. A blood screen reveals a salicyclate level of 8.4 mmol/l and the child lapses into coma.
106. A 23-year-old girl is brought to the A&E after having collapsed in a night club. She is thought to have taken Ectasy (3-4 Methylenedioxymethamphetamine). Initial resuscitation has been done buther temperature is now 39.5°C .
107. A 43-year-old chemist is thought to have swallowed cyanide and is brought in to the A&E Department confused. His pulse rate is 100 beats/min and 50 ml of 50 % dextrose is given intravenously.
108. A 24-year-old male homosexual patient with heart failure takes an overdose of his medication. On questioning he says he sees yellow-green visual haloes and his pulse is irregular.

Eleven

Ethics

THEME: 1
ETHICAL ISSUES REGARDING PRACTICE OF MEDICINE IN UK

Options

a. Resuscitate without consent and cervical smear, as this may be the only opportunity.
b. Resuscitate even without consent.
c. Wait for relatives before you begin resuscitation.
d. Transfuse with blood.
e. Do not transfuse with blood even if the patient is serious.
f. Inform relevant health authority.
g. Respect the patient's confidentiality, don't inform the health authority.
h. Respect the patient's confidentiality don't tell the lawyer.
i. Tell lawyer about her condition.
j. Ask for consent again.
k. Needn't ask for consent again.

For each of the situations/conditions given below, choose the one most appropriate/discriminatory option from above. The options may be used once, more than once, or not at all.

Questions

1. A 17-year-old boy is brought into A&E unconscious, following an RTA.
2. You are treating a surgeon for Hepatitis B. You ask him to inform the NHS Trust where he is working but he refuses.
3. A 32-year-old woman is brought into A&E by her husband drifting in and out of consciousness, following an RTA.

She is in shock and you decide she needs immediate blood transfusion. Her husband objects saying that they are devout Jehovas Witness and age against blood transfusion. Her condition is deteriorating.

4. A 50-year-old wealthy widow has terminal breast cancer and she has only days to live. She has confided in you before that her daughters are threatening to kill each other, over who inherits her estate and her enormous wealth. She has not made her will and her lawyer requests that you tell him whether her condition is terminal so he can convince her to sign the will. Informing her about her worsening condition has caused significant deterioration in her condition before.
5. You are treating a 56-year-old woman who had an acute MI. Her condition is not improving and you want your medical secretary to type a referral letter. The secretary asks for patient's medical records so that she can type the letter.

THEME: 2
ETHICAL ISSUES REGARDING PRACTICE OF MEDICINE IN UK

Options

a. Report him to trust managers
b. Don't do anything
c. Call police and inform them at once
d. Give her pills after explaining risks to her and disregard her mother completely.
e. Carryout termination even without parent's knowledge
f. Carryout operation to save at least first baby
g. Respect parent's decision and let nature take its course.
h. Carryout sterilisation.
i. Tell her you cannot give her pills without her mother's consent.
j. Giver her pills and inform her mother.
k. Tell the parents and carryout termination only after their consent

l. Get partner's written and informed consent before sterilising.
m. Inform health minister
n. Seek a judicial review

For each of the situations/conditions given below, choose the one most appropriate/discriminatory option from above. The options may be used once, more than once, or not at all.

Questions

6. You are the SHO on the psychiatry ward. Your consultant is having a sexual relationship with a widow he has been treating for depression. The lady is getting better and awaiting discharge next week.
7. A 34-year-old woman wants to have a sterilisation. Her last-born child has cerebral palsy and her partner strongly objects to the procedure. They are married.
8. A mother has Siamese twins. One of the twins has no heart and liver and depends on the other for survival and as such without an operation to save the one with major organs they will both perish. Since having the operation means certain death of one of the babies, the parents who are staunch Christians oppose the operation. What should be done?
9. A 12-year-old girl wants OC pills. She does not want her parents to know bout this.
10. A 19-year-old girl wants to have a termination of pregnancy. She is 14 weeks pregnant. The procedure to terminate is not without complications. She does not want her mother informed about the termination.

THEME: 3
PRINCIPLES OF THE DUTIES OF A DOCTOR REGISTERED WITH THE GMC

Options

a. Make the care of your patient your first concern.
b. Treat every patient politely and considerately
c. Respect patients' dignity and privacy

d. Listen to patients and respect their views
e. Give patients information in a way they can understand
f. Respect the right of patients to be fully involved in decisions about their care.
g. Keep your professional knowledge and skills up to date
h. Recognise the limits of your professional competence
i. Be honest and trustworthy
j. Respect and protect confidential information
k. Make sure that your personal beliefs do not prejudice your patients' care
l. Act quickly to protect patients from risk if you have good reason to believe that you or a colleague may not be fit to practice.
m. Avoid abusing your position as a doctor
n. Work with colleagues in the ways that best serve patients' interests.

For each of the situations/conditions given below, choose the one most appropriate/discriminatory option from above. The options may be used once, more than once, or not at all.

Questions

11. A 22-year-old Indian woman requests a female doctor to perform a pelvic exam.
12. A 55-year-old man who is being admitted for a total knee replacement states that he is a Jehovah's witness and therefore refuses any blood products.
13. A 16-year-old girl informs you that she may be pregnant, and her parents are unaware.
14. A 30-year-old man is offered the choice of whether he would like to receive interferon injections for multiple sclerosis.
15. A 60-year-old diabetic sees you for a neurological opinion and asks if you would renew his insulin prescription as a favour.
16. Your patient reports feelings of depression. You seek a psychiatric opinion.
17. You ask a patient to undress to examine the abdomen. You remember to cover the patients groin.

18. You are asked to examine a patient at his bedside. You remember to pull the curtain around the bed to ensure privacy.
19. You see an overworked colleague struggle with his duties. You intervene and offer assistance.

THEME: 4
ETHICAL ISSUES REGARDING PRACTICE OF MEDICINE IN UK

Options

a. Tell the police
b. Don't tell the police
c. Ask the girl to come with parent or guardian
d. Talk to the girl about the importance of telling her parents, if she refuses go ahead with the procedure.
e. Offer the contraception only with parent's consent.
f. Offer contraception if risks are discussed even without parental consent.
g. Consult with senior managers of NHS Trust
h. Tell partner of patient's illness
i. Don't tell the partner as the patient is against it.
j. Consult with social services.

For each of the situations/conditions given below, choose the one most appropriate/discriminatory option from above. The options may be used once, more than once, or not at all.

Questions

20. A 13-year-old girl is pregnant and requires a termination of pregnancy. She tells you emphatically that at no point should you consider informing her parents.
21. An armed robber is injured during an exchange of gunfire with the police and comes to A&E and naturally requests your silence.
22. A 13-year-old girl is having unprotected sex with her 17-year-old boyfriend and asks that she be given the OC pill.

23. A 32-year-old man is found to be HIV positive. He is against condom use and after having a lengthy talk with you, he still refuses to accept the need to tell his wife.
24. A 30-year-old man is pulled over while driving for suspected driving in an aberiated condition. A breath test proves negative and the patient say it's probably the medication you prescribed that is to blame. The police call you and request you to tell them what the medication you prescribed for the man. The man then calls and tells you not to tell the police.

Twelve

Pharmacology

THEME: 1
PRESCRIBING FOR PAIN RELIEF

Options

a. A bolus of intravenous opiate
b. A subcutaneous opiate infusion
c. Acupuncture
d. Carbamazepine
e. Corticosteroids
f. Hypnotherapy
g. Intramuscular non-steroidal anti-inflammatory drugs
h. Oral non-steroidal anti-inflammatory drugs
i. Oral opiates
j. Proton pump inhibitors (eg. Omeprazole)
k. Selective serotonin re-uptake inhibitor eg Fluoxetine
l. Simple analgesics
m. Transcutaneous electrical nerve stimulation (TENS) machine
n. Tricyclic antidepressant

For each of the situations/conditions given below, choose the one most appropriate/discriminatory option from above. The options may be used once, more than once, or not at all.

Questions

1. A 70-year-old woman presents with severe, retrosternal chest pain and sweating. An ECG shows acute infero-lateral myocardial infarction.
2. A 65-year-old woman with inoperable gastric cancer causing obstruction, and multiple liver metastases, is taking a large dose of oral analgesia. Despite this, her pain is currently unrelieved.

3. A 28-year-old woman has just been diagnosed with having rheumatoid arthritis and her rheumatologist has just begun giving her gold injections. She continues to complain of joint pain and stiffness, particularly for the first two hours of each day.
4. A 55-year-old obese woman with a known hiatus hernia, presents with recurrent, severe, burning retrosternal chest pain associated with acid regurgitation and increased oral flatulence.
5. A 70-year-old woman reports severe paroxysms of knife-like or electric shock-like pain, lasting seconds, in the lower part of the right side of her face.
6. A 30-year-old man presents with an 8-year-history of back pain, worse in the morning and one episode of uveitis.

THEME: 2
SIDE EFFECTS OF ANTIEPILEPTIC DRUGS

Options

a. Carbamazepine
b. Sodium valproate
c. Phenytoin
d. Phenobarbitone
e. Benzodiazepines
f. Gabapentin
g. Vigabatrin
h. Lamotrigine
i. Ethosuximide
j. Tiagabine
k. Topiramate
l. Amitriptyline
m. Paraldehyde

For each of the situations/conditions given below, choose the one most appropriate/discriminatory option from above. The options may be used once, more than once, or not at all.

Questions

7. A 50-year-old woman has been on anti-epileptic drugs for 5 years. She now presents with nystagmus, unsteady movements and hyperplasia of the gums.

8. A 30-year-old woman on anti-epileptic medication now presents with ankle swelling, tremor, weight gain and hair thinning.
9. An 18-year-old girl who first presented with episodes of 'absences' at school has been on anti-epileptics for 2 years. She now presents with ataxia, drowsiness, gum hypertrophy and swelling of the tongue.
10. An 18-year-old girl was treated for status epilepticus with Intramuscular anti-epileptics now presents with a sterile abscess at the site of injection.
11. A 15-year-old boy diagnosed with West syndrome (infantile spasms) has been on anti-epileptics for 3 month now presents with diplopia and nausea. He is found to have marked visual field defects.
12. A 25-year-old man is on treatment for epilepsy. A full blood count shows the following: MCV – 110 fl MCHC – 27 g/dl.
13. A 30-year-old woman on treatment for epilepsy complains of anorexia and nausea and general fatigue. She has no body swelling. Blood investigations show Na is 124 mmol/L, K is 4 mmol/L. Plasma osmolality is 200 mmol.

THEME: 3
INVESTIGATION OF DRUG SIDE EFFECT

Options

a. Urea and electrolytes
b. Liver function tests
c. Full blood count
d. Chest X-ray
e. Thyroid function tests
f. Serum electrolytes
g. ECG
h. Arterial blood gases
i. Activated thromboplastin time
j. Bleeding time
k. Prothrombin time
l. Typothyroidism

For each of the situations/conditions given below, choose the one most appropriate/discriminatory option from above. The options may be used once, more than once, or not at all.

Questions

14. A 18-year-old boy has swallowed 40 aspirin tablets.
15. A 60-year-old woman has taken all the Warfarin tablets in the container at one time 3 hours ago.
16. A 39-year-old woman is taking Digoxin but now has developed nausea, abdominal pain and palpitations.
17. A 20-year-old boy who is taking oral theophylline for asthma presents with symptoms.
18. A 45-year-old woman has been taking Amiodarone for the past 3 years for a rhythm disturbance. For the past 3 months she has been complaining of lethargy and being depressed.

THEME: 4
DRUG OF CHOICE

Options

a. None
b. Benzylpenicillin
c. Amoxycillin
d. Cefotaxime
e. Gentamicin
f. Metronidazole
g. Ciprofloxacin
h. Erythromycin
i. Trimethoprim
j. Doxycycline
k. Co-amoxiclav
l. 2 or more antibiotics together

For each of the situations/conditions given below, choose the one most appropriate/discriminatory option from above. The options may be used once, more than once, or not at all.

Questions

19. A 34-year-old woman complains of severe burning on passing urine like 'passing a broken glass'. She also has a urethral discharge. Gram stain of the urethral swab is negative.

20. A 20-year-old student develops bloody diarrhoea after eating a reheated chicken.
21. A 43-year-old man has cough, fever and mild dyspnoea. He has reduced air entry and is dull to percussion at the left lung base. He is neither systemically unwell nor hypoxic. He has a documented penicillin allergy.
22. A 42-year-old man presents with malaise and low-grade fever for 2 weeks. He recently had treatment for a dental abscess. On examination he has splinter haemorrhages and an early diastolic murmur.
23. A 4-year-old child presents with acute fever, drowsiness, stridor and drooling. She looks shocked and unwell.
24. A 56-year-old female smoker presents with severe dyspnoea, dry cough and fever. She is unwell, tachycardic and cyanosed.

THEME: 5
OVER THE COUNTER MEDICATIONS

Options

a. Paracetamol
b. Aspirin
c. Loperamide
d. Cimetidine
e. Chlorpheniramine
f. Loratidine
g. 1% hydrocortisone cream
h. Topical clotrimazole
i. Xylometazoline nasal spray
j. Sodium cromoglycate nasal spray
k. Aluminium hydroxide/magnesium trisilicate
l. Malathion lotion
m. Should be investigated first

For each of the situations/conditions given below, choose the one most appropriate/discriminatory option from above. The options may be used once, more than once, or not at all.

Questions

25. A 25-year-old woman complains of vulval itching and a white vaginal discharge.

26. A 34-year-old woman complains of heartburn, indigestion and reflux with water bash.
27. A 4-year-old boy is ferbrile and irritable with a generalised vesicular rash. He has a history of a febrile convulsion in the past.
28. A 20-year-old student suffers with hay fever. She is due to take her final exams and is worried that the hay fever will affect her performance. However, she is also worried that medication may make him drowsy.
29. A 50-year-old woman has a 2 month history of epigastric pain after meals.

THEME: 6
PRESCRIBING FOR ALCOHOL AND DRUG ABUSE

Options

a. Acamprosate
b. Admit and give Benzodiazepines
c. Benzodiazepine
d. Disulfiram
e. Electroconvulsive therapy
f. Hematinics
g. Heroin
h. High potency vitamins
i. Insulin coma therapy
j. Lithium
k. Liver extract
l. Methadone
m. Multivitamins
n. Naltrexone
o. Refer to substance misuse team
p. Vitamin K

For each of the situations/conditions given below, choose the one most appropriate/discriminatory option from above. The options may be used once, more than once, or not at all.

Questions

30. A 50-year-old woman presents to the clinic with a history of shakes for 12 hours, which started after she woke up following a 36 hour binge of alcohol at a party.

31. A 35-year-old unemployed woman has been in hospital for a period of detoxification due to alcohol. She is ready for discharge but wants to remain abstinent after discharge.
32. A 30-year-old man wants help in coming off heroin. He attends the A&E. He has been injecting heroin intermittently for the 6 months. His partner is not a drug user and very supportive.
33. A 50-year-old filmmaker presents with making up stories to fill the memory gaps. She shows global amnesia on testing and there is no impairment of consciousness. She gives a history of alcohol abuse and has been hearing voices. She is already taking vitamin supplements.
34. A 40-year-old man has been admitted to the medical ward with jaundice and a past history of alcohol abuse. He is now seeing ants crawling over him and is becoming disturbed and restless.

THEME: 7
SIDE-EFFECTS OF COMMON DRUGS

Options

a. Impotence
b. Wasting
c. Deep vein thrombosis
d. Bronchospasm
e. Pseudomembranous colitis
f. Haemorrhagic cystitis
g. Constipation
h. Retrobulbar neuritis
i. Endometrial carcinoma
j. Steven-Johnson syndrome
k. Retroperitoneal fibrosis

For each of the situations/conditions given below, choose the one most appropriate/discriminatory option from above. The options may be used once, more than once, or not at all.

Questions

35. Cimetidine

36. Cyclophosphamide
37. Diamorphine
38. Amoxycillin
39. Oral contraceptive pill
40. Aspirin
41. Ethambutol
42. Tamoxifen
43. Methysergide

THEME: 8
DRUG OF CHOICE

Options

a. Diamorphine IV
b. Diamorphine IM
c. Salbutamol nebulisation
d. Nebulised steroids
e. Protamine sulphate
f. Carbamazepine
g. Donepezil
h. Methadone
i. Naltrexone
j. Vigabatrin
k. Sulphasalazine
l. Carbimazole
m. Fluoxetine

For each of the situations/conditions given below, choose the one most appropriate/discriminatory option from above. The options may be used once, more than once, or not at all.

Questions

44. A 60-year-old woman with no previous history is brought to A&E by her husband who says that she has become progressively forgetful and tends to have mood swings.
45. A 30-year-old 13 weeks pregnant woman complains of heat intolerance. She has lost weight despite a good appetite.

46. A 40-year-old woman develops a crushing chest pain associated with nausea and profuse sweating. The pain is still present when she arrives in hospital an hour later.
47. A 15-year-old known asthmatic is brought to A&E breathless. His pulse is 56. No wheezing is heard.
48. A 35-year-old woman has been treated for morphine dependence. She wants to stay off the drug.
49. A 40-year-old woman is suffering from ulcerative colitis.
50. A 44-year-old woman complains of morning stiffness of both her knees. On examination they are found to be swollen and tender. She has lost weight.
51. A 30-year-old woman has lost weight since the death of her husband 3 years ago. She is withdrawn and has a bleak view of the future.

THEME: 9
DRUG OVERDOSE

Options

a. Lithium
b. Aspirin
c. Ethanol
d. Benzodiazepine
e. Tricyclic antidepressants
f. LSD overdose
g. Beta blocker
h. Paracetamol
i. Methanol
j. Amphetamine
k. Digoxin

For each of the situations/conditions given below, choose the one most appropriate/discriminatory option from above. The options may be used once, more than once, or not at all.

Questions

52. A 20-year-old student was admitted to A&E with pyrexia and sweating. His pulse was 120 and BP was 100/60. He also complained of deafness and tinitus.

53. A 35-year-old woman was admitted to A&E unconscious. Her temperature was 37.7°C pulse was 130 and BP 95/65. Neurological examination showed bilateral extensor plantars. Her pupils were dilated. ECG showed sinus tachycardia and occasional ventricular ectopics.
54. A 62-year-old woman presented with drowsiness and confusion. Her pulse was 50 and his BP was 100/70. ECG showed first-degree heart block and widening of QRS interval.
55. A 70-year-old man presented with nausea, vomiting and diarrhoea. He also complained of blurring vision and flashes of light. On examination, he was slightly confused and his pulse was slow and regular.
56. A 38-year-old man with long-standing psychiatric illness was admitted with polyuria, diarrhoea, vomiting and coarse tremor involving both hands.
57. A 25-year-old waiter developed jaundice, right hypochondrial pain and tenderness, hypoglycaemia and oliguria 2 days after an overdose.

THEME: 10
DRUG INTERACTIONS

Options

a. Loop diuretics
b. Allopurinol
c. NSAIDs
d. Alcohol
e. Erythromycin
f. Amitriptyline
g. Thiazide diuretic
h. Ranitidine
i. Cimetidine
j. Verapamil
k. Amiodarone
l. Chloramphenicol
m. Omeprazole

For each of the situations/conditions given below, choose the one most appropriate/discriminatory option from above. The options may be used once, more than once, or not at all.

Questions

58. A 35-year-old manic depressive is noted to have high serum levels of lithium and profound hypokalemia. Her GP has started her on an antihypertensive.
59. A 44-year-old woman on carbamazepine for trigeminal neuralgia now presents with severe dizziness. She was recently started on an antibiotic course.
60. A 45-year-old man taking phenytoin for epilepsy now presents with ataxia, slurred speech and blurred vision. His medications include carbamazepine, tagamet and allopurinol. Which among these 3 drugs is responsible for the interaction with phenytoin?
61. A 50-year-old diabetic on metformin presents with lactic acidosis. His medication includes erythromycin and paracetamol. He also drinks heavily.

THEME: 11
MANAGEMENT OF DRUG DEPENDENCY

Options

a. Disulfiram
b. Methadone
c. Needle exchange programme
d. IV vitamin B_{12} and thiamine
e. Gradual reducing course of diazepam
f. Outpatient referral to drug dependency team
g. Chlormethiazole
h. Chlordiazepoxide
i. Naloxone
j. Group psychotherapy
k. Inform police
l. Hospital admission

For each of the situations/conditions given below, choose the one most appropriate/discriminatory option from above. The options may be used once, more than once, or not at all.

Questions

62. A 70-year-old woman has taken 20 mg of temazepam at night for the last 30 years. She has begun to suffer with falls and has agreed that temazepam might be contributing to this.
63. A 26-year-old heroin addict is worried because her partner has been diagnosed as having HIV. She is HIV negative. She does not feel able to stop using heroin at the present times.
64. A 40-year-old man has become increasingly dependent on alcohol since his wife died last year. He admits that he has a problem and wishes to stop drinking. He does not wish to take anti-depressants.
65. A 30-year-old builder was admitted for an elective anterior cruciate ligament repair. He admits to drinking at least 60 units of alcohol per week and has no desire to stop. You are keen to prevent him from developing withdrawal symptoms as this may impair his recovery from the operation.
66. A 63-year-old retired surgeon is admitted with a short history of bizarre behaviour. He claims that the GMC are investigating him for murder and have hired a private detective to follow him. He has evidence of coarse tremor, horizontal nystagmus and an ataxic gait. His wife says the story about GMC is not true but says her husband has been drinking a lot since retirement.
67. A 37-year-old retired professional footballer admits to using cocaine and heroin for the last 3 years. He has recently signed a contract to present a sports show on television and wishes to 'clean his life up' first. His wife and family are supportive of this.

THEME: 12
WARNINGS FOR SPECIFIC DRUGS

Options

a. Must be taken with food.
b. Must be taken on an empty stomach
c. Must avoid alcoholic drinks

d. This drug may colour urine
e. Not to be stopped without doctor's advice
f. Avoid exposure of the skin to sunlight
g. Take a full glass of water at least 30 minutes before breakfast and remain upright until after breakfast
h. May reduce effect of OC pills
i. May cause blue tinted vision
j. Not to be taken with antacids
k. Not to be taken with iron tablets

For each of the situations/conditions given below, choose the one most appropriate/discriminatory option from above. The options may be used once, more than once, or not at all.

Questions

68. Sulfasalazine
69. Chlorpropamide
70. Sildenafil
71. Alendronate
72. Ampicillin
73. Phenytoin

THEME: 13
IMPORTANT DRUG INTERACTIONS

Options

a. OC pills and erythromycin
b. Warfarin and rifampicin
c. Cyclosporin A and phenytoin
d. Captopril and triamterene
e. Propanolol and verapamil
f. Theophylline and erythromycin
g. Lithium and bendrofluazide
h. Digoxin and frusemide
i. Warfarin and amiodarone
j. Metformin and cimetidine
k. Phenytoin and isoniazid
l. Pencillamine and tetracycline

For each of the situations/conditions given below, choose the one most appropriate/discriminatory option from above. The options may be used once, more than once, or not at all.

Questions

74. An elderly man on treatment for an irregular heart rate develops ankle edema for which he is given a new drug. 2 weeks later he develops complete heart block, nausea and complains of seeing 'yellow'
75. A patient on treatment for a psychiatric disorder is noted to have hypertension for which she is prescribed a new drug. Within a week she develops tremor, agitation and 4 weeks later presents with heart block, seizures and a raised creatinine of 400.
76. A young career woman is treated by her GP for a respiratory infection. A week later she develops irregular bleeding. One month after this, a pregnancy test is positive.
77. A man develops a persistent arrhythmia for which DC cardioversion is planned. He is commenced on appropriate treatment for 4 weeks leading to cardioversion. He plans a holiday during which he contacts tuberculosis. One week after starting ATT he develops sudden onset left sided weakness.
78. A young woman is on maximal therapy for rheumatoid arthritis. She is also on treatment for acne. At routine follow-up, her urea is 30 and her creatinine 600.

THEME: 14
INVESTIGATION OF DRUG OVERDOSE

Options

a. Bleeding time
b. Prothrombin time
c. APTT
d. ECG
e. Serum urea and electrolytes
f. Full blood count

g. Phenytoin levels
h. Peak flow measurement
i. Spirometry

For each of the situations/conditions given below, choose the one most appropriate/discriminatory option from above. The options may be used once, more than once, or not at all.

Questions

79. A 25-year-old girl who has ingested 25 tablets of paracetamol
80. A 16-year-old girl who has ingested 20 tricyclic antidepressants. She tells you she wanted to end her life.
81. A 25-year-old asthmatic who was on oral theophyllines at home was given IV phenytoin on the ward.
82. An 18-year-old nightclub dancer was given a 'pill' by a friend. This was to help her relax so she could enjoy the night.

THEME: 15
PRESCRIBING AND LIVER FAILURE

Options

a. Spironolactone 100 mg/day PO
b. Frusemide 100 mg/day PO
c. Paracentesis
d. Paracentesis with albumin infusion
e. Ciprofloxacin 250 mg PO
f. Flucloxacillin 500 mg/day PO
g. Chlorpheniramine 75 mg PO
h. Cholestyramine 4 g/8h PO
i. Tetracycline 250 mg/8h PO
j. Stop warfarin
k. Increase warfarin dosage
l. Decrease warfarin dosage
m. Bedrest, salt and fluid restriction

For each of the situations/conditions given below, choose the one most appropriate/discriminatory option from above. The options may be used once, more than once, or not at all.

Questions

83. A 32-year-old chronic alcoholic is in liver failure. He has severe pruritus.
84. A 30-year-old chronic alcoholic is on warfarin following an acute MI he suffered 3 months ago. He now develops liver cirrhosis.
85. A 32-year-old man has had hepatitis B for the last 1-year- and now presents with a grossly distended abdomen and other stigmata of liver disease. You are worried he may develop spontaneous bacterial peritonitis.
86. A 30-year-old woman presents with a mildly distended abdomen, yellowing of the mucus membranes. She is found to have spider naevi on her chest.

THEME: 16
PRESCRIPTION AND DISEASE

Options

a. Vancomycin
b. Benzylpenicillin
c. Erythromycin
d. Actinomycin
e. Metronidazole
f. Amoxycillin
g. Glyceryl trinitrate
h. Co-trimoxazole
i. Zidovudine
j. Ondansetron
k. Fluconazole
l. Imidazole
m. Verapamil
n. IV immunoglobulins
o. Piperacillin
p. Trimethoprim

For each of the situations/conditions given below, choose the one most appropriate/discriminatory option from above. The options may be used once, more than once, or not at all.

Questions

87. Meningococcal Meningitis
88. Tetanus
89. *Trichomonas vaginalis*
90. Vincent's angina
91. Uncomplicated UTI
92. Pseudomembranous colitis (patient is allergic to vancomycin)
93. Sinusitis in patient allergic to penicillin
94. Acute otitis media
95. Acute streptococcal sore throat
96. Pneumocystis
97. Amoebiasis

THEME: 17
ADVERSE EFFECTS OF MEDICATIONS

Options

a. Nifedepine
b. Carbimazole
c. Rifampicin
d. Ampicillin
e. Propanolol
f. Captopril
g. Co-trimoxazole
h. Simvastatin
i. Thiazide diuretic
j. Isoniazid
k. Propyl thiouracil

For each of the situations/conditions given below, choose the one most appropriate/discriminatory option from above. The options may be used once, more than once, or not at all.

Questions

98. A 50-year-old alcoholic was diagnosed to have tuberculosis. He was started on some medications then a few months later developed numbness and tingling in both feet.

99. A 65-year-old diabetic was prescribed a medication for newly diagnosed hypertension. She did not tolerate the medication because of persistent dry cough.
100. A 14-year-old boy presented to his GP with fever, rash and sore throat. The GP diagnosed tonsillitis and started him on an antibiotic. He later developed a blotchy purpuric rash all over his body.
101. A 52-year-old man who had a triple bypass, complained of myalgia a few weeks after starting a new medication. His liver function tests were abnormal.
102. A 68-year-old man was started on medication for hypertension. He presented later with a tender swollen right first metatarsal joint.
103. A 48-year-old woman was recently diagnosed thyrotoxic presented with fever and sore throat.

THEME: 18
SIDE EFFECTS OF DRUGS

Options

a. Danazol
b. Clomifene citrate
c. Methotrexate
d. GnRH agonists
e. Oxytocin
f. Bromociptine
g. Progestrogens
h. HRT
i. Prednisolone
j. NSAIDs

For each of the situations/conditions given below, choose the one most appropriate/discriminatory option from above. The options may be used once, more than once, or not at all.

Questions

104. Weight gain, acne, growth of facial hair, voice changes, decreased breast size, atrophic vaginitis and dyspareunia.

105. Osteoporosis in cases of prolonged use, hot flushes, decreased libido and vaginal dryness.
106. Breakthrough bleeding, weight gain, depression, prolonged amenorrhoea after starting treatment.
107. Visual disturbances, ovarian hyperstimulation, hot flushes, headache, weight gain, depression and abdominal discomfort.
108. May increase the risk of breast carcinoma and deep vein thrombosis. Side-effects include weight gain, abdominal discomfort, depression and jaundice.
109. Headache, postural hypotension and Raynaud's phenomenon. High doses may cause retroperitoneal fibrosis.

THEME: 19
PRESCRIBING FOR PAIN RELIEF

Options

a. Paracetamol
b. Aspirin
c. Co-proxamol
d. Ibuprofen
e. Diclofenac
f. Tramadol
g. Morphine
h. Diamorphine
i. Nitrous oxide
j. Pethidine
k. Carbamazepine
l. Topical ketoprofen

For each of the situations/conditions given below, choose the one most appropriate/discriminatory option from above. The options may be used once, more than once, or not at all.

Questions

110. A 12-year-old boy has a dental extraction and is complaining of a painful jaw.
111. A 70-year-old woman has bone pain from metastatic breast disease. Simple analgesia has been ineffective.

112. A 35-year-old man is admitted with an acutely painful abdomen. He has epigastric tenderness. His amylase is elevated.
113. A 50-year-old woman has severe shooting pains in the left side of her face following an attack of shingles.
114. A 21-year-old man has dislocated the terminal phalanx of his left little finger in a fight. There does not appear to be a fracture and you wish to give him analgesia to allow reduction of the dislocation.

THEME: 20
SIDE EFFECTS OF DRUGS

Options

a. Amiodarone
b. Aspirin
c. Atenolol
d. Carbimazole
e. Chlorpromazine
f. Erythromycin
g. L-Dopa
h. Lisinopril
i. Lithium
j. Metformin
k. Sulphasalazine
l. Verapamil

For each of the situations/conditions given below, choose the one most appropriate/discriminatory option from above. The options may be used once, more than once, or not at all.

Questions

115. Cold hands and feet, fatigue and impotence
116. Peripheral neuropathy, pulmonary fibrosis, hyperthyroidism
117. Postural hypotension, involuntary movements, nausea, discolouration of the urine.
118. Thirst, polyuria, tremor, rashes hypothyroidism
119. Sore throat, rash, pruritus and nausea.

Thirteen

Dermatology

THEME: 1
DIAGNOSIS OF SKIN DISEASE

Options

a. Fungal infections.
b. Erythema multiforme.
c. Granuloma annulare.
d. Basal cell carcinoma.
e. Psoriasis.
f. Discoid eczema.
g. Pityriasis rosea.
h. Impetigo.
i. Pityriasis alba.
j. Freckles.
k. Seborrheic keratoses.
l. Pityriasis versicolor.

For each of the situations/conditions given below, choose the one most appropriate/discriminatory option from above. The options may be used once, more than once, or not at all.

Questions

1. Herald patch, oval red lesions with scaly edge.
2. Superficial slightly scaly infection with the yeast M. furfur.
3. Posteczema hypopigmentation, often on children's face.
4. Active erythematous scaly edge with central scarring.
5. Well defined red patches, covered with honey colored crusts.
6. Pinkish papules forming a ring.
7. Brown macules, related to sun exposure.
8. Pearly papules with central ulcer.

THEME: 2
DIAGNOSIS OF SKIN DISORDERS

Options

a. Multiple petechiae in both axillae.
b. Draining sinus on lateral chest wall.
c. Purplish submucosal lesion on the hard palate.
d. Exuberant violaceous nodules over the nose and malar areas.
e. Black pigmented nodules along folds of skin in axillary and perineal areas.

For each of the situations/conditions given below, choose the one most appropriate/discriminatory option from above. The options may be used once, more than once, or not at all.

Questions

9. A 24-year-old homosexual man with fever, weightloss, and diffuse alveolar infiltrates on chest roentgenogram.
10. A 31-year-old man with confusion and dyspnea 24 hours after fracturing his femur at a skin resort.
11. A 52-year-old black woman with hypercalcemia and interstitial fibrous of the lung.
12. A 69-year-old man with confusion, fever, dense consolidation with cavitation in the right lower lobe.
13. A 74-year-old man with hemoptysis and right hilar mass on chest roentgenogram.

THEME: 3
DIAGNOSIS OF SKIN CONDITION

Options

a. Lichen planus.
b. Seborrheic dermatitis.
c. Erythema chronicum migrans.
d. Pyoderma gangrenosum.
e. Vitiligo.
f. Acne.
g. Thrombophlebitis migrans.
h. Dermatitis herpetiformis.

i. Acanthosis nigricans.
j. Nerobiosis lipoidica.
k. Erythema marginatum.
l. Erythema multiforme.

For each of the situations/conditions given below, choose the one most appropriate/discriminatory option from above. The options may be used once, more than once, or not at all.

Questions

14. Itchy grouped blisters on knees, elbows and scalp in a patient with chronic diarrhea.
15. Successive crops of tender nodules along blood vessels in a patient with pancreatic cancer.
16. Yellowish, shiny skin with telangiectasia, on the skin of a diabetic.
17. Circular lesions with central blisters, widespread—including palms and soles with ulcers in the mouth and genitalia.
18. Pigmented, dark, rough, thickened skin in axillae and groins.

THEME: 4
DIAGNOSIS OF SKIN LESIONS

Options

a. Vitiligo
b. Melanoma
c. Rodent ulcer
d. Benign naevus
e. Keratoacanthoma
f. Pyoderma gangrenosum
g. Erythema marginatum
h. Dermatitis herpetiformis
i. Tophi
j. Necrobiosis lipoidica
k. Granuloma annulare
l. Erythema migrans
m. Erythema nodosum
n. Erythema ab igne

For each of the situations/conditions given below, choose the one most appropriate/discriminatory option from above. The options may be used once, more than once, or not at all

Questions

19. A young oil engineer complains of painful red lesions on his thighs. Physical examination determines them to be nodular. He has recently been vaccinated for travel to Asia.
20. A young woman complains of mark on her abdomen. Initially it was purple and then it enlarged and faded in the centre. Over the past few weeks it has multiplied outwards.
21. A middle-aged woman presents with a lesion on her calf. It is an ulcerated nodule with a red and necrotic border. It is very tender.
22. A 52-year-old man complains of a large white patch on his back. It is geographic with a hyperpigmented border. He has just come back from a beach holiday and it is physically irritating him.
23. A 28-year-old woman with a heart condition has a rash on her lower arms. It is pink or red and ring like. It moves up and down her arms and she can't get rid of it.

THEME: 5
DIAGNOSIS OF SKIN LESIONS

Options

a. Eczema herpetiformis
b. Morbiliform rash
c. Erythema multiforme
d. Erthema marginatum
e. Dermatitis herpetiformis
f. Maculapapular rash
g. Generalized urticaria
h. Lichen planus
i. Erythema chronicum migrans
j. Erythema nodusum

For each of the situations/conditions given below, choose the one most appropriate/discriminatory option from above. The options may be used once, more than once, or not at all

Questions

24. A 24-year-old man visited a forest area 2 weeks ago and developed a flu like illness. He now has a stiff neck, sore throat and arthralgia.
25. A 14-year-old boy has had a pyrexia, rash, raised ESR. Subcutaneous nodules and a generalized rash is noted on her trunk.
26. A 15-year-old girl has difficulty swallowing and large circular lesions (target lesion) are noted around her mouth, the inside of her mouth is swollen with crustation of the gingival.
27. A 6-year-old girl presents with failure to thrive and a rash is noted, the child dislikes gluten-based foods.
28. A 14-year-old boy has haematuria, hypertension, abdominal pain and a rash is noted on the flexor surfaces of his lower limbs.

THEME: 6
DIAGNOSIS OF SKIN INFECTIONS

Options

a. Cellulitis
b. Shingles
c. Pityriasis versicolor
d. Molluscum contagiosum
e. Ringworm
f. Necrotizing fascitis
g. Impetigo
h. Scabies
i. Leprosy
j. Seconday syphilis

For each of the situations/conditions given below, choose the one most appropriate/discriminatory option from above. The options may be used once, more than once, or not at all

Questions

29. A 30-year-old man complains of a painless rash on his trunk. He has 3 pale, pink, scaly circular lesions with central clearing, which measure between 3 and 8cm in diameter.
30. A 60-year-old man complains of a 2-day history of pain in the left side of his chest. He now has a blistering rash in a vertical band of skin on his left side.
31. A 35-year-old woman from Nigeria has a number of depigmented patches of skin on her legs. They are painless with reduced skin sensation.
32. A 28-year-old businessman returned from a trip to Thailand 2 months ago. He now has a faint paplar rash, which includes is palms and soles. He did have a painless ulcer on his penis but this resolved weeks ago.
33. A 25-year-old woman from Ghana has a painless rash on her trunk of multiple scaly patches measuring between 1 and 3 cm in diameter.
34. A 38-year-old man presents with a 12 hour history of a painful swollen right arm. He has parasthesiae in his fingers. He is febrile and the arm is tender with dusky skin.

THEME: 7
DIAGNOSIS OF SKIN INFECTIONS

Options

a. Infected sebaceous cyst
b. Furunculosis
c. Cellulitis
d. Herpes zoster
e. Carbuncle
f. Erysipelas
g. Hidradenitis suppurativa
h. Infected sinus
i. Skin necrosis
j. Scrofula

For each of the situations/conditions given below, choose the one most appropriate/discriminatory option from above. The options may be used once, more than once, or not at all

Questions

35. A 55-year-old non-insulin dependent diabetic man presents with chronics recurrent tender swelling in his groin. These red swellings eventually discharge pus.
36. A 45-year-old gardener presents with fever and swelling over his left cheek. The left side of his face is red, hot and tender with a raised border.
37. A 60-year-old obese insulin dependent diabetic woman presents with red papules and vesicles along the left preauricular region and mandible. It was preceded by fever.
38. A 70-year-old man with peripheral vascular disease present with a pinprick sized hole in the centre of his groin wound following a aorto-bifemoral graft. The discharge is serous.
39. A 50-year-old woman presents with a tender 1.5 cm swelling in the preauricular region. There is a puncture seen in the centre. The swelling is tense and smooth and attached to the skin.

THEME: 8
DIAGNOSIS OF SKIN LESIONS

Options

a. Lichen planus
b. Psoriasis
c. Pityriasis versicolor
d. Pityriasis rosea
e. Acne vulgaris
f. Allergic contact dermatitis
g. Acanthosis nigrans
h. Herpes zoster
i. Erythema nodosum
j. Dermatitis herpetiformis
k. Pemphigus vulgaris
l. Pemphigoid

For each of the situations/conditions given below, choose the one most appropriate/discriminatory option from above. The options may be used once, more than once, or not at all.

Questions

40. A 80-year-old man presents with itching followed by large, tense bullae on the limbs that do not rupture easily. Nikolsky's sign is negative.
41. A 50-year-old man presents with brownish scaly lesions of varying size on his trunk. Depigmentation after treatment lasts for several months.
42. A 30-year-old female presents with an itch painful rash over the lobes of both pinna. Her earlobes are pierced.
43. A 50-year-old man presents with a rash consisting of discrete purple shiny polygonal papules with fine white lines in previous scratch marks on his forearm. He is also noted to have a white lacy network of lesions on the buccal mucosa.
44. A 60-year-old man presents with brown pigmented plaques in the axilla. He underwent prostatectomy recently.

THEME: 9
DIAGNOSIS OF SKIN LESIONS

Options

a. Erythema nodosum
b. Erythema multiforme
c. Henoch-schonlein purpura
d. Eczema
e. Psoriasis
f. Necrobiosis lipoidica
g. Ringworm
h. Shingles
i. Urticaria
j. Pemphigus
k. Pemphigoid

For each of the situations/conditions given below, choose the one most appropriate/discriminatory option from above. The options may be used once, more than once, or not at all.

Questions

45. A 65-year-old woman has a 3-day history of painful blistering rash on her left outer thigh. She has recently been diagnosed with breast cancer.

46. A 25-year-old woman was recently started on Co-trimoxazole for a UTI. She is now complaining of painful. Red, raised lesions on both shins.
47. A 30-year-old builder has developed pink scaly patches on both knees. He has similar lesions on his elbows and scalp.
48. A 65-year-old woman has developed extensive blistering particularly involving her legs. The blisters are fragile and seem to spread under the skin surface when pressed. She feels generally unwell but has no other symptoms.
49. A 16-year-old girl presents with small purple lesions on her buttocks and shins. She also has painful joints and abdomen. Urinalysis reveals proteinuria.
50. A 60-year-old man who has had diabetes for several years, has developed a waxy yellow patch on his left shin, which is showing signs of inflammation and ulceration.

THEME: 10
DIAGNOSIS OF SKIN LESIONS

Options

a. Seborrhoeic Keratosis
b. Malignant melanoma
c. Café au lait parch
d. Haemangioma
e. Cambell de Morgan spor
f. Keratpecanthoma
g. Solar keratosis
h. Basal cell carcinoma
i. Squamous cell carcinoma
j. Bowen's disease
k. Marjolin's ulcer

For each of the situations/conditions given below, choose the one most appropriate/discriminatory option from above. The options may be used once, more than once, or not at all.

Questions

51. A 60-year-old man presents with a persistent itchy ulcer on his right cheek. He has had this ulcer for years. The

edges are rolled with a central scab that falls off and reforms. The local lymph nodes are not enlarged.

52. A 65-year-old farmer presents with a grey thickened patch of skin on the rim of his left ear. The 1 cm lesion is painless, raised, firm and has not changed in size over many years.
53. A 40-year-old woman presents with a rapidly growing 1cm lump in the skin of her wrist. The lump is the same colour as her skin but the centre is necrotic. It is freely mobile and rubbery in consistency with a hard core.
54. A newborn baby presents with several, 2cm pale brown macules on the back.
55. A 20-year-old man presents with a chronic paronychia. On examination, there is an expanding brown pigmentation present beneath the toe-nail with enlargement of the local lymph nodes.

THEME: 11
SKIN DISEASE IN CHILDREN

Options

a. Erythema chronicum migrans
b. Erythema infectiosum
c. Erythema multiforme
d. Erythema nodosum
e. Exanthema subitum
f. Purpura fulminans
g. Tinea corporis

For each of the situations/conditions given below, choose the one most appropriate/discriminatory option from above. The options may be used once, more than once, or not at all

Questions

56. A nine-months old child is nonspecifically unwell for three days with a fever. The rash subsides and the child breaks out in maculopapular rash over its body.
57. Following a course of Septrin for a bacterial infection, a five-year-old child breaks out in a widespread macular rash with target lesions.

58. A four-year old boy has a runny nose and mild fever and develops bright red cheeks and reticular rash on forearms.
59. Following a tick bite on holiday in a forested area, a seven-year-old boy develops an erythematous macule at the site of the bite which then spreads into an annular lesion with a clear central area.

THEME: 12
INVESTIGATION OF SKIN LESIONS

Options

a. Full blood count
b. Kveim test
c. ANCA
d. ESR
e. Antibodies to double stranded DNA
f. Skin biopsy
g. Skin biopsy for Ziehl Neelsen straining for acid-fast bacilli
h. Fasting cholesterol and triglyceride levels
i. Anti-Ro antibodies
j. Serum pancreativ gluganon
k. Muscle biopsy
l. Serum glucose

For each of the situations/conditions given below, choose the one most appropriate/discriminatory option from above. The options may be used once, more than once, or not at all

Questions

60. A 38-year-old man presents with malaise and arthralgia. He is noted to have various skin lesions, including a purple bulbous nose and tender red raised nodules on his anterior shin.
61. A 70-year-old woman presents with mid-facial disfigurement. The nose appears to have been gnawed off by a condition. The cutaneous lesion shows grandulomas with central caseation.
62. A 50-year-old woman presents with fleshy co loured papules over the right distal interphalangeal joint of her thumb and a brown waxy plaque over her right shin.

63. A 50-year-old woman present with weakness in her upper arms. She has difficulty combing her hair. On examination she is noted to have ragged cuticles and nail fold capillary dilatation.
64. A 60-year-old woman presents with crops of yellow papules on her elbows and knees. Her serum glucose is normal.

THEME: 13
INVESTIGATION OF DERMATOLOGICAL LESIONS

Options

a. Skin scrapings
b. Skin biopsy
c. Wood's light
d. Patch test
e. Urine testing for glucose
f. Full blood count
g. Immunoflourescent staining of skin sample
h. Antinuclear antibodies
i. Clotting screen
j. Chest X-ray
k. Kveim test
l. Mantoux test
m. ESR

For each of the situations/conditions given below, choose the one most appropriate/discriminatory option from above. The options may be used once, more than once, or not at all

Questions

65. A 7-year-old girl presents with an itchy rash in her elbow creases and behind her knees. Lichenification is seen in both the elbow and knee flexures.
66. A 10-year-old boy presents with areas of scaling and hair loss. On examination, there are areas of crusting on the scalp and matting of the hair.
67. A 33-year-old female presents with a facial rash and a rash on the back of her hands. She is notes to have a

maculopapilar rash over her forehead, nose and cheeks and a blue-red discolouration of the back of her hands.

68. A 40-year-old man presents with areas of erythema and scaling of the skin of the groin and perianal region.
69. A 65-year-old man presents with irritation and erythema of the skin and blister formation. The blisters are over the legs and are tense.

THEME: 14
INVESTIGATION OF ALLERGIES

Options

a. Skin prick testing
b. Patch testing
c. Serum IgE levels
d. RAST
e. Oral challenge testing
f. Measure C1 and C4 levels
g. IM adrenaline 1:1000+piriton treatment
h. Inspect for nasal polyps.

For each of the situations/conditions given below, choose the one most appropriate/discriminatory option from above. The options may be used once, more than once, or not at all

Questions

70. A 30-year-old man presents with nasal blockage and watery nasal discharge. He states that symptoms are worse at work. The floors are carpeted, and there is central heating. On examination, he has oedematous and pale nasal inferior turbinates.
71. A 20-year-old female is started on penicillin for acute tonsillitis. She develops stridor and generalised rash.
72. A 10-year-old boy presents with abdominal pain and bloating after eating shellfish.
73. A 12-year-old boy with cystic fibrosis complains of bilateral nasal blockage and mouth breathing.
74. A 30-year-old woman presents with recurrent attacks of cutaneous swelling of her face. These episodes seem to be triggered by stress. There is no associated urticaria or pruritis.

THEME: 15
THE TREATMENT OF SKIN CONDITIONS

Options

a. Topical coal tar
b. Topical steroids
c. Clotrimazole
d. Erythromycin
e. Adrenaline
f. Oral prednisolone
g. Dapsone
h. Oxytetracycline
i. Cetrimide
j. Acyclovir
k. Oral nystatin

For each of the situations/conditions given below, choose the one most appropriate/discriminatory option from above. The options may be used once, more than once, or not at all

Questions

75. A 24-year-old man presents with multiple silver-scaly lesions over the extensor surfaces of his elbows and knees. He also has nail pitting and arthropathy of the terminal interphalangeal joints.
76. An 18-year-old female presents with an itch rash along the flexor surfaces of her elbows and knees. Scaling and weeping vesicles are features.
77. A 23-year-old female with Hodgkin's disease presents with small, white mucosal flecks in the mouth that can be wiped off.
78. A 50-year-old man presents with flaccid bullae over the limbs and trunk following a course of pencillamine for his rheumatoid arthritis.
79. A 20-year-old hairdresser presents with itchy vesicles on her palms.

THEME: 16
SKIN AND SYSTEMIC DISEASES

Options

a. Generalised vitiligo.
b. Localized vitiligo.
c. Telangiectasia.
d. Erythroderma.
e Papulosquamous lesions of palms and soles.
f. Scarring alopecia.
g. Yellow coloured papules.
h. Acanthosis nigricans.
i. Folliculitis.
j. Pyderma gangrenosum.
k. Photosensitivity.
l. Cutaneous vasculitis.

For each of the situations/conditions given below, choose the one most appropriate/discriminatory option from above. The options may be used once, more than once, or not at all.

Questions

80. SLE.
81. Diabetes mellitus.
82. Tuberculoid leprosy.
83. Scleroderma.
84. Sulfa drugs.
85. Hyperlipoproteinemia.
86. Secondary syphilis.
87. Obesity.
88. Rheumatoid arthritis.
89. Henoch-Schonlein purpura.

THEME: 17
ASSOCIATION OF SYSTEMIC DISEASE AND SKIN LESIONS

Options

a. Erythema chronicum migrans
b. Erythema multiforme

c. Pretibial myxoedema
d. Dermatitis herpetiformis
e. Livedo (a cutaneous vasculitis)
f. Dermatomyositis
g. Bazin's disease
h. Dermatitis artefacta
i. Alopecia areata
j. Mycosis Fungoids
k. Bowen's disease
l. Paget's disease
m. Rodent ulcer
n. Café au lait spots

Questions

90. Addison's disease
91. Cutaneous T-cell lymphoma
92. Coeliac disease
93. Hyperthyroidism
94. Tuberculosis
95. Polyarteritis nodosa
96. Mycoplasma pneumonia
97. Lyme disease
98. Von Recklinghausen disease
99. Bronchial carcinoma

THEME: 18
DIAGNOSIS OF SKIN MANIFESTATIONS OF SYSTEMIC DISEASES

Options

a. Erythema nodosum
b. Erythema multiforme
c. Erythema marginatum
d. Erythema chronicum migrans
e. Vitiligo
f. Pyoderma gangrenosum
g. Acquired icthyosis
h. Necobiosis lipoidica

i. Dermatitis herpetiformis
j. Acanthosis nigricans
k. Pretibial muxoedema

For each of the situations/conditions given below, choose the one most appropriate/discriminatory option from above. The options may be used once, more than once, or not at all

Questions

100. A 53-year-old female presents with proptosis, heat intolerance and red oedematous swellings over the lateral malleoli which progress to thickened oedema.
101. A 45-year-old man presents with a shiny area on his shins with yellowish skin and telangiectasia. He also suffers from areas of fat necrosis.
102. A 55-year-old female who is advised to eat a gluten free diet presents with itchy blisters in groups on her knees, elbows and scalp.
103. A 30-year-old man suffering from Crohn's disease presents with a pustule on his leg with a tender red-blue necrotic edge.
104. A 15-year-old female presents with fever and mouth ulcers. She is also noted to have target lesions with a central blister on her palms and soles.

THEME: 19
ASSOCIATION OF SKIN LESIONS AND SPECIFIC DISEASE

Options

a. Hyperthyroidism
b. Diabetes Mellitus
c. Liver disease
d. Ceoliac disease
e. Hypogonadism
f. Carcinoma of tail of pancreas
g. Measles
h. Deep vein thrombosis
i. Psoriasis

j. Leptospirosis
k. Borrelia duttoni infection

Questions

105. A fit 55-year-old gentleman complains of recurrent episodes of seeing visible veins on his body which are tender. He has started to loose weight and attributes this to his diarrhoea. The consultant dermatologist thinks he has thrombophlebitis migrans.
106. A 49-year-old woman complains of itchy blisters .which are occurring in groups on her knees and elbows.The itch is becoming unbearable and she is contemplating suicide. She responds to 180 mg Dapsone within 48 hours of treatment.
107. A Welsh farmer with malaise and arthralgia is increasingly anxious about a skin lesion which started as a paule (Diameter approx 1 mm)which has progressed to a red ring(Diameter approx 50 mm) with central fading.
108. A 42-year-old man who reports a loss in weight presents with a shiny erythematous lesion on her shin. Its edges appear yellowish and are beginning to ulcerate with undermining. She says it started as a pustule sometime ago. Her blood glucose is 5.3 mmol/l.
109. A 32-year-old woman complains of palpitations and is found to have red oedematous swellings above both lateral malleoli which are beginning to affect her feet. She is found to have digital cluubing and periorbital puffiness.

THEME: 20
CUTANEOUS LESIONS ASSOCIATED WITH GASTROINTESTINAL CONDITION

Options

a. Carcinoid.
b. Glucagonoma.
c. Crohn's disease.
d. Gluten enteropathy.
e Ulcerative colitis.

f. Acute pancreatitis.
g. Malabsorption syndrome.
h. Gastric adenocarcinoma.

For each of the situations/conditions given below, choose the one most appropriate/discriminatory option from above. The options may be used once, more than once, or not at all.

Questions

110. Erythema nodosum.
111. Pyoderma gangrenosum.
112. Acanthosis nigricans.
113. Nodular fat necrosis.
114. Dermatitis herpetiformis.

THEME: 21
SIDE EFFECTS OF DRUGS ON SKIN

Options

a. Dystrophic nail changes.
b. Gram-negative folliculitis.
c. Black pigmentation of face.
d. Erythema nodosum.
e. Morbilliform eruption in patients with AIDS.
f. Gingival hyperplasia.
g. Reactions in patients with nasal polyps.

For each of the situations/conditions given below, choose the one most appropriate/discriminatory option from above. The options may be used once, more than once, or not at all.

Questions

115. Bleomycin.
116. Chloroquine.
117. Birth control pills.
118. Tetracycline.
119. Sulfamethoxazole and trimethoprim.

THEME: 22
DIAGNOSIS OF ERYTHEMA

Options

a. Erythema ab igne.
b. Rosacea.
c. Erythema annulare centrifugum.
d. Erythema nodosum.
e. Dermato myositis.
f. Erythema induratum.

For each of the situations/conditions given below, choose the one most appropriate/discriminatory option from above. The options may be used once, more than once, or not at all.

Questions

120. Associated with tuberculosis and present symmetrical deep seated painless red nodules on the legs.
121. Appears on extensor surfaces of legs/arms and Streptococcal infection, barbiturate and sulphonamide ingestion are some of the causes.
122. Appears on legs of women due to prolonged exposure to heat.
123. Follows bite by Ixodes.
124. Commonly associated over telangiectasia.

THEME: 23
DIAGNOSIS OF BLISTERING

Options

a. Trauma
b. Impetigo
c. Herpes zoster
d. Erythema multiforme
e. Insect bites
f. Fixed drug eruption
g. Dermatitis herpetiformis
h. Porphyria cutanea tarda

i. Epidermolysis bullosa
j. Pemphigoid
k. Pemphigus
l. Steven-Johnson syndrome

For each of the situations/conditions given below, choose the one most appropriate/discriminatory option from above. The options may be used once, more than once, or not at all

Questions

125. A 65-year-old woman has multiple tense blisters with underlying erythema, which started on her arms and legs and now involves her trunk. Skin biopsy shows a split at the level of the basement membrane.
126. A 25-year-old man with a history of diarrhoea and weight loss has a blistering rash on his buttocks and elbows with marked pruitus.
127. A 55-year-old woman was recently diagnosed with breast cancer. She now has a 2-day history of painful blistering eruption, which effects a band of skin on the left side of her back.
128. An 18-year-old man with diabetes has a 2-day history of painful blisters on his left cheek. When the blisters heal they leave a yellow crust on the skin.
129. A 25-year-old man has had a recent sore throat for which he was given a course of antibiotics. He now has multiple blisters on his limbs. The blisters have central pallor and there is pruritus. His mouth is unaffected.
130. A 68-year-old Asian woman has multiple blisters on her trunk and a few on her limbs. The blisters are fragile and most have ruptured, leaving erthematous scaly patches. Pressure on an intact blister seems to cause it to spread.

THEME: 24
FACIAL APPEARANCE

Options

a. Acne rosacea
b. Addison's disease

c. Chloasma
d. Discoid lupus erythamatosus
e. Lupus pernio
f. Lupus vulgaris
g. Mitral stenosis
h. Peutz-Jeghers syndrome
i. Rhinophyma
j. Sarcoidosis
k. Seborrhoeic determatitis
l. Systemic lupus erythematosus

For each of the situations/conditions given below, choose the one most appropriate/discriminatory option from above. The options may be used once, more than once, or not at all

Questions

131. A 25-year-old man with excessive dandruff and a pruritic erythematous rash affecting his eyebrows, ears scalp and lateral margins of the nose.
132. A 35-year-old woman with a malar butterfly rash complains of a dry mouth and joint pains.
133. A 40-year-old woman with a diffuse, purple-red infiltration if the nose and cheeks. She has had a persistent dry cough, mild dyspnoea, weight loss and malaise for over a year. Chest examination appears normal.
134. A patient presents to the A&E department with recurrent colicky abdominal pain. There are a number of small brownish-black macules affecting the perioral skin and oral mucosa.
135. A 45-year-old man presents with a persistent reddish papulopustular rash affecting the cheeks, nose, forehead and chin. The nose appears bulbous and craggy.

THEME : 25
DIAGNOSIS OF SCALES AND PLAQUES

Options

a. Psoriasis.
b. Eczema.

c. Fungal.
d. Seborrhoeic dermatitis.
e Seborrhoeic keratosis.
f. Erythema multiforme.
g. None of the above.

For each of the situations/conditions given below, choose the one most appropriate/discriminatory option from above. The options may be used once, more than once, or not at all.

Questions

136. A 29-year-old develops multiple plaques, which are not well demarcated. The lesions are markedly itchy and symmetrical.
137. A 54-year-old woman develops generalised plaques. The lesions are well demarcated and symmetrical. There is no itch.
138. Active erythematous scaly edge with central scarring.

THEME: 26
PRURITUS

Options

a. Chronic renal failure
b. Dermatitis herpetiformis
c. Eczema
d. Iron deficiency
e. Lichen planus
f. Liver disease
g. Lymphoma
h. Old age
i. Polycythaemia
j. Pregnancy
k. Scabies
l. Thyroid disease

For each of the situations/conditions given below, choose the one most appropriate/discriminatory option from above. The options may be used once, more than once, or not at all.

Questions

139. A 55-year-old woman presents complaining of oral soreness exacerbated by spicy foods and a pruritic, cutaneous rash principally affecting her shins and the flexor surfaces of her wrists.
140. A 30-year-old man presents with groups of small intensely itchy vesicles affecting the skin on his knees, elbows, buttocks and scalp.
141. A 55-year-old woman presents with recurrent headaches, intermittent visual disturbances, angina and Raynaud's phenomenon. She has been troubled by a generalized itch that is worse after a hot bath. Examination reveals splenomegaly and bruises.
142. A 19-year-old man is seen in clinic with painless cervical lymphadenopathy initially noticed by his girlfriend. He has been feeling lethargic for some time with nigh sweats and itchy skin.
143. A 70-year-old woman complains of generalized itch, tiredness and shortness of breath on exercise. On examination she appears pale, and thin with brittle, spoon shaped nails.

THEME: 27
HAIR LOSS

Options

a. Alopecia areata
b. Androgentic alopecia
c. Colchicine
d. Hypothyroidism
e. Iron deficiency
f. Lichen planus
g. Lupus erythematosus
h. Malnutrition
i. Scalp ringworm
j. Secondary syphilis
k. Telofen effluvium
l. Traumatic

For each of the situations/conditions given below, choose the one most appropriate/discriminatory option from above. The options may be used once, more than once, or not at all.

Questions

144. A 55-year-old woman is complaining about patchy hair loss with localised areas of erythema scaling and scarring affecting the scalp. She has a sore mouth and a skin rash affecting the flexor surfaces of her wrists and shins.
145. A 20-year-old man presents with sharply defined non-erythematous patches of baldness on his scalp. His eyebrows and beard are all affected and examination of the individual hairs show that they taper towards the scalp.
146. Three months after experiencing a severe illness with high fevers an 18-year-old man notices excessive numbers of hair in hairbrush and on his pillow.
147. A 50-year-old woman notices some diffuse thinning of her hair with bitemporal recession.
148. A 65-year-old woman presents with thinning hair, loss of the outer third of her eyebrows and lethargy.

THEME: 28
DIAGNOSIS OF PREMALIGNANT DISEASE

Options

a. Erythroplasia of querat
b. Marjolins ulcer
c. Malignant melanoma
d. Pytriasis versicolor
e. Dermatofibroma
f. Lentigo maligna
g. Basal cell carcinoma
h. Porokeratosis
i. Squamous cell carcinoma
j. Solar keratosis
k. Pyogenic granuloma
l. Lupus vulgaris

m. Psoriasis
n. Seborrhoiec keratosis
o. Bowen's disease

Questions

149. A 56-year-old man who works in Australia for most of the year presents with cutaneous scaling on his arms and forehead. There is no history of progression, induration and no obvious ulceration is seen on examination.
150. A retired 55-year-old man who worked in an arsenic factory presents with a flat scaly, red crusted plaque on his right hand. He says it is progressively increased in size.
151. A 45-year-old woman presents with multiple marked brown lesions on the forehead and limbs.
152. A 36-year-old woman presents with multiple scaly lesions on the upper trunk and back,, which seem to disappear and recur.
153. A 56-year-old man presents with a shallow ulcerative lesion on the right cheek. It has pearly rolled margins.
154. A 65-year-old uncircumcised man is found to have a red scaly lesion on his penis. The consultant dermatologist confirms it is Bowen's disease.

THEME: 29
INVESTIGATION OF SKIN NODULES

Options

a. Curettage
b. Antinuclear antibodies
c. Microscopy
d. Chest X-ray
e. Biopsy
f. None; only clinical features
g. HbSAg
h. Renal angiogram
i. Mesenteric angiogram
j. Full blood count

k. Bone marrow biopsy
l. Serum uric acid
m. Lipid profile
n. Serology

For each of the situations/conditions given below, choose the one most appropriate/discriminatory option from above. The options may be used once, more than once, or not at all.

Questions

155. A 53-year-old man complains of reddish brown nodules on both his elbows.
156. A middle-aged man complains of swellings in his ear. On physical examination you find numerous white lesions, some of which are ulcerated and discharging a cheesy white material.
157. A middle-aged housewife presents with persistent non-tender white nodules on her back.
158. A 42-year-old woman complains of nodule on her face. Initially it was small and round. It has since grown into a pearly and translucent papule.
159. A 38-year-old man presents with fever, arthralgia and hypertension. He complains of numbness in his legs. You note erythematous ulcerating nodules along the line of various arteries.

THEME: 30
MANAGEMENT OF SKIN COMPLAINTS

Options

a. Topical steroids
b. Vascular exploration
c. Surgical stripping
d. Swiss roll operation
e. Cyclophosphamide
f. Combination chemotherapy
g. Radiotherapy
h. Azathioprine
i. Benzylpenicillin

j. Penicillin-V
k. Phrophylactic penicillin G
l. Good personal hygiene
m. Avoidance of trauma
n. Intermittent compression

For each of the situations/conditions given below, choose the one most appropriate/discriminatory option from above. The options may be used once, more than once, or not at all

Questions

160. A healthy young woman complains of swelling in the right leg. At first the swelling was only noticeable after exercise, but recently it has become more permanent. On examination you find the lower right leg to be larger and firmer than the left.
161. You are called to examine an immigrant family form East Africa. An adolescent boy has an enormous facial swelling. He also complains of back pain, leg pain and painful micturition.
162. A 74-year-old man complains of back pain and fatigue. His Hb is low, his ESR high and his urine contains abnormal proteins.
163. A young man presents with chronic fever and malaise. He has a fish like scaly rash over his upper abdomen. His cervical lymph nodes are painless, rubbery and discrete.
164. A middle-aged naturist complains of a swollen and painful right leg. The leg first bothered her after a beach holiday in the summer. You find numerous calf nodes to be tender and enlarged.

Fourteen

Surgery

THEME: 1
DIAGNOSIS OF SHOCK

Options

a. Cardiogenic shock
b. Hypovolemic shock
c. Anaphylactic shock
d. Adreno cortical failure
e. Vasovagal faint
f. Septic shock

For each of the statements/situations given below, choose the one most appropriate/discriminatory option.

Questions

1. Extremities may be warm and will perfused.
2. Drug of choice is adrenaline.
3. Patient on treatment for meningococcal meningitis suddenly develops shock.
4. Patient goes into shock while doing paracervical block during labor.
5. Cardiac index < 2 liters/minute/m^2.
6. High incidence of pulmonary failure.
7. Icterus is common.
8. Hypotension with high cardiac output.
9. Cardiac index (litres/minutes/m^2) 2.2
   BP (mm Hg) 80/55
   Pulse 140
   CVP (cm water) 1.5
   Blood Lactate (mg/100 mg) 19

	Blood pH	7.1
	PCO_2 (torr)	38
	PCV	36
10.	Cardiac index (litres/minutes/m^2)	5.2
	BP (mm Hg)	80/55
	Pulse	140
	CVP (cm water)	6.0
	Blood Lactate (mg/100 mg)	16
	Blood pH	7.7
	PCO_2 (torr)	29
	PCV	42

THEME: 2
RISK FACTORS FOR DEEP VEIN THROMBOSIS

Options

a. Dehydration
b. Hormone replacement therapy
c. Immobility
d. Inherited clotting abnormality
e. Malignancy
f. Multiple myeloma
g. Polycythaemia rubra vera
h. Pregnancy
i. Varicose veins

For each of the situations/conditions given below, choose the one most appropriate/discriminatory option from above. The options may be used once, more than once, or not at all.

Questions

11. A 60-year-old man presents with malaise and back pain which has been present for three months. He is found to have significant proteinuria
12. A 30-year-old woman presents with a three month history of amenorrhoea.
13. A 60-year-old man with a plethoric appearance presents with pleuritic chest pain. He has a palpable splenomegaly.
14. A 70-year-old man presents with back pain and jaundice.

15. A 25-year-old woman with a family history of deep vein thrombosis was prescribed a combined oral contraceptive pill six months ago and has not missed any tablets.

THEME: 3
PROGRESSION OF BREAST CARCINOMA

Options

a. Asthma
b. Axillary recurrence
c. Bonemarrow infiltration
d. Bony metastasis
e. Cerebral
f. Hyper calcemia
g. Left ventricular failure
h. Liver metastasis
i. Local occurrence
j. Lymphagitis carcinomatosis
k. Peritoneal recurrence
l. Pleural effusion
m. Spinal cord compression

For each of the situations/conditions given below, choose the one most appropriate/discriminatory option from above. The options may be used once, more than once, or not at all.

Questions

16. A 56-year-old woman who underwent mastectomy for a breast tumour four-year-oldago now complains of increasing breathlessness. On examination of her respiratory system she is noticed to have decreased movement of the left hemithorax which is dull to percussion and has absent breath sounds.
17. A 60-year-old woman is admitted to the Accident& Emergency Department having fallen in the street. She is complaining of pain in the right hip and the right lower limb is lying in external rotation. She had breast conserving surgery6 months back.

18. A 43-year-old woman treated two-year-oldago for grade 3 axillary node positive breast carcinoma presents with increasing confusion, headache and vomiting. On examination she is drowsy but has no focal neurological signs. She does have blurring of optic disc margins.
19. A 35-year-old woman treated one-year-ago for abreast cancer with 12/20 nodes positive presents with a two day history of increasing confusion. She is drowsy and disoriente. Her husband reports that she has been complaining of severe thirst for past week.

THEME: 4
DIAGNOSIS OF THROMBOEMBOLISM

Options

a. Inferior vena cava obstruction
b. Superior vena cava obstruction
c. Lymph oedema
d. Deep vein thrombosis
e. Pneumonia
f. Bronchiectasis
g. Aortic stenosis
h. Mitral stenosis
i. Pulmonary embolism
j. Ruptured Baker's cyst
k. Venous insufficiency

For each of the situations/conditions given below, choose the one most appropriate/discriminatory option from above. The options may be used once, more than once, or not at all

Questions

20. A 26-year-old female patient security who has been taking the combined oral contraceptive pill for six months. There is no calf tenderness but the skin over her legs is itchy and pigmented.
21. A 31-year-old woman who has been taking the oral contraceptive pill for six months is brought to the Accident & Emergency Dept. in a state of collapse. Her blood pressure is 70/40 and her neck veins are distented.

22. A 40-year-old woman who has complained of joint pain, stiffness and swelling that are worse in the morning for 5-year-oldand is receiving steroids for her illness. She has been off the pill for one-year but now presents with a sudden onset severe right calf pain.
23. A 30-year-old woman who has been taking oral contraceptive pill for six months presents with palpitations and on examination a mid diastolic murmur is found.
24. A 23-year-old woman who has been taking the combined oral contraceptive pill for six months presents with a hiustory of cough producing green sputum and fever over the last two or three days.

THEME: 5
INVESTIGATION OF THROMBOEMBOLIC DISEASE

Options

a. Chest X-ray
b. Coagulation screen
c. Contrast spiral CT scan
d. Digital subtraction angiography
e. Echocardiography
f. Femoral duplex scan
g. MRI scan
h. Platelet count
i. Selective arteriogram
j. Ventilation-perfusion scan

For each of the situations/conditions given below, choose the one most appropriate/discriminatory option from above. The options may be used once, more than once, or not at all.

Questions

25. A 29-year-old woman who has been taking the OC pull for 6 months is brought to A&E in a state of collapse. Her blood pressure is 70/40 and she has raised neck veins.
26. A 23-year-old woman, who has been taking the OC pill for 6 months, presents with bilateral ankle oedema and a tender calf.

27. A 20-year-old woman, who has been taking the OC pill for 5 months present with history of cough, producing green sputum and fever, over the last 2-3 days.
28. A 22-year-old woman, who has been taking the OC pill for 5 months presents with palpitations and on examination has a diastolic murmur and a thrill.

THEME: 6
PREVENTION AND TREATMENT OF THROMBOTIC DISEASE

Options

a. Aspirin
b. Compression stockings
c. Early mobilization
d. Foot pump
e. Subcutaneous unfractioned heparin
f. Subcutaneous LMW heparin
g. IV heparin
h. Warfarin (INR 2-3)
i. Warfarin (INR 3-4.5)
j. Phenindione
k. Thrombolysis
l. Nothing

For each of the situations/conditions given below, choose the one most appropriate/discriminatory option from above. The options may be used once, more than once, or not at all.

Questions

29. A 30-year-old woman is 16 weeks pregnant and develops a painful swollen leg. A femoral vein thrombosis is diagnosed with Doppler ultrasound. She has already been started on IV heparin.
30. A 50-year-old man is admitted for an elective total hip replacement. He has a history of peptic ulcer disease and takes lansoprazole. He is otherwise well. What prophylaxis against thrombosis is indicated?

31. A 70-year-old man is in atrial fibrillation secondary to rheumatic heart disease. Echocardiogram shows a dilated left atrium and mild mitral stenosis only. He has developed a sever rash with Warfarin in the past.
32. A 22-year-old man is admitted for an elective hemorrhoidectomy. He has no other medical problems
33. A 28-year-old woman has had 4 spontaneous abortions, 2 deep vein thrombosis and suffers with migraine. Blood test confirms the presence of anticariolipin antibodies.
34. A 30-year-old woman is 25 weeks pregnant and has collapsed at home, having painful swollen leg for 2 days. She is breathless and cyanosed despite receiving 60% oxygen via a facemask. Her pulse is 130/min, BP 80/40. An urgent echocardiogram shows thrombus in the left pulmonary artery and evidence of heart failure.

THEME: 7
MANAGEMENT OF THROMBOEMBOLIC DISEASE

Options

a. Phlegm microscopy and culture
b. Echocardiography
c. Blood culture
d. Blood transfusion
e. Duplex scan
f. IV bolus of warfarin
g. 20 mg aspirin 12 hourly
h. Coronary Angiography
i. Counselling
j. Streptokinase
k. Protamine sulphate
l. Diathermy
m. Positrol emission tomography
n. Cervical smear
o. Abdominal USG
p. Dilatation and curettage

For each of the situations/conditions given below, choose the one most appropriate/discriminatory option from above. The options may be used once, more than once, or not at all.

Questions

35. A 30-year-old woman who has been taking her OC pills for 9 months is brought to A&E in a state of collapse. Her blood pressure is low and has a loud P2 on auscultation.
36. A 31-year-old woman is being treated for a thromboebolic tendency. The nurse administers dose of subcutaneous heparin and she begins to bleed form the nose and other injection sites.
37. A 26-year-old obese woman present with palpitations. On examination she is febrile and has nail bed flucctuance. He has previously presented with a diastolic murmur of mitral stenosis.
38. A 25-year-old woman, who has been taking the OC pill for 2 months, present with a 3-months history of cough with sputum, fever and night sweats. Her partner dies of RTA.
39. A 16-year-old woman who has been taking the OC pill for 6 months present with complaints of bleeding every month in her pill free days. Her mother died of cervical carcinoma.

THEME: 8
MANAGEMENT OF DEEP VEIN THROMBOSIS

Options

a. Therapeutic heparin (10000 unit intravenous loading dose and 1000 units hourly thereafter as continuous intravenous drip)
b. Prophylactic mini-dose heparin (5000 units subcutaneously every 12 hours).
c. Ligation of the inferior vena cava and gonadal veins.
d. Insertion of a vena caval umbrella.
e. Pulmonary embolectomy by means of cardiopulmonary bypass.

For each of the situations/conditions given below, choose the one most appropriate/discriminatory option from above. The options may be used once, more than once, or not at all.

Questions

40. A 79-year-old woman with a history of phlebitis who is under going hip replacement.
41. A 58-year-old patient with congestive failure who has a pulmonary infarction convincingly shown by perfusion lung scan.
42. A 26-year-old para 9, postpartum female who has sepsis and is producing emboli in spite of therapeutic doses of heparin.
43. A desperately ill 72-year-old man who is producing emboli in spite of heparin therapy, he has a grossly infected abdominal incision six days after right colectomy.
44. A 32-year-old woman who had a massive embolism to right lung 28 hours prior to angiography, when her right ventricular pressure was 30/0.

THEME: 9
CAUSES OF VARICOSE VEINS

Options

a. Pregnancy
b. Ovarian cyst
c. Fibroids
d. Arteriovenous fistula
e. Intra-abdominal malignancy
f. Iliac vein thrombosis
g. Ascites
h. Klippel-Trenaunay syndrome
i. Abdominal lymphandenopathy
j. Retroperitoneal fibrosis
k. Deep vein thrombosis

For each of the situations/conditions given below, choose the one most appropriate/discriminatory option from above. The options may be used once, more than once, or not at all.

Questions

45. A 60-year-old man complains of pain and swelling in the whole of his right leg. Forced plantar flexion of the leg increases the pain. He is noted to have hard muscles of the leg and lipodermatosclerosis.
46. A 30-year-old woman on oral contraceptives presents with dilated tortuous veins crossing her abdomen to join the tributaries of the superior vena cava.
47. A 40-year-old man presents with varicose veins in the lower extremity. He recently underwent orchidectomy for seminoma.
48. A 10-year-old boy presents with tortuous, dilated veins on the lateral side of his left leg. The left leg is slightly longer the right leg.
49. A 55-year-old man complains of a dull ache in the calves, relieved by lying down. He presents with tortuous, dilated veins on the medial aspect of his lower extremities. He is noted to have splenomegaly, clubbing of his fingers, and small testes.

THEME: 10
SIDE EFFETS OF GASTRIC SURGERY

Options

a. Gastrojejunostomy
b. Bilateral truncal vagotomy and hemigastrectomy
c. Total gastrectomy
d. Parietal cell vagotomy
e. Truncal vagotomy and pyloroplasty
f. Selective gastric (total) vagotomy and pyloroplasty
g. Distal hemigastrectomy

For each of the situations/conditions given below, choose the one most appropriate/discriminatory option from above. The options may be used once, more than once, or not at all.

Questions

50. High incidence of vitamin B_{12} malabsorption.
51. Highest incidence of recurrent ulceration.

52. Surgical management of an 80-year-old man with bleeding duodenal ulcer.
53. Necrosis of part of the stomach occurs as complications.
54. Ulcer recurrence rate of less than 1 percent.

THEME: 11
COMPLICATIONS OF TRANSPLANTATION SURGERY

Options

a. Acute tubular necrosis
b. Hyperacute rejection
c. Accelerated acute rejection
d. Acute rejection
e. Chronic rejection

For each of the situations/conditions given below, choose the one most appropriate/discriminatory option from above. The options may be used once, more than once, or not at all.

Questions

55. Occurs at about 7 to 28th day postoperative and is due reduced immunosuppression.
56. No crossmatch compatibility.
57. Effectively treated with high-doses of prednisolone, antilymphocyte globulin.
58. This condition is characterized by progressive vasculopathy in the graft, causing slow decline in function over months or years.
59. Usually temporary, lasting 1-10 days and related to the harvest and preservation of the kidney.
60. Second-set immune response that occurs within the first week of transplantation.

THEME: 12
DIAGNOSIS OF NECK SWELLINGS

Options

a. Squamous cell carcinoma of the larynx
b. Papillary carcinoma

c. Hodgkin's lymphoma
d. Atypical mycobacteria
e. Infected thymic cyst
f. Cystic hygroma
g. Laryngoceles
h. Branchial cyst
i. Dermoid cyst
j. Chordorma
k. Thyroid mass
l. Thyroglossal cyst
m. Chemodectoma
n. Cervical rib

For each of the situations/conditions given below, choose the one most appropriate/discriminatory option from above. The options may be used once, more than once, or not at all.

Questions

61. If 25-year-old female presents with a swelling on the side of the neck since birth. The swelling is situated along the anterior border of the sternocliedomastoid muscle and it is cystic in consistency.
62. Enlarged cervical node, fever, malaise and weight loss.
63. Inflamed mass or draining sinus in the head or neck.
64. Cystic midline swelling over the front of the neck which moves on deglutition and swallowing.
65. Hoarseness, cough and stridor.
66. A midline swelling is felt in the front of the neck in the sub mental triangle. This swelling is soft, indentable and nontransilluminant.
67. Slow growing painless neck mass associated with prior radiation exposure.
68. Patient comes with swelling in the posterior triangle of neck and also complains of pain in the ulnar border of arm.
69. Firm mass felt anterior to sternocleidomastoid muscle which may be pulsatile.
70. Twenty four-year-old male comes with bony hard swelling in front of neck in midline.

THEME: 13
MANAGEMENT OF SKIN TRAUMA

Options

a. Exploration and primary suture
b. Wound excision and primary suture of skin
c. Wound excision and delayed primary grafting
d. Primary grafting
e. Wound excision and primary grafting
f. Wound excision and left open

For each of the situations/conditions given below, choose the one most appropriate/discriminatory option from above. The options may be used once, more than once, or not at all.

Questions

71. Incised wound.
72. Penetrating wounds.
73. Lacerated wounds with skin loss.
74. Crushed and devitalised wounds.
75. Muscle injuries.
76. Lacerated wounds without skin loss.
77. Clean incised wounds with skin loss.

THEME: 14
EXAMINATION OF URINE

Options

a. 1st glass is hazy but 2nd glass is clear.
b. 1st glass is clear but 2nd glass is cloudy.
c. Both glasses are cloudy.
d. 1st glass contains thread.

For each of the situations/conditions given below, choose the one most appropriate/discriminatory option from above. The options may be used once, more than once, or not at all.

Questions

78. Gonorrhea.

79. Urethritis.
80. Diverticulitis.
81. Cystitis.
82. Prostatitis.

THEME: 15
GENITAL ULCER

Options

a. Syphilis.
b. Granuloma inguinale.
c. Genital herpes.
d. Traumatic ulcer.
e. Squamous cell carcinoma.
f. Chancroid.
g. Lymphogranuloma inguinale.

For each of the situations/conditions given below, choose the one most appropriate/discriminatory option from above. The options may be used once, more than once, or not at all.

Questions

83. Painful ulcer with buboes.
84. Firm, indurated, painless ulcer.
85. Painless ulcer with suppurative painful buboes.
86. Punched out ulcer.
87. Raised everted edge.
88. Rolled elevated ulcer.
89. Onset immediately after sexual activity.

THEME: 16
DIAGNOSIS OF ULCERS

Options

a. Ischaemic ulcer
b. Basal cell carcinoma
c. Squamous cell carcinoma
d. Syphillis
e. Tuberculosis

f. Trophic ulcer
g. Venous ulcer
h. Barret's ulcer
i. Behcet's disease
j. Aphthous ulcers

For each of the situations/conditions given below, choose the one most appropriate/discriminatory option from above. The options may be used once, more than once, or not at all.

Questions

90. A 60-year-old man presents with a superficial leg ulcer. The ulcer has a sloping edge, and the skin around the edge is red-blue and almost transparent.
91. A 70-year-old man presents with an ulcer on the right pinna with palpable neck nodes. The edges of the ulcer are everted.
92. A 50-year-old man presents with an ulcer on the left side of his nose. The edges are rolled.
93. A 60-year-old man presents with painful ulcers in the oral mucosa. He underwent cholecystectomy a week prior. The edges are erthematous.
94. A 30-year-old woman presents with painful ulcers of the labia and mouth. She also suffers from arthritis.

THEME: 17
THYROID SWELLING

Options

a. Anaplastic carcinoma.
b. Papillary carcinoma.
c. Medullary carcinoma.
d. Follicular carcinoma.
e. Colloid goitre.
f. Lymphoma.
g. Hashimoto's thyroiditis.
h. Riedel's thyroiditis.
i. De–quervain's thyroiditis.
j. Nodular goitre.
k. Graves' disease.

For each of the situations/conditions given below, choose the one most appropriate/discriminatory option from above. The options may be used once, more than once, or not at all.

Questions

95. Most common cause of thyroid enlargement.
96. Woody hard thyroid swelling, patient was also diagnosed to have primary sclerosing cholangitis, about 1 month back.
97. Patient with history of radiations to neck about 10-year-oldback, now comes with multiple discrete swelling in front of neck.
98. Patient comes with swelling in front of neck which is rapidly progressing. His brother and mother also have neck swelling present for the last 6 years.
99. A 20-years-old girl who had viral URI about 1 month back, now comes with swelling in front of neck. On palpation, the swelling is firm and tender.
100. Patient with a large thyroid swelling. He also complains of diarrhea. His mother died of thyroid cancer.
101. Patient presents with thyroid swelling which has been rapidly progressing for the past 2 months and for last 15 days also complains of dysphagia and hoarseness.
102. Smooth, firm goitre with myxoedema.

THEME: 18
DIAGNOSIS OF SWELLING OF SALIVARY GLANDS

Options

a. Chronic recurrent sialadenitis.
b. Pleomorphic adenoma.
c. Adenolymphoma.
d. Acute bacterial parotitis.
e. Carcinoma of salivary gland.
f. Miculicz disease.
g. Adenoid cystic carcinoma.

For each of the situations/conditions given below, choose the one most appropriate/discriminatory option from above. The options may be used once, more than once, or not at all.

Questions

103. A patient presents with history of swelling in the region of submandibular gland, which becomes prominent and painful on chewing. He also gives history of sour taste in the month on pressing the swelling.
104. A 70-year-old patient comes with swelling in the parotid region for the last 10 years. On palpation the swelling is soft and cystic.
105. A 70-year-old patient comes with swelling in the region of parotid gland for past 18 months. On palpation the swelling is hard.
106. A 70-year-old male patient comes with swelling in parotid region for the last 10 years. On examination swelling involves the lower pole of the gland and is firm in consistency.
107. A patient comes with 6 months history of bilateral parotid swelling which has been progressively increasing. On routine chest X-ray was also found to have perihilar lymphoadenopathy.
108. A 70-year-old male patient comes with 1 month history of facial palsy. O/E a small hard parotid swelling is felt.

THEME: 19
DIAGNOSIS OF RENAL MASS

Options

a. Wilm's tumor.
b. Grawitz tumor.
c. Carcinoma of renal pelvis.
d. Hydronephrosis.
e. Polycystic disease of kidney.
f. Neuroblastoma.

For each of the situations/conditions given below, choose the one most appropriate/discriminatory option from above. The options may be used once, more than once, or not at all.

Questions

109. A 50-year-old male comes with history of hematuria for last 2 months. On examination, a renal mass is felt and left varicocele is also present.
110. A 4-year-old child comes with bilateral abdominal masses. He is otherwise well. On examinations, the masses are tense and cystic.
111. A 3-year-old child comes with bilateral abdominal masses and mild weight loss. On examination, he is also found to be hypertensive.
112. A 50-year-old male comes with history of bilateral abdomen masses. Patient's father who died of an accident also had the same problem.

THEME: 20
TREATMENT OF RENAL CALCULI

Options

a. Percutaneous nephrolithostomy
b. Extracorporeal shockwave lithrotripsy
c. Alkaline diureses
d. Nephrectomy
e. Percutaneous nephrostomy
f. Expectant management
g. Acid diuresis
h. Intravenous antibiotics
i. Peritoneal dialysis

For each of the situations/conditions given below, choose the one most appropriate/discriminatory option from above. The options may be used once, more than once, or not at all.

Questions

113. A 30-year-old pregnant woman present with septicaemia and abdominal pain. Investigations reveal an obstructed right kidney due to a 2 cm calculus. She is commenced on intravenous antibiotics.
114. A 40-year-old man presents with left side renal colic. Intravenous urography show a 1 cm calculus in the upper

third of the ureter. There is no complete obstruction. His symptoms fail to resolve on medical therapy

115. A 20-year-old man presents with renal colic secondary to a 1 cm cystine calculus.
116. A 30-year-old man presents to A&E with a right-sided renal colic. IVU shows a 4 mm calculus in the distal part of the ureter with no complete obstruction.
117. A 40-year-old woman if found to have a staghorn calculus in a non-functioning kidney.
118. A 60-year-old man presents with frequent attacks of left sided renal colic due to a 2.5 cm calculus in the renal pelvis. He has a cardial pacemaker and is known to have a 6 cm aortic aneurysm.

THEME: 21
DIAGNOSIS OF INGUINAL/SCROTAL SWELLING

Options

a. Ectopic testes.
b. Undescended tastes.
c. Inguinal hernia.
d. Hydrocele.
e. Cyst of epididymis.
f. Testicular tumor.
g. Genital tuberculosis.

For each of the situations/conditions given below, choose the one most appropriate/discriminatory option from above. The options may be used once, more than once, or not at all.

Questions

119. Swelling present only on coughing and straining.
120. Cystic scrotal swelling with no palpable testes.
121. Cystic scrotal swelling and testes is felt separately.
122. Testes palpable in inguinal canal.
123. Testes palpable in superficial inguinal pouch.
124. Main complication is trauma.
125. Main complication is cryptorchidism.
126. Solid scrotal swelling, confined to testes.
127. Solid scrotal swelling, involving epididymis.

THEME: 22
ANTIBIOTIC PROPHYLAXIS OF SURGICAL PATIENTS

Options

a. Angiography
b. Bronchoscopy
c. Colles fracture
d. Dental treatment of a cardiac patient
e. Dislocated shoulder
f. Emergency appendicectomy
g. Heart valve replacement
h. Sigmoid colectomy
i. Splenectomy
j. Thyroidectomy

For each of the situations/conditions given below, choose the one most appropriate/discriminatory option from above. The options may be used once, more than once, or not at all.

Questions

128. 3 gm sachet of amoxycillin one hour before the procedure.
129. Three days of intravenous broad spectrum antibiotics beginning with induction of anaesthesia.
130. Clear fluids by mouth and two sachets of sodium picosulphate on the day before the operation plus broad spectrum intravenous antibiotics at induction.
131. Long-term oral penicillin and immunisation against pneumococcal infection.
132. One dose of metronidazole.

THEME: 23
PROPHYLACTIC ANTIBIOTIC REGIMENS

Options

a. Ampicillin 500 mg Q 8h IV x 3 doses.
b. Metronidazole suppository 1 gm Q 8h x 3 doses
   And
   Cefuroxime 1.5 gm Q 8h IV x 3 doses.

c. Metronidazole iv 1 gm Q 8h x 3 doses
And
Cefuroxime 1.5 gm Q 8h IV x 3 doses.
d. Co-amoxiclav 1.2 gm IV x 1 dose.

For each of the situations/conditions given below, choose the one most appropriate/discriminatory option from above. The options may be used once, more than once, or not at all.

Questions

133. Vascular surgery.
134. Appendicectomy.
135. Biliary surgery.
136. Colorectal surgery.

THEME: 24
DIAGNOSIS OF DERMAL TUMORS

Options

a. Capillary hemangioma.
b. Salmon pink patch.
c. Strawberry nevus.
d. Port wine stain.
e. Campbell–de–morgan spots.
f. Cavernous hemangioma.
g. Sclerosing angioma.
h. Hemangio sarcoma.
i. Hereditary hemorrhagic telengiectasia.

For each of the situations/conditions given below, choose the one most appropriate/discriminatory option from above. The options may be used once, more than once, or not at all.

Questions

137. Blemish on head or neck of a newborn child which rapidly disappears spontaneously.
138. Pigmented tumor of skin which results from fibrosis of capillary hemangioma. On palpation, it is hard in consistency.

139. Number of bluish red or dark blue nodules scattered over extremities. Nodules spread centrally along the limb may ulcerate and can metastasise to liver and lung.
140. Congenital capillary malformations usually present at birth.
141. Dark red stain present from birth, flush with the skin of face, lips and buccal mucosa. This lesion has no tendency to regress.
142. Vasculo endothelial malignant tumor. It may also involve liver in workers exposed to vinyl chloride.
143. Malignancy aggressive tumor of blood vessels associated with early metastats and poor prognosis.
144. A 70-year-old male comes with bright red aggregates of dilated capillaries which can be emptied on pressing.

THEME: 25
DIAGNOSIS OF DERMAL SWELLINGS

Options

a. Epidermoid cyst (Sebaceous cyst).
b. Cock's peculiar tumor.
c. Pott's puffy tumor.
d. Dermoid.
e. Verruca vulgaris.
f. Keratoacanthoma (Molluscum sebaceum).
g. Ganglion.
h. Meningocele.

For each of the situations/conditions given below, choose the one most appropriate/discriminatory option from above. The options may be used once, more than once, or not at all.

Questions

145. Soft, cystic scalp swelling of 6 months duration. Fluctuation is present. The centre of the swelling is adherent to the skin with a bluish punctum.
146. A 50-year-old male with a rapidly growing nodule with a characteristic central crater filled by a Keratin plug.

147. A 50-year-old male with a long standing swelling over the scalp. The swelling has undergone recent increase in size with ulceration over the surface. The swelling is cystic in consistency.
148. Swelling in the occipital region of a 2 months old child. This swelling is transilluminant and becomes prominent on crying.
149. Cystic, subcutaneous swelling on the flexor aspect of fingers.
150. Patient with history of fever, headache and swelling over the scalp. On examination there is a diffuse swelling with redness over the scalp.

THEME: 26
DIAGNOSIS OF EPIDERMAL TUMORS

Options

a. Papilloma.
b. Seborrheic keratosis (basal cell papilloma).
c. Senile keratosis.
d. Bowen's disease.
e. Squamous cell carcinoma (epithelioma).
f. Basal cell carcinoma (rodent ulcer).

For each of the situations/conditions given below, choose the one most appropriate/discriminatory option from above. The options may be used once, more than once, or not at all.

Questions

151. Very slow growing, red scaly plague. It represents carcinoma-in-situ. It may be mistaken for psoriatic plague.
152. Ulcer with raised everted edges and central scab.
153. Pendunc, papillary lesion often pigmented with melanin.
154. A 70-year-old male with small, hard, brown scaly tumor on forehead.
155. Lesion with raised and rolled edges which grows slowly with central ulceration and scabbing.

THEME: 27
CUTANEOUS MANIFESTATIONS OF CARCINOMA BREAST

Options

a. Elephantiasis chirugens.
b. Skin ulceration.
c. Paget's disease.
d. Peau de orange.
e. Cancer en cuircasse.
f. Nipple retraction.
g. Skin dimpling.
h. Lymphangio sarcoma.

For each of the situations/conditions given below, choose the one most appropriate/discriminatory option from above. The options may be used once, more than once, or not at all.

Questions

156. Involment of the lactiferous ducts by the tumor cells.
157. Lymphedema of the upper extremity following radical mestectomy and radiotherapy.
158. Involvement of the ligaments of Cooper.
159. Tethering of the skin by the ducts of the involved sweat glands along with cutaneous lymphatic edema.
160. Multiple metastatic nodules on the chest wall.

THEME: 28
INVESTIGATIONS

Options

a. CT scan brain.
b. Skull X-rays.
c. S. calcium.
d. Blood glucose.
e. S. amylase.
f. Urine pregnancy test and U/S pelvis.
g. U/S abdomen.

h. CT abdomen.
i. FBC.
j. Plain X-ray abdomen—erect.
k. Plain X-ray abdomen—supine.

For each of the statements/situations given below, choose the one most appropriate/discriminatory option. The options can be used once, more than once, or not at all.

Questions

161. A 12-year-old child with right lower abdomen pain since morning and is refusing to eat his favorite breakfast meals—developed vomiting and diarrhea since midmorning and was brought to the hospital at 4 p.m. On examination furred tongue, foetor present. There is tenderness in the right iliac fossa.
162. A 24-year-old lady with history of irregular periods with sudden onset of severe lower abdomen pain and pain at the shoulder tips. Her LMP was 6 weeks ago.
163. A 50-year-old man, known diabetic and alcoholic, was brought to the A&E with h/o sudden onset gastric pain for 8 hours following an alcoholic binge. On examination alert, BP is 100/70, PR 110/m. Abdomen—signs of peritonism present.
164. A 20-year-old man who was brought to the A&E, with history of fall from twowheeler 2 hours ago. He was drowsy and disoriented for 5-10 minutes after the fall. On examination BP 130/80, PR 68/m, GCS 15/15, small hematoma over the left temporoparietal region.
165. A 60-year-old man with history of abdominal pain, vomiting, abdominal distention, rebound tenderness present. Bowel sounds sluggish.
166. 23-year-old, known IDDM patient—underwent operation for papillary carcinoma of thyroid at 7.30 a.m. in the morning. During ward rounds at 8.00 p.m., she is drowsy but well oriented. On tapping over the parotid region, the facial muscles twitch.

THEME: 29
COMPLICATIONS OF THYROID SURGERY

Options

a. Thyroid storm.
b. Unilateral recurrent laryngeal nerve palsy.
c. Hypocalcemia.
d. Reactionary hemorrhage.
e. External laryngeal nerve palsy.
f. Bilateral recurrent nerve palsy.
g. Tracheomalacia.

For each of the statements/situations given below, choose the one most appropriate/discriminatory option. The options can be used once, more than once, or not at all.

Questions

167. A 60-year-old patient recovering from a surgery of toxic goitre is found to be hypotensive, cyanosed in the recovery room. On examination her neck is tense. There is oozing of blood from the drain.
168. There is sudden onset of breathlessness and stridor within a few minutes of extubation after thyroidectomy. The patient had a long standing goitre for which he had undergone surgery. The cords were moving well at the time of extubation.
169. A 40-year-old patient follows up in the consulting room of a surgeon complaining of tingling numbness, paresthesias, inspiratory stridor and involuntary spasm of the upper extremities. She has undergone surgery for carcinoma thyroid a week ago.
170. After undergoing a hemithyroidectomy, a 30-year-old patient complains of hoarseness of voice. IDL examination reveals an immobile vocal cord on one side.
171. A 20-year-old pop singer complains of inability to raise the pitch of her voice. She attributes this to the thyroid surgery she underwent a few months back.

THEME: 30
COMPLICATIONS OF SPLENECTOMY

Options

a. Acute gastric dilatation.
b. Reactionary hemorrhage.
c. Overwhelming postsplenectomy infection.
d. Subphrenic abscess.
e. Hemetemesis.
f. Deep vein thrombosis.
g. Left lower lobe atelectasis.

For each of the statements/situations given below, choose the one most appropriate/discriminatory option. The options can be used once, more than once, or not at all.

Questions

172. On the third postoperation day after splenectomy, patient develops bronchospasm, dyspnea and oxygen saturation is decreased. The air entry on the left side is reduced.
173. A 26-year-old male has been operated for abdominal trauma, splenectomy was done. On the third pos-t operation day the patient developed acute abdominal pain and upper abdominal distention, with hypotension. On insertion of a ryles tube 2 liters of coffee ground fluid was aspirated.
174. A 25-year-old patient was operated for staging laparotomy for lymphoma few months back. He presents with high fever, dyspnea, tachynea and hypotension. Sputum examination reveals pneumococcal organisms.
175. A splenectomised patient develops fever on the sixth post operation day and is noted to have swelling in the lower limbs.
176. Patient has undergone splenectomy complains of fever on the sixth postoperation day. This fever is persistent and is associated with upper abdominal pain. On examination, there is intercostal tenderness and redness over the left side chest wall.

THEME: 31
COMPLICATIONS OF ACUTE PANCREATITIS

Options

a. Pseudocyst.
b. ARDS.
c. Fat necrosis.
d. Coagulopathy.
e. Colonic necrosis.
f. Hemetemesis.
g. Pancreatitis abscess.
h. Chronic pancreatitis.

For each of the statements/situations given below, choose the one most appropriate/discriminatory option. The options can be used once, more than once, or not at all.

Questions

177. Patient admitted to the ICU with acute pancreatitis starts developing abdominal distension, pain and high fever. His abdomen is tender and there is absence of peristaltic sounds. His total count is 30,000 with polymorpho leucocystosis. CT abdomen reveals irregularity over the pancreas with gas shadows in the phlegmon.
178. Patient with acute pancreatitis has persistent tachycardia, abdominal distention and ileus. His total WBC counts are raised. X-ray of the abdomen reveals free gas under diaphragm.
179. A 60-year-old alcoholic presents with acute pancreatitis. On admission to the ICU his oxygen saturation is persistently low. His pO_2 fails to rise inspite of positive pressure ventilation. His chest X-ray reveals multiple fluffy shadows.
180. A 50-year-old alcoholic presents with history of recurrent episodes of abdominal pain and anorexia precipitated by alcohol binges. Five-year-oldago he was diagnosed to have acute pancreatitis.

181. A patient of pancreatitis after recovery from his acute attack presents with a large epigastric swelling which shows transmitted pulsations. He has a persistently raised amylase levels.
182. Often requires urgent operation.
183. Operative internal drainage contraindicated.

THEME: 32
COMPLICATIONS OF GALLSTONES

Options

a. Obstructive jaundice.
b. Acute pancreatitis.
c. Emphysematous cholecystitis.
d. Carcinoma of gallbladder.
e. Mucocele.
f. Gallstone ileus.
g. Chronic pancreatitis

For each of the statements/situations given below, choose the one most appropriate/discriminatory option. The options can be used once, more than once, or not at all.

Questions

184. A 50-year-old patient presents with acute onset of pain in the upper abdomen with vomiting. His abdomen is tender and guarding present and there is periumbilical echymoses.
185. A 34-year-old female patient presents with a smooth globular lump in the right hypochondrium of a weeks duration. She gives history of attacks of pain in the right hypochondrium. Ultrasound examination reveals an impacted stone in the Hartmann's pouch.
186. A 30-year-old lady presents with history of dark coloured urine and pale stools. There is history of colicky upper abdominal pain for the past few weeks. On examination, there is mild hepatomegaly and the gallbladder is not palpable. Serum alkaline phosphatase levels are raised.

187. A 50-year-old diabetic patient presents with a sudden onset of upper abdominal pain, fever and vomiting. On examination he was severe tachycardia, abdominal tenderness and distension. X-ray abdomen shows presence of gas in the biliary tree.
188. A 50-year-old patient with symptoms of colicky abdominal pain, vomiting and constipation for couple of days. X-ray reveals multiple air fluid levels and abdomen shows gallstones.

THEME: 33
DIFFERENTIAL DIAGNOSIS OF LUMP IN RIGHT ILIAC FOSSA

Options

a. Ileocecal tuberculosis.
b. Actinomycosis.
c. Ovarian mass.
d. Appendicular lump.
e. Ectopic kidney.
f. Carcinoma cecum.
g. Undescended testes presents with a freely mobile ballotable lump in the right lower abdomen.
h. Ectopic pregnancy.

For each of the statements/situations given below, choose the one most appropriate/discriminatory option. The options can be used once, more than once, or not at all.

Questions

189. A 30-year-old female presents with a freely mobile ballotable lump in the right lower abdomen.
190. A 30-year-old female presents with a lump in the right iliac fossa for the past 3 weeks. She gives a history of pain over the iliac fossa which lasted for 5 days and was treated conservatively. On examination, there is a minimally tender lump in the RIF.
191. A 45-year-old female patient presents with complaints of malena, weight loss and abdominal pain. On examination

there is a hard fixed lump in the right iliac fossa. Stool examination reveals occult blood. A barium enema revealed irregular filling defect in the cecum.

192. A 40-year-old female presents with lump in the right iliac fossa. This lump has been noted since childhood and there has been no change in size. On examination this lump is fixed, firm in consistency. The sonologist could not locate the right kidney in the renal fossa.
193. A 40-year-old Asian female presents with a lump in the right iliac fossa. She also gives a history of chronic colicky abdominal pain, altered bowel habits and weight loss. Barium meal follow through shows an irregular cecum which is pulled up with widening of the ileocecal angle.

THEME: 34
CAUSES OF HEPATOMEGALY

Options

a. Hydatid cyst.
b. Amoebic liver abscess.
c. Metastases in liver.
d. Hepatoma.
e. Congenital liver cyst.
f. Gaucher's disease.

For each of the statements/situations given below, choose the one most appropriate/discriminatory option. The options can be used once, more than once, or not at all.

Questions

194. A 40-year-old farmer presents with a lump in the right hypochondrium. The lump is cystic in nature and a thrill is felt on percussion.
195. A 50-year-old alcoholic presents with a rapid enlarging lump in the right hypochondrium. There is a sudden deterioration in his liver function tests. Ultrasound examination reveals a large echogenic mass in the right lobe of liver.

196. A 60-year-old patient with upper abdominal lump. The lump is nodular and nontender. He also gives a history of constipation alternating with diarrhoea. Stool examination shows occult blood.
197. A 40-year-old patient presents with a tender lump in the right hypochondrium. There is a history of fever with chills. On examination there is inter costal tenderness and tender hepatomegaly. X-ray abdomen reveals tenting of the right dome of diaphragm.
198. A 30-year-old female develops sudden onset tender massive hepatomegaly with rapidly increasing ascites. She gives a history of diarrhea a few weeks ago. There is also history of oral contraceptive intake.

THEME: 35
DIAGNOSIS OF MASS IN RIGHT ILIAC FOSSA

Options

a. Appendicular mass
b. Tuberculosis
c. Crohn's disease
d. Ulcerative colitis
e. Caecal carcinoma
f. Lymphoma
g. Ectopic kidney
h. Tubo-ovarian mass
i. Ectopic pregnancy
j. Intussusception
k. Volvulus

For each of the situations/conditions given below, choose the one most appropriate/discriminatory option from above. The options may be used once, more than once, or not at all.

Questions

199. A 20-year-old Somali man presents with a 2-month history of weight loss, fever and mass in the right iliac fossa (Hb 10, WCC 13000/mm^3, ESR 90 mm/hr)

200. A 20-year-old Greek man presents with a 4-month history of weight loss, fever, night sweats and right-sided abdominal pain. The pain usually follows alcohol intake. Clinical examination reveals a mass in the right iliac fossa.
201. A 70-year-old woman presents with nausea, increasing dyspepsia and a mass in the right iliac fossa (Hb 9.8 MCV 65 fl)
202. A 25-year-old man is found to have a mobile mass in the right iliac fossa during a routine medical examination for insurance purposes.
203. A 25-year-old man presents with a 3-month history of central abdominal pain associated with occasional vomiting and diarrhoea. A barium follow through demonstrates the string sign of the terminal ileum and clinical examination reveals a mass in the right iliac fossa.

THEME: 36
CAUSES OF ABDOMINAL MASSES

Options

a. Psoas abscess
b. Appendicitis
c. Tuberculosis
d. Crohn's disease
e. Diverticulitis
f. Carcinoma in the simoid colon
g. Carcinoma of the caecum
h. Obstruction of the common bile duct by a calculus
i. Carcinoma of the pancreas
j. Ovarian cyst
k. Mesenteric cyst

For each of the situations/conditions given below, choose the one most appropriate/discriminatory option from above. The options may be used once, more than once, or not at all.

Questions

204. A 40-year-old man presents with fever, painless jaundice and a palpable gallbladder.

205. A 30-year-old woman presents with colicky abdominal pain and distension. On examination, a smooth, mobile, spherical mass is palpated in the centre of her abdomen. A fluid thrill is elicited, and the mass is dull to percussion.
206. A 20-year-old man presents with fever, abdominal and back pain and a mass in the right iliac fossa. The swelling is soft tender, dull and compressible. It extends below the groin. He denies nausea, vomiting, or diarrhoea.
207. A 50-year-old man presents with a dull ache in the right iliac fossa and diarrhoea. A freely mobile mass is palpated in the right iliac fossa. The rectum is normal and thee faeces contains blood.
208. A 55-year-old man presents with severe, left iliac fossa pain, nausea, and chronic constipation. A tender, sausage-shaped mass is palpated in the left iliac fossa.

THEME: 37
DIAGNOSIS OF ABDOMINAL MASS

Options

a. Mestothelioma
b. Gastric carcinoma
c. Pancreatic carcinoma
d. Bowel carcinoma
e. Endometrial carcinoma
f. Chronic appendicitis
g. Pseudomyxoma peritonei
h. Cold abscess
i. Mesenteric cyst
j. Omental torsion
k. Umbilical hernia
l. Femoralhernia
m. Pelvic abscess
n. Acute appendicitis

For each of the situations/conditions given below, choose the one most appropriate/discriminatory option from above. The options may be used once, more than once, or not at all.

Questions

209. A 33-year-old woman presents with fever and abdominal pain. She also has diarrhoea. Per rectal examination discloses a tender boggy swelling anteriorly.
210. An elderly man is brought into A&E with acute abdominal pain. He has been vomiting. On examination you find a tender central abdominal mass.
211. A shipyard worker complains of lump in his abdomen and increasing girth. Over the past few months he has felt unwell and had to let out his trousers. On physical examination you find a bulky and discrete epigastric mass and evidence of shifting dullness.
212. A middle-aged woman was operated on for acute appendicitis. At operation a mucocele was discovered. Since her operation she has suffered from repeated bouts of abdominal pain and constipation. She also complains of weight loss.
213. A healthy young woman complains of a painless abdominal swelling. On physical examination you find a non-tender lower right swelling. The swelling is tense and mobile, but only vertically.

THEME: 38
DIAGNOSIS OF LUMP IN THE GROIN

Options

a. Inguinal hernia
b. Femoral hernia
c. Saphenovarix
d. Spigelian hernia
e. Hydrocoele
f. Inguinal lymphedenopathy
g. Haematocoele
h. Femoral artery aneurysm
i. Pantaloon hernia

For each of the situations/conditions given below, choose the one most appropriate/discriminatory option from above. The options may be used once, more than once, or not at all.

Questions

214. A 40-year-old woman presents with a lump in left groin. The lump is not reducible and lies below and lateral to the pubic tubercle.
215. A 40-year-old woman who underwent varicose vein surgery recently presents with a lump in the groin. The lump appears on lying down and transmits on cough impulse. It lies just below the groin crease and medial to femoral pulse.
216. A 60-year-old man presents with a swelling in the groin and the scrotum. Clinical examination reveals a scrotal swelling and you cannot get above it.
217. A 30-year-old man presents with a reducible groin lump lying above the medial to the pubic tubercle.

THEME: 39
TREATMENT OF OLIGURIA

Options

a. Percutaneous nephrostomy
b. Suprapubic cystostomy
c. Urethral catheterisation
d. Blood transfusion
e. Fluid challenge
f. 500 ml of IV mannitol
g. Walk around

For each of the situations/conditions given below, choose the one most appropriate/discriminatory option from above. The options may be used once, more than once, or not at all.

Questions

218. Following an elective herniorraphy , a small 67-year-old man is unable to pass urine, when a nurse hands him a small bottle for microscopic studies. He is otherwise well.
219. A 34-year-old woman presents with right sided loin pain and oliguria. An intravenous urogram shows right sided dilated calyces and hydroureter.

220. A man involved in a mining accident presents with oliguria and passing dark brown urine.
221. A 45-year-old man sustained a pelvic fracture and now presents with oliguria, A pulse rate of 120 beats/min and blood pressure of 70/50 mmHg.
222. A 23-year-old man who sustained a pelvic fracture is unable to pass urine . On examination he has abdominal tenderness and fullness and blood on the urethral meatus.

THEME: 40
CAUSES OF DYSPHAGIA

Options

a. Foreign body.
b. Scleroderma.
c. Achlasia cardia.
d. Lye stricture.
e. Carcinoma of esophagus.
f. Plummer Vinson syndrome.
g. Peptic stricture.
h. Presbyesophagus.
i. Zenker's diverticulum.

For each of the statements/situations given below, choose the one most appropriate/discriminatory option. The options can be used once, more than once, or not at all.

Questions

223. A 60-year-old female presents with gradual progressive dysphagia initially for solids and later on for fluids too. There has been progressive weight loss.
224. A 60-year-old female presents with anemia and dysphagia. There is a feeling of something get stuck in the throat. The esophagus could not be negotiated beyond the cricopharynx.
225. A 30-year-old female presents with complaints of dysphagia for liquids only. She has also suffered from repeated episodes of pneumonia in the past few months.

226. A 30-year-old male presents with slow progressive onset of dysphagia. There is a past history of retrosternal burning pain and he has been treated with prokinetics and h2 receptor blockers for GE reflux.
227. A 50-year-old male presents with sudden onset dysphagia for one day. He can neither swallow liquids nor solids. The patient also seems to have misplaced his dentures.

THEME: 41
MANAGEMENT OF DYSPHAGIA

Options

a. Endoscopic snaring.
b. Negus ballon dilatation.
c. Bougie dilatation of the esophagus.
d. Cardiomyotomy.
e. Esophagus resection.
f. Endoscopic stenting.
g. Laser luminisation.

For each of the statements/situations given below, choose the one most appropriate/discriminatory option. The options can be used once, more than once, or not at all.

Questions

228. Peptic stricture.
229. Foreign body in esophagus.
230. Esophageal carcinoma.
231. Achlasia cardia.
232. Tracheo–esophageal fistula following malignancy.

THEME: 42
CHEST TRAUMA

Options

a. Surgical emphysema.
b. Tension pneumothorax.
c. Dissecting aneurysm of aorta.
d. Diaphragmatic tear.

e. Flail chest.
f. Pericardial tamponade.
g. Fracture ribs.

For each of the statements/situations given below, choose the one most appropriate/discriminatory option. The options can be used once, more than once, or not at all.

Questions

233. A football player collapses on the field after a midfield collision. On examination, his pulse is thready, hypotensive and cyanosed. The air entry on the right side is absent and there is shift of mediastinum.
234. A 40-year-old patient involved in a RTA presents with hypotension, tachypnea and chest pain. On examination the air entry on the left side of the chest is reduced and peristaltic sounds are heard in the left chest.
235. A 25-year-old male presents with right sided chest pain after assault. On examination, there is a localised area of tenderness over the right seventh rib. The pain becomes worse on coughing. The air entry is equal.
236. The above patient after a few hours develops swelling on the chest wall which spreads upto the neck above and to the anterior abdominal wall.
237. A 50-year-old patient presents with a parasternal stab injury. On examination, his pulse is thready. BP is 80 mm systolic and JVP is raised.

THEME: 43
CAUSES OF PORTAL HYPERTENSION

Options

a. Postnecrotic cirrhosis.
b. Noncirrhotic portal hypertension.
c. Budd-Chiari syndrome.
d. Left sided portal hypertension.
e. Biliary cirrhosis.
f. Alcoholic cirrhosis.

For each of the statements/situations given below, choose the one most appropriate/discriminatory option. The options can be used once, more than once, or not at all.

Questions

238. A 60-year-old chronic alcoholic presents with hemetemesis. On examination, the liver is shrunken. Spleen is enlarged and there are signs of liver cell failure.
239. 60-year-old female patient who underwent cholecystectomy. There is history of jaundice, fever with chills since surgery. LFT reveals a raised alkaline phosphatase levels, hyperbilirubinemia.
240. A 6-year-old boy presents with a history of hemetemesis. There is a history of umbilical sepsis in the neonatal period. On examination, the spleen is enlarged. The liver biopsy is normal.
241. A 60-year-old patient who underwent surgery for coronary artery by pass grafting 15-year-oldback presents with hemetemesis. His upper GI endoscopy reveals varices. Anti hepatitis C antibody levels are raised.
242. A 60-year-old alcoholic presents with repeated episodes of acute abdominal pain in the epigastrium. These episodes of pain were related to the intake of alcohol. His upper GI endoscopy examination reveals large esophageal and gastric varices. His liver biopsy is normal.

THEME: 44
DIAGNOSIS OF COMPLICATIONS OF ABDOMINAL SURGERY

Options

a. Mesenteric adenitis
b. Pulmonary embolism
c. Bilary peritonitis
d. Acute mesenteric thrombosis
e. Subphrenic abscess
f. Cholestastis
g. Small bowel obstruction

h. Posterior MI
i. Splenic rupture
j. Deep vein thrombosis
k. Wound dehiscence
l. Incisional hernia
m. Anterolateral MI
n. Inferior MI

For each of the situations/conditions given below, choose the one most appropriate/discriminatory option from above. The options may be used once, more than once, or not at all.

Questions

243. Ultrasound shows intra-abdominal free fluid.
244. Blood pressure is 80/60 mmHg and pulse is 110/min
245. ECG show Q waves and ST elevation in leads III and aVF.
246. Liver function tests show raised alkaline phosphataase, raised bilirubin, normal albumin and normal hepatocellular enzymes.
247. A 5 days following cholecystectomy, incision wound is noted to have a serous discharge.
248. A 3 days following bowel resection, a 45-year-old man presented with chest pain on inspiration and haemoptysis, JVP is raised and the P2 is loud on auscultation.

THEME: 45
LOW URINE OUTPUT AFTER SURGERY

Options

a. Acute tubular necrosis
b. Acute urinary retention
c. Blocked catheter
d. Chronic renal impairment
e. Intravascular depletion

For each of the situations/conditions given below, choose the one most appropriate/discriminatory option from above. The options may be used once, more than once, or not at all.

Questions

249. An 80-year-old man who is normally hypertensive; postoperative day 1 following a right hemicolectomy. He has epidural analgesia and his blood pressure is 125/70 mmHg
250. A 65-year-old man has undergone a hernia repair as a day-case. He has not passes urine since the procedure and on examination a suprapublic mass is palpable.
251. A 76-year-old man has undergone a TURP (transurethral resection of the prostrate gland) in spite of irrigation his urine is heavily blood stained and he is passing 20 ml hour.
252. A 35-year-old man has had a subtotal colectomy for ulcerative colitis. He has been given gentamicin antibiotic prophylaxis and diclofenac sodium for analgesia. It is the firs postoperative day and his urine output has tailed off to 10 ml/hour.

THEME: 46
POSTOPERATIVE FEVER

Options

a. Basal lung collapse
b. CMV line infection
c. Sulphrenic abscess
d. Urinary tract infection
e. Wound infection

For each of the situations/conditions given below, choose the one most appropriate/discriminatory option from above. The options may be used once, more than once, or not at all.

Questions

253. A 75-year-old man is discharged for the ICU after major abdominal surgery. He has a prolonged ileus, so TPN is commenced. On the 7th postoperative day he develops a temperature of 38.5°C
254. An obese 45-year-old woman undergoes and open cholecystectomy for gallstones. She is slow to mobiles and on the second day develops a temperature of 37.9°C.

255. A 76-year-old man undergoes an Hartman's procedure for stercoral perforation. On the 8th postoperative day he develops a high spiking fever.
256. A 15-year-old boy undergoes an emergency appendectomy for a perforated gangrenous appendix. On the 5th postoperative day he develops a temperature of 37.8°C and a thin serosanguineous discharge is noted on the wound dressing.

THEME: 47
POSTOPERATIVE COMPLICATIONS

Options

a. Acute tubular necrosis
b. Cardiac failure
c. Chest infection
d. Deep vein thrombosis
e. Myocardial infarction
f. Pulmonary embolism
g. Pelvic abscess
h. Secondary haemtrrhage
i. Septicaemia
j. Transfusion reaction
k. Urinary retension
l. Urinary tract infection
m. Wound dehiscence
n. Wound infection

For each of the situations/conditions given below, choose the one most appropriate/discriminatory option from above. The options may be used once, more than once, or not at all.

Questions

257. A 50-year-old woman underwent an anterior resection for carcinoma of the rectum one week ago. She has a low grade pyrexia (37.5°C) and is complaining of pain in the left calf. She has pitting oedema of the left ankle.
258. A 24-year-old man underwent an appendicectomy six days ago for a perforated appendix. He appeared to be making a good recovery but has developed intermittent

pyrexia (up to 39°C). On clinical examination there is no obvious cause for this pyrexia .He is tender anteriorly on rectal examination.

259. A 69-year-old man underwent an emergency repair of an abdominal aortic aneurism .He had been severely hypotensive before and during surgery. Following surgery his blood pressure was satisfactory but his urinary output was only 5ml hr in the first two hours.
260. A 60-year-old woman has undergraduate eft hemicolectomy for carcinoma of the colon. On the fourth pos-operative day she became hypotensive (BP 60/40 mmHg) , pulse 130 beats /min.She has a pyrexia (38.5°C) with warm hands and feet.
261. An 80-year-old woman underwent emergency laparotomy for peritonitis. On the fourth postoperative day she was noticed to have a serosanguinous discharge from the wound.

THEME: 48
THE TREATMENT OF POSTOPERATIVE PAIN

Options

a. Aspirin tablets
b. Diclofenac suppositories
c. Dihydrocodeine analgesia
d. Patient controlled analgesia (PCA) with morphine
e. Intercostal nerve blocks
f. Epidural analgesia
g. Carbamazepine
h. Paracetamol tablets
i. Diamorphine
j. Intramuscular pethidine

For each of the situations/conditions given below, choose the one most appropriate/discriminatory option from above. The options may be used once, more than once, or not at all.

Questions

262. A 33-year-old man requires analgesia following an exploratory laparotomy and splenectomy

263. A 55-year-old woman with terminal metastatic breast carcinoma requires long-term analgesia following radical mastectomy.
264. A 40-year-old man complains of phantom limb pain following below-knee amputation
265. A 25-year-old man underwent excision of a sebaceous cyst under local anaesthesia. He uses salbutamolinhaler on a regular basis.
266. A 60-year-old man requires analgesia following a total thyroidectomy.

THEME: 49
INVESTIGATIONS OF POSTOPERATIVE COMPLICATIONS

Options

a. Chest X-ray
b. Serum calcium
c. 12-lead electrocardiogram
d. Ultrasound abdomen
e. Serum glucose
f. Mid-streak specimen of urine
g. Thyroid function tests
h. Pulmonary angiogram
i. Bladder ultrasound
j. Serum haemoglogulin

For each of the situations/conditions given below, choose the one most appropriate/discriminatory option from above. The options may be used once, more than once, or not at all.

Questions

267. A 55-year-old man post thyroidectomy presents with tetany. Upon tapping the preauricular region, the facial muscles begin to twitch.
268. A 50-year-old man postcoronary artery bypass graft surgery presents with fever and sever epigastric pain.
269. A 70-year-old woman post dynamic hip screw for a right neck of femur fracture presents with pallor, tachycardia,

and hypotension. Her oxygen saturation is 90%. The rest of her examination is normal.

270. A 65-year-old man 10 days post right total hip replacement, presents with sudden breathlessness and collapses. On examination, here is noted to have a pleural rub, increased JVP, and a swollen right leg.
271. A 35-year-old primigravida post Caesarian section complains of inability to void. She denies dysuria but complains of fullness. She was treated with an epidural for analgesia.

THEME: 50
THE MANAGEMENT OF POSTOPERATIVE COMPLICATIONS

Options

a. Intravenous calcium gluconate
b. Insolin in dextrose
c. Potassium replacement
d. Intravenous saline and frusemide
e. Check serum area and creatine
f. Check full blood count
g. Obtain KUB film
h. Obtain chest X-ray
i. Mid – stream urine for culture
j. Intravenous hydrocortisone

For each of the situations/conditions given below, choose the one most appropriate/discriminatory option from above. The options may be used once, more than once, or not at all.

Questions

272. A 40-year-old woman started on gentamicin in the recovery room suddenly stops breathing. She had received a neuromuscular blocking agent.
273. A 50-year-old man develops postoperative hypotension and oliguria following bowel surgery. An ECG shows prolonged PR interval and QRS interval, loss of P waves, and depression of the ST segment.

274. A 70-year-old man develops tinnitus and deafness after surgery. His medications include gentamicin and frusemide.
275. A 40-year-old woman has undergone intestinal bypass surgery for gross obesity. She now present with pain in the lumbar region and haematuria. She is apyrexial.
276. A 40-year-old woman with systemic lupus erythematosus develops nausea, vomiting and sever pain following cholecystectomy. She becomes hypotensive and tachycardic. She is noted to have an irregular tan and denies sunexposure.

THEME: 51
THE MANAGEMENT OF POSTOPERATIVE COMPLICATIONS

Options

a. Intravenous dantrolene sodium
b. Intravenous calcium gluconate
c. Blood transfusion
d. Blood cultures
e. Obtain Chest X-ray
f. Midstream urine collection for culture
g. Intravenous broad-spectrum antibiotics
h. Insulin in dextrose
i. Foley catherisation
j. Obtain abdominal X-ray
k. Check full blood count

For each of the situations/conditions given below, choose the one most appropriate/discriminatory option from above. The options may be used once, more than once, or not at all.

Questions

277. A 30-year-old female postappendectomy develops high fever of 42°C, hypotension and mottled cyanosis in the recovery room. She received halothane inhalation gas in surgery. She was noted to have trismus during intubation.

278. A 40-year-old man complains of circumoral numbness following thyroidectomy. Tapping over the preauricular region elicits facial twitching.
279. A 50-year-old man postnephrectomy becomes febrile, confused tachpnoeic and tachycardiac. He was recently advanced to a soft diet. He has no bowel sounds
280. A 60-year-old man postcholesytectomy complains of lower abdominal pain. On examination, his bladder is palpable at the umbilicus.
281. A 70-year-old woman posttotal hip replacement becomes tachynoeic. She is pale and hypotensive.

THEME: 52
ACUTE ABDOMEN

Options

a. Acute salphingitis
b. Adhesive small bowel obstruction
c. Appendicitis
d. Leaking aortic aneurysm
e. Mesenteric ischaemia
f. Pancreatitis
g. Perforated peptic ulcer
h. Ureteric colic

For each of the situations/conditions given below, choose the one most appropriate/discriminatory option from above. The options may be used once, more than once, or not at all.

Questions

282. A 60-year-old man with epigastric pain and brief collapse at home is now alert with some mild back pain and tachycardia.
283. A 45-year-old man has been taking fibrobrufen for persistent abdominal pain. He has been brought to A&E after a sudden collapse, and an erect chest film shows gas under the diaphragm.
284. A 36-year-old woman has been brought to A&E by her husband with very sever left-sided abdominal pain. Her

husband states that she has been pacing around the bedroom all night, unable to find a comfortable position, and the patient describes the pain as being 'worse that a labour pain'

285. An 87-year-old woman is admitted with rigid abdomen. A careful history reveals she has been having pain after meals and has stopped eating very much. Her blood gas assay reveals a metabolic acidosis. Her amylase level is within normal limits.
286. A 23-year-old woman; presents with right iliac fossa pain for days, associated with nausea but no omitting. A dipstick urine test is normal and careful history reveals an offensive vaginal discharge.

THEME: 53
DIAGNOSIS OF ACUTE ABDOMEN

Options

a. Acute pancreatitis
b. Acute Cholecystitis
c. Acute myocardial infarction
d. Pyloric stenosis
e. Intestinal obstruction
f. Appendicular abscess
g. Acute appendicitis
h. Acute pyelonephritis
i. Possible rupture aortic aneurysm
j. Aortic dissection
k. Possible twisted ovarian cyst
l. Oesophageal varices

For each of the situations/conditions given below, choose the one most appropriate/discriminatory option from above. The options may be used once, more than once, or not at all.

Questions

287. A 74-year-old man with a previous history of pain in his calves while walking, is bought to A&E after having collapsed in the street. He is complaining of abdominal pain radiating to his back.

288. A 24-year-old woman presents to the A&E with a sudden onset of left iliac fossa pain. She is pale and has a pulse of 120 with a BP of 105/65. On examination of her abdomen she is tender in her left iliac fossa.
289. A 36-year-old woman present with a 12 hour history of severe epigastric pain associated with several episodes of vomiting. She drinks about 40 units of alcohol per week. She is tender with guarding in the epigastrium. Plain radiography shows no evidence of free gas.
290. A 40-year-old man is admitted with a history of 244 hours of colicky central abdominal pain and bile stained vomiting. His only past medical history is an appendectomy when he was 8. On examination his abdomen is distended, but there is no tenderness. Bowel sounds are increased.
291. A fit 18-year-old man present with 12 hour history of central abdominal pain radiating to his right iliac fossa. He is pyrexial with tenderness, guarding and rebound in the right iliac fossa.

THEME: 54
DIAGNOSIS OF ACUTE ABDOMEN

Options

a. Acute gastroenteritis
b. Acute pancreatitits
c. Acute appendicitis
d. Bilary colic
e. Acute cholecystitis
f. Ectopic pregnancy
g. Mesenteric thrombosis
h. Perforated peptic ulcer
i. Renal colic
j. Acute salphingitis
k. Spontaneous abortion
l. Strangulated hernia
m. Torsion ovarian cyst
n. Ulcerative colitis
o. Urinary tract infection

For each of the situations/conditions given below, choose the one most appropriate/discriminatory option from above. The options may be used once, more than once, or not at all.

Questions

292. A 20-year-old married woman present to A&E with the onset of acute lower abdominal pain. Her last menstrual period was 6 weeks earlier. She has pain radiating to the left shoulder.
293. A 15-year-old girl presents with a 24 hour history of ventral abdominal pain, followed by the right iliac fossa pain, worse on coughing . She has fever and rebound in the right iliac fossa.
294. A 30-year-old woman has severe colic and upper abdominal pain radiating to her right scapula and is vomiting.
295. A 12-year-old girl has central abdominal pain and is vomiting. On examination her abdomen is found to be distended with no rebound and a tender lump in the right groin.
296. A 31-year-old woman has severe colic and upper abdominal pain. She is febrile and vomiting. Haematological investigations shows moderate leukocytes.
297. A 31-year-old woman presents with acute severe abdominal pain. Her BP is 100/60 and no abdominal signs are found. Hb is 17g g/dl and the plasma amylase is only mildly raised.

THEME: 55
CAUSES OF ACUTE ABDOMINAL PAIN

Options

a. Acute appendicitis
b. Acute pancreatitis
c. Perforation
d. Bowel obstruction
e. Diverticulitis
f. Acute salphingitis
g. Ruptured ectopic pregnancy

h. Pyelonephritis
i. Urinary tract infection
j. Renal/ureteric colic
k. Ruptured aortic aneurysm
l. Acute cholecystitis

For each of the situations/conditions given below, choose the one most appropriate/discriminatory option from above. The options may be used once, more than once, or not at all.

Questions

298. A 33-year-old woman has collapsed with severe abdominal pain. She is apyrexial, pulse 140, and BP 90/40. Abdomen is rigid and tender with guarding. She says she cannot be pregnant as she had an IUCD in-situ.
299. A 28-year-old woman has a 24 hour history of sever constant loin pain and vomiting. She has had rigors and sweats. Urinalysis reveals blood and protein
300. A 20-year-old man has 24 hour history of abdominal pain, which started in the para-umbilical area but seems to have moved to his right iliac fossa. He is tender in this area with guarding and rebound tenderness.
301. A 60-year-old man who has had a previous laparotomy for a perforated duodenal ulcer has a 24 hour history of colicky abdominal pain, absolute constipation and vomiting. He has a distended resonant abdomen and high-pitched bowel sounds.
302. A 35-year-old woman has a 2-day history of severe abdominal pain and profuse vomiting. She has previous had episodes of right upper quadrant pain particularly after fatty meals. She is jaundiced and mildly tender in her epigastrium. Pulse is 120 and BP is 90/50 mmHg
303. A 70-year-old man who has a long history of hypertension and a recent history of intermittent back pain, has collapsed with severe central abdominal pain, which radiates to his back. His abdomen is tender and he has pulsatile mass in the midline.

THEME: 56
DIAGNOSIS OF ABDOMINAL PAIN

Options

a. Acute appendicitis
b. Diverticular disease
c. Abdominal aortic aneurysm
d. Perforated peptic ulcer
e. Crohn's disease
f. Ulcerated colitis
g. Acute pancreatitis
h. Chronic active hepatitis
i. Acute viral hepatitis
j. Pseudo-obstruction
k. Acute cholecystits
l. Acute diverticulitis

For each of the situations/conditions given below, choose the one most appropriate/discriminatory option from above. The options may be used once, more than once, or not at all.

Questions

304. A 20-year-old man presents with colicky per umbilical pain which shifts to the right iliac fossa, fever, and loss of appetite.
305. A 48-year-old man presents with severe epigastric pain radiating to the back. He is noted to have some bruising in the flanks.
306. A 42-year-old woman presents with anorexia, abdominal pain, and increasing jaundice. She is asthmatic and takes methyldopa for hypertension.
307. A 50-year-old man presents with left sided colicky iliac fossa pain, change in bowel habits and rectal bleeding. A thickened mass is palpated in the region of the sigmoid colon. His full blood count is normal.
308. A 78-year-old woman with stable angina presents with massive abdominal distension 10 days following a total hip replacement.

THEME: 57
DIAGNOSIS OF ACUTE ABDOMINAL PAIN

Options

a. Acute intermittent porphyria
b. Acute pancreatitis
c. Ischaemic colitis
d. Sigmoid calculus
e. Intussusception
f. Familial Mediterranean fever
g. Acute appendicitis
h. Paroxysmal nocturnal haemoglobinuria
i. Diverticulitis
j. Meckel's diverticulitis
k. Perforated peptic ulcer
l. Inflammatory bowel disease

For each of the situations/conditions given below, choose the one most appropriate/discriminatory option from above. The options may be used once, more than once, or not at all.

Questions

309. A 63-year-old man presented with vomiting, bloody diarrhoea and acute pain in the left iliac fossa. He had had a similar episode, which followed a heavy meal, and he had 2 MI over the last 10 yrs. On examination his temperature was 37.7 and his left iliac fossa was tender with no guarding.
310. A 72-year-old woman presented with sudden severe left-sided abdominal pain while straining to pass stools. She had had a long history of constipation. On examination she was afebrile. Her abdomen was distended, particular on the left and tender and tympanitic with increased bowel sounds.
311. A 24-year-old Cypriot student presented with sever abdominal pain, fever and a tender swollen left knee. 4 weeks ago he also suffered from a similar swelling in his right ankle. On examination his temperature was 39.9°C and his abdomen was diffusely tender. Urinalysis showed protein +++, blood negative and glucose negative.

312. A 34-year-Old Spanish lawyer presented with severe colicky central abdominal pain radiating to the back. She had recently been started on barbiturates for convulsions and insomnia. On examination her temperature was 38.1c and there was a laparotomy scar with no evidence of organomegaly.
313. A 13-year-old girl presented with a 6 hour history of pain in the right iliac fossa and fresh bleeding per rectum. On examination her temperature was 36.5°C, blood pressure 100/60 and pulse was 120. Oral mucosa was normal. Abdomen was soft, with no organomegaly. All investigations were normal including full blood count, clotting profile, urea and electrolytes, gastroscopy and Sigmoidoscopy.

THEME: 58
INVESTIGATION OF ACUTE ABDOMEN

Options

a. Serum amylase
b. White cell count
c. Creactive protein
d. Abdominal ultrasound
e. Erect chest X-ray
f. Supine abdominal X-ray
g. Diagnostic peritoneal lavage
h. CT abdomen + contrast
i. Diagnostic laparoscopy
j. Beta HCG
k. Gastrograffin enema
l. Immediate laparotomy

For each of the situations/conditions given below, choose the one most appropriate/discriminatory option from above. The options may be used once, more than once, or not at all.

Questions

314. A 25-year-old woman presents in a state of collapse. She has a painful, tender rigid abdomen. Pulse is 120, BP 80/50. Bowel sounds are scanty.

315. A 52-year-old man presents with onset of severe abdominal pain over an hour. He has a history of epigastric pain over the last 3 months. He is acfebrile, tachycardic and normontensive. He has generalized tenderness with guarding and absent bowel sounds.
316. A 42-year-old obese woman complains of a 24 hour history of severe epigastric pain and profuse vomiting. On examination she is tachycardiac and mildly jaundiced. She has mild tenderness in the left upper quadrant and normal bowel sounds.
317. A 45-year-old builder fell from scaffolding to the ground earlier in the day. He landed on his left side and initially had pain in his lower left chest. He has now developed severe abdominal pain. He is becoming increasingly tachycardic and is hypotensive. His abdomen is tender with guarding and he is tender over his left 10th and 11th ribs.
318. A 70-year-old woman has developed an increasingly painful and swollen abdomen over a period of 24 hrs. She has not opened her bowels for 3 days and begun to vomit today. On examination she has a distended tender abdomen with scanty bowel sounds. She has an exquisitely tender mass at the top of her right thigh.
319. A 70-year-old man presents with sudden central abdominal pain and collapsed. He is severely shocked. He has a tender, rigid abdomen and there is an expansile, pulsatile mass in the upper abdomen.

THEME: 59
MANAGEMENT OF ABDOMINAL PAIN

Options

a. Colonic irrigation
b. Metronidazole
c. Codeine phosphate
d. Formal resection
e. Transfusion
f. Sigmoid colectomy
g. Propantheline

h. Diathermy
i. Haemorrhoidectomy
j. Fluids
k. High fibre diet

For each of the situations/conditions given below, choose the one most appropriate/discriminatory option from above. The options may be used once, more than once, or not at all.

Questions

320. A middle-aged woman complains of chronic abdominal pain especially on the left side. She has had diarrhoea for 2 weeks and wonders if she has eaten something recently although she says her system has always been sensitive.
321. A 54-year-old man who has suffered recurrent hours of abdominal pain and deadhead for 10 years is brought in exhausted. A barium enema demonstrates muscle thickening and gross multiple diverticula
322. An elderly man complains of diarrhoea with mucus. He is dehydrated and weak. On Sigmoidoscopy you find an area of bowel with a granular and plum coloured appearance. You also detect induration.
323. A young woman presents with abdominal pain, tenderness and fever. She goes to the bathroom 10 times a day. She says she doesn't have diarrhoea, but her stools are always soft and sometimes a little bloody.
324. A pal young man complains of bleeding per rectum. You find a rectal mucosa thick and boggy on rectal examination. On Sigmoidoscopy you find the bowel wall to be erthematous and grandular. Inspection leads to light bleeding.

THEME: 60
MANAGEMENT OF ABDOMINAL PAIN

Options

a. Sigmoidoscopy
b. Permanent ileostomy
c. Stool culture
d. Colectomy

e. Antibiotics
f. Antipyretics
g. Plain abdominal X-ray
h. Laxitives
i. High-dose of steroids
j. Blood transfusion
k. IV line
l. Sulphasalazine
m. Bowel resection with end to end anastomosis

For each of the situations/conditions given below, choose the one most appropriate/discriminatory option from above. The options may be used once, more than once, or not at all.

Questions

325. A 54-year-old man with a long history of abdominal pain present with acute left-sided abdominal pain. At times the pain is colicky and at times the pain is relieved by defecation.
326. A 50-year-old man complains of acute constipation and left sided abdominal pain. Over the past 10 years he has had a numerous bowel operations and his health has declined steadily.
327. A young woman complains of persistent mild fever and diarrhoea. She says her stools appear almost normal, but that they contain blood.
328. A 32-year-old man has just returned form holiday. He complains of sever abdominal pain, vomiting and blood diarrhoea. He has a high fever and is sweating.

THEME: 61
TREATMENT OF INTESTINAL OBSTRUCTION

Options

a. Right hemicolectomy
b. Urgent herniography
c. Sigmoid colectomy
d. Nasogastric aspiration and electrolyte replacement
e. Subtotal colectomy and ileorectal anastomosis

f. Anterior resection
g. Exploratory laparotomy and Hartman's procedure
h. Abdominaoperineal resection with end colostomy
i. Transverse colectomy
j. Proximal loop colostomy

For each of the situations/conditions given below, choose the one most appropriate/discriminatory option from above. The options may be used once, more than once, or not at all.

Questions

329. A 60-year-old man presents with abdominal pain in the right iliac fossa and distension. X-ray shows a single dilated loop of bowel of 12 cm in diameter with convexity under the left hemi diaphragm.

330 A 70-year-old man present with bowel obstruction and pain in rectum. Rectal examination and biopsy confirm an obstructing carcinoma of the rectum.

331. A 50-year-old man complains of constant groin pain associated with nausea and vomiting. On examination he has a positive cough impulse. A tender tense lump is palpitated and is not reducible.

332. A 60-year-old man presents with fever, vomiting and intense left iliac fossa pain. On examination he has a rigid distended abdomen with rebound tenderness on the left. Erect check X-ray reveals air under the diaphragm.

333. An 80-year-old man presents with abdominal distension and pain. Sigmoidoscopy and barium enema confirm an obstructing carcinoma of the recto sigmoid.

THEME: 62
ACUTE MANAGEMENT OF SURGICAL CONDITIONS

Options

a. IV fluids and nasogastic tube
b. Intramuscular pethidine
c. Immediate surgical exploration
d. Conservative management
e. Reduction and internal fixation

f. External fixation
g. X-ray
h. Sedation
i. IV fluid resuscitation
j. Plaster of Paris replacement

For each of the situations/conditions given below, choose the one most appropriate/discriminatory option from above. The options may be used once, more than once, or not at all.

Questions

334. A 25-year-old athlete presents to hospital after injuring his knee. He now complains of sever pain in the left shin. X-ray show no fractures; serum hyperkalemia detected.
335. A 65-year-old man with known atherosclerosis has abdominal pain and is hypotensive on admission
336. A 40-year-old man presents with severe pain in the loin, which radiates round the flank to his groin. The pain is episodic and severe every few minutes.
337. A 78-year-old lady slips on the ice and stretches her hand out to avoid the fall. X-ray shows an undiscplaced Cilles' fracture.
338. A 32-year-old chronic alcoholic presents with acute vomiting and retrosternal pain, which radiates to the back.

THEME: 63
INVESTIGATION OF PATIENT WITH ACUTE ABDOMEN

Options

a. Angiography
b. Arterial blood gases
c. Blood glucose concentration
d. Computed tomography
e. Diagnostic laproscopy
f. Erect chest X-ray
g. Full blood count

h. Gastroscopy
i. Plain radiography of the abdomen
j. Pregnancy test
k. Serum amylase activity
l. Sigmoidoscopy
m. USG abdomen
n. Urgent operation
o. Urine dipstick and culture
p. Water soluble contrast enema

For each of the statements/situations given below, choose the one most appropriate/discriminatory option. The options can be used once, more than once, or not at all..

Questions

339. A 71-year-old man with a previous history of pain in his calves on walking is brought to the A&E department after having collapsed in the street. He is complaining of abdominal pain radiating to his back.
340. A 22-year-old woman presents with a sudden onset of left iliac fossa pain. She is pale and has a pulse rate of 120 beats /min with a BP of 105/65 mmHg . On examination of her abdomen she is tender in her left iliac fossa.
341. A 35-year-old woman presents with a 12 hour history of severe epigastric pain associated with several episodes of vomiting. She drinks 30 units of alcohol per week. She is tender with guarding in the epigastrium . Plain radiography shows no evidence of free gas.
342. A 45-year-old man is admitted with a history of 24 hours of colicky central abdominal pain and bile stained vomiting. His only past medical history is an appendicectomy when he was 12. On examination his abdomen is distended ,but there is no tenderness. Bowel sounds are increased.
343. A fit 17-year-old man presents with a 12 hour history of central pain localising to his right iliac fossa. He is pyrexial with tenderness, guarding and rebound tenderness in the right iliac fosa.

THEME: 64
THE TREATMENT OF ABDOMINAL PAIN

Options

a. ERCP and endoscopic sphinectomy
b. Laparoscopic cholecytectomy
c. IV fluid, IV antibiotics and analgesia
d. Subtotal colectomy, mucous fistula and permanent ileostomy
e. Laparotomy
f. Mesalazine
g. Panprotocolectomy
h. Hartmann's procedure

For each of the situations/conditions given below, choose the one most appropriate/discriminatory option from above. The options may be used once, more than once, or not at all .

Questions

344. A 20-year-old female present with recurrent bloody diarrhoea and crampy abdominal pain. Sigmoidoscopy and biopsy confirm ulcerative colitus
345. A 25-year-old man involved with an RTA sustains blunt trauma to his upper abdomen. He complains of left shoulder pain and diffuse abdominal pain. He becomes increasing tachycardic and hypotensive and develops peritoneal signs.
346. A 40-year-old woman presents with pyrexia and right upper quadrant abdominal pain. The white cell count is 14 with elevated neutrophils. Both the chest X-ray and the abdominal X-ray are unremarkable.
347. A 50-year-old man presents with fever, right upper quadrant pain and jaundice. Ultrasound reveals a dilated common bile duct.
348. A 30-year-old man present with sever, intractable abdominal pain. He is pyrexia tachycardiac and has marked abdominal distension. On X-ray the colon is noted to have a transverse diameter of 7 cm.

THEME: 65
INVESTIGATIONS OF SURGICAL DISEASE

Options

a. Gastrograffin swallow
b. Upright chest X-ray
c. Abdominal x-ray
d. Full blood count
e. Mesenteric arteriogram
f. Computed tomography of the abdomen
g. Technetium 99 radioactive scan
h. Abdominal ultrasound
i. Serum urea and electrolytes
j. Stool culture

For each of the situations/conditions given below, choose the one most appropriate/discriminatory option from above. The options may be used once, more than once, or not at all.

Questions

349. A 60-year-old man postoperative rigid oesophagoscopy and removal of a foreign body, now present with substernal pain, fever and tachypnoea.
350. A 65-year-old man with a history of cirrhosis, present with massive rectal bleeding, and right lower quadrant pain. NG tube lavage reveals no blood in the stomach. Colonoscopy reveals no varices. You suspect angiodysplasia of the caecum.
351. A 20-year-old man presents with passage of frank blood and clots from his rectum. His blood tests, barium enema, and upper GI series are all normal.
352. A 60-year-old man with lung cancer is noted to have elevated liver function tests. You suspect metastatic disease.
353. A 65-year-old alcoholic now presents with a tender, palpable midline mass. He was recent hospitalised for acute pancreatits 2 weeks prior. He has a raised amylase. You now suspect he has a pancreatic pseudocyst.

THEME: 66
DIAGNOSIS OF TRAUMATIC INJURIES

Options

a. Pulmonary embolus
b. Fat embolism
c. Haemothorax
d. Neurogenic shock
e. Cerebral compression
f. Perforated peptic ulcer
g. Haemobilia
h. Airway obstruction
i. Cerebral injury
j. Small bowel perforation
k. Cardiac tamponade
l. Tension pneumothorax

For each of the situations/conditions given below, choose the one most appropriate/discriminatory option from above. The options may be used once, more than once, or not at all .

Questions

354. A 20-year-old man is thrown off his motorbike in an RTA and sustains an open femur fracture. He did not lose conciousness. On examination, he becomes confused and short of breath. He is noted to have cutaneous and mucous membrane petechiae.
355. A 25-year-old man presents with massive haematemesis. He has a stab wound in the right side of his chest. Endoscopy demonstrates clear oesophagus and stomach with gushing of blood in the duodenum and a drop in pulse.
356. A 20-year-old man is thrown out of his car in an RTA and arrives incubated with a large gaping temporal scalp wound. His BP is 80/50 with a pulse rate of 115. His pupils are equal and respond sluggishly. However, he does not move his extremities. C-spine shows a fracture of C5. His chest is clear to auscultation and the abdomen is soft. He has no externa signs of injury to his limbs. His CVP is 3.

357. A 30-year-old woman with sever maxillofacial injuries becomes confused and agitated.
358. A 20-year-old man is stabbed in the anterior left cheek. He becomes dyspnoeic and hypotensive. On examination, he has distended neck veins and faint heart sounds. His pulse volume drops greater than 10 mmHg with inspiration

THEME: 67
MANAGEMENT OF TRANSFUSION REACTIONS

Options

a. Stop the transfusion, check patient identify against unit, inform hematologist and send unit and fresh blood samples to lab.
b. Slow the transfusion. Maintain airway and give oxygen. Give in adrenaline and salbutamol.
c. Stop the transfusion. Monitor closely and give paracetamol.
d. Slow the transfusion. Monitor closely and give chlorpheniramine.
e. Stop the tranfusion. Maintain airway, give oxygen and a diuretic. Consider exchange transfusion.

For each of the statements/situations given below, choose the one most appropriate/discriminatory option. The options can be used once, more than once, or not at all.

Questions

359. Urticaria and itch.
360. Bronchospasm, cyanosis, hypotension.
361. Dyspnea, hypoxia, tachycardia.
362. Shivering and fever (less than 40 degree celsius), 30-60 minutes after starting transfusion.
363. Agitation and fever (more than 40 degree celsius) within minutes of starting transfusion, hypotension, chest pain.

THEME: 68
INVESTIGATION OF AN ISCHAEMIC LIMB

Options

a. Ventilation perfusion (V/Q) scan
b. Electrocardiography

c. Ultrasound
d. Femoral duplex scan
e. Femoral arteriography
f. Venography
g. Ankle–brachial index measurement
h. Digital subtraction angiography
i. Coagulation prifile
j. None of the above

For each of the statements/situations given below, choose the one most appropriate/discriminatory option. The options can be used once, more than once, or not at all.

Questions

364. A 36-year-old man complains of pain at rest in his calves.
365. A 34-year-old man complains of pain in the calves on walking .The pain is absent on resting.
366. A 55-year-old patient is scheduled to go femoral bypass surgery. Doctor wants to know the exact site of block.
367. A 46-year-old woman is brought to the A & E Deptt. Breathless and complaining of chest pain. He has a two month history of leg pain.

THEME: 69
TREATMENT OF LOWER LIMB ISCHAEMIA

Options

a. Femoro-popliteal bypass
b. Percutaneous balloon angioplasty
c. Femoro-distal bypass
d. Intra-arterial t-PA infusion
e. Below knee amputation
f. Fasciotomy
g. Lumbar sympathectomy
h. Aorto-femoral bypass
i. Axillo-femoral bypass
j. Femoro-femoral crossover graft

For each of the situations/conditions given below, choose the one most appropriate/discriminatory option from above. The options may be used once, more than once, or not at all.

Questions

368. A 65-year-old man present with intermittent claudication of the left calf. The claudication distance is 100 m. Angiography demonstrates a 1.5 cm stenosis of the left superficial femoral artery.
369. A 73-year-old diabetic woman presents with critical ischaemia of the right leg. Angiography reveals extensive disease of the superficial femoral, popliteal and tibial arteries. Pulse generated run-off in the posterior tibial artery.
370. A 72-year-old man presents with a 4 hour history of acute ischaemia of left leg. Clinical examination reveals signs of acute ischaemia with no evidence of gangrene. There is no neurological deficit. An urgent arteriogram reveals a complete occlusion of the distal superficial femoral artery most likely caused by thrombosis.
371. A 57-year-old smoker present with intermittent claudication of the right calf. The claudication distance is 70m. Angiography reveals a 12 cm stenosis in the proximal superficial femoral artery.
372. A 21-year-old motorcyclist present with multiple injuries following a RTA. Clinical examination reveals a critically ischaemic right lower leg. The right dorsalis pedis pulse is feeble. The right calf is tense and swollen. The intracompartmental pressure is 55 mmHg. Angiography shows no discontuity of the arterial tree.

THEME: 70
DIAGNOSIS OF BREAST SWELLING

Options

a. Fibro adenosis.
b. Cyst formation.
c. Sclerosing adenosis.

d. Plasma cell mastitis.
e. Fibro adenoma.
f. Serocystic disease of brodie.
g. Medullary duct carcinoma.
h. Paget's disease.
i. Scirrhous carcinoma.
j. Atrophic scirrhous carcinoma.
k. Inflammatory carcinoma.

For each of the statements/situations given below, choose the one most appropriate/discriminatory option. The options can be used once, more than once, or not at all.

Questions

373. Firm, encapsulated, breast mouse.
374. Diffuse lumpiness best palpated using fingers.
375. Intraepithelial neoplasia with underlying duct carcinoma.
376. Fulminating form most often seen during or immediately after pregnancy.
377. Well circumscribed mass. Histologically has prominent lymphocytic infiltrate with pseudocapsule.
378. Discrete lumps of short history seen in perimenopausal women. Swelling is smooth, tense and may be fluctuant.
379. Swelling is usually bilateral and is due to aberrant duct involution . This condition is also called duct ectasia.
380. Firm, mobile lump, associated mastalgia. Mammography may show speckled calcification.
381. Firm, encapsulated lump with ulceration of overlying skin by pressure nercosis. Lump is mobile and well cicumscribed. Pateint is otherwise well.

THEME: 71
INVESTIGATION OF BREAST DISEASE

Options

a. Open biopsy
b. Fine needle biopsy
c. Ultrasound
d. Reassurance

e. Mammography
f. Wide excision
g. Computed tomography
h. Magnetic resonance imaging
i. Lymphagiography

For each of the statements/situations given below, choose the one most appropriate/discriminatory option. The options can be used once ,more than once or not at all.

Questions

382. A 35-year-old woman comes to the clinic for screening of her breasts.
383. A 45-year-old woman presenrs with a mass in her right upper quadrant of her right breast. A round smooth mass is found in the axilla.
384. A 36-year-old woman comes with ahard mass in her breast. The skin is tethered. Ultrasound and mammography were inconclusive. The patient wants to be satisfied that this is not malignant.
385. A 36-year-old woman presents with itching of her left nipple. On examination, no ulceration is seen, but a scaly lesion around the nipple is observed.
386. A 23-year-old woman says she feels lumps in her breasts during the time of her periods. She also feels anxious and irritable.

THEME: 72
DIAGNOSIS OF VASCULAR DISEASE

Options

a. Thromboangitis obliterans.
b. Ruptured Baker's cyst.
c. Deep vein thrombosis.
d. Atherosclerosis.
e. Embolus.
f. Varicose veins.
g. Cellulitis.
h. Sciatica.

For each of the statements/situations given below, choose the one most appropriate/discriminatory option. The options can be used once, more than once, or not at all.

Questions

387. A 60-year-old diabetic, complains of pain in thigh and gluteal region on walking up the stairs for the last six months. She is a smoker and has ischemic heart disease.
388. A 45-year-old is admitted to casualty with excruciating pain in the right leg. On examination limb is pale and dorsalis pedis and posterior tibial pulse is absent. Pulse is 88/min, irregular and he has a pansystolic murmur at apex.
389. An obese 40-year-old lady, developed a painful leg on 10th postoperation day following emergency surgery for a ruptured ectopic pregnancy.
390. A 28-year-old shipyard worker admitted for pain in calf while work which has been increasing over last 3 months. There is no history of hypertension or diabetes but he is a smoker. On examination, he has loss of posterior tibial and dorsalis pedis pulsations along with a non-healing ulcer at the base of right 1st MCP joint.
391. A 50-year-old policemen comes with generalized aches on his lower limbs.on examination, pigmentation around both ankles is seen and a swelling appears below left ingiunal ligament when he coughs.

THEME: 73
INVESTIGATION OF AORTIC ANEURISM

Options

a. Abdominal Ultrasound
b. Chest X-ray
c. Barium meal
d. Transoesophageal echocardoigraphy
e. Endoscopic studies
f. Barium swallow
g. Computed tomography of head
h. Echo cardiography

i. Spiral computed tomography
j. Lower limb angiography
k. Coronary angiography
l. Plain abdominal X-ray

For each of the statements/situations given below, choose the one most appropriate/discriminatory option. The options can be used once, more than once, or not at all.

Questions

392. A man presents with abdominal pain radiating to the back.He is found to have pulsatile mass in the abdominal pain. He is haemodynamically stable.
393. A 67-year-old man is being prepared for the repair of an aortic aneurysm.Exercise ECG reveals ischaemia .There is claudication in the legs.
394. This patient is due for repair of aneurysm of aorta , wants to know about the extension of the aneurysm to the renal artery.
395. An obese, 34-year-old man complains of retrosternal pain associated pain associated with water brash.

THEME: 74
CAUSES OF PAIN IN THE LOWER EXTREMITIES

Options

a. Buerger's disease
b. Varicose veins
c. Leriche syndrome
d. Femoral-popliteal disease
e. Acute arterial occlusion of the lower limb
f. Post-traumatic vasomotor dystrophy
g. Raynaud's phenomenon
h. Phlebitis
i. Anterior tibial compartment syndrome
j. Osteomyelitis
k. Deep venous thrombosis

For each of the situations/conditions given below, choose the one most appropriate/discriminatory option from above. The options may be used once, more than once, or not at all.

Questions

396. A 30-year-old marathon runner presents with intense pain in his anterolateral calf. On examination, he has a swollen leg with pain on dorsiflexion and numbness in the first dorsal web space.
397. A 50-year-old woman presents with pain in the calves after prolonged standing. On examination, she has mild ankle oedema, paper-thin skin, and an ulcer over the medial molleolus and lipodermatosclerosis.
398. A 60-year-old man with a history of myocardial infarction now presents with a painful left leg. On examination, the left is cold. Peripheral pulses cannot be palpated. He cannot lift his leg and complains of pins and needles in the leg.
399. A 55-year-old man presents with buttock and thigh pain. He is impotent.
400. A 60-year-old man complains of pain in the calves, severe enough to limit his mobility. The pain is now in his feet and worse at night in bed. He hangs his leg over the side of the bed to relieve the pain. Beurger's test is positive.

THEME: 75
DIAGNOSIS OF PERIPHERAL VASCULAR DISEASE

Options

a. Acute ischaemia of the legs
b. Chronic ischaemia of the legs
c. Intermittent claudication
d. Raynaud's phenomenon
e. Ischaemic foot
f. Dissecting aortic aneurysm
g. Takayasu's syndrome
h. Kawasaki's disease
i. Thromboangiitis obliterans
j. Cardiovascular syphilis
k. Abdominal aneurysm

For each of the situations/conditions given below, choose the one most appropriate/discriminatory option from above. The options may be used once, more than once, or not at all.

Questions

401. A 23-year-old female present with paresthesias and loss of distal pulses in her arms. She is noted to be hypertensive. She describes feeling unwell a month prior with fever and night sweats.
402. A 20-year-old male smoker is noted to have intense tumor of the feet absent foot pulses. On examination, he has an amputated right second toe.
403. A 25-year-old female complains of intermittent pain in her fingers. She describes episodes of numbness and burning of the fingers. She wears gloves whenever she leaves the house.
404. A 60-year-old smoker presents with cramp-like pain in the calves relieved by rest and non-healing ulcers. On examination, her has cold extremities with lack of hair around the ankles and absent distal pulses.
405. A 70-year-old man presents with an acutely painful, pale, paralysed pulse less left leg. He is noted to atrial fibrillation.

THEME: 76
MANAGEMENT OF VARICOSE VEINS

Options

a. Graduated compression stocking
b. Crepe bandage
c. X-ray
d. Skin graft
e. Doppler Ultrasound
f. Elevation of the leg
g. Sclerosant
h. Lose weight

For each of the statements/situations given below, choose the one most appropriate/discriminatory option. The options can be used once, more than once, or not at all.

Questions

406. A middle-aged man with bilateral leg varicose veins is to fly to New York for a abusiness meeting. He comes to you for advice. His father died of embolism .He is scared of surgical operations.
407. An obese woman has bilateral leg varicose veins. Her BMI is 30 and she is found to have Lipodermosclerosis. around her shins.
408. A 54-year-old man presented with varicose veins which developed following a compound fracture of the left lower limb a couple of weeks ago and have persisted.
409. A 45-year-old woman with a BMI of 33 presents with bilateral varicose veins. No treatment has been attempted.

THEME: 77
DIAGNOSIS OF HYPOTHYROIDISM

Options

a. Cretinism.
b. Adult hypothyroidism.
c. Myxodema coma.
d. Hashimoto's goitre.
e. Vascular damage to pituitary glands.

For each of the statements/situations given below, choose the one most appropriate/discriminatory option.The options can be used once, more than once, or not at all.

Questions

410. A 32-year-old female presented with menstrual disturbance, constipation and tiredness after work. On examination she had median nerve palsy in right hand and slow relaxation of ankle jerk. ECG showed flattened T waves.
411. A 3-year-old child presented with failure of growth. On examination he revealed to be having a paraumbilical hernia, pot belly and protruding tongue. Face is pale and puffy.
412. A 40-year-old lady was admitted to A&E with history of LOC since one hour. There is no history of trauma nor is she a diabetic. On examination she had bloated face, pouting lips and core temperature is 30°C.

413. A 30-year-old lady c/o intolerance to cold and weight gain and also c/o pain in the neck. On examination there is no thyromegaly. Blood tests showed the presence of thyroid antibodies. There is a family history of pernicious anemia.
414. A 28-year-old lady developed complications during pregnancy. She had abruptio placenta, i.e. shock which was treated. Nine months later she complained of menorrhagia, her weight gain was quite significant and atrophy of breast shooted.

THEME: 78
DIAGNOSIS OF THYROID CONDITION

Options

a. Retrosternal goiter.
b. Primary thyrotoxicosis
c. Secondary thyrotoxicosis.
d. Carcinoma thyroid.

For each of the statements/situations given below, choose the one most appropriate/discriminatory option.The options can be used once, more than once, or not at all.

Questions

415. A 40-year-old man who has a goiter since 2-year-old c/o hoarseness of voice and swelling overscalp. He suffered a fracture of arm few months ago. On examination there is cervical lymphadenopathy. IDL showed paralysis of laryngeal nerve.
416. A 30-year-old man comes with unexplained diarrhea and wt less since 5 months. On examination there is a goitre and he has proximal myopathy. Sleeping PR is 120/mt.
417. A 40-year-old man c/o a cervical swelling which has appeared recently, followed by this he also complained of breathlessnes at night. On examination there are distended neck veins.
418. A 30-year-old man who is having a neck swelling since a long time, presented with dyspnea. Eye signs are not prominent.
419. A 35-year-old man c/o neck swelling, rapidly growing in size. On examination he is found to have a thrill over the swelling. PR 110/mt and a fine tremor of hands is present.

THEME: 79
DIAGNOSIS OF THYROID SWELLINGS

Options

a. Thyrotoxicosis factitia.
b. Jod Bardew thyrotoxicosis.
c. Thyrotoxic crisis (storm).
d. Lingual thyroid.
e. Thyroglossal cyst.
f. Thyroglossal fistula.

For each of the statements/situations given below, choose the one most appropriate/discriminatory option.The options can be used once, more than once, or not at all.

Questions

420. A thyrotoxic patient underwent thyroidectomy recently, developed hyperpyrexia, restlessness and dehydration.
421. Patient presented with swelling in midline which moves on protruding his tongue and swallowing.
422. A 30-year-old man c/o swelling in midline and relevent surgery followed by which he developed discharge of mucus at operation site.
423. Large doses of iodides given to a hyperthyroidism endemic goitre produced temporary hyperthyroidism.
424. A Hypothyroid patient having L–thyroxine develops hyperthyrodism.
425. A 30-year-old man c/o dysphasia noticed recent change in his speech. Sometimes he feels choking. On examination thus is a round swelling at the back of tongue.

THEME: 80
ADRENAL AND PARATHYROID GLANDS

Options

a. Hypoparathyroidism.
b. Hyperparathyroidism.
c. Waterhouse-Frederichson syndrome.
d. Phaeochromocytoma.

e. Conn's syndrome.
f. Nephroblastoma.
g. Wilm's tumor.

For each of the statements/situations given below, choose the one most appropriate/discriminatory option. The options can be used once, more than once or not at all.

Questions

426. A 20-year-old female c/o tiredness, restlessness with personality change. She has a past history of peptic ulcer. X-ray abdomen showed a stone in the right kidney.
427. A 3-year-old child brought with complaints of abdominal swelling. On examination swelling is knobby and extending across the midline.
428. A 35-year-old man c/o vomiting, sweating and breathlessness. On examination he is found to be having BP of 180/110. There is a lump in right hypochondium. His blood sugar is 12 mmol/l.
429. A 30-year-female c/o muscular weakness and polyuria and polydypsia. On examination BP is 160/100 mm Hg. Her plasma Na^+ K^+ and plasma angiotensin levels are low.
430. A 3-year-old child had meningoccocal septicemia, cyanosis and vomiting. There are petechial hemorrhages on the skin and purple blotches.
431. A 25-year-old lady c/o tingling and numbness in fingers and toes. On examination toes are plantar flexed and ankle joint is hyperextended.

THEME: 81
CAUSES OF NECK LUMPS

Options

a. Bronchial cyst
b. Ludwig's angina
c. Parotitis
d. Thyroglossal cyst
e. Dermoid cyst
f. Parapharyngeal abscess

g. Thyroid swelling
h. Sialectaisis
i. Larygooele
j. Pharyngeal pouch
k. Reactive lymphadenitis

For each of the situations/conditions given below, choose the one most appropriate/discriminatory option from above. The options may be used once, more than once, or not at all.

Questions

432. A 45-year-old clarinet player present with a neck swelling that expands with forced inspiration.
433. A 4-year-old boy present with a small midline neck swelling that moves on swallowing. It is painless, mobile, transilluminates and fluctuats.
434. A 26-year-old man following a trip to the dentist for toothache presents with a tender neck swelling, pyrexia and pain on swallowing. His tonsils are not inflames.
435. A 30-year-old male presents with a 5 cm neck swelling anterior to the sterno-mastoid muscle on the left side in its upper third. He states that the swelling has been treated with antibiotics for infection in the past.
436. A 20-year-old man presents with a painful swelling under his jaw. On examination, he has trismus and is dribbling saliva.

THEME: 82
INVESTIGATION OF LUMP IN THE NECK

Options

a. Ultrasound
b. Technetium scan
c. Iodine uptake scan
d. FNAC
e. Excision biopsy
f. Paul Bunnel test
g. Thyroid function tests
h. Doppler ultrasound
i. Digital subtraction angiography

j. Sialogram
k. Nasapharynogoscopy

For each of the situations/conditions given below, choose the one most appropriate/discriminatory option from above. The options may be used once, more than once, or not at all.

Questions

437. A 53-year-old woman presents with a 6-month history of mass below the angle of the jaw on the right. It is gradually increasing in size and is mobile and firm to touch. There is no associated pain or facial weakness.
438. A 67-year-old man presents with a mass in the anterior triangle of the neck. It has increased in size over the last 2 months. It is soft, pulsatile and has an associated bruit.
439. A 38-year-old woman presents with a 2-month history of a swelling in the anterior part of the neck, left of the midline. The swelling is not painful and she feels otherwise well. On examination she has a solitary thyroid nodule in the left lobe of the thyroid. She is clinically euthyroid.
440. A 46-year-old woman presents with diffuse welling in the anterior part of the neck. She also describes a hoarse voice. On examination she has a diffuse multinodular goitre, bradycardia and slow relaxing reflexes.
441. A 27-year-old man describes intermittent painful swelling below his jaw. The pain and swelling is worse on eating. He is otherwise well. On examination there is a small tender swelling in the left submandibular region.
442. A 72-year-old man present with a hard painless swelling in the anterior triangle of the neck. He has had hoarse voice for 2 months. He is a lifelong smoker and drinks heavily.

THEME: 83
THE TREATMENT OF NECK LUMPS

Options

a. Incision and drainage
b. Intravenous antibiotics

c. Sistrunk's operation
d. Endoscopic diverticulotomy
e. External excision
f. Antituberculous chemotherapy
g. Submandibular gland excision
h. Total thyroidectomy
i. Excisional biopsy
j. Thryoid lobectomy

For each of the situations/conditions given below, choose the one most appropriate/discriminatory option from above. The options may be used once, more than once, or not at all.

Questions

443. A 20-year-old man presents with a mobile midline neck swelling that moves when he sticks out his tongue.
444. A 50-year-old man presents with a right neck swelling that is discharging malodorous cheesy discharge. Chest X-ray shows patchy shadows in the left apex.
445. A 30-year-old woman presents with a 4 cm cystic swelling over the anterior third of her left sternomastoid muscle.
446. A 40-year-old man presents with a midline neck swelling. The swelling has grown to 5 cm over 6 weeks and moves upon swallowing. Fine needle aspiration shows anaplastic cells.
447. A 60-year-old smoker presents with a 6 cm neck lump in the posterior triangle. The fine needle aspirate is inconclusive.

THEME: 84
DIAGNOSIS OF BREAST DISEASE

Options

a. Fibroadenoma
b. Fibrocytic disease
c. Galactocele
d. Intraductal papilloma
e. Mammary duct ectasia
f. Breast cancer

g. Cystosarcoma phylloids
h. Breast abscess
i. Fat necrosis
j. Paget's disease
k. Eczema of the nipple

For each of the situations/conditions given below, choose the one most appropriate/discriminatory option from above. The options may be used once, more than once, or not at all.

Questions

448. A 28-year-old female presents with a solitary 3 cm freely mobile painless nodule. She also complains of a serious nipple discharge and axillary lymphadenopathy.
449. A 36-year-old female with multiple and bilateral cystic breast swellings which are notes to be particular painful and tender premenstrually. She states that during pregnancy the symptoms improved.
450. A 50-year-old woman presents with nipple discharge, nipple retraction, dilation of ducts, and chronic intraductal and periductal inflammation. The diagnosis is confirmed by breast biopsy, and no further treatment is required.
451. A 50-year-old woman presents with an eczematoid appearance to her nipple and areola. It is associated with a discrete nodule that is attached to the overlying skin.
452. A 33-year-old lactating female presents with a 1-week history of a painful, erythematous breast lump and pyrexia. She has tried a course of antibiotics to no avail.

THEME: 85
DIAGNOSIS OF BENIGN BREAST DISEASE

Options

a. Breast abscess
b. Benign mammary dysplasia
c. Fibroadenoma
d. Periductal mastitis
e. Silicon granulomas
f. Leaking breast implant

g. Sebaceous cyst
h. Duct papilloma
i. Lipoma
j. Fat necrosis
k. Duct extais
l. Rupruted breast implant
m. Cystic disease

For each of the situations/conditions given below, choose the one most appropriate/discriminatory option from above. The options may be used once, more than once, or not at all.

Questions

453. A 33-year-old female is found to have rippling of the lower margins of her breast implants.
454. A 30-year-old female presents with a smooth , firm 3 cm breast mass that is not attached to skin. FNAC shows no malignant cells.
455. A 20-year-old female complains of breast lumpiness and breast pain prior to her periods. On examination, her breast are tender in the outer quadrants with some nodularathy. FNAC shows fibrosis, adenosis and cystic changes.
456. A 50-year-old woman presents with multiple discrete smooth breast lumps. Yellow fluid is obtained on aspiration. FNAC shows no malignant cells.
457. A 40-year-old woman presents with persistent cheesy nipple discharge. She is noted to have nipple retraction and no discrete lumps. Mammogram shows duct thickening.

THEME: 86
DIAGNOSIS OF BREAST LUMPS

Options

a. Duct ectasia.
b. Traumatic fat necrosis.
c. Mondors disease.
d. Fibroadenosis.
e. Duct papilloma.
f. Acute mastitis.
g. Tubercular abscess

For each of the statements/situations given below, choose the one most appropriate/discriminatory option. The options can be used once, more than once, or not at all.

Questions

458. A 30-year-female presented with painless swelling in breast for six months on examination. edges are level but has a soft centre. There is discharge of pus on pressing the nipple. Axillary lymph nodes are enlarged. The count is normal.
459. A 35-year-old lady c/o swelling in upper part of breast. On examination swelling is hard, irregular fixed to skin. There are no enlargement of axillary lymph nodes. She gives h/o of vehicular accident 6 months back.
460. A 25-year-old lady presented with guttering over the surface of breast. On examination there is an indurated cord and a grove like structure along it's side in subcutaneous plane.
461. A 30-year-old presented with a swelling extending from the nipple with a multi colored discharge per nipple. On examination there is pain and tenderness and a mass.
462. A 20-year-old presenting with blood stained discharge per nipple. On examination found to be having a cystic swelling beneath the nipple. Pressure on it causes discharge from the nipple.

THEME: 87
DIAGNOSIS OF BREAST CONDITION

Options

a. Fibroadenoma.
b. Fibroadenosis.
c. Paget's disease of nipple.
d. Retromammary abscess.
e. Eczema.
f. Cancer-en-cuircasse.
g. Cystosarcoma phylloids.

For each of the statements/situations given below, choose the one most appropriate/discriminatory option. The options can be used once, more than once, or not at all.

Questions

463. A 45-year-old female complains of premenstrual pain and tenderness in both breasts On examination there is a dark green discharge per nipple and fine nodularity of both breasts.
464. A 25-year-old lady presented with swelling of breasts. On examination firm, well defined, lobulated extremely mobile lump felt.
465. A 30-year-old lady presented with swelling of breast. On examination afebrile, count high. Breast palpation revealed no abnormality. X-ray showed erosion of third rib.
466. A 30-year-old lady presented with eczematous condition of right nipple and over a period of time nipple got eroded. Histology showed foamy cells and atypical nuclei.
467. A 30-year-old lady with a hard lump in right breast of size 7.5 cm presented with non pitting oedema of right arm as well as there are nodules over the chest wall.
468. A 40-year-old lady c/o large swelling of right breast, On examination ulceration over skin, bosselated surface, mobile over the chest wall.

THEME: 88
INVESTIGATION OF BREAST DISEASE

Options

a. FNAC
b. Sterotype cone biopsy
c. Wide excision
d. Mammography
e. Ultrasound
f. CT scan
g. MRI
h. Family history
i. Ductulography

For each of the situations/conditions given below, choose the one most appropriate/discriminatory option from above. The options may be used once, more than once, or not at all.

Questions

469. A 28-year-old woman who presents with a mass in the upper lateral quadrant of her breast. On examination, she has a discreet 2 cm mass, which is mobile, non tender and does not involve the axilla. She has a morbid fear of needles.
470. A 24-year-old woman presents with a diffuse nodular breast swelling, which seems to increase in size during her periods. There is no axillary involvement and it disappears after her menses.
471. A 59-year-old woman has a mass in the upper lateral quadrant of her left breast. The skin is pulled in and there is no axillary involvement.
472. A 34-year-old woman had a mammography done. It showed diffuse calcification. She wants to know for sure that she has no malignancy.

THEME: 89
TREATMENT OF BREAST CANCER

Options

a. Chemotherapy, LHRH & biphosphonates
b. Simple mastectomy
c. Tamoxifen
d. Radiotherapy
e. Patey's mastectomy
f. Wide local excision combined with axillary dissection + radiotherapy Tamoxifen.
g. Radical mastectomy
h. Expectant management
i. Excision biopsy and cytology

For each of the situations/conditions given below, choose the one most appropriate/discriminatory option from above. The options may be used once, more than once, or not at all.

Questions

473. A 70-year-old woman presents with a 2 cm lump in the upper outer quadrant of the right breast. The lump does

not involve the skin and is mobile/ FNAC reveals malignant cells. Mammography shows a speculate lesion corresponding to the lump.

474. A 40-year-old woman is found to have a widespread microcalcification during screening mammography. A sterotactic cone biopsy reveals a low-grade ductal carcinoma in situ.
475. A 35-year-old woman presents with a 4 cm carcinoma of the left breast and multiple bone metastases in the pelvis.
476. A 95-year-old woman presents with a locally advanced carcinoma of the left breast. The tumour is ER positive.

THEME: 90
DIAGNOSIS OF RECTAL BLEEDING

Options

a. Carcinoma of the colon
b. Proctitis
c. Carcinoma of the rectum
d. Haemorrhoids
e. Ulcerative colitis
f. Diverticular disease
g. Peptic ulceration
h. Fissure-in-ano
i. Carcinoma of the anus
j. Fistulae in Crohn's disease

For each of the situations/conditions given below, choose the one most appropriate/discriminatory option from above. The options may be used once, more than once, or not at all.

Questions

477. A 30-year-old man presents with painless rectal bleeding mixed with mucus. He has a history if intermittent diarrhoea. On examination there is no evidence of perianal disease.
478. A 40-year-old man presents with painless melena. On examination, the anus and rectum are normal. He denies weight loss. He drinks and smokes heavily.

479. A 25-year-old man present with anal pain, bloody discharge and mucus. On examination there are multiple puckered scars around the anus.
480. A 50-year-old man passes 500 ml of fresh blood from his rectum. He describes a need to defecate but instead of passing stool, he passed blood. He has chronic, left sided abdominal discomfort. He denies weight loss and has no palpable masses.
481. A 70-year-old man presents with painless rectal bleeding. The blood is streaked on his stool. He complains of tenesmus. A soft, fixed mass is palpated on digital rectal examination. There are no palpable inguinal lymph nodes.

THEME: 91
DIAGNOSIS OF ANORECTAL DISEASE

Options

a. Fistulo-in-ano
b. Anorectal abscess
c. Pilonidal sinus
d. Perianal haematoma
e. Perianal warts
f. Fissure-in-ano
g. Carcinoma of the rectum
h. Haemorrhoids
i. Diverticular disease
j. Proctlgia fugax
k. Prolapsed rectum
l. Intussusception

For each of the situations/conditions given below, choose the one most appropriate/discriminatory option from above. The options may be used once, more than once, or not at all.

Questions

482. A 90-year-old female presents with a large lump in her anus. It appeared after defecation. The lump is red with concentric folds of mucosa around a central pit and is nontender.

483. A 50-year-old woman present to her GP with severe rectal pain. It is worse at night and last minutes to hours. The rectal examination is normal.
484. A 39-year-Old Italian man present to his GP with a painful bottom. On examination, the gluteal cleft over the midline of the sacrum , and coccyx is red and tender.
485. A 30-year-old man presents with anal pain, discharge and itching. On examination there are multiple opening 2 cm behind and to the right of the anus.
486. A 29-year-old mother of two present with pain on defecation with blood staining of the toilet paper. On examination, she has a split in the skin posterior to the anus and a small skin tag at the lower end.

THEME: 92
DIAGNOSIS OF PENILE CONDITIONS

Option

a. Phimosis
b. Paraphimosis
c. Priapism
d. Penile warts
e. Peyronie's disease
f. Squamous cell carcinoma of the penis
g. Erythroplasia of Queyrat
h. Impotence
i. Balanitis xerotica obliterans

For each of the situations/conditions given below, choose the one most appropriate/discriminatory option from above. The options may be used once, more than once, or not at all.

Questions

487. A 40-year-old man presents to casualty with a painful penis. On examination, the foreskin is retracted behind the glans with glandular swellings.
488. A 12-year-old boy with a history of UTIs presents with difficult urinating. On examination, the opening of the foreskin is pinhole in size.

489. A 50-year-old man with a history of chronic renal failure presents with a painful penis. On examination, the corpus cavernosa are erect, and the corpus spongiosum is flaccid.
490. A 40-year-old man with Reidel's throiditis complaints that intercourse is painful. He provides a photo that shows dorsal curvature of the erect penis.
491. A 55-year-old man complains that he is unable to obtain erection. He had undergone abdominal aortic aneurysm repair recently.

THEME: 93
DIAGNOSIS OF TESTICULAR PAIN

Options

a. Orchitis
b. Epididymitis
c. Testicular torsion
d. Varicocoele
e. Inguinal hernia
f. Testicular tumour

For each of the statements/situations given below, choose the one most appropriate/discriminatory option. The options can be used once, more than once, or not at all.

Questions

492. An 18-year-old boy develops sudden pain in her left testis while cycling to school.
493. A 24-year-old complaints of pain in his right testis. He also reports pain on opening his mouth.
494. A 54-year-old male complains of pain in his left testis on standing for a long-time.
495. A middle-aged man complains of severe testicular pain. On examination it's relieved by elevation of the testis.

THEME: 94
CAUSES OF SCROTAL SWELLINGS

Options

a. Hydrocele

b. Varicocele
c. Epididymal cyst
d. Seminoma
e. Teratoma
f. Chronic epididymitis
g. Mumps orchitis
h. Acute epididymitis
i. Torsion of the testis
j. Inguinal hernia
k. Testicular gumma
l. Scrotal haematoma

For each of the situations/conditions given below, choose the one most appropriate/discriminatory option from above. The options may be used once, more than once, or not at all.

Questions

496. A 30-year-old man presents with a swelling within the left scrotum, which aches when he stands. On examination the swelling is not tender and feels like 'a bag of worms'
497. A 25-year-old present with pyrexia, headache and painful swelling of his face and testes.
498. A 35-year-old man presents with a swelling of his left testis, which is gradually increasing in size. On examination the swelling is hard, nontender and doesn't illuminate.
499. A 45-year-old man presents with a painless swelling in his scrotum. His left testis cannot be felt. The swelling transilluminates.
500. A 20-year-old man presents with an acute onset of vomiting and pain in the lower abdomen after playing football. His abdomen is soft but he has a very tender, swollen right testis, which lies high within the scrotum.
501. A 40-year-old man presents with a painless swelling in his scrotum, which is fluctuant and transilluminant. Both the testes are easily palpable.

THEME: 95
THE TREATMENT OF TESTICULAR SWELLINGS

Options

a. Surgical exploration of the scotum

b. Injections of chronic gonadotropin
c. Surgical fixation of the testes in the scrotum
d. Orchidectomy alone
e. Orchidectomy followed by radiotherapy
f. Orchidectomy followed by chemotherapy
g. Bedrest and the appropriate antibiotic
h. Surgical removal of the cyst
i. No treatment is required
j. Aspiration of fluid
k. Inguinal herniorrhaphy

For each of the situations/conditions given below, choose the one most appropriate/discriminatory option from above. The options may be used once, more than once, or not at all.

Questions

502. A 14-year-old boy present with an acutely swollen and painful testis and also pain in the lower abdomen. On examination, the testis lies high in the scrotum.
503. A 35-year-old man presents with a solid testis and abdominal lymph nodes. He has a history of undescended testes as a child.
504. A 20-year-old man presents with a solid testis this is markedly cystic in appearance and lymph node deposits.
505. A 18-year-old man presents with fever, leukocytes, and a very painful swelling in the testis. Examination of the urine reveals the presence of pus cells.
506. A 60-year-old man presents with a large scrotal swelling that gets in the way of his clothes. On examination, the swelling is fluctuant, and the testis is palpable separately from the swelling.

Fifteen

Radiology

THEME: 1
X-RAY SPINE

Options

a. Ankylosing spondylitis.
b. Rheumatoid arthritis.
c. Osteoporosis.
d. Osteomalacia.
e. Scheurmann's disease.
f. Spondylosis.

For each of the situations/conditions given below, choose the one most appropriate/discriminatory option from above. The options may be used once, more than once, or not at all.

Questions

1. 'Scottie dog'.
2. Bamboo spine.
3. Rugger jersey spine.
4. Apophysitis.

THEME: 2
PLAIN SKULL X-RAY

Options

a. Diffuse increase in vault density.
b. Diffuse increase in thickness.
c. Localized increase in bone density.
d. Lucent areas.
e. Tram like calcification.

f. Ring calcification.
g. Erosion of the posterior clinoid.
h. Erosion of the lamina dura of the dorsum sella.

For each of the situations/conditions given below, choose the one most appropriate/discriminatory option from above. The options may be used once, more than once, or not at all.

Questions

5. Osteomyelitis.
6. Fluorosis.
7. Trauma.
8. Sturge-Weber syndrome.
9. Thalassemia.
10. Increased intracranial pressure.
11. Old aneurysm.

THEME: 3
HAND X-RAY

Options

a. Sarcoid.
b. Early hyperparathyroidism.
c. Lipoidoses.
d. Scleroderma.

For each of the situations/conditions given below, choose the one most appropriate/discriminatory option from above. The options may be used once, more than once, or not at all.

Questions

12. Coarse trabeculations.
13. Erosion of terminal phalangeal tuft.
14. Pseudo clubbing.
15. Subperiosteal erosions.

THEME: 4
CARDIOVASCULAR ULTRASOUND

Options

a. M-Mode echocardiography.
b. 2D–echocardiography.
c. Duplex doppler.

For each of the situations/conditions given below, choose the one most appropriate/discriminatory option from above. The options may be used once, more than once, or not at all.

Questions

16. Real time images of anatomy and spatial relationships.
17. Colour coding of flow directions.
18. Measurement of chamber size.
19. Assessment of valve and wall motion.

Sixteen

Biochemistry

THEME: 1
PLASMA ENZYMES

Options

a. ALT (SGPT).
b. AST (SGOT).
c. Aldolase.
d. Alpha amylase.
e. Creatine kinase.
f. LDH.

For each of the situations/conditions given below, choose the one most appropriate/discriminatory option from above. The options may be used once, more than once, or not at all.

Questions

1. Uremia.
2. Pulmonary embolism.
3. Liver disease.
4. Pancreatitis.
5. Hemolysis.

THEME: 2
PORPHYRIAS

Options

a. Acute intermittent porphyria.
b. Variegate porphyria.
c. Porphyria cutanea tarda.

For each of the situations/conditions given below, choose the one most appropriate/discriminatory option from above. The options may be used once, more than once, or not at all.

Questions

6. Increased urinary porphobilinogin only during attacks.
7. Increased fecal porphyrins.
8. Precipitated by drugs.
9. Cutaneous photosensitivity in the main feature.
10. Increased urinary porphobilinogen during and also in between attacks.

THEME: 3
WHEN TO TREAT HYPERLIPIDEMIA

Options

a. Above 4.8 m mol/lit.
b. Above 5.0 m mol/lit.
c. Above 5.2 m mol/lit.
d. Above 5.5 m mol/lit.
e. Above 6.0 m mol/lit.
f. Above 6.8 m mol/lit.
g. Above 7.8 m mol/lit.
h. Above 11.2 m mol/lit.

For each of the situations/conditions given below, choose the one most appropriate/discriminatory option from above. The options may be used once, more than once, or not at all.

Questions

11. Patient with ischemic heart disease, but otherwise asymptomatic.
12. Normal adult male.
13. Normal old aged male.
14. Patient with just angina.
15. Patient with past history of myocardial infarction.
16. Hypertensive patient.

THEME : 4
DIAGNOSIS OF HYPERLIPIDEMIA

Options

a. Lipoprotein lipase deficiency.
b. Familial defective Apo protein B.
c. Polygenic hypercholesterolemia.
d. Familial combined hyperlipidemia.
e. Remnant particle disease.
f. Familial hypertriglyceridemia.

For each of the situations/conditions given below, choose the one most appropriate/discriminatory option from above. The options may be used once, more than once, or not at all.

Questions

17. Cholesterol 7.5-16 m mol/lit and triglyceride level < 2.3 m mol/lit and raised LDL. On examination patient has tendon xanthomas, arcus and xanthelesma.
18. Both cholesterol and triglyceride levels 9-14 m mol/lit and raised LDL. Patient has palmar striae and tuberous xanthoma.
19. Cholesterol < 6.5 m mol/lit, triglycerides 10-30 m mol/lit and raised chylomicrons.
20. Commonest primary hyperlipidemia.
21. Cholesterol 6.5-10 m mol/lit and triglycerides 2.3-10 m mol/lit, both LDL and VLDL raised. Patient is found to have arcus and xanthelesma.

THEME : 5
MANAGEMENT OF HYPERLIPIDEMIA

Options

a. No specific treatment required.
b. Statin.
c. Fibrate.
d. Statin and fibrate.
e. Dietary advice.

f. Cholestyramine.
g. Nicotinic acid.
h. Treat secondary cause first.

For each of the situations/conditions given below, choose the one most appropriate/discriminatory option from above. The options may be used once, more than once, or not at all.

Questions

22. A 72-year-old man has suffered an acute MI. He is found to have a total serum cholesterol level of 5 mmol/l and triglyceride of 2.5 mmol/l on discharge from hospital.
23. A 40-year-old man was admitted with acute pancreatitis. After recovering from this, he was found to have a triglyceride level of 7.4 mmol/l. His cholesterol is 6.7 mmol/l. He admits to drinking 4 cans of strong beer everyday.
24. A 50-year-old man has peripheral vascular disease and angina. He has no secondary causes for dyslipidemia. His total cholesterol is measured at 5.8 mmol/l and his triglyceride level is 3.4 mmol/l
25. A 38-year-old woman has symptomatic primary biliary cirrhosis. Her total cholesterol is 7.8 mmol/l and triglyceride level is 2.1 mmol/l.
26. A 55-year-old woman has recently been diagnosed with type 2 diabetes and is found to have a fasting total cholesterol level of 4.9 mmol/l and triglyceride of 4.0 mmol/l. After 6 months of dietary treatment, her diabetes is well controlled but her triglyceride is still 3.8 mmol/l

THEME: 6
SIDE EFFECTS OF CHOLESTEROL LOWERING DRUGS

Options

a. Porphyrias.
b. Cholelithiasis.
c. Flushing.
d. Constipation.

For each of the situations/conditions given below, choose the one most appropriate/discriminatory option from above. The options may be used once, more than once, or not at all.

Questions

27. Nicotinic acid.
28. Statins.
29. Cholestyramine.
30. Fibrates.

THEME: 7
ELECTROLYTE IMBALANCE

Options

a. Hypernatremia.
b. Hyponatremia.
c. Hypokalemia.
d. Hyperkalemia.
e. Hypercalcemia.
f. Hypocalcemia.
g. Deficiency of zinc.
h. Deficiency of selenium.
i. Hypoglycemia

For each of the situations/conditions given below, choose the one most appropriate/discriminatory option from above. The options may be used once, more than once, or not at all.

Questions

31. ECG shows tall tented T-waves, small p-waves, wide QRS complexes.
32. Can cause red crusted skin lesions around nostrils and corners of mouth.
33. Causes paresthesias, tetany, depression and prolongs QT interval.
34. Causes confusion, fits anorexia and muscle weakness and may be caused as a complication of SIADH.
35. Sweating, palpitations, tremors, drowsiness and fatigue.

36. Muscle weakness and ectopic beats. ECG shows flattened or inverted T-waves.
37. Severe abdominal pain, nausea, vomiting, constipation, polyuria and polydipsia.

THEME: 8
INVESTIGATIONS OF MINERAL DISORDERS

Options

	Ca^{2+}	PO_4^{3-}	*Alkaline Phosphate*
a.	N	N	N
b.	D	D	I
c.	N	N	I
d.	I	I/N	N
e.	I	I/N	I
f.	I	D/N	N/I
g.	D	I	N
h.	D	I	N/D

Key: N-Normal; I-Increased; D-Decreased

For each of the situations/conditions given below, choose the one most appropriate/discriminatory option from above. The options may be used once, more than once, or not at all.

Questions

38. Primary hyperparathyroidism.
39. Osteomalacia.
40. Myeloma.
41. Paget's disease.
42. Osteoporosis.
43. Renal failure.
44. Hypoparathyroidism.
45. Bone metastases.

THEME: 9
BONE BIOCHEMICAL DISORDERS

Options

a. Osteoporosis.
b. Paget's disease.
c. Osteomalacia.

For each of the situations/conditions given below, choose the one most appropriate/discriminatory option from above. The options may be used once, more than once, or not at all.

Questions

46. Normal bony tissue but reduced mineral content.
47. Reduced bone density.
48. Increased bone turnover with localized bone enlargement.

THEME : 10
DIAGNOSIS OF HYPERCALCEMIA

Options

a. Primary hyperparathyroidism.
b. Secondary hyperparathyroidism.
c. Metastatic prostate cancer.
e. Hypoparathyroidism.
f. Tertiary hyperparathyroidism.
g. Hyperthyroidism.
h. Sarcoidosis.
i. Multiple myeloma.
j. Paget's disease of the bone.
k. Thiazide diuretics.
l. Hyperparathyroid with ectopic PTH.

For each of the situations/conditions given below, choose the one most appropriate/discriminatory option from above. The options may be used once, more than once, or not at all.

Questions

49. A 28-year-old woman with breathlessness: Calcium 2.9, phosphate 0.9, ALP 70, PTH low normal, 25-OH vitamin D low-normal, !,25-OH vitamin D high.
50. A 65-year-old woman who has recently become wheelchair bound due to hip pain: calcium 2.95, phosphate 0.9, ALP 750, PTH normal, 25-OH vitamin D normal
51. A 55-year-old man with back pain: calcium 3.1, phosphate 0.6, ALP 70, albumin 28g/l, total protein 91g/l, Hb 10g/l.
52. A 60-year-old man presented with following reports on a routine screen: calcium 2.85, phosphate 0.8, ALP 110, PTH raised, 25-OH vitamin low-normal.
53. A 40-year-old woman with bone pain, drowsiness and thirst: calcium 3.3, phosphate 0.75, ALP 190, PTH low-normal, PTH high, glucose 6 mmol/l.

THEME: 11
ABG ABNORMALATIES

Options

a. Diabetic hyperosmolar coma.
b. Metabolic alkalosis due to diuretic.
c. Barter syndrome.
d. Renal failure.
e. Severe failure.
f. Severe asthma requiring reassurance and oxygen.
g. Metabolic alkalosis needs in NaCl therapy.
h. Renal tubular acidosis.
i. Diabetic keto acidosis.

For each of the situations/conditions given below, choose the one most appropriate/discriminatory option from above. The options may be used once, more than once, or not at all.

Questions

54. A 30-year-old male, a known asthmatic is admitted to causalty, looking very tired. P_H – 7.34, PO_2 – 6.5, PCO_2 – 6, HCO_3 – 16.

55. A 20-year-old known patient of IDDM is admitted with acute abdominal pain and dyspnea. P_H – 7.04, PO_2 – 13, PCO_2 – 1.2, HCO_3 – 3, Na – 138, K – 6.1, Cl – 103, anion gap – 32, Blood glucose – 18.
56. A 50-year-old male recovering from a myocardial infection sustained 14 days ago, on diuretics for hypertension. P_H – 7.54, PO_2 – 8, PCO_2 – 4.5, HCO_3 – 30.
57. A 50-year-old lady with long standing history of dyspepsia is now admitted with complaints of vomiting. P_H – 7.52, PO_2 – 12, PCO_2 – 6.5, HCO_3 – 40, K – 2.1. The patient also complains of sever generalized weakness.

THEME: 12
ABG ABNORMALITIES

Options

a. Septicemia.
b. Lactic acidosis.
c. Respiratory acidosis due to COPD.
d. Pickwickian syndrome.
e. Salicylate poisoning.
f. Respiratory alkalosis.
g. Mixed respiratory alkalosis with metabolic acidosis.
h. Uremic acidosis.
i. Methyl alcohol poisoning.

For each of the situations/conditions given below, choose the one most appropriate/discriminatory option from above. The options may be used once, more than once, or not at all.

Questions

58. A 70-Year-old diabetic lady on regular OHA's is now admitted with breathlessness. P_H – 7.1, PO_2 – 12, Na – 138, Cl – 101, PCO_2 – 2.5, HCO_3 – 5, K – 4.1, anion gap –32, blood glucose – 10.
59. A 25-year-old collegiate male was brought to causalty with severe breathlessness. His girlfriend has recently left him. P_H – 7.48, PCO_2 – 3, PO_2 – 10, HCO_3 – 20.

60. A 60-year-old chronic smoker complains of dyspnea. P_H –7.15, PO_2 – 8, PCO_2 – 10, HCO_3 – 30.
61. An obese 25-year-old male complains of drowsiness throughout the day and often falling asleep in his office. P_H – 7.35, PO_2 – 9, PCO_2 – 7.8, HCO_3 – 32.

THEME: 13
CAUSES OF HYPOKALEMIA

Options

a. Lower gastrointestinal losses.
b. Prior use of diuretics.
c. Renal tubular acidosis (RTA).
d. Current use of diuretics.
e. Malignant hypertension.
f. Primary hyperaldosteronism.
g. Glucocorticoid excess.

For each of the situations/conditions given below, choose the one most appropriate/discriminatory option from above. The options may be used once, more than once, or not at all.

Questions

62. Normal blood pressure urine K^+ 15 m mol/L bicarbonate above normal.
63. Hypertension, low plasma renin, low-plasma aldosterone.
64. Normal blood pressure, urine K^+ 40 m mol/L, low serum bicarbonate.
65. Hypertension, low-plasma renin, high plasma aldosterone.
66. Normal blood pressure, urine K^+ 15 m mol/L, bicarbonate low.

Seventeen

Pediatrics

THEME: 1
DIAGNOSIS OF FEVER WITH RASH

Options

a. Measles.
b. German measles.
c. Roseola infantum.
d. Erythema infectiosum.
e. Enterovirus infection.
f. Hand foot mouth disease.
g. Smallpox.
h. Mumps.
i. Chickenpox.

For each of the situations/conditions given below, choose the one most appropriate/discriminatory option from above. The options may be used once, more than once, or not at all.

Questions

1. Bathing suit rash, centrifugal evolution. Multilocular vesicles umbilication. Lesions show same stage of development.
2. Macular/maculopapular rash appears at the end of the disease, from 3rd or 4th day. Rash starts in the trunk and then involves extremities. Rash is sparse over face and legs and fades in a few hours.
3. Vesicles on palms and soles which heal without scarring.
4. Crops of vesicles of different ages seen on back, which start appearing on the 3rd day of fever. Rash has a centripetal evolution.

5. Top to toe rash, progress rapidly in 1-2 days and fades quickly from 3rd day onwards.

THEME: 2
PHYSICAL EXAMINATION OF CHILDREN

Options

a. Newborn.
b. Early infancy (2 weeks to 6 months).
c. Late infancy (6 months to 2 years).
d. Preschool years (2 to 5 years).
e. School age years (5 – 12 years).

For each of the situations/conditions given below, choose the one most appropriate/discriminatory option from above. The options may be used once, more than once, or not at all.

Questions

6. Measurement of the thigh-foot angle to determine tibial torsion.
7. Elicitation of the tonic neck reflex.
8. Examination of the permanent dentition for decay and occlusion.
9. Fundoscopic examination for a bilateral red reflex.

THEME: 3
CARDIOVASCULAR MANIFESTATIONS OF CONGENITAL DISORDERS

Options

a. Marfan's syndrome.
b. Glycogen storage disease.
c. Down's syndrome.
d. Turner's syndrome.
e. Noonan's syndrome.
f. William's syndrome.
g. Rubella syndrome.
h. Trisomy 18 syndrome.

For each of the situations/conditions given below, choose the one most appropriate/discriminatory option from above. The options may be used once, more than once, or not at all.

Questions

10. Endocardial cushion defect.
11. Patent ductus arteriosis.
12. Aortic aneurysm.
13. Aortic coarctation.
14. Supraventricular aortic stenosis.
15. Hypertrophic cardiomyopathy.
16. Ventricular septal defect.
17. Pulmonary stenosis.

THEME: 4
CAUSES OF DEFECTS IN THE NEWBORN FROM MATERNAL INFECTIONS

Options

a. Hepatitis B
b. Rubella
c. Cytomegalovirus
d. Toxoplasmosis
e. Rubeola
f. Varicella zoster
g. Listeria
h. Neisseria gonorrhoea
i. Chlamydia trachomatis
j. Group B *Streptococcus*
k. Group B coxsackie virus

For each of the situations/conditions given below, choose the one most appropriate/discriminatory option from above. The option may be used once, more than once, or not at all.

Questions

18. A newborn baby is born with cataracts, cardiac defects, and deafness.

19. A newborn is noted to have microcephaly, epileptic fits and chorioretinitis.
20. A stillbirth is also noted to have microcephaly and hepatosplenomegaly and jaundice.
21. A newborn is noted to eye abnormalities, skin scarring and limb hypoplasia.
22. A newborn develops fatal encephalomyocarditis.

THEME: 5
DIAGNOSIS OF CHILDHOOD SEIZURES

Options

a. Grand mal
b. Infantile spasm
c. Febrile convulsions
d. Status epilepticus
e. Petit mal
f. Temporal lobe seizure
g. Jacksonian seizure
h. Tuberous sclerosis
i. Neurofibromatosis
j. Sturge-Weber syndrome
k. Benign paroxysmal vertigo

For each of the situations/conditions given below, choose the one most appropriate/discriminatory option from above. The option may be used once, more than once, or not at all.

Questions

23. A 9-year-old boy is bought to the GP for daydreaming at school. The attack is reproduced by encouraging the child to hyperventilate. The child becomes inattentive for 5 seconds, and the eyes roll up.
24. A 10-year-old boy presents to the GP with worsening seizures. The attacks begin with a cry and continuous muscle spasm, followed by jerking and tongue biting. The child then drifts into unconsciousness.
25. A 3-year-old girl presents to the GP with earache and seizures. She is apyrexial and on examination, has acute

otitis media. The seizure is described as lasting for 5 minutes with jerky movemements of the limbs.

26. A 12-year-old boy presents to his GP with convulsions that are described to start in his thumb and progress along the same side of his body.
27. An 8-year-old boy presents with a history of epilepsy and mental retardation. He is noted to have butterfly distribution of warty lesions over his nose and cheeks.

THEME: 6
DIAGNOSIS OF GENETIC DISORDERS AND BIRTH DEFECTS

Options

a. Fetal alcohol syndrome
b. Fragile X syndrome
c. Margan's syndrome
d. Trisomy 21
e. Turner's syndrome
f. Trisomy 13
g. Hurler syndrome
h. Homosystinuria
i. Phenylketonuria
j. Klinefelter's syndrome
k. Neurofibromatosis

For each of the situations/conditions given below, choose the one most appropriate/discriminatory option from above. The option may be used once, more than once, or not at all.

Questions

28. A 6 week old infant presents with irritability. He is in the 2nd percentile for weight and length. On examination, he has a small midface and a long philtrum. He has clinodactyly of the fifth finger and cervical vertebral fusion.
29. An 8-year-old girl presents to her GP with scoliosis. She is in the 100th percentile for her height. She wears glasses for myopia and is of normal intelligence. On examination,

she is noted to have a mid-systolic click and a late systolic murmur. She also has hypermobile joints.

30. A 10-year-old boy presents with chest pain and is diagnosed with acute myocardial infarction. He is tall with long limbs and digits. He has dislocated lens and is mildly mentally retarded.
31. A 10-year-old boy presents with progressive mental retardation. He is in the 5th percentile for his height. He has a large head and coarse faeces. He is noted to have hepatomegaly.
32. A 15-year-old girl presents to her GP, as she has not started to menstruate and has no breast development. She is in the 3rd percentile for her height. She has learning difficulties at school. On examination she has a mid-systolic ejection murmur on auscultation and multiple pigmented skin naevi.

THEME: 7
HEART DISEASE IN CHILDHOOD

Options

a. Aortic stenosis
b. AV septal defect
c. Dilated cardiomyopathy
d. Innocent murmur
e. Patent ductus arteriosis
f. Tetralogy of Fallot

For each of the situations/conditions given below, choose the one most appropriate/discriminatory option from above. The option may be used once, more than once, or not at all.

Questions

33. A 4-week-old baby needed ventilatory support for 4 days and is weaned off air. Two days later he becomes tachypnoeic with poor feeding and has three episodes of apnoea. There is an increase in weight. Clinically peripheral perfusion is poor in the CVS, the pericardium is active and the peripheral pulses are bounding. A loud systolic murmur is heard in the pulmonary area. Chest X-ray shows pulmonary oedema.

34. A 9-month-old recovers from a respiratory infection but increasingly gets breathless firs on excertion and subsequently at rest. He is tachycardiac. The apex beat was on the left anterior axillary line in the 6th intercostals space. Liver is 3 cm below costal margin. A gallop rhythm was present with a panysystolic murmur at the apex. ECG shows widened QRS complexes and LV preponderance. Chest X-ray shows gross cardiomegaly.
35. A 16-week-old baby is noted to get 'blue discoloration' of the arms and legs intermittently with no associated dyspnoea. The baby was pink at birth and subsequent clinical examinations were normal. On examination the baby's growth was found to be within normal limits. No cyanosis is noted. Peripheral pulses are normal. No cardiac enlargement. A thrill is felt in the pulmonary area with a rough ejection systolic murmur best heard in the same area. P2 was single and quiet. ECG shows RV hypertrophy with a right QRS axis. CXR shows oligaemic lungs. O2 saturation is 89-92% on air.
36. An 8-year-old boy develops faintness associated with central chest pain while playing football. This has recently been restricting him due to discomfort by the has not been breathless. On examination peripheral pulses felt well. BP 126/78 mmHg. Hyperactive apex. Systolic thrill felt suprasternally. Harsh systolic murmur at apex and aortic area. ECG: left ventricular hypertrophy.
37. A 4-month-old baby with breathlessness and failure to thrive. A cardiac murmur was first noted around 6 weeks of age. No cyanosed but tachypnoeic and tachycardiac. Hyperdynamic apex beat, loud P2. Loud panysystolic murmur at left sternal edge. ECG RA enlargement, QRS + 230, RV hypertrophy. CXR: Enlarged heart, prominent pulmonary artery and pulmonary plethora.

THEME: 8
FITS AND FAINTS IN CHILDREN

Options

a. Benign paroxysmal vertigo

b. Breath-holding attacks (cyanotic spells)
c. Complex partial seizure
d. Congenital heat block
e. Reflex anoxic seizure (pallid spells)
f. Suprabentricular tachycardia
g. Syncope

For each of the situations/conditions given below, choose the one most appropriate/discriminatory option from above. The option may be used once, more than once, or not at all.

Questions

38. A 10-year-old had three episodes of loss of consciousness, the first two at school and the last on a shopping outing at a crowded summer sale. She was well prior to the attacks (all having occurred when she had been standing among a crowd). She had felt dizzy, nauseated and become pale and sweaty before loosing consciousness for about 2 minutes. There was no incontinence but twitching of the fingers was noted. On recovery she felt tired.
39. A 2.5-year-old had three episodes of vomiting and sudden onset of ataxia over the past 6 months. The attacks were rather short (5–10 minutes) but during which he appeared frightened and pale and had to lie down. After the attack he was back to normal. It was mentioned that he keeps his eyes down or closed when travelling by car of lift.
40. A 15-month-old girl has had recurrent episodes of loss of consciousness precipitated by temper tantrums. She is developmentally within normal limits. When upset she starts with a shrill cry, goes floppy and blue, losing consciousness for about 1 minute during which a few jerky movement of limbs may occur.
41. A 7-year-old boy has had four episodes of loss of consciousness over the past 6 months. Two occurred in the morning soonafter he woke up when he was noticed to be in a 'dreamlike state' with his head turned to the right and doing 'pill rolling' movements with his hand. This was followed by loss of posture and a generalised seizure lasting 3-4 minutes.

42. A 3-year-old with a history of attacks of loss of consciousness associated with minor trauma such as knocking of his head or injury to his finger. He becomes pale, loses consciousness and goes floppy, sometimes twitching slightly. During one attack he had a heart rate of 30 beats per minute, which rapidly recovered. He regained consciousness rapidly each time.

THEME: 9
DIAGNOSIS OF DIAPER DERMATITIS

Options

a. Ammonia dermatitis.
b. Candida dermatitis.
c. Seborrheic eczematous dermatitis.
d. None of the above.

For each of the situations/conditions given below, choose the one most appropriate/discriminatory option from above. The options may be used once, more than once, or not at all.

Questions

43. Diffuse, red, shiny rash extending into skin folds.
44. Red, desquamating rash, sparing skin folds.
45. Isolated psoriasis like scaly plaques.
46. Most common type of nappy rash.

THEME: 10
DIAGNOSIS OF DISORDERS OF CHROMOSOMAL NUMBER

Options

a. Cri-du-chat syndrome.
b. Turner syndrome.
c. Down syndrome.
d. Edward syndrome.
e. Patau syndrome.
f. Klinefelter's syndrome.

For each of the situations/conditions given below, choose the one most appropriate/discriminatory option from above. The options may be used once, more than once, or not at all.

Questions

47. Abnormal ear and facies, flared fingers, growth deficiency, rocker bottom feet.
48. Short stature webbed neck, normal intelligence, cubitus valgus and infertility.
49. Cleft lip palate, polydactyly, scalp defects mental deficiency, microophthalmia.
50. Microcephaly, dysmorphic features,mental retardation, abnormal cry.
51. Mental deficiency,hypotonia,duodenal atresia, simian crease, Brush field's spots on iris, mongloid facies.

THEME : 11
DIAGNOSIS OF NEUROCUTANEOUS SYNDROMES

Options

a. Tuberous sclerosis.
b. Neurofibromatosis.
c. Sturge-Weber syndrome.
d. Ataxia telangiectasia.
e. von Hippel-lindau syndrome.

For each of the situations/conditions given below, choose the one most appropriate/discriminatory option from above. The options may be used once, more than once, or not at all.

Questions

52. Mental retardation, choreoathetosis, posterior column demyelination.
53. Megaloencephaly, peripheral nerve tumors.
54. Ataxia, retinal detachment.
55. Intracranial calcification, convulsions.

THEME: 12
DIAGNOSIS OF JAUNDICE IN A CHILD

Options

a. ABO incompatibility.
b. Alpha antitrypsin deficiency.
c. Biliary atresia.
d. Breastfeeding jaundice.
e. Breast milk jaundice.
f. Choledochal cyst.
g. Cholelithiasis.
h. Crigler-Najjar syndrome.
i. Cystiofibrosis.
j. Dubin-Johnson syndrome.
k. Erythroblastosis (Rh incompatibility).
l. Galactosemia.
m. G6PD deficiency.
n. Hepatitis.
o. Hereditary spherocytosis.
p. Hypothyroidism.
q. Physiologic Hyperbilirubinemia.
r. Sepsis.
s. Down's syndrome.
t. Intrauterine TORCH infections.

For each of the situations/conditions given below, choose the one most appropriate/discriminatory option from above. The options may be used once, more than once, or not at all.

Questions

56. A 3-day serum, healthy infant is noted to be jaundiced. Physical examination is otherwise normal. Laboratory values: Hb. 16.8 g/dl; reticulocytes 1.0 percent; bilirubin unconjugated 8.5 mg/dl, conjugated 0.8 mg/dL.
57. A weakend infant has been jaundiced for about 2 weeks. He has been asymptomatic and physical examination otherwise normal. Laboratory values Hb 14.2 gdL; reticulocytes 1.2 percent; bilirubin unconjugated 4.5 mg/dL. Conjugated 5.5 mg/dl;ALT 25 IU/l, AST 5IU/l.

Abdominal ultrasound examination revealed normal sized liver; P a gallbladder is not visualized.

58. An otherwise well 4-week-old infant has remained jaundiced since day 3 of life despite two exchange transfusions and continuous phototherapy. Laboratory values HB 14g/dl; reticulocytes 1.0 percent bilirubin unconjugated 16 mg/dl, conjugated 0.2mg/dl: ALT 15 IU/l, AST 40 IU/l. A Coomb's test prior to first exchange transfusion was negative. Ultrasound examinations reveals a normal liver and gallbladder.
59. Jaundice detected at the age of 12 hours (total serum bilirubin 10.5 mg/dl indirect 9.9 mg/dl) born to a para 2, gravida 2 mother whose blood group is A negative.
60. A 3-day-old term neonate, small for gestation age, lethargic and disinterested in feeds. Serum bilirubin 14.2, direct 1.6 mg/dl, has hepatosplenomegaly.
61. 5 day baby born to a primigravida who had prolonged rupture of membrane. The baby has hypotension, petechial rash serum bilirubin14 mg/dl, direct 0.9 mg/dl.
62. A 18-day-old baby who had delayed passage of meconium,with serum bilirubin of 12 mg/dl with a direct of 0.8 mg/dl.

THEME: 13
INVESTIGATION OF NEONATAL JAUNDICE

Options

a. ABO haemolytic disease of newborn
b. Biliary atresia
c. G6PD deficiency
d. Galactosaemia
e. Hypothyroidism
f. Neonatal hepatitis
g. Neonatal sepsis

For each of the situations/conditions given below, choose the one most appropriate/discriminatory option from above. The option may be used once, more than once, or not at all.

Questions

63. A 5-day-old baby born at 36 weeks weighing 3 kg becomes lethargic and has gone off feeds. The mild icterus noted on the 3rd day has deepened and clinically the baby looks ill. Investigations were as follows. WBC 18000, neutrophils 13500 NA 131 mmol urea 9.8 mmol CRP 90 S bilirubin 220 micromol ART pH 7.26 base deficit – 14.2 mmol.
64. A 4-day-old baby is noted to have mild icterus when seen by the midwife in the morning. Birth was at 40 weeks by normal delivery, weight being 3.850kg. She was breast-fed and had been feeding well. The baby was brought to hospital 8 hours later as her jaundice had rapidly worsened. Investigations were serum bilirubin 380 micromol (95% unconjugated) Hb 7.2 g/l both mother and baby are group A Rh +ve. The parents are of Mediterranean origin.
65. A 6-day-old infant develops vomiting followed by a prolonged convulsion. She had been irritable lethargic. Examination revealed an ill infant with moderate jaundice and significant liver enlargement, investigations were serum bilirubin 180 micromol, blood glucose 1.0 mmol Hb 14 gm% WBC 13000 normal differential count CRP 15 ALT 80 units CGT 120 units urine reducing substances positive (clinitest).
66. A 6-week-old baby presents with persistent jaundice since birth. The mother delivered the baby as an emergency, having arrived in the UK from an Asian country. The birth weight was 3.4 kg with normal Apgar scores. The baby is snuffly and develops a cough. Examination: respiratory rate 50/min liver 3 cm below costal margin. Investigations: total bilirubin 120 mmol, conjugated bilirubin 65 mmol free thyroxine 14.2 pmol TSH 6.2 ulU ALT 70 units CGT 110 units alk phosphatase 800 units. The chest X-ray was clear but the right humerus showed a periostial region.

THEME: 14
THE MANAGEMENT OF PAEDIATRIC GASTROINTESTINAL DISORDERS

Options

a. Vancomycin
b. Panproctocolectomy
c. Gluton-free diet
d. Pancreatic enzyme supplementation
e. Barium enema
f. Rectal biopsy
g. D penicillamine and avoidance of chocolates, nuts and shell fish
h. Diverting colostomy
i. Loperamide

For each of the situations/conditions given below, choose the one most appropriate/discriminatory option from above. The option may be used once, more than once, or not at all.

Questions

67. A 2-year-old girl presents with failure to thrive and diarrhoea. She is found to have iron deficiency anaemia. Small bowel biopsy shows flattened villi, elongate crypts and loss of columnar cells.
68. A 12-year-old boy is being treated for osteomyelitis. He has been on intravenous antibiotics for 2 weeks. He now has diarrhoea. On Sigmoidoscopy, there are multiple patchy yellowish areas of necrotic mucosa.
69. A 6-month-old baby boy presents with repeated bouts of vomiting and abdominal distension. He is normal between attacks. A sausage shaped mass is palpated in his abdomen.
70. A 2-month-old baby girl presents with failure to thrive. She has frequent episodes of vomiting with abdominal distension. The abdominal X-ray shows proximal bowel dilation and no faeces or gas in rectum.
71. A 12-year-old boy presents with liver disease. A slit lamp examination reveals Kayser-Fleischer rings in the cornea. His urinary copper level is high.

THEME: 15
HAEMATURIA IN CHILDREN

Options

a. Acute glomerulonephritis
b. Benign recurrent haematuria
c. Haemolytic uraemic syndrome
d. Nephroblastoma
e. Renal venous thrombosis
f. Urinary tract infection

For each of the situations/conditions given below, choose the one most appropriate/discriminatory option from above. The option may be used once, more than once, or not at all.

Questions

72. A four-year-old child has an upper respiratory tract infection followed two week later by haematuria associated with oliguria and periorbital oedema.
73. A three-year-old girl has itching, frequency and pain on urination.
74. A child of four months presents with an abdominal mass and investigation shows displacement of the right kidney and there is microscopic haematuria.
75. A six-year-old child presents with number of episodes of painless macroscopic haematuria, with no evidence of UTI and a normal IVU.

THEME: 16
SEPSIS IN CHILDHOOD

Options

a. *Escherichia coli*
b. Group B *Streptococcus*
c. Mycoplasma pneumoniae
d. Pneumocystis carinii
e. Pseudomonas aeruginosa
f. Salmonella typhimurium

g. *Staphylococcus* aureus
h. *Staphylococcus* epidermidis

For each of the situations/conditions given below, choose the one most appropriate/discriminatory option from above. The option may be used once, more than once, or not at all.

Questions

76. An 8-year-old girl treated for acute lymphoblastic leukaemia who is in remission develops high fever 3 days after the last course of chemotherapy. Otherwise she was asymptomatic and clinically no focus of sepsis was found. The WBC was 1100/ml with a neutrophil count of 650. The blood culture taken via the portacath grew a pure growth of an organism.
77. A 9-year-old girl originally diagnosed at the age of 7 months with cystic fibrosis has had multiple admissions with recurrent chest infections over the past 2 years needing intravenous antibiotic therapy. There has been rapid deterioration of her lung function during this period with the persistence of an organism in the sputum that was difficult to irradiate.
78. A 14-year-old Nigerian boy presents with fever and painful swelling of his left knee joint soonafter returning from holiday in Nigeria. He has sickle cell disease and during the last week of his stay in Africa developed an acute gastroenteritis which is now settling. Aspiration of the joint yielded a purulent fluid that grew an organism.
79. A 2-day-old baby is transferred from the maternity unit because of increasing respiratory distress, lethargy and poor feeding. The delivery was normal at 37 weeks with no immediate problems. Clinically the baby appears ill with peripheral circulatory failure and respiratory distress. The chest X-ray reveals bilateral inflammatory changes. The blood culture and the mother's high vaginal swab grew the same organism.
80. A 12-year-old develops fever with rigors and painful swelling of the right ankle and was seen in hospital 3 days later. There was a tender swelling of the lower leg and

ankle and marked tenderness. Investigation revealed a leucocytosis with a high neutrophil count and high ESR and CRP levels. X-rays of the ankle and lower tibia are normal. A blood culture grew an organism.

81. A 10-month-old baby develops high-fever with rigors and vomiting and has stopped feeding. At presentation she is in shock with cold peripheries needing fluid resuscitation. She is commenced on antibiotics immediately as septic shock is suspected. Her blood and urine cultures both grew the same organism. Subsequent imaging revealed bilateral vesico-ureteric reflux.

THEME: 17
DIAGNOSIS OF VOMITING IN CHILDREN

Options

a. Urinary tract infection.
b. Intracranial space occupying lesion.
c. Hypertensive encephalopathy.
d. Manchausen syndrome by proxy.
e. Migraine.
f. Reflux oesophagitis.
g. Viral gestroenteritis.
h. Intussusception.
i. Cyclical vomiting.
j. Congenital hypertrophic pyloric stenosis

For each of the situations/conditions given below, choose the one most appropriate/discriminatory option from above. The options may be used once, more than once, or not at all.

Questions

82. A 7-month-old infant brought to casualty with vomiting, high fever and abdominal colic since 3 days. She had been failing to thrive since the last two months.
83. A 4-year-old girl brought with signs of mild dehydra .on. She has been vomiting, passing 6-7 watery stools since morning. On examination no abnormalities detected.

84. A 6-year-old boy has been having projectile vomiting on and off associated with non-specific headache since 3 weeks. He has suffered double vision since last week.
85. A 6-year-old girl has been suffering from episodes of severe unilateral headache with vomiting since severe months.
86. A 4-week-old infant was brought to casualty with history of forceful nonbilious since 3 days.
87. A 1-year-old infant brought to casualty with episodes of screaming and drawing up his knees. He has been vomiting since a day.

THEME: 18
DIAGNOSIS OF MALABSORPTION AND DIARRHOEA IN CHILDREN

Options

a. Lactose intolerance
b. Chronic disease
c. Acrodermatitis Enteropathica
d. Chronic nonspecific diarrhoea
e. Coeliac disease
f. Ulcerative colitis
g. Giardia Lamblia infection
h. Enterobius Vermicularis infection
i. Ascaris Lumbricoides
j. Hirshsprungs disease
k. Intussuseption
l. Irritable Bowel Syndrome
m. Endometriosis#
n. Acute on chronic appendicitis
o. Endometriosis

For each of the situations/conditions given below, choose the one most appropriate/discriminatory option from above. The options may be used once, more than once, or not at all.

Questions

88. A 4-year-old Irish girl looks wasted and apppears short for his age. The mother reoports the daughter has been

vomiting on several occasions in the past with associated diarrhoea. The SHO thinks he has an enteropathy and on serology IgA gliadin and endomysial antibodies are found.

89. A mother brings her 5-year-old son who has been passing bloody stools associated with severe abdominal pain. On examination he is found to have mildly swollen tender wrists and red tender nodular lesions were found on her forearms.
90. A 8-year-old girl has got repeated episodes of diarrhoea. On each occasion the stool contains segments of undigested food .The paediatrician recommends restricting fluids to meal times. The girls condition improves and she is thriving.
91. A mother and her daughter have just returned from a tropical holiday and is concerned that her daughter has an STD since she complains of constant perianal and vulval irritation . There is no associated vaginal discharge. She has worms coming out of her bottom at night.
92. A 15-year-old girl complains of episodic diarrhoea which typically starts in the morning with an urge to go to the toilet on walking and after breakfast.She says there is abdominal pain in the right iliac fossa releived by defecation or flatus. She has had the symptoms for three months.

THEME: 19
INVESTIGATIONS OF PAEDIATRIC EMERGENCIES

Options

a. Full blood count (FBC)
b. Serum glucose
c. Skull X-ray
d. Chest X-ray
e. Urinanalysis
f. ESR
g. Serum urea and e8lectrolytes
h. Computed tomography scan of the head
i. Lateral soft-tissue neck X-ray

For each of the situations/conditions given below, choose the one most appropriate/discriminatory option from above. The option may be used once, more than once, or not at all.

Questions

93. An 8-month-old baby is bought to casualty by her mother after falling off the sofa onto her head. On examination, she is irritable and alert with no literalising signs. There is a haematoma over the left occiput.
94. A 6-year-old girl is brought to casualty by her mother after falling off a climbing frame in the school playground. On examination she has no deformity or swelling on her extremities. Instead of she has bruising of various colours over her arms and she has tender ribs to palpation.
95. A 2-year-old girl is brought to casualty by her father after falling down the stairs. She is drowsy and has vomited twice. On examination she has a swelling over her occiput. Her pupils are sluggish to respond. Her blood pressure is 120/70 and her pulse rate is 60.
96. A 2-year-old boy has swallowed a 50 pence coin and points to his throat. He is not distressed.
97. A 16-year-old girl presents to casualty with an uncontrollable spontaneous nosebleed. She has bruising of various ages over her extremities.

THEME: 20
DIAGNOSIS OF CHILDHOOD RESPIRATORY DISEASES

Options

a. Bronchiolitis
b. Croup
c. Asthma
d. Cystic fibrosis
e. Epiglottitis
f. Obstructive sleep apnoea
g. Chlamydia trachomatis infection
h. Pneumonia

i. Allergic rhinitis
j. Influenza
k. Rectronsillar abscess
l. Gonorrhoeal infection

For each of the situations/conditions given below, choose the one most appropriate/discriminatory option from above. The option may be used once, more than once, or not at all.

Questions

98. A 2-year-old boy presents with coughing and wheezing. Other members of the family are also suffering from an upper respiratory tract infection. On examination, he has flaring of the nostrils and audible expiratory wheezes.
99. A 10-year-old thin boy presents with chronic cough. Chest X-ray reveals bronchiectasis. He also suffers from steatorrhoea.
100. A 4-year-old boy presents to the GP for night terrors and loud snoring. On examination, he is a mouth breather with large tonsils that meet at the midline.
101. A 2-week-old infant presents with staccato cough and purulent conjunctivitis. On examination, he is apyrexial with diffuse rales on auscultation of the chest.
102. A 2-year-old boy presents with a 3-day history of noisy breathing on ispiration and a barking bough worse at night. He has a low-grade fever and is hoarse.

THEME: 21
DIAGNOSIS OF RESPIRATORY DISTRESS IN CHILDREN

Options

a. Laryngomalacia.
b. Respiratory distress syndrome.
c. Congenital diaphragmatic hernia.
d. Asthma.
e. Cardiac failure.
f. Tetralogy of Fallot.
g. Pneumonia.

h. Foreign body aspiration.
i. Epiglottitis.
j. Bronchiolitis.

For each of the situations/conditions given below, choose the one most appropriate/discriminatory option from above. The options may be used once, more than once, or not at all.

Questions

103. A 7-year-old girl was brought to casualty with sudden onset of high fever, respiratory distress and drooling of saliva.
104. A 9-month-old infant with respiratory distress, has been unable to complete feeds and is sweating a lot, is tachypnoeic and tachycardiac.
105. A 3-month-old female infant having noisy breathing since day five. Wheezing is more while child is feeding and diminishes during sleep.
106. A 5-year-old girl with history of bouts of respiratory distress and cough which has had a variable course over one year.
107. A 5-year-old girl was brought with history of bouts of cough and breathlessness since 3 months. The episodes are not relieved by bronchodilators but the child is well in between episodes.

THEME: 22
TREATMENT OF ASTHMA IN CHILDHOOD

Options

a. As required oral bronchodilator
b. Adrenaline
c. Desensitisation
d. Inhaled long acting bronchodilator
e. Inhaled sodium cromoglycate
f. Inhaled steroid
g. Intermittent inhaled bronchodilator
h. Intravenous (IV) aminophylline
i. Milk free diet
j. Oral steroids

k. Nebulised bronchodilator
l. Oral theophylline
m. Regular inhaled bronchodilatior
n. Regular oral bronchodilator

For each of the situations/conditions given below, choose the one most appropriate/discriminatory option from above. The options may be used once, more than once, or not at all.

Questions

108. A 9-year-old boy has a mild cough and wheeze after playing football in the cold weather.
109. A 6-year-old girl with asthma uses her bronchodilator twice a day to relieve her mild wheeze. Her parents refuse to give her any treatment containing corticosteroids.
110. A 9-year-old girl with chronic asthma presents to the A&E department with rapidly worsening wheeze not relieved with inhaled bronchodilators. Steroids have been given orally.
111. A 4-year-old boy with eczema and recurrent wheeze whenever gets a viral infection has now developed night cough,there has been no improvement in spite of using inhaled bronchodilators twice each night.
112. A 14-year-old boy,with well controlled asthma,using inhaled steroids and a bronchodilator comes to the A&E department. with breathlessness and swollen lips after eating a peanut butter sandwich.

THEME: 23
DRUG TREATMENT IN CHILDHOOD

Options

a. Co-trimoxazole
b. Dexamethasone
c. Digoxin
d. Enalapril
e. Indomethacin
f. Prostaglandin E
g. Rifampicin

h. Sodium valproate
i. Vancomycin
j. Vigabatrin

For each of the situations/conditions given below, choose the one most appropriate/discriminatory option from above. The option may be used once, more than once, or not at all.

Questions

113. An 18-month-old child known to be HIV positive has had a chronic cough of over three-month duration. Chest X-ray showed bilateral infiltrates and a granular pattern and tracheal aspirates are positive for pneumocystis carinii.
114. An 11-month-old presents with multiple fits, mostly absences, and a few major tonic/chlonic fits within a period of 2 months. Clinically there is an ash leaf skin lesion but no neurological deficit. The CT scan shows three small subependymal tubers.
115. A 2-month-old baby develops increasing breathlessness, cough and poor feeding. Examination reveals a baby failing to thrive and tachypnoeic. There is no cyanosis. The apex is hyperdynamic. A loud pansystolic murmur and a short mid-diastolic rumble are heard over the precordium. P2 is loud and split. Liver is 4cm below the costal margin. Has been on Frusemide and spironlactone with no improvement.
116. Two siblings aged 5 and 9-year respectively of a child with a confirmed case of meningicoccal disease present for prophylactic antibiotic therapy.
117. A 10-day-old baby born at 32-week needs IPPV for 6 days and is successfully weaned off when she redevelops respiratory distress. Clinically the pulses are bounding and there is a loud continuous murmur in the pulmonary area. Fluid restriction and diuretics are not helpful.
118. A 6-month-old baby presents with frequent attacks of head nodding and flexion of limbs over the past 6 weeks. The baby has become more lethargic and appears to have regression in his activities and synchronous pattern.

119. A 2-week-old neonate born at 28 weeks and having a central line becomes ill and 'septic' blood culture grows multiresistant *Staphylococcus aureus*. The baby has been on penicillin and gentamicin for 5 days postnatally for prolonged rupture of membranes.

THEME: 24
AETIOLOGICAL FACTORS IN DEVELOPMENTAL DELAY AND MENTAL HANDICAP

Options

a. Birth asphyxia
b. Duchenne's muscular dystrophy
c. Coeliac disease
d. Fetal alcohol syndrome
e. Familial predisposition
f. Tay-Sachs disease
g. Bacterial meningitis
h. Klinefelter's syndrome
i. Phenylketonuria
j. Normal finding
k. Fragile X syndrome

For each of the situations/conditions given below, choose the one most appropriate/discriminatory option from above. The options may be used once, more than once, or not at all.

Questions

120. A 10-year-old boy is getting very poor grades at school and according to the headteacher seems to think like a 2-year-old .The mother also says the son has a very short temper. On examination unusually large-large testes are found. The boy's elder brother and uncle had similar complaints.
121. A 5-year-old girl was born after a normal delivery has been developing normally. After an acute illness a regression of milestones has been noticed.
122. A 2-year-old girl was born weighing 4 kg after a labour that lasted 18 hours in a mother of 2. She is able to stand but yet to walk. The mother says her other child had similar problems.

123. A 6-year-old boy with a birth head circumference of 29 cm and short palpebral fissure is found to be mentally retarted. The boys mother is on acamprostate.
124. A 25-year-old bartender gives birht to a 2.9 kg baby boy. The baby is found to have a head circumference of 32 cm. She has had her job for the last 6 years.

THEME: 25
DIAGNOSIS OF NORMAL DEVELOPMENTAL MILESTONES

Options

a. 3 months
b. 6 months
c. 9 months
d. 12 months
e. 18 months
f. 2 years
g. 3 years
h. 4 years
i. 5 years
j. 6 years
k. 7 years

For each of the situations/conditions given below, choose the one most appropriate/discriminatory option from above. The option may be used once, more than once, or not at all.

Questions

125. A child is asked to copy figures. She can successfully draw a square and triangle but has difficulty with copying a diamond.
126. A mother is concerned that her baby is not walking yet. He is sitting unsupported and babbling contentedly. He holds a pencil in a scissor grasp and transfers the pencil between his hands prior to placing it in his mouth.
127. A child is asked to copy figures. She can only copy a circle. She can climb upstairs on foot per stop and builds a tower of 9 cubes.

128. A child is asked to copy figures. She can copy a circle and a cross. She can stand on one foot for 5 seconds and climbs up and downstairs one foot per step.
129. A mother is concentred that her baby is not talking yet. He walks around furniture and can stand-alone for a few seconds. He holds objects in a pincer grasp.

THEME: 26
INVESTIGATION OF CHILDHOOD ENDOCRINE AND METABOLIC DISORDERS

Options

a. Full blood count (FBC)
b. Serum electrolytes
c. Serum ADH levels
d. Serum growth hormone levels
e. Detection of phenylkestones in the urine
f. Thyroid function tests
g. Detection of galactose in the urine
h. Serum ACTH levels
i. High-serum blood glucose
j. Low-serum blood glucose
k. Detection of cystine in the urine
l. Plasma corisol levels

For each of the situations/conditions given below, choose the one most appropriate/discriminatory option from above. The option may be used once, more than once, or not at all.

Questions

130. A 1-month-old baby presents with poor feeding and lethargy. On examination he has an umbilical hernia and an enlarged tongue.
131. A newborn female is note to have an enlarged clitoris and fused labia.
132. A 13-year-old obese girl with a history of asthmA&Eczema presents with amenorrhoea. Her blood pressure is noted to be 130/80.
133. A 1-month-old baby presents with vomiting, jaundice and hepatomegaly. The baby is worse after feeding.

134. An 8-year-old boy presents to the GP with short stature. He complains of constant thirst and is noted to pass huge volumes of colourless urine.

THEME: 27
DIAGNOSIS OF COMMON GENETIC DISORDERS

Options

a. Klinefelter's syndrome
b. Patau syndrome
c. Down' s syndrome
d. Turner's syndrome
e. Cri-du-chat syndrome
f. Fragile X syndrome
g. Sickle cell disease
h. Sickle cell trait
i. Betathalassemia
j. William's syndrome
k. Prader-Willi syndrome
l. Di George syndrome
m. Acute myeloid leukaemia
n. Edward's syndrome

For each of the situations/conditions given below, choose the one most appropriate/discriminatory option from above. The option may be used once, more than once, or not at all.

Questions

135. A 15-year-old boy has very poor grades at school despite being attentive and hard working. His mother reckons it because he is teased at school because his breast look like a girls. On further examination he is found to have a small testis. He is mildly asthmatic.
136. A 5-year-old South African boy is bought into the A&E deeply jaundiced. He is found to have mildly swollen, tender feet and hands. His mucosae are pale.
137. A 6-year-old Asian boy gets regular blood transfusion for his haematological abnormality. His mucosae are pale

and skull is grossly bossed. Hematoligical investigations were done and are as follows:
MCHC 25g/dl
Hb 8g/dl
MCV 74fl

138. A 10-year-old boy is brought into A&E with a swollen right arm. His temperature is 38.5°C and is unable to move the arm due to severe pain. Blood cultures confirm salmonella osteomyelitis. This is his second presentation this month and earlier presented with an acute onset hepatospenomegaly associated with sever pallor. The SHO does a sodium metabisulphite test on the patient's blood, which turns out to be positive.
139. A 39-year-old male is getting progressively forgetful and is later found to have Alzheimer's disease. He has small ears and an IQ score of 67.

THEME: 28
GENETIC DEFECTS

Options

a. Angelman's syndrome
b. Beckwith-Wiedemann syndrome
c. Down's syndrome
d. Edward's syndrome
e. Klinefelter's syndrome
f. Noonan's syndrome
g. Russell-Silver syndrome
h. Turner's syndrome

For each of the situations/conditions given below, choose the one most appropriate/discriminatory option from above. The option may be used once, more than once, or not at all.

Questions

140. A newborn male who is hypotonic and noted to have brachcephaly and recurrent vomiting due to duodenal atrsia.

141. A 14-year girl of normal intelligence who is short for her age and has not ye t started to menstruate.
142. A small for dates newborn with mall chin, severe mental retardation and abnormally shaped soles of the feet.
143. A 5-year-old girl with short stature and hypertrophy of her left sided limbs and mild mental retardation.

THEME: 29
DIAGNOSIS OF ABNORMAL CHILDHOOD DEVELOPMENT

Options

a. Klinefelter's syndrome
b. Turner's syndrome
c. Testicular feminisation syndrome
d. Marfan's syndrome
e. Adrenogenital syndrome
f. Homocystinuria
g. Achondroplasia
h. Down's syndrome
i. Duchenne muscular dystrophy
j. Spina bifida
k. Cerabral palsy
l. Osteogenesis imperfecta
m. Acromegaly

For each of the situations/conditions given below, choose the one most appropriate/discriminatory option from above. The option may be used once, more than once, or not at all.

Questions

144. An 18-month-old boy presents to the GP for late walking and difficulty climbing stairs. On examination, the boy has lumber lordosis and calf hypertrophy.
145. A 14-year-old girl presents to the GP for absence of periods. On examination she is petite with no breast development. Other noted features include pterygium colli and cubitus value.
146. A 15-year-old boy presents to his GP with a sore throat. He is tall for his age and is noted to have long limbs and small testicles.

147. A 16-year-old girl presents to her GP with flat feet. She is tall for her age and is noted to have a high arched palate and a long-arm span.
148. A 6-year-old boy presents to his GP with short stature. He has a large skull, prominent forehead, and a saddle shaped nose. The back is lordotic.

THEME: 30
INVESTIGATION OF LOSS OF CONSCIOUSNESS IN A CHILD

Options

a. Full blood count (FBC)
b. Serum electrolytes
c. Serum glucose
d. Urinanalysis
e. Serum hepatic enzymes and ammonia level
f. Computed tomography of the head
g. Toxicology screens
h. Lumbar puncture
i. Serum calcium
j. Thyroid function tests
k. Chest X-ray
l. Blood cultures

For each of the situations/conditions given below, choose the one most appropriate/discriminatory option from above. The option may be used once, more than once, or not at all.

Questions

149. A 10-month-old baby is bought into casualty after a fall. He is irritable and drowsy. On examination he is noted to have bruising behind the ears and blood in the ear canal. His blood pressure is labile.
150. A 10-year-old boy presents with delirium and emesis following an upper respiratory tract infection. He had been treated with paracetamol and aspirin. On examination, he is apyrexial. His bowel habits are normal.

151. A 10-year-old boy is brought into casualty somnolent. On examination, he is noted do have dry mucous membranes and is notes to be breathing in a deep, sighing manner. The mother explains that he has been complaining of abdominal pain.
152. A 14-year-old girl presents to casualty in a coma. On examination, papilloedema is noted. Her parents report that she had been complaining of headaches.
153. A 10-month-old baby girl presents with pallor, hypotonia and listlessness. On examination she is noted to have a full anterior fontanelle.

THEME: 31
DIAGNOSIS OF CHILDHOOD ILLNESSES

Options

a. Measles
b. Rubella
c. Varicella zoster
d. Mumps
e. Erythema infectiosum
f. Infectious mononucleosis
g. Tuberculosis
h. Typhus
i. Kawasaki syndrome
j. Pneumococcal meningitis
k. Haemophilus influenzae epiglottitis
l. Streptococcal throat infection

For each of the situations/conditions given below, choose the one most appropriate/discriminatory option from above. The option may be used once, more than once, or not at all.

Questions

154. A 15-year-old girl presents with fever, cough, coryza, and conjuctuvutus 9 days after exposure. On examination, she has blue-white punctate lesions on the buccal mucosa.
155. A 17-year-old boy presents with fever, stridor and trismus. He is noted to be drooling saliva. On examination, he has

palpable neck nodes. He fails to respond to a course of penicillin.

156. A 7-year-old girl presents with a low-grade fever and a 'slapped cheek' erythematous eruption on her cheeks.
157. A 4-year-old boy presents with an acute onset of fever and a vesicular eruption, following an incubation period of 12 days. The vesicles evilve into pustules and crust over.
158. A 1-year-old baby boy presents with a 5-day history of fever, strawberry tongue and erythema of the palms and soles. He also has an enlarged 2 cm lymph node.

THEME: 32
SMALL STATURE

Options

a. Congenital adrenal hyperplasia
b. Constitutional delay in puberty
c. Early onset puperty (idiopathic/constitutional puberty)
d. Familial (genetic) short stature
e. Growth hormone difficiency
f. Small-for –dates (at birth)

For each of the situations/conditions given below, choose the one most appropriate/discriminatory option from above. The option may be used once, more than once, or not at all.

Questions

159. A 12-year-old boy is referred because of not growing for the past 2-year. His classmates have overtaken him in stature though in the early years. He was the tallest in the class and he needed changes of shoes and clothing frequently at the time. History reveals that he developed public hair at 7-8-year-old of age and his voice changed around the same time.
160. A healthy 6-year-old has 'not grown' for the past 2–3 years. Born at term following a normally deliver he weighed 3.2 kg at birth. His genital frown has been satisfactory and developmental progress normal. The child's height is on 0.4th centile and mid-parental centile for height lay

between 50th and 75th centiles. Over the past year he has grown 2.3 cm.

161. Parents are concerned about their 14-year-old son who has 'stopped growing' over the past 2–3 years and has been overtaken by the rest of his classmates. He is getting bullied and dropped out of the school football team. Clinical examination was normal, the height lying on the 5th centile. No axillary or pubic hair is noted and the testicular volume is 2 ml. The bone age is reported as 11.4 years. Mid–parental centile for height is between the 25th and 50th centiles.
162. A 13-year-old white boy is referred by his GP because of short stature. He has always been the smallest in the class, but is an active child with no previous history of illness. Birth history was normal with a weight of 3.7 kg at birth. His present height is 144 cm (4'9") on the 9th centile and he has proceeded on this line for the last 5 years. The father is 5'6" and the mother is 5'1" tall. The bone age is 12.5 years.
163. A 13.5-year-old Asian girl is brought by her adoptive English parents because of their concern regarding her growth. She was adopted and brought to the UK at the age of 3 years. Her initial growth was normal, proceeding on the 25th to 50th centile until 11 yrs, and then slowed and has crossed to the 3rd centile. She has her menarche at 9.2 years.

THEME: 33
INVESTIGATION OF FAILURE TO THRIVE

Options

a. Full blood count (FBC)
b. Sweat test
c. Urinanalysis
d. Serum electrolytes
e. Bone films
f. Thyroid function tests
g. Buccal smear (females)
h. Stool culture
i. Echocardiogran

j. Fasting blood glucose
k. Abdominal untrasound

For each of the situations/conditions given below, choose the one most appropriate/discriminatory option from above. The option may be used once, more than once, or not at all.

Questions

164. A small 6-year-old boy on regular salbutamol inhaler presents with nasal obstruction and persistent cough. On examination, he is found to have nasal polyps.
165. A 2-year-old boy presents with anorexia, impaired growth, abdominal distension, abnormal stools, and hypotonia. He is irritable when examined.
166. A 14-year-old girl presents with anorexia. She reports that her appetite is food but cannot seem to gain weight. Her parents describe her as hyperactive and emotional. Her blood pressure is noted to be 130.80 and her pulse rate 108/min.
167. A 5-year-old boy presents with weight loss and nocturnal enuresis. His parents describe him as having profound mood swings. They have attempted to limit his fluid intake at night.
168. A 6-week-old boy presents with failure to thrive. The mother reports that he takes one hour for feeding with frequent rests. On examination he is noted to be tachycardic, tachypneic and have an enlarged liver.

THEME: 34
DIAGNOSIS OF ACUTE VOMITING IN CHILDREN

Options

a. Acute appendicitis
b. Cyclical vomiting
c. Duodenal atresia
d. Gastroesophageal reflux
e. Gastroenteritis
f. Meconium ileus
g. Meningitis

h. Mesenteric adenitis
i. Overfeeding
j. Pancreatitis
k. Pyschogeic vomiting
l. Pyloric stenosis
m. UTI
n. Whooping cough

For each of the situations/conditions given below, choose the one most appropriate/discriminatory option from above. The option may be used once, more than once, or not at all.

Questions

169. A 2-day-old breast-fed male infant vomiting after each feed. Abdominal X-ray demonstrated a "double bubble"
170. A 6-week-old breast-fed boy has had projectile vomiting after every feed for the past two weeks. He is now lethargic, dehydrated and tachypnoeic
171. A 4-month-old boy who is thriving has persistent vomiting, which is occasionally blood stained and is associated with crying.
172. An 8-year-old girl shows signs of moderate dehydration. She has vomited all fluids for 24 hours and the vomit is not bile stained. Her abdomen is now soft and non- tender. She has had 2 similar episodes in the past year.

THEME: 35
DIAGNOSIS OF ACUTE ABDOMINAL PAIN AND VOMITING IN CHILDREN

Options

a. Hirchsprung's disease
b. Pyloric stenosis
c. Acute cholecysititis
d. Duodenal atresia
e. Intussusception
f. Wilm's nephroblastoma
g. Mesenteric thrombosis
h. Gastroesophageal reflux

i. Meningitis
j. Meconium ileus
k. Cyclical vomiting
l. Necrotizing enterocolitis
m. Psychogenic vomiting
n. UTI
o. Acute pancreatitis
p. Gastroenteritis

For each of the situations/conditions given below, choose the one most appropriate/discriminatory option from above. The option may be used once, more than once, or not at all.

Questions

173. A 5-month-old baby presents with vomiting, following a 2 hours history of abdominal pain associated with drawing of legs. The mother says her baby has passed reddish stool.
174. A 12-year-old girl presents with fever, flank pain. An abdominal mass is found on examination. Urine microscopy shows no haematuria.
175. An 8-year-old girl shows signs of moderate dehydration. She is vomiting all fluids for 24 hours and the vomit is not bile stained. Her abdomen is now soft and non-tender. She has had 2 similar episodes in the past year.
176. A 6-week-old breast fed girl has projectile vomitng after ever feed for the last 2 weeks. She is now lethargic, dehydrated and tachypnoeic.
177. A 1 day old breast fed infant is vomiting after each feed. Abdominal X-ray shows a double bubble sign.
178. A 6-year-old febrile child is drowsy and vomiting. She is being treated for otits media by her GP.
179. 8 days after a premature birth, a mother notices her baby crying excessively and has passed blood and mucus per rectum. The infant is still in the special care baby unit.
180. A 15-year-old boy who is thriving has a mild abdominal pain and is assign 'rice water' stools. He had been at a 'mates' birthday party the night before.

THEME: 36
CHRONIC DIARRHOEA IN INFANCY AND CHILDHOOD

Options

a. Cystic fibrosis
b. Giardiasis
c. Gluten enteropathy
d. Hirschsprung disease
e. Milk protein intolerance
f. Toddlers diarrhoea
g. Ulcerative colitis or chronic inflammatory bowel disease

For each of the situations/conditions given below, choose the one most appropriate/discriminatory option from above. The option may be used once, more than once, or not at all.

Questions

181. A 15-year-old boy has had abdominal pain and diarrhoea intermittently for the past 2 years. Recently the frequency of his complaints has increased with passage of blood and mucus in the stools and loss of weight. He also suffers from intermittent fever and joint pains and on examination is noted to have erythema nodosum lesions on his shins.
182. An 18-month-old boy has had frequent loose motions for the past 6-8 months. Frequency varied from 4-8 stools per day. Loose to watery. No blood or mucus but has undigested vegetable matter in the stool. He feeds well and is gaining weight satisfactorily. Repeatedly, stool examination and investigations are normal.
183. A 7-month-old girl has been passing large offensive stools since 3 months of age. She feeds well but her weight has gradually fall across the centiles form the 75th to the 9th. She has had persisitednt'chestiness' needing frequent antibiotics.
184. A 1-year-old girl presents because of 'failure to thrive' and diarrhoea. Having initially grown well the child has gradually dropped below. The 2nd centile in weight over

the last 6 months. Clinically she is wasted anaemic and has abdominal distension. Stools are described as 'large, loose, offensive and difficult to flush'. An Iga antiendomysial antibody in serum was positive.

185. A 3-month-old male infant presents with abdominal distension and alternating diarrhoea and constipation since 4 weeks of age. The stools vary between hard small pellets and loose motions with mucus. There is a history of delay in passage of meconium after birth for 3 days.

THEME: 37
PETECHIAL RASH IN A CHILD

Options

a. Acute lymphoblastic leukaemia
b. Henoch-Schonlein purpura
c. Idiopathic thrombocytopaenic purpura
d. Meningococcaemia
e. Traumatic petechiae or echhymoses

For each of the situations/conditions given below, choose the one most appropriate/discriminatory option from above. The option may be used once, more than once, or not at all.

Questions

186. A 6-month-old baby presents with a history of paroxysmal cough of 4 days duration. The Gp is concerned when examination reveals fine purpuric eruptions around her eyes and neck. The baby missed the DVP vaccination due to 'recurrent colds'.

187. A 5-year-old gild develops colicky pain that is intermittent. The next day she has painful swelling of both her ankles and feet. Examination also reveals a palpable pupuric rash on the lefts and larger confluent ecchymoses on the back of the thighs and buttocks.

188. A 12-year-old boy presents with fever of 12 hours duration when he develops headache and vomiting. The parents are concerned when he becomes lethargic and develops some spots on his limbs and chest. On examination he

looks ill and is febrile. BP 90/45 mmHg and a tachycardia at 140/min. He has poor capillary refill and sparse petechiae on upper and lower limbs.

189. A 3-year-old girl has been 'unwell' for the past 10-14 days, being off colour, lethargic and with a poor appetite. Over the previous 48 hours she has developed bruised over the trunk and limbs. She is rather pale and has generalised enlargement of lymph nodes.
190. A healthy 4-year-old boy develops bruises on his body over a period of 24 hours. This was also accompanied by a nosebleed for the first time. He has an upper respiratory infection with a low-grade fever 2 weeks earlier.

THEME: 38
CAUSATIVE ORGANISMS OF MENINGITIS

Options

a. *Neisseria meningitidis.*
b. *H. Influenza.*
c. *Streptococcus pneumoniae.*
d. *E. coli.*
e. Group B hemolytic *Streptococcus.*
f. *Listeria monocytogenes.*

For each of the situations/conditions given below, choose the one most appropriate/discriminatory option from above. The options may be used once, more than once, or not at all.

Questions

191. A 1-day-old infant incessant crying, sudden onset fever.
192. A 2-year-old child presents with fever, vomiting. Also complains of headache, earache and ear discharge.
193. A 5-year-old child developed fever, arthritis and was generally unwell presents with mild headache. LP done was normal. Comes 3 days later with sudden increase in headache, vomiting and seizures.
194. A 4-year-old child develops sudden onset fever, headache, seizures. Child is also suffering from cough and productive sputum.

THEME: 39
DIAGNOSIS OF PAEDIATRIC NEUROLOGICAL DISORDERS

Options

a. Platybasia.
b. Duchenne's muscular dystrophy
c. Brain abscess
d. Syringomyelia
e. Glioblastoma multiforme
f. Ageneisi of corpus callosum
g. Arnold-Chiari malformation
h. Cerebral lymphoma
i. Klippel-Feil syndrome
j. Medulloblastoma
k. Tuberous sclerosis

For each of the situations/conditions given below, choose the one most appropriate/discriminatory option from above. The option may be used once, more than once, or not at all.

Questions

195. A 7-month-old infant with spasms and delayed milestones.
196. A 19-year-old student presented with loss of pinprick and temperature sensation over her shoulders and upper arms. MRI of the spine showed a fluid filled cystic cavity in the cervicothoracic cord.
197. A 3-week-old infant with meningomyelocoele presented with progressive head enlargement since birth.
198. A 6-year-old boy presented with clumsiness, abnormal gait and repeated falls. On examination he had prominent calf muscles and lumbar lordosis. He waddled slightly while walking. Deep tendon reflexes were depressed at the ankles.
199. A previously health 5-year-old girl presented with a 3 week history of morning headaches and unsteady gait. CT shows a lesion in the cerebrellar vermis.
200. A 9-year-old boy presented with learning difficulties. On examination he is found to have axillary freckles and multiple café-ay-lait spots.

THEME: 40
ACUTE ABDOMINAL PAIN IN CHILD

Options

a. Constipation.
b. Sickle cell disease.
c. TB.
d. Lead toxicity.
e. Renal colic.
f. Volvulus.
g. Hirschsprung's disease.
h. Appendicitis.
i. Gastroesophageal reflux.
j. Abdominal migraine.
k. Choose one of the above as the cause for the following scenarios.

For each of the situations/conditions given below, choose the one most appropriate/discriminatory option from above. The options may be used once, more than once, or not at all.

Questions

201. A 10-year-old girl complains of acute onset abdominal pain felt in the right side – with no relief on rest or any particular position remained at constant intensity for 6 hours and then automatically subsided completely. Her mother complains that she had treated with antibiotics many times in the past.
202. A 7-day-old child with crying spells with more crying on touching his tummy. Has passed stools only once after birth and that time also hard stool.
203. One and a half-day-old boy found to have anemia. Mother has recently noticed pica in this child. Now child has developed some abdominal pain with no other problem.
204. Mother comes with a well looking 5-year-old child in your clinic and says that the child complains of abdominal pain on and off for last 2 years which subsides on its own. Her elder son died of a injury six months ago but also had similar complaints.

THEME: 41
CAUSES OF RECTAL BLEEDING IN CHILDREN

Options

a. Meckel's diverticulum
b. Eosinophilic colitis
c. Intussusception
d. Hemolytic-uraemic syndrome
e. Lymphonodular hyperplasia
f. Juvenile polyps
g. Ulcerative colitis
h. Crohn's disease
i. Hemorrhoids
j. Hirschsprung's disease
k. Anal fissure

For each of the situations/conditions given below, choose the one most appropriate/discriminatory option from above. The option may be used once, more than once, or not at all.

Questions

205. A 15-month boy is admitted to A&E shocked. There is no history of diarrhoea, but he has been passing large amounts of melanotic stools. On examination he is anaemic.
206. A 4-year-old girl present with bloody diarrhoea and crampy abdominal pain. Blood tests show anaemia and thrombocytopenia.
207. A 5-week-old infant present with scanty streaks of fresh blood mixed with normal coloured stools.
208. A 7-year-old boy presents with streaks of fresh blood on the side of normal coloured stools and drops of fresh blood in the toilet. There is no history of abdominal pain or rectal pain.
209. A 3-year-old boy is admitted to A&E after passing several grossly bloody stools. There is no history of abdominal pain, fever or vomiting. On examination her is markedly pale.

210. A 12-year-old girl presented with a 4-week history of rectal bleeding and frequent loose motions. She reported lower abdominal cramping during defecation but denied fever, weight loss, arthritis or vomiting. Investigations showed anaemia but normal ESR, albumin and liver enzymes.

THEMEL: 42
LRI IN CHILDREN

Options

a. Acute bronchiolitis.
b. Pneumonia.
c. Whooping cough.
d. Bronchiectasis.
e. Lung abscess.
f. Tuberculosis.

For each of the situations/conditions given below, choose the one most appropriate/discriminatory option from above. The options may be used once, more than once, or not at all.

Questions

211. A 2-year-old girl child develops cough, fever is looking generally unwell. Brought to your clinic by her mother. Her father died of HIV one year ago.
212. A 4-month-old boy child develops nasal discharge and coughing, sneezing and also develops acute onset fever. In the last 2 days, you have seen 3 children from the same locality with same complaints.
213. A 5-year-old girl from lower socioeconomic status with high grade fever, cough, holds her right chest while coughing.

THEME: 43
PAROXYSMAL COUGH IN CHILDHOOD

Options

a. Allergic rhinitis
b. Asthma

c. Cystic fibrosis
d. Foreign body inhalation
e. Gastro-oesophagela reflux
f. Pertussis

For each of the situations/conditions given below, choose the one most appropriate/discriminatory option from above. The option may be used once, more than once, or not at all.

Questions

214. A 2-year-old boy is seen with a history of paroxysmal cough of sudden onset 2 days previously. He had been well before the onset and has been playing with his 5-year-old brother in the house. He also has a mild intermittent wheeze since the onset of the cough. He is not in any respiratory distress. Examination revealed diminution of air entry to the right chest posterior and the chest X-ray shows emphysema of the right lower lobe.
215. A 3-year-old girl has had a paroxysmal nocturnal cough intermittently for the past 6-8 months. She is well during the day with only a tendency to cough on exertion. The mother complains that each time she gets a cold ' it goes to her chest' and she has had frequent antibiotic treatment. There is a history of mild eczema. Clinically, except for a dry skin no abnormalities were noted.
216. An 18-month-old girl has had a paroxysmal nocturnal cough associated with a 'persistent cold' that has not cleared for several weeks. She starts to cough as she goes to sleep and may retch and vomit on some occasions. The cough is not severe during the day but she sounds 'rattly'. There is a strong history of atophy in the family.
217. A 5-week-old baby was admitted with cough and vomiting of 1 weeks duration. Cough was paroxysmal sometimes associated with choking and transient cyanosis. Clinical examination reveals tachypnoea of 45/minutes with good bilateral air entry and conducted sounds. The older sibling also has a less severe cough for the past 6 weeks and has not completed her immunisation.

THEME: 44
DIAGNOSIS OF PULMONARY DISEASES IN CHILDREN

Options

a. Pulmonary sequestration
b. Asthma
c. Tuberculosis
d. Bronchopulmonary dysplasia
e. Bronchogenic cyst
f. Cystic fibrosis
g. Pulmonary arteriovenous fistula
h. Larygomalacia
i. Massive pulmonary embolism
j. Tracheo-oesophageal fistula
k. Pulmonary hemosiderosis

For each of the situations/conditions given below, choose the one most appropriate/discriminatory option from above. The option may be used once, more than once, or not at all.

Questions

218. A 4-year-old girl presents with a history of recurrent pneumonia and failure to gain weight. On examination wheezes and crepitations were heard and fingers showed clubbling.
219. A 7-week-old infant presents with a 6-week history of noisy breathing. It is inspiratory in nature and increases when the baby is crying or during respiratory infections. It disappears completely when the baby is asleep.
220. A 5-year-old child presents with a history of chronic left lower lobe pneumonitis. On contrast bronchography the area involved fails to fill, outlined by bronchi that are filed.
221. A 4-year-old child presents with a history of dyspnoea, cyanosis, clubbing, haemoptysis and epistaxis. On examination there is generalized telangiectasia. Blood tests show polycythaemia.
222. A 1-year-old with presents with a history of coughing, especially with feeds and recurrent chest infection.
223. A 6-year-old boy presents to A&E with dyspnoea, wheezing and cough. On examination, he is slightly cyanosed. His respiratory rate is 30 BP is 100/60 and pulse is 110.

THEME: 45
INVESTIGATING PULMONARY DISEASE IN CHILDREN

Options

a. Barium swallow
b. Pulmonary angiography
c. Chest radiography
d. Contrast bronchography
e. CT chest
f. Fibre-optic Bronchoscopy
g. Chest ultrasonagraphy
h. ECG
i. Venous cineangiography
j. Sweat test
k. Echocardiography

For each of the situations/conditions given below, choose the one most appropriate/discriminatory option from above. The option may be used once, more than once, or not at all.

Questions

224. To guide needle thoracocentesis to sample a pleural effusion.
225. To assess an infant with apnea.
226. To evaluate a child with chronic cough and wheezing.
227. To differentiate a mediastinal mass from a collapsed lung.
228. To rule out pulmonary arterio – venous fistula.
229. To rule out laryngomalacia.

THEME: 46
CAUSES OF RESPIRATORY SYMPTOMS IN CHILDREN

Options

a. Asthma
b. Bronchiolitis
c. Croup
d. Pneumonia

e. Whopping cough
f. Epiglottitis
g. Diphtheria
h. Inhaled foreign body
i. Trachy-esophageal fistula
j. Cystic fibrosis
k. Cardiac disease
l. Respiratory distress syndrome

For each of the situations/conditions given below, choose the one most appropriate/discriminatory option from above. The option may be used once, more than once, or not at all.

Questions

230. A 2-year-old girl has been unwell for 2 months with difficulty in breathing. She has a barking bough with no sputum. The cough is worse at night and after feeding. Sometimes the bouts of coughing end with vomiting. There is no wheeze.
231. A 3-year-old boy has had a chronic cough for 3 months. He has had several chest infections and has required several courses of antibiotics. On examination he has a monophonic wheeze heard in the right lower lung field. He is systematically well.
232. A 6-year-old refugee is unwell with a high fever, sore throat and harsh cough. She has some difficulty swallowing and has a hoarse voice. There is thick grey exudates on the tonsils.
233. A 5-month-old baby has been tired and irritable for a few days with a runny nose. She now has a cough and is wheezy. On examination her temperature is 37.8°C and she has nasal flaring, intercostals recession and cyanosis.
234. A 1-month-old baby has had a chronic cough since birth and has been treated for 2 episodes of pneumonia. He becomes cyanosed when feeding. He is on the 3rd percentile of weight despite abdominal distension. When coughing he produces copious amounts of secretions and appears to ' blow bubbles'.

THEME: 47
DIAGNOSIS OF PERINATAL INFECTIONS

Options

a. Coxsackie B virus
b. Varicella zoster virus
c. Cytomegalovirus
d. Herpes simplex type 2
e. Toxoplasmosis
f. Mumps
g. Hepatitis A
h. Syphilis
i. Malaria
j. Rubella virus

For each of the situations/conditions given below, choose the one most appropriate/discriminatory option from above. The option may be used once, more than once, or not at all.

Questions

235. Only very rarely leads to congenital infection before 16 weeks gestation, but is know to infect all infants born to women with recent infection.
236. Causes birth defects when a mother is infected with a primary infection as opposed to recurrent infection.
237. Surviving infants exhibit cardiac malformation, hepatitis, pancreatitis and adrenal necrosis.
238. Surviving infants suffer from microcephaly, persisted PDA, pulmonary artery stenosis, ASD, cataract or microphthalmia.
239. The characteristic triad of abnormalities includes chorioretinitis, microcephaly and cerebral calcifications.
240. Not strictly teratogenic, but infants may suffer from endocardial fibroelastosis, urogenital abnormalities and ear and eye malformations.

THEME: 48
INVESTIGATION OF CONGENITAL DISEASES IN CHILDREN

Options

a. Blood films
b. Haemoglobin electrophoresis
c. Direct and indirect bilirubin
d. Sweat test
e. Heel-prick test
f. Urinary homocysteine
g. Karyotyping
h. Genetic testing
i. Echocardiography
j. Immunoglobulin levels
k. Specific enzyme levels
l. Clinical diagnosis only

For each of the situations/conditions given below, choose the one most appropriate/discriminatory option from above. The option may be used once, more than once, or not at all.

Questions

241. A 1-week-old baby is permanently sleepy and floppy and rarely feeds or cries. He has an excessively large tongue and is jaundiced, brachycardic and hyporeflexic.
242. A 3-year-old girl is admitted with painful swellings of her hands and feet. She has prolonged jaundice after birth but has developed normally. On examination she has splenomegaly and is jaundiced and pale.
243. A 4-year-old boy has had recurrent chest infections since birth and has now developed intermittent diarrhoea. He is failing to gain weight or height normally. A recent sputum culture grew *Staphylococcus aureus*.
244. A 14-year-old girl has not yet begun to menstruate. She gets teased for being the shortest girl in her class. On examination she has delayed breast development with wide-space nipples. There is a systolic murmur heard at the left sternal edge.

245. A 12-year-old boy had a protracted attack of gastro-enteritis during which he became jaundiced. No both the jaundice and gastroenteritis have settled. His mother says that he became jaundiced as a younger boy when he had a chest infection.
246. A 20-month girl has failed to thrive soonafter birth. She is very pale and appears breathless. She has frontal bossing of the skull and splenomegaly.

THEME: 49
CARDIAC CATHETER FINDINGS

Options

a. RV pressure up, pulmonary artery pressure down.
b. RV pressure up, RV O_2 > R atrial O_2.
c. Right atrial pressure and oxygenation up compared to IVC.
d. RV pressure up, pulm artery O_2 > RV O_2.
e. Pulm artery pressure > RV. RV O_2 and PaO_2 down.
f. RV pressure up, pulmonary artery pressure down, right atrial pressure up, PaO_2 down.

Match the above findings with the given conditions.

For each of the situations/conditions given below, choose the one most appropriate/discriminatory option from above. The options may be used once, more than once, or not at all.

Questions

247. ASD.
248. Patent ductus.
249. Fallot's tetrology.
250. VSD.
251. Pulmonary stenosis + foramen ovule.
252. Pulmonary stenosis.

THEME: 50
TREATMENT OF UTI IN CHILDREN

Options

a. Trimethoprim 1-2 mg/Kg/single dose

b. Trimethoprim 3 mg/Kg/bd
c. Amoxycillin
d. Amoxycillin 500 mg/8 hr
e. Gentamicin 10 mg/Kg/day
f. Ciprofloxacillin 500 mg stat
g. Metronidazole 500 mg/Kg/day
h. Co-amoxiclav 20-45 mg/kg/day
i. Nalidixic acid 50 mg/Kg/day

For each of the situations/conditions given below, choose the one most appropriate/discriminatory option from above. The options may be used once, more than once, or not at all.

Questions

253. A 2-year-old boy presents with frequency and dysuria shown to have vesico-ureteric reflux. He is treated for acute infection and you want him to stay healthy untill surgical intervention.
254. A 6-year-old girl presents with a fever , freqency, dysuria and abdominal pain.
255. A 5-year-old boy presents with dysuria, fever, frequency and vomiting. Abdominal ultrasound shows no abnormalities.
256. Almost 50% of all *E. coli* infections are unresponsive to this.

THEME: 51
DRUGS IN CHILDHOOD

Options

a. Aminophylline
b. Aspirin
c. Azithromycin
d. Benzylpenicillin
e. Brufen
f. Ceftotaxime
g. Cisapride
h. Isoniazid
i. Tetracyclines

For each of the situations/conditions given below, choose the one most appropriate/discriminatory option from above. The option may be used once, more than once, or not at all.

Questions

257. Is recommended as first line empirical therapy in bacterial meningitis where cause of infection is not known.
258. Is not recommended for analgesic with antifungal agents.
259. Causes arthythmias in association with antifungal agents.
260. Should not be given to children under 12 years of age as it can cause staining and malformation of teeth.

THEME: 52
DIAGNOSIS OF PAINFUL JOINTS IN CHILDREN

Options

a. Transient synovitis (Irritable Hip)
b. Slipped upper femoral epiphyses
c. Congenital hip dislocation
d. Juvenile rheumatoid arthritis
e. Ankylosing spondylitis
f. Perthes' disease
g. Septic arthritis

For each of the situations/conditions given below, choose the one most appropriate/discriminatory option from above. The option may be used once, more than once, or not at all.

Questions

261. A 5-year-old boy presents with a painful knee joint. His mother notices that he has started to limp. On examination all the movements of the hip joint are limited. X-ray of the femoral head shows patchy density.
262. A 3-year-old girl is bought to hospital by an anxious mother, who says the child is taking too long to walk normally. On examination her perineum appears wide and the lumbar lordosis appears to be increased. She complains of occasional hip pain and is seen to have a waddling gait.

263. A 5-year-old boy present with painful right hip and is seen to be limping. There is no history of trauma. The SHO in-charge admits the boy and 24 hours later; the boy has no complaints and is discharged. X-ray of the right hip appears normal and no other joints are involved.

THEME: 53
DIAGNOSIS OF CHILDHOOD EXTREMITY PAIN

Options

a. Non-accidental injury
b. Chondromalacia patella
c. Slipped femoral disease
d. Osgood – Schlatter disease
e. Sickle cell disease
f. Juvenile rheumatoid arthritis
g. Influenza
h. Reactive arthritis
i. Transient synovitis of the hick
j. Growing pains
k. SLE

For each of the situations/conditions given below, choose the one most appropriate/discriminatory option from above. The option may be used once, more than once, or not at all.

Questions

264. A 15-year-old female presents with fever, arthritis, weight loss and fatigue. Urinalysis reveals proteins, red blood cells and casts. Lab results reveal the presence of antinuclear antibodies to dsDNA.
265. A 4-year-old girl presents with a 3-month history of arthritis involving the knees and ankles. She is noted to have irodocyclitis on slit lamp examination. The ANA is positive and the rheumatoid factor is negative.
266. An 8-year-old girl presents with recurrent extremity pain. On examination she is found to have yellow green bruises on her calf and a 1 cm circular scar on her palm.

267. An 15-year-old boy presents with a limp and pain in the knee. On clinical examination the leg is externally rotated and 2 cm shorter. There is limitation of flexion, abduction and medial rotation. As the hip is flexed, external rotation is increased.
268. A 13-year-old girl presents with a painful and swollen knee. There is no history of injury. A tender lump is palpitated over the tibial tuberosity.

THEME : 54
NONACCIDENTAL INJURY

Options

a. Elderly abuse
b. Child physical abuse
c. Child sexual abuse
d. Emotional abuse
e. Henoch schonlein purpura
f. Immune thrombocytopenic purpura
g. Child neglect
h. Coelic disease
i. Osteogenesis imperfecta
j. Osteoporosis
k. Sickle cell anaemia
l. Senile purpura
m. Precocious puberty

For each of the situations/conditions given below, choose the one most appropriate/discriminatory option from above. The options may be used once, more than once, or not at all.

Questions

269. A mother of 16-year brings her baby for immunisation .The notices the baby has multiple bruises along both arms and legs and is crying excessively. The house officer notices multiple fractures and that the baby has blue sclerae.
270. A 70-year-old man is receiving treatment for Alzheimer's disease. He is looked after by a 23-year-old grand daughter. He has recently developed faecal incontinence. The SHO notices bruises on both wrists and back.

271. A 14-year-old girl asthamatic is brought into the chest clinic for regular check up. The H.Officer notices blue discolorations of the skin in the back abdomen further examination reveals more areas with similar lesions especially on the buttocks . The mother who is Afro-carribean fails to explain their occurrence.
272. An anxious mother brings her 6-year-old daughter who is bleeding per vagina. 6 months prior to this psesentation the girl had a confirmed *Streptococcal* sore throat infection but is otherwise normal.
273. A 12-year-old girl with a body mass index (BMI) of 16 is brought by her auntie to hospital. The girl has been staying with her stepmother and is found to be unkept and smelly.The auntie is worried that the girl has taken an overdose of paracetamol.

Eighteen

Orthopedics

THEME: 1
DIAGNOSIS OF ORTHOPEDIC CONDITIONS

Options

a. Sudeck's osteodystrophy.
b. Radial nerve injury.
c. Axillary nerve injury.
d. Fat embolisation.
e. Tennis elbow.
f. Sebaceous cyst.
g. Ganglion.
h. Triggler finger.
i. Dequervan's syndrome.
j. Volkmann's ischemic contracture.
k. Dupuytren's contracture.
l. Carpal tunnel syndrome.
m. Mallet finger.

For each of the situations/conditions given below, choose the one most appropriate/discriminatory option from above. The options may be used once, more than once, or not at all.

Questions

1. A 20-year-old boy who has closed fracture of surgical neck humerus 4 weeks back, which was treated by sling and body bandage. He is unable to abduct his shoulder.
2. A 20-year-old female who noticed a smooth round swelling on dorsum of wrist, which increases in size, following excessive work. The swelling is painless and firm. It decreases many times in size.

3. A 20-year-old typist who developed pain in right hand with tingling and numbness in thumb and lateral 2 fingers. She wakes up many times in night because of pain and tingling. On examination, she has mild weakness of abductor policies brevis.
4. A 45-year-old male manual worker has pain in forearm and on lateral side of elbow. He has tenderness on lateral humeral epicondyle.
5. A 50-year-old male had a road traffic accident and sustained fracture pelvis and fracture femur. He was operated on second day for fracture femur. On 4th day he suddenly developed confusion, dyspnea and fever. On examination, he has petechiae on neck, chest and abdomen.
6. A 45-year-old male who is on carbamazepine for epilepsy developed thickness in the palm and flexion deformity of little humerus.
7. A 30-year-old male who has humerus fracture developed ipsilateral wrist drop. Fracture in forearm 6 weeks back, for which he was given plaster cast. He has edema of hand and fingers with shiny skin and restricted painful movement of fingers and shoulder on removal of cast.
8. A 70-year-old timid male who has had fracture in forearm 6 weeks back, for which he was given plaster cast. He has edema of hand and fingers with shiny skin and restricted painful movement of fingers and shoulder. X-ray shows patchy osteoporosis on removal of cast.
9. A 35-year-old male who has pain in palm radiating to index finger. On examination tenderness present at metacarpophalangeal joint of index finger with firm nodule palpable. The finger can be flexed but it straightens with resistance and audible click which is painful. X-ray of the hand is normal.
10. A 23-year-old male has had plaster cast for closed supracondylar fracture of humerus. On removing the cast, he was found to have swollen fingers and atrophied forearm muscles. Passive stretching of fingers is painful.
11. A 20-year-old male sustained injury on right index finge while playing baseball. On examination, there was active

flexion at distal interphalangeal joint but no extension. X-ray of hand was normal.

THEME : 2
DIAGNOSIS OF BONY SWELLINGS

Options

a. Osteosarcoma.
b. Osteomyelitis.
c. Septic arthritis.
d. Tuberculosis arthritis.
e. Exotosis.
f. Painful hip in children.
g. Juvenile rheumatoid arthritis.
h. Ewing's sarcoma.
i. Osteoarthritis.
j. Multiple myeloma.
k. Osteoid osteoma.
l. Secondaries.
m. Giant cell tumors.
n. Aneurysmal bone cyst.
o. Neurofibroma.

For each of the situations/conditions given below, choose the one most appropriate/discriminatory option from above. The options may be used once, more than once, or not at all.

Questions

12. A 4-year-old child presents with pain of spontaneous onset knee for 2 days. He developed mild fever on second day. He can walk but has a limp. On examination, he has painful restriction of right hip rotations.
13. A 70-year-old chronic alcoholic with uncontrolled diabetes has developed limping for 3 months. He is not able to squat. He has low-grade fever and decreased appetite for last one month.
14. A 16-year-old male presents with fever and pains in right lower thigh for 1 month. On examination lower third of his thigh is red, hot tender new bone formation.

15. A 10-year-old boy who complains of pain in his legs which settles with aspirin.
16. A 60-year-old lady complains of backache has anemia and raised ESR.
17. A 14-year-old boy has fever and swelling of left arm with a wrist drop.
18. A 15-year-old male noticed swelling on left knee following a fall while playing. Swelling has not subsided after 2 weeks of rest and not subsided after 2 weeks of rest and analgesics. On examination, he has full knee movements without much pain. He has painless left ingiunal lymph nodes enlargement.
19. A 12-year-old male presents with right foot drop. On examination, he has bony swelling on the side of knee.
20. A 12-year-old male presents with pain and swelling of left leg with fever of 15 days duration.
21. A 65-year-old man with cough, hemoptysis and pathological fracture of the femur.
22. Pseudoarthritis of the tibia.

THEME: 3
THE TREATMENT OF FRACTURES AND DISLOCATIONS

Options

a. Kocher's method
b. AO cannulated screws
c. Bedrest
d. Open reduction and Kirschner wire
e. Buddy strapping
f. Reconstructive surgery with internal graft or implant augmentation
g. Physiotherapy for strengthening exercises
h. Austin Moore Hemiarthroplasty
i. Dynamic hip screw
j. Total hip replacement
k. Open reduction and internal fixation

For each of the situations/conditions given below, choose the one most appropriate/discriminatory option from above. The options may be used once, more than once, or not at all.

Questions

23. A 50-year-old fit man presents with a right hip fracture. On X-ray, the fracture line is sub-capital.
24. A 20-year-old athlete twists his knee on holiday while skiing. On examination, he has a positive drawer sign with the tibia sliding anteriorly.
25. A 70-year-old woman presents with a left hip fracture. On X-ray, the fracture line is intertrochanteric.
26. A 40-year-old woman sprains her wrist. She complains of persistent pain and tenderness over the dorsum distal to Lister's tubercle. X-ray shows a large gap between the scaphoid and the lunate. In the lateral view, the lunate is tilted dorsally and the scaphoid anteriorly.
27. A 30-year-old basketball player presents with severe pain in his shoulder. He is holding his arm with the opposite hand. He explains that he fell on an outstretched hand. The X-ray shows overlapping shadows of the humeral head and glenoid fossa, with the head lying below and medial to the socket. There is also a fracture of the neck of the humerus.

THEME: 4
MANAGEMENT OF LOWER LIMB FRACTURES

Options

a. Traction
b. Below-knee plaster
c. Above-knee plaster
d. Dynamic hip screw
e. Intramedullary nail
f. Hemi-arthroplasty
g. Total Hip Replacement
h. Open reduction and internal fixation
i. External fixation
j. Dynamic condylar screw
k. Bedrest only
l. Analgesia and active mobilisation

For each of the situations/conditions given below, choose the one most appropriate/discriminatory option from above. The options may be used once, more than once, or not at all.

Questions

28. A 78-year-old woman is admitted with an intertrochanteric fracture to her proximal femur. She has dementia and cardiac failure, which is reasonably well controlled. She lives in a nursing home and usually uses a Zimmer frame to walk short distances.
29. An 84-year man is admitted with a painful left hip after a fall at home. He has a fracture of his left inferior and superior pubic rami but his femur appears intact. He has pain on standing. He has no significant medical history.
30. An obese 32-year-old woman tripped on the road with eversion of her right foot. She has a displaced fracture of medial malleolus and fracture of fibula above the level of the tibio-fibular joint.
31. A 14-year-old boy fell from a stolen moped and sustained an open comminuted fracture of the distal third of his femur.
32. A 65-year-old woman with a history of osteoporosis is admitted with a displaced subcapital fracture of the right femoral neck. She has no other medical problems and is usually mobile without walking aids.

THEME: 5
TREATMENT OF FEMORAL FRACTURES

Options

a. Dynamic hip screw (DHS)
b. Gallows traction
c. Hemiarthroplasty
d. Intramedullary nailing
e. Multiple cannulated hip screws
f. Open reduction and internal fixation (ORIF)
g. Skeletal traction
h. Total hip replacement

For each of the situations/conditions given below, choose the one most appropriate/discriminatory option from above. The options may be used once, more than once, or not at all.

Questions

33. A 78-year-old lady with a displaced subcapital (Garden IV) fracture of the left femoral neck.
34. A 24-year-old motorcyclist with a closed fracture of the right femoral shaft.
35. A nine month old child with a spiral fracture of the femoral shaft.
36. A 57-year-old lady with an undisplaced fracture of the right femoral neck.
37. An 83-year-old lady with a displaced intertrochanteric fracture.

THEME: 6
COMPLICATIONS OF TOTAL HIP REPLACEMENT (THR)

Options

a. Anterior dislocation
b. Cellulitis
c. Chest infection
d. Deep infection
e. Deep vein thrombosis (DVT)
f. Haematoma
g. Posterior dislocation
h. Pulmonary embolism (PE)

For each of the situations/conditions given below, choose the one most appropriate/discriminatory option from above. The options may be used once, more than once, or not at all.

Questions

38. A 73-year-old man complains of swelling and discoloration of the right leg seven days after a right THR. He has tenderness behind the right knee on palpation.

39. An 81-year-old lady develops a pyrexia of 38 °C three weeks after her left THR. Her wound is oozing and her blood tests reveal a CRP of 150 mg/l and an ESR of 96 mm/hour.
40. A 67-year-old lady develops swelling and bruising of the left thigh four days after her left THR. Blood tests are normal.
41. A 77-year-old man develops sudden chest pain and breathlessness five days after his left THR. His pulse oximetry readings are 82% on air.
42. A 75-year-old lady develops sudden severe pain in her right hip whilst sitting down three weeks after her right THR. She is unable to stand and her right leg is internally rotated, flexed and adducted at the hip.

THEME : 7
MANAGEMENT OF ORTHOPEDIC CONDITIONS

Options

a. Plaster of Paris cast.
b. Closed reduction and plaster cast.
c. External fixation.
d. Local application of ice and crepe bandage.
e. Internal fixation.
f. Debridement and external fixation.
g. Bone grafting and internal fixation.
h. Wait and watch with periodic X-ray assessment.
i. Closed reduction and Thomas's splint.
j. Joint replacement.

For each of the situations/conditions given below, choose the one most appropriate/discriminatory option from above. The options may be used once, more than once, or not at all.

Questions

43. 60-year-old lady with Colle's fracture.
44. 65-year-old was treated by internal fixation. He has now developed pain in the hip with limping and X-ray shows collapsed head of femur but united fracture.

45. 35-year-old healthy male who has Galleazzi fracture dislocation.
46. 35-year-old male who has closed transverse fracture of humerus shaft and was treated by closed reduction and plaster cast for last 3 months comes with nonunion.
47. 20-year-old male who has had fracture humerus 3 months back and was treated by internal fixation. At present X-ray shows no callus formation.
48. 3-year-old child which closed fracture of shaft of femur.
49. 10-year-old child with undisplaced fracture of radius and ulna.

THEME: 8
MANAGEMENT OF ORTHOPEDIC CONDITIONS

Options

a. Local ice analgesics.
b. Plaster cast (POP).
c. Local steroid injury.
d. Physiotherapy.
e. Decompression.
f. Manipulation/reduction and POP.
g. Closed reduction and POP.
h. Internal fixation.
I. Hemiarthroplasty

For each of the situations/conditions given below, choose the one most appropriate/discriminatory option from above. The options may be used once, more than once, or not at all.

Questions

50. A 50-year-old male hypertensive with ischemic heart disease presents with pain and restricted movements of left shoulder with failed analgesic treatment.
51. A 70-year-old male sustained wrist fracture following fall.
52. A 20-year-old young girl sprained her ankle while climbing down the stairs.
53. A 65-year-old man with fractured hip.
54. A 7-year-old child with fracture of both bones of forearm.

THEME: 9
DIAGNOSIS OF FRACTURES

Options

a. Colles' fracture
b. Femoral neck fracture
c. Calcaneum fracture
d. Scaphoid fracture
e. Smith's fracture
f. Monteggia fracture disclosure
g. Galeazzi fracture disclosure
h. Anterior shoulder dislocation
i. Mallet finger
j. Bennett's fracture dislocation
k. Posterior shoulder dislocation

For each of the situations/conditions given below, choose the one most appropriate/discriminatory option from above. The options may be used once, more than once, or not at all.

Questions

55. A 27-year-old epileptic man falls onto his outstretched hand and now holds his arm in abduction. The deltoid appears hollow.
56. A 70-year-old female resident of a nursing home is brought into casualty after falling out of bed. On examination, her leg is shortened, adducted and externally rotated. The hip is tender to palpation, and she is unable to weight-bear.
57. A 40-year-old man falls from a tree and lands on his feet. He now presents with painful and swollen heels. His soles are bruised.
58. A 12-year-old presents with a fracture of the lower one third of the radius. She has also sustained a dislocation of the inferior radio-ulnar joint.
59. A 30-year-old cricketer presents with painful phalanx. He cannot actively extend the terminal phalanx of his middle finger.

THEME: 10
DISORDERS OF THE KNEE JOINT

Options

a. Anterior cruciate ligament injury
b. Gout
c. Meniscal injury
d. Osgood Schlatter's disease
e. Osteoarthritis
f. Osteosarcoma of the proximal tibia
g. Patella bursitis
h. Patella fracture
i. Rheumatoid arthritis
j. Septic arthritis

For each of the situations/conditions given below, choose the one most appropriate/discriminatory option from above. The options may be used once, more than once, or not at all.

Questions

60. A 33-year-old nurse was running for the bus when she tripped and fell over an uneven paving slab. She felt something crack and afterwards was unable to bare weight on the leg. In A&E considerable bruising around the knee is noted. She is unable to lift her leg off the couch.
61. A 13-year-old boy presents to his GP with a 6 month history of pain and swelling at the front of his knee. His symptoms are exacerbated by exercise and relieved by rest. There is now a prominent lump anteriorly over the proximal tibia. There is no specific history of trauma. His friend has recently been treated for leukaemia.
62. A 55-year-old ex-footballer presents to his GP with a long history of aches and pains in various joints. He has had previous meniscectomies of both knees and since he took part in a charity match last weekend he has been aware of considerable pain and swelling in his right knee. He can barely walk. Examination confirms a large tense effusion within the joint and significant restriction in joint movement. He is otherwise well.

63. A 55-year-old publican presents to his GP with a 24 hour history of acute pain and swelling in his left knee. He has been unable to sleep. Examination confirmed a large effusion in his knee and considerable tenderness. He is known to have a recent history of congestive cardiac failure but no significant musculoskeletal symptoms had been documented previously.

THEME: 11
FRACTURE COMPLICATIONS

Options

a. Acute Ischaemia
b. Compartment syndrome
c. Growth plate disturbance/damage
d. Malunion
e. Muscle haematoma
f. Nerve compression
g. Sudeck's atrophy – Reflex sympathetic dystrophy
h. Tendon rupture

For each of the situations/conditions given below, choose the one most appropriate/discriminatory option from above. The options may be used once, more than once, or not at all.

Questions

64. A 15-year-old boy notes a deformity of his right wrist two weeks following the removal of his plaster for a fracture of the distal radius.
65. A 35-year-old lady presents with severe pain and stiffness of her fingers and hands two weeks following removal of her plaster cast for management of an undisplaced distal, radial fracture. She would not allow the doctors to touch her hand, which was noted to be well perfused.
66. A 21-year-old male came into A&E at 3 am complaining of severe agonising pain in his forearm. He would not let anyone move his fingers. He was in a backslab for a displaced fracture of the radius and ulna and had been due for admission late that day for an open reduction and internal fixation.

THEME: 12
INVESTIGATION OF TRAUMA

Options

a. Chest X-ray
b. CT head scan
c. Lateral cervical spine X-ray
d. Lumbar spine X-ray
e. MRI thoraco-lumbar spine
f. Shoulder X-ray
g. Skull X-ray
h. Ultrasound scan abdomen

For each of the situations/conditions given below, choose the one most appropriate/discriminatory option from above. The options may be used once, more than once, or not at all.

Questions

67. A 32-year-old boxer who complains of left-sided weakness 24 hours after a boxing match.
68. A 19-year-old man who has sustained stab wounds to his abdomen and trunk. His respiratory rate is 23 breaths/minutes, his breath sounds appear normal and his pulse is 142/minutes and his BP is only 80/40.
69. A 47-year-old woman complains of left shoulder and neck pain after falling off her bicycle. She has a graze on her forehead and also complains of tingling in her left ring finger and little fingers (digits IV and V).
70. A 27-year-old motorcyclist has been involved in an accident and complains of loss sensation below the umbilicus and paralysis of both legs. His BP is 80/50 mmHg with a pulse rate of 72/minutes.
71. A 54-year-old roofer complains of lower back pain radiating into the right leg having fallen from a scaffold. He has no loss of power or sensation when examined.

THEME: 13
MULTIPLE TRAUMA

Options

a. Fractured os calcis and thoraco-lumbar vertebrae

b. Fractured pelvis, femur, and cervical spine
c. Fractured right humerus, right femur and pelvis
d. Head/facial injury, fractured sternum, tibial fractures
e. Respiratory distress and facial burns

For each of the situations/conditions given below, choose the one most appropriate/discriminatory option from above. The options may be used once, more than once, or not at all.

Questions

72. A 37-year-old driver of a car struck by a van on the driver's side.
73. A 25-year-old roofer falling 7 metres to the ground, landing feet first.
74. A 43-year-old man involved in an explosion at a petrochemical plant.
75. The driver of a car involved in a head-on-collision whilst not wearing a seat belt.
76. A 19-year-old motorcyclist thrown 19 metres from his bike.

THEME: 14
THE TREATMENT OF FRACTURES

Options

a. Collar and cuff sling
b. Broad arm sling
c. Open reduction and internal fixation
d. Closed reduction and plaster immobilisation
e. Hemiarthroplasty
f. Skeletal traction
g. Skin traction
h. External fixation
I. Balanced traction

For each of the situations/conditions given below, choose the one most appropriate/discriminatory option from above. The options may be used once, more than once, or not at all.

Questions

77. A 12-year-old boy is injured in Rugby. He sustained a blow to his chest. He complains of pain around the shoulder. X-ray reveals a fracture of the middle-third of the clavicle with displacement.

78. A 6-year-old girl falls onto the side of her left arm and now complains of left shoulder pain. On examination, she has numbness over the 'regimental badge' area. X-ray reveals a greenstick fracture of the proxial humerus.
79. A 55-year-old woman presents with pain in her upper arm without a history of trauma. Examination reveals intact radial nerve and brachial artery. X-ray demonstrates a transverse fracture of the humerus with a lytic lesion at the fracture site.
80. A 60-year-old woman with a history of breast carcinoma presents with pain in her right thigh. X-rays reveals a transverse fracture of the femur.
81. An 18-month-old baby is brought to casualty after a fall unable to weight-bear. X ray reveals a spiral fracture of the femur.

THEME: 15
THE TREATMENT OF SHOULDER REGION

Options

a. Broad arm sling
b. Collar and cuff sling
c. Rest and analgesia then mobilise
d. Injection of local anaesthesia and steroids
e. Manipulation under anaesthesia
f. Traction on the arm in 90 degrees of abduction and externally rotate the arm
g. Hippocratic technique
h. Kocher's technique
i. Surgical repair

For each of the situations/conditions given below, choose the one most appropriate/discriminatory option from above. The options may be used once, more than once, or not at all.

Questions

82. A 20-year-old man presents with shoulder pain and decreased range of movement after being struck in the upper back. X-ray reveals fracture of the scapula.

83. A 60-year-old builder presents with pain in the upper arm. On examination, he has a low bulge of the muscle belly of the long head of biceps.
84. A 50-year-old man complains of pain in his shoulder. The pain is elicited in abduction between an arc of 60 and 120 degrees. He reports that he has always had shoulder trouble.
85. A 20-year-old Rugby player falls onto the point of his shoulder and complains of shoulder tip pain. The lateral end of the clavicle is very prominent.
86. A 30-year-old hiker falls onto his outstretched hand and injures his right shoulder. On examination, there is loss of the rounded shoulder contour with prominence of the acromion. On palpation, there is a gap beneath the acromion and the humeral head is palpable in the axilla. The nearest hospital is 6 hours hike away and you are alone with him upon the mountain. You cannot obtain a signal on your mobile phone. You decide to treat the patient.

THEME: 16
CAUSES OF PAINFUL KNEE

Options

a. Reiter's syndrome
b. Meniscal tear
c. Rupture of the patellar tendon
d. Osgood-Schlatter's syndrome
e. Septic arthritis
f. Ankylosing sponditis
g. Osteoarthritis
h. Gout
i. Rheumatoid arthritis
j. Posterior cruciate
k. Anterior cruciate
l. Collateral ligament injury
m. Tumour of the bone and cartilage
n. Osteomyelitis

For each of the situations/conditions given below, choose the one most appropriate/discriminatory option from above. The options may be used once, more than once, or not at all.

Questions

87. A 20-year-old female presents with a painful locked knee following a twisting injury. There is no immediate haemarthrosis.
88. A 30-year-old female passenger strikes her shin against the car dashboard in an RTA and now complains of severe knee pain. On examination, she has profound haemarthrosis. The knee is immobilised in plaster to prevent flexion.
89. A 30-year-old female twists her knee while skiing and now presents with an acutely painful swollen knee. Aspiration of the haemarthrosis eases the pain and you are able to examine the knee. With the knee flexed at 90 degrees you are able to pull the tibia forwards on the femur by 1 cm.
90. A 10-year-old boy on prednisolone presents with a painful swollen knee. He recently had a chest infection. He is now unable to move the knee at all. There is a joint effusion present.
91. A 50-year-old woman presents with myalgia, fever and a painful swollen knee. She denies trauma. She has a raised ESR and CRP. X-ray shows some bony erosion.

THEME: 17
DIAGNOSIS OF ORTHOPEDIC DISORDERS

Options

a. Paget's disease.
b. Osteoporotic fracture vertebrae.
c. Secondaries.
d. Multiple myeloma.
e. PID.
f. Myofascial pain.
g. Ankylosing spondylosis.
h. Spondylosis.

For each of the situations/conditions given below, choose the one most appropriate/discriminatory option from above. The options may be used once, more than once, or not at all.

Questions

92. A 60-year-old female presented with acute onset bone and backpain following a rough journey in car. On examination, she has tenderness at midthoracic vertebrae. With spasm. She feels better on bending forward.
93. A 24-year fit man suddenly developed severe backpain (lower lumbar) as getting up from bed is the morning analgesics.
94. A 60-year-old man brought to casualty with fractured lip. He is deaf and has billeted pedal oedema. X-ray shows siderotic bone.
95. A 70-year-old man has been brought to casualty with acute asset paraplegia following trivial fall. He was treated for prostatic malignancy in the past.

THEME: 18
MOST COMMON SITE OF INVOLVEMENT

Options

a. Hip.
b. Knee.
c. Pelvis.
d. Humerus.
e. Tibia.
f. Skull.
g. Femur.

For each of the situations/conditions given below, choose the one most appropriate/discriminatory option from above. The options may be used once, more than once, or not at all.

Questions

96. Osteoma.
97. Aneurysmal bone cyst.
98. Paget's disease.

99. Osteoarthritis.
100. Fibrous dysplasia.
101. Syphilitic osteoperiostitis.
102. Pseudoarthritis.

THEME: 19
DEFORMITIES DUE TO ORTHOPEDIC TRAUMA

Options

a. Dinner fork deformity.
b. Gamekeeper's thumb.
c. Coxa vara.
d. Gibbus.
e. Cubitus valgus.
f. Mallet finger.
g. Gunstock deformity.
h. Garden spade deformity.
i. Genu valgum

For each of the situations/conditions given below, choose the one most appropriate/discriminatory option from above. The options may be used once, more than once, or not at all.

Questions

103. Colle's fracture.
104. Smith's fracture.
105. Avulsion of extensor tendon from distal phalanx.
106. Rupture of ulnar collateral ligament of metacarpophalangeal joint of thumb.
107. Wedge compression of vertebrae.
108. Supracondylar fracture humerus.
109. Intertrochanteric fracture.
110. Condylar fracture of tibia.

THEME: 20
CONDITIONS OF THE HAND

Options

a. Volkman's ischaemic contracture
b. Dupuytren's contracture

c. Carpal tunnel syndrome
d. Claw hand
e. Raynaud's phenomenon
f. Scleroderma
g. Rheumatoid arthritis
h. Paronychia
i. Psoriasis
j. Koilonychia
k. Glomus tumour
l. Subungual haematoma

For each of the situations/conditions given below, choose the one most appropriate/discriminatory option from above. The options may be used once, more than once, or not at all.

Questions

111. A 20-year-old female presents with a painful fingertip that throbs and has kept the patient up all night. The skin at the base and side of the nail is red, tender and bulging.
112. A 30-year-old female presents with a painful fingernail. On examination, there is a small purple red spot beneath the nail. She denies history of trauma to the finger.
113. A 60-year-old man with acromegaly presents with pins and needles in the index finger and the middle fingers of his right hand worse at night.
114. A 20-year-old man presents with fingers that are permanently flexed in his right hand. However, the deformity is abolished by flexion of the wrist. He admits to trauma to his elbow recently. He also complains of pins and needles sensation.
115. A 20-year-old female complains of intermittent pain in her fingertips. She describes the fingers undergoing colour changes from white to blue and then to red. The symptoms are worse in the winter.

THEME: 21
THE TREATMENT OF UPPER HAND INJURIES

Options

a. Sling
b. Kocher's method

c. Collar and Cuff
d. Open reduction and Kirschner wire fixation
e. Buddy strapping
f. Open reduction and internal fixation
g. Traction on the arm in abduction followed by rotation of the arm laterally with pressure on the humeral head.
h. Closed reduction and cast immobilisation
i. Open reduction and plating
j. Plaster cast immobilisation alone
k. Splinting in a plaster cast

For each of the situations/conditions given below, choose the one most appropriate/discriminatory option from above. The options may be used once, more than once, or not at all.

Questions

116. A 40-year-old man with a history of epilepsy presents with right shoulder pain. The arm is held in medial rotation with a flat shoulder. The anteroposterior film shows a humeral head like an electric light bulb and an empty glenoid sign.
117. An 8-year-old boy presents with a painful and swollen elbow. He fell onto his outstretched hand. The lateral X-ray shows an undisplaced supracondylar fracture line running obliquely downwards and forwards.
118. A 70-year-old female with osteoporosis falls onto the back of her hand. She presents with wrist pain. The X-ray shows a fracture through the distal radial metaphysics, and the distal fragment is displaced and tilted anteriorly.
119. A 3-year-old child presents with a painful, dangling arm after having her arm jerked. The forearm is held in pronation. There are no X-ray changes.
120. A 25-year-old man presents with a swollen tender finger. X-ray shows a transverse, undisplaced fracture of the proximal phalanx.

THEME: 22
DIAGNOSIS OF HAND INJURIES

Options

a. Mallet finger

b. Bennett's fracture
c. Median nerve injury
d. Radial nerve injury
e. Ulnar nerve injury
f. Boutonniere deformity
g. Flexor digitorum profundus
h. Flexor digitorum superficialis injury
i. Ulnar collateral ligament injury

For each of the situations/conditions given below, choose the one most appropriate/discriminatory option from above. The options may be used once, more than once, or not at all.

Questions

121. A 40-year-old woman presents with drooping of the terminal phalanx of her middle right finger. She was making the bed at the time of injury. She is now unable to extend the tip of her finger.
122. A 45-year-old man presents with lacerations to the hand from cut glass. You hold all three uninjured fingers in extension and ask him to flex the lacerated finger. He is unable to comply.
123. A 20-year-old man with a history of depression presents with slashed wrists. You ask the patient to place the back of his hand flat on the table and have him point his thumb to the ceiling against resistance. He is unable to comply.
124. A 40-year-old man presents with numbness in his palm after falling and hitting the heel of his hand against the pavement. The distribution of numbness is over the palmar aspect of the 4th and 5th digits.
125. A 30-year-old woman sustains injury to her hand while skiing. She complains of pain around the metacarpophalangeal joint of her thumb and has difficulty abducting her thumb. She has loss of pincer ability.

THEME: 23
DEFORMATION DUE TO NERVE INJURIES

Options

a. Claw hand.

b. Wrist drop.
c. Foot drop.
d. 'Z' deformity of thumb.
e. Volkmans ischemic contracture.
f. Pointing index.
g. Swan neck deformity.
h. Shoulder drop.

For each of the situations/conditions given below, choose the one most appropriate/discriminatory option from above. The options may be used once, more than once, or not at all.

Questions

126. Fracture shaft humerus.
127. Colle's fracture.
128. Fracture of neck of fibula.
129. Young man who had a cardiac catheterisation through the antecubital vein.
130. Fracture head of radius.
131. Valgus injury to the elbow.

THEME: 24
DIAGNOSIS OF NERVE INJURIES ASSOCIATED WITH FRACTURES

Options

a. Axillary nerve.
b. Radial nerve.
c. Ulnar nerve.
d. Median nerve.
e. Sciatic nerve.
f. Gluteal nerve.
g. Facial nerve.
h. Musculocutaneous nerve.

For each of the situations/conditions given below, choose the one most appropriate/discriminatory option from above. The options may be used once, more than once, or not at all.

Questions

132. Fracture neck of humerus.
133. Fracture neck of fibula.
134. Fracture lateral condyle.
135. Fracture of head of radius.
136. Fracture of shaft of humerus.
137. Dislocation of shoulder.
138. Fracture neck of femur.
139. Colles fracture.
140. Fracture medial epicondyle humerus.
141. Supracondylar fracture of humerus.

THEME: 25
INVESTIGATIONS FOR BONE DISEASES

Options

a. Rheumatoid factor.
b. Serum-uric acid.
c. HLA B 27
d. Serum-protein-electrophoresis.
e. Bone densitometry.
f. Istope bone scan.
g. MRI scan.
h. 3D CT scan.
i. Ultrasound.

For each of the situations/conditions given below, choose the one most appropriate/discriminatory option from above. The options may be used once, more than once, or not at all.

Questions

142. Low backpain with left sided sciatica.
143. A 70-year-old man with paraplegia.
144. A 30-year-old man has pain and deformities of both hands.
145. A 30-year-old man has backache and limited chest expansion.
146. A 40-year-old man. Woke up with pain in his great toe.

THEME: 26
DIAGNOSIS OF HEAD INJURIES

Options

a. Basal skull fracture
b. Depressed skull fracture
c. Compound skull fracture
d. Diffuse axonal injury
e. Concussion
f. Subdural haematoma
g. Intracerebral haemorrhage
h. Extradural haemorrhage
i. Open skull fracture
j. Brain concussion

For each of the situations/conditions given below, choose the one most appropriate/discriminatory option from above. The options may be used once, more than once, or not at all.

Questions

147. A 30-year-old female involved in an RTA is brought by ambulance to A&E. She is noted to have bruising of the mastoid process and periorbital haematoma. On otoscopic examination she has bleeding behind tympanic membrane.
148. A 60-year-old man was kicked in the head a week ago. He is brought to A&E in an unconscious state. He smells of alcohol. On examination he has a rising BP and unequal pupils.
149. A 40-year-old man was struck in the head by a cricket ball. He had an episode of loss of consciousness lasting 5 minutes. The patient now complains of headache. He has no lateralizing signs on neurological examination.
150. A 50-year-old man with a history of epilepsy has a fit and strikes the side of the head on the edge of the bathtub. He is dazed and complains of headache. Skull X-ray reveals a linear fracture of the parietal area. His level of consciousness diminishes.

151. A 60-year-old man is struck in the head with a dustbin lid and presents with an open scalp wound. Skull X-ray confirms an underlying skull fracture. The dura is intact.

THEME: 27
DIAGNOSIS OF BACKPAIN

Options

a. Discitis
b. Prolapsed lumbar disc
c. Senile kyphosis
d. Tuberculosis
e. Pyogenic spondylitis
f. Adolescent kyphosis (Scheuermann's disease)
g. Lumbar spondylosis
h. Spinal stenosis
i. Spondylolisthesis
j. Osteoarthritis
k. Scoliosis

For each of the situations/conditions given below, choose the one most appropriate/discriminatory option from above. The options may be used once, more than once, or not at all.

Questions

152. A 30-year-old female presents with back pain and pain in the buttock and lower limb. She was moving house and lifting heavy objects. She stands with a slight list to one side. Straight leg raise is restricted and painful.
153. A 60-year-old man presents with longstanding back pain and ill-health. On examination, he has a hunchback. The X-ray shows destruction of the front of the vertebral bodies and calcification of a psoas abscess.
154. A 13-year-old female presents with a convexity of 70 degrees in her thoracic spine.
155. A 12-year-old female presents with backache and fatigue. On examination, she has rounded shoulders with a hump and a lumbar lordosis.

156. A 50-year-old female presents with chronic backache. On examination, the buttocks are flat, the sacrum appears to extend to the waist, and the transverse loin creases are seen. A step can be felt when the fingers are run down the spine.

THEME: 28
THE TREATMENT OF BACK PAIN

Options

a. Physiotherapy
b. Rest, weight loss and analgesia
c. Surgical removal of a prolapsed disc
d. Nerve root decompression
e. Spinal decompression with laminectomy
f. Lateral mass fusion
g. Calcitonin
h. Chemotherapy
i. Radiotherapy
j. Excision of the nidus

For each of the situations/conditions given below, choose the one most appropriate/discriminatory option from above. The options may be used once, more than once, or not at all.

Questions

157. A 30-year-old man presents with bone pain around the knee. X-ray shows bony destruction and periosteal elevation with subperiosteal new bone formation. Chest X-ray reveals nodules.
158. A 70-year-old man presents with low back pain, aching and numbness in his thighs and legs. He prefers to walk uphill than downhill. His activities are now severely restricted. X-ray reveals a trefoil-shaped lumbar spinal canal and osteoarthritic changes.
159. A 60-year-old man presents with chronic back pain. On examination he has a large head and bowed shins. He is hard of hearing. X-rays show sclerosis and osteoporosis. His blood tests show an elevated alkaline phosphatase.

160. A 70-year-old woman presents with chronic back pain. On examination, she is tender along her shoulders, ribs and back. Blood tests reveal a high calcium and high urea. X-rays show osteolytic lesions.
161. A 20-year-old man presents with a painful shin. Aspirin seems to relive the pain. On X-ray there is a localised osteolytic lesion surrounded by a rim of sclerosis.

THEME: 29
CAUSES OF BACK PAIN

Options

a. Multiple Myeloma
b. Secondary prostate disease
c. Osteomyelitis
d. Ankylosing spondylitis
e. Sarcoidosis
f. Lupus
g. Reiter's disease
h. Lumbar prolapse and sciatica
i. Spondylolisthesis
j. Spinal Stenosis
k. Paget's disease

For each of the situations/conditions given below, choose the one most appropriate/discriminatory option from above. The options may be used once, more than once, or not at all.

Questions

162. A 30-year-old female complains of sudden and severe back pain. Her back has 'gone'. She walks with a compensated scoliosis. On examination, she has pain from the buttock to her ankle and sensory loss over the sole of her left foot and calf.
163. A 50-year-old man presents with back pain radiating down both his legs. The pain is aggravated by walking and relieved by resting or leaning forward. On examination, he has limited straight leg raise and absent ankle flexes.

164. A 50-year-old woman presents with backache. She is noted to have a normocytic, normochromic anaemia and a high erythrocyte sedimentation rate.
165. A 60-year-old man presents with lumbar spine bone pain and pain in his hips. He is noted to have an elevated serum alkaline phosphatase of 1000 IU/l. The calcium and phosphate levels are normal. He is hard of hearing.
166. A 20-year-old man complains of lower back pain radiating down the back of both his legs. On X-ray, the vertebrae are square and tramline. His ESR is elevated.

THEME: 30
THE MANAGEMENT OF BACK PAIN

Options

a. Obtain chest X-ray
b. Bedrest for two weeks
c. Rest for two days with analgesia
d. Physiotherapy
e. Urinanalysis
f. Investigate for underlying tumour or other bone pathology
g. Urgent orthopaedic referral for surgical decompression
h. Routine orthopaedic referral for decompression of nerve root
i. Abdominal ultrasound.

For each of the situations/conditions given below, choose the one most appropriate/discriminatory option from above. The options may be used once, more than once, or not at all.

Questions

167. A 40-year-old man complains of lower back pain after moving heavy furniture. He has no associated nerve root findings.
168. A 50-year-old female complains of back pain worse at night. X-ray of her spine shows crush fractures of two vertebrae. She denies trauma.
169. A 60-year-old man presents with back pain radiating bilaterally below the knees. On examination, he has saddle anaesthesia, urinary incontinence and loss of anal tone.

170. A 50-year-old female complains of chronic lower back pain radiating into her buttocks. There is no evidence of nerve root entrapment.
171. A 30-year-old man complains of back pain radiating below the knee. On examination, he has sensory loss over the lateral aspect of the right calf and medial aspect of the right foot. He is unable to dorsiflex his great toe. He has tried bedrest for 6 weeks.

THEME: 31
THE MANAGEMENT OF NECK INJURIES

Options

a. Repeat C-spine X-ray
b. Skull traction
c. Cervical collar
d. Surgical decompression and stabilisation
e. Anti-inflammatories and physiotherapy
f. Reduction and immobilisation in a halo-body cast
g. Immobilisation in a halo-body cast.

For each of the situations/conditions given below, choose the one most appropriate/discriminatory option from above. The options may be used once, more than once, or not at all.

Questions

172. A 30-year-old female complains of headache and painful stiff neck following whiplash injury sustained 24 hours ago. She has no neurological findings. X-ray shows loss of the normal lordotic curve of the spine.
173. A 25-year-old female involved in an RTA is found to have an unstable fracture of C1 with disruption of the arch.
174. A 30-year-old man involved in an RTA is sent to X-ray wearing a hard cervical collar with sandbags secured on either side of his head. The cervical X-ray shows no abnormalities of all 7 vertebrae down to the C6/C7 junction. He has no neck pain. He has no focal neurological signs.

175. A 19-year-old man involved in a high-velocity RTA is found to have a displaced fracture of the odontoid peg.
176. A 25-year-old female sustains head injuries going through the windshield of a car in a high-speed RTA. X-ray shows undisplaced fracture of the pedicle of C2.

THEME: 32
DIAGNOSIS OF LOWER LIMB FRACTURES

Options

a. Pelvic fracture
b. Sacrococcygeal fracture
c. Femoral neck fracture
d. Supracondylar fracture
e. Femoral condyle fracture
f. Intertrochanteric fracture
g. Tibial plateau fracture
h. Femoral shift fracture
i. Fracture of the proximal fibula
j. Fractured patella
k. Fractured tibial spine

For each of the situations/conditions given below, choose the one most appropriate/discriminatory option from above. The options may be used once, more than once, or not at all.

Questions

177. A 20-year-old cyclist was struck in an RTA and brought into casualty. His perineum and scrotum are swollen and bruised. He is unable to pass urine and there is a streak of blood at the external meatus.
178. A 70-year-old woman catches her toe in the carpet and falls twisting her hip into external rotation. On examination, her leg is in lateral rotation and appears short. She is able to take some steps.
179. An 80-year-old woman presents to casualty after a fall directly onto her hip and is now unable to weight-bear. The leg is shorter and externally rotated. She cannot lift her leg.

180. A 20-year-old female was roller-blading when she fell. She is now unable to weight-bear. On examination, her leg is rotated externally and shorter. The thigh is swollen and bruised.
181. A 10-year-old child twisted his knee and now presents with a swollen immobile knee. The joint is tense, tender and doughy. Aspiration reveals a haemarthrosis. Examination under anaesthesia shows that extension is blocked.

THEME: 33
DIAGNOSIS OF ANKLE AND FOOT DEFORMITIES

Options

a. Hallux rigidus
b. Hallux valgus
c. Pes cavus
d. Hammer toe
e. Mallet toe
f. Rheumatoid arthritis
g. Morton's Metatarsalgia
h. Stress fracture
i. Osteoarthritis
j. Ruptured tendo Achilles
k. Diabetic foot
l. Gout
m. Plantar fasciitis

For each of the situations/conditions given below, choose the one most appropriate/discriminatory option from above. The options may be used once, more than once, or not at all.

Questions

182. A 45-year-old man complains that he is unable to tiptoe. He feels as though he has been struck above the heel. Plantarflexion is weak. With the patient prone, the foot remains still when the calf is squeezed.
183. A 60-year-old man is noted for bilateral foot deformities. He has swollen, painless feet, claw toes, and plantar

ulceration over the metatarsal heads. He also has an amputated 5th toe digit.

184. A 50-year-old woman complains of sharp pain in the forefoot radiating to the toes. Tenderness is elicited in the third inter-digital space, and sensation is diminished in the cleft.
185. A 40-year-old woman presents with a second toe deformity. The proximal joint is fixed in flexion, and the metatarsophalangeal joint is extended. She has a painful callous on the dorsum of the toe and under the metatarsal head.
186. A 50-year-old woman presents with pain on walking. On examination, the metatarsophalangeal joint is enlarged and tender, with a callosity under the medial side of the distal phalanx. Dorsiflexion is restricted and painful.

THEME: 34
ANKLE INJURIES

Options

a. Elastic bandage and physiotherapy
b. External fixation
c. External fixation and wound debridement
d. Manipulation under anaesthesia (MUA) and POP application
e. Open reduction and internal fixation (ORIF)
f. Plaster of Paris (POP) immobilisation
g. Suture repair

For each of the situations/conditions given below, choose the one most appropriate/discriminatory option from above. The options may be used once, more than once, or not at all.

Questions

187. A 26-year-old man complains of sudden onset pain at the back of his heel and calf whilst playing squash. He has calf tenderness and is unable to stand on his toes; X-rays are normal.

188. A 54-year-old woman sustains a twisting injury to the left ankle whilst stepping off a kitchen ladder. She has swelling and tenderness over the lateral aspect of the ankle. X-rays show an undisplaced fracture of the distal fibula.
189. A 23-year-old motorcyclist involved in an RTA has a compound (open) fracture of the left tibia with extension into the ankle joint.
190. A 31-year-old footballer sustains an injury to the right ankle in a tackle. There is swelling and tenderness over both medial and lateral aspects of the ankle. X-rays show a displaced fracture of the distal fibula (Weber type C) with evidence of talar shift.
191. A 43-year-old window cleaner falls off his ladder injuring his left heel. X-rays confirm an extra-articular fracture of the calcaneum.

THEME: 35
CAUSES OF PAINFUL FOOT

Options

a. Morton's Neuroma
b. Stress fracture
c. Avulsion fracture
d. Jones fracture
e. Hallux fracture
f. Plantar fasciitis
g. Freiberg's disease
h. Metatarsalgia
i. Kohler's disease
j. Bunion
k. Gout

For each of the situations/conditions given below, choose the one most appropriate/discriminatory option from above. The options may be used once, more than once, or not at all.

Questions

192. A 50-year-old presents with pain over the medial calcaneum and pain on dorsiflexion and eversion of the forefoot.

193. A 60-year-old man complains of continuous pain in his forefoot worse when walking. X-rays shows widening and flattening of the second metatarsal head and degenerative changes in the metatarsophalangeal joint.
194. A 50-year-old woman complains of painful shooting pains in her right foot when walking. She is tender in the 3rd/4th interdigital space.
195. A 30-year-old soldier complains of pain in the foot when bearing weight. X-ray shows no fracture. He is tender around the proximal 5th metatarsal bone.
196. A 20-year-old man complains of pain over the lateral aspect of his right foot. X-ray shows a transverse fracture of the basal shaft of the 5th metatarsal bone.

Nineteen

Psychiatry

THEME: 1
DIAGNOSIS OF MOOD DISORDER

Options

a. Bipolar disorder.
b. Major depression.
c. Dysthymia.
d. Cyclothymia.
e. Atypical depression.
f. Mania.
g. Postpartum depression.
h. Post-traumatic stress disorder.

For each of the situations/conditions given below, choose the one most appropriate/discriminatory option from above. The options may be used once, more than once, or not at all.

Questions

1. A 36-year-old Vietnam War veteran is brought into the emergency department in an anxious, tremulous and diaphoretic state. While coming out of a bar, he attempted to grab a police officer's revolver after hearing a car backfire. He was shouting incoherently about "the enemy".
2. Initial episode in-patient who later develops bipolar disorder.
3. A change in personality in adolescence.
4. Uninhibited spending.
5. A tendency to experience more health problems than most people.
6. Delusions of grandeur.

7. Decreased rapid eye movement latency.
8. Sleeplessness.
9. Carbamazepine treatment.
10. Congestive heart failure.
11. Pseudodementia.
12. Lithium is the drug of choice.
13. A 42-year-old man is brought to the emergency department by his family after becoming threatening when they confronted him about his excessive spending. He bought rupees 5000 worth of clothing in the preceding week and then gave it away. He explains that this is a part of his presidential campaign, which he has been working on night and day for several weeks.

THEME: 2
DIAGNOSIS OF PERSONALITY DISORDERS

Options

a. Antisocial.
b. Passive aggressive.
c. Schizoid.
d. Histrionic.
e. Borderline.
f. Avoidant.
g. Multiple personality.
h. Narcissistic.

For each of the situations/conditions given below, choose the one most appropriate/discriminatory option from above. The options may be used once, more than once, or not at all.

Questions

14. A 35-year-old female presents to the GP with chronic feelings of boredom and depression. She shops excessively and is sexually promiscuous. She has cut herself in past to relieve her anxiety.
15. A 30-year-old man has no close friends. He avoids social situations. He is unable to express tender emotions. He has no overt signs of hallucination or delusional behaviour.

16. A 28-year-old female presents to her GP. She suffers from low self esteem and does not take risks in life. She seems extremely sensitive to criticism.
17. A 15-year-old boy is brought to his GP by his parents for abusive behaviour. He is delinquent from school and has been arrested for assault and for theft.
18. A 25-year-old man believes he is perfect. He is unable to empathise and manipulates people and situations. He sees everyone else as flawed. His relationships are shallow.

THEME: 3
TREATMENT OF DEPRESSION.

Options

a. Electroconvulsive therapy
b. Flupenthixol
c. Psychodynamic psychotherapy.
d. Cognitive therapy.
e. Behavioural Therapy
f. Marital therapy.
g. Lithium prophylaxis.
h. imipramine
i. No action.
j. Psychosurgery
k. Hypnotherapy
l. Ab-reaction
m. Counselling

Questions

19. A 20-year-old first time mother presents with severe weight loss, anorexia and believes that her husband is interested in killing her and their baby son and feels completely worthless.
20. A 40-year-old man has been treated for depression for 6 months. He is now beginning to lose weight and gertting suicidal thoughts more frequently than before.
21. A 29-year-old woman presents with inability to sleep and aggressiveness and increased libido. Her husband says prior to this she was markedly withdrawn and blamed

herself for her daughter's death due to cancer. She also has suicidal thoughts.

22. A 12-year-old boy refuses to go to school because of constant failure to get grade A. He is threatening to starve himself to death.
23. A 16 year girl with a BMI of 16 complains of 3 month history of amennorrhoea. She is not on the pill and the pregnancy test is negative. She Aspires to be a model.

THEME: 3
DIAGNOSIS OF ALCOHOL RELATED SYNDROME

Options

a. Delirium tremens.
b. Intoxication.
c. Hallucinosis.
d. Korsakoff's psychosis.
e. Wernicke's encephalopathy.

For each of the situations/conditions given below, choose the one most appropriate/discriminatory option from above. The options may be used once, more than once, or not at all.

Questions

24. Visual and tactile hallucinations.
25. Blackouts.
26. Confabulation.
27. Dehydration.
28. A 20-year-old man is brought to the emergency department after tearing up a restaurant and assaulting his companions. He is confused and agitated. His friends deny any history of violence or prior psychiatric history. They state that he had become violent quite suddenly and that they have been unable to calm him.

THEME : 4
DIAGNOSIS OF PSYCHIATRIC DISORDERS

Options

a. Brief reactive psychosis

b. Bipolar disorder.
c. Panic disorder.
d. Delusional disorder.
e. Dysthmia
f. Pica
g. Agarophobia
h. Fugue
i. Cocaine intoxication
j. Drug toxicity.
k. Suicidal risk
l. Dementia
m. Panic attacks
n. Opiod abuse
o. Schizophrenia.

For each of the situations/conditions given below choose the one most appropriate/discriminatory option from above. The options may be used once, more than once, or not at all.

Questions

29. A 40-year-old man insists that his wife is unfaithful and sleeping with the entire neighborhood. He is hypertensive, argumentative, and litiginous. His wife has left him due to his behaviour. He functions well at work.
30. A 25-year-old woman presents with personality changes. She is noted by friends initially to be anxious, irritable, and an insomniac and weeks later, she becomes profoundly depressed with low self esteem and contemplates suicide. In consultation, she has pressured speech with boundless energy .
31. A 20-year-old woman has a "mental breakdown". She has recently broken up with her boyfriend. She has dramatic mood swings, memory loss ,and incoherent speech. This lasts for a month.
32. A 20-year-old woman presents to her GP complaining of feeling depressed ever since she can remember. Her parents died in a car crash 10 years ago. She sees herself as a failure but functions well at work. She has trouble falling asleep.
33. A 50-year-old woman complains of sudden episodes of impending doom. During these episodes she feels choked and sweats profusely.

34. A 70-year-old retired engineer experiences changes in personality and impaired social skills. This is corroborated by his family, who describe him as forgetful and not sharp. There are no objective features of depression.
35. A 20-year-old man is noted to be withdrawn, isolated, and "peculiar". He experiences persecutory delusions and auditory hallucinations.
36. A 60-year-old widow is noted to by her family to be restless, disorganized, crying, and frequently expresses her wish to join her deceased partner.
37. a 40-year-old Irishman complains of frequent episodes of chest pain, sweating, palpitations, a sense of impending doom, and trembling that lasts for minutes at a time.
38. A 25-year-old man presents with miosis, slurred speech, disoriented, and respiratory depression.
39. A 2-year-old boy presents with anaemia and abdominal pain. His mother states that she has seen him peeling paint chips off the wall and wonders if he has been eating this.
40. A 23-year-old woman becomes afraid to leave her home. She functions normally except will not step outside her house.
41. An 18-year-old man presents with nausea, vomiting and diaphorisis. His pupils are dilated, and his blood pressure is elevated. He has a history of drug addictaion.
42. A 30-year-old woman is found in an amnestic state. Her husband reports that she had been missing for a few days after she had been served with divorce papers.
43. A 30-year-old man with bipolar disorder is taking lithium. He was recently started on thiazide for mild hypertension. He is now confused with ataxia,blurred vision, and a coarse tremor.

THEME: 5
WITHDRAWAL SYMPTOMS OF PSYCHOTROPIC DRUGS

Options

a. Benzodiazepines.
b. Monoamine oxidase inhibitors.

c. Tricyclic compounds.
d. Phenothiazines.

For each of the situations/conditions given below, choose the one most appropriate/discriminatory option from above. The options may be used once, more than once, or not at all.

Questions

44. Cholinergic actions, insomnia, restlessness and anxiety.
45. Acute anxiety and psychotic symptoms with hyperactivity.
46. Orofacial dystonias.
47. Panic, shaking, sweating and nausea.

THEME: 6
MENTAL HEALTH AND SOMATOFORM DISORDERS

Options

a. Ulcerative colitis.
b. Cardiovascular disease.
c. Migraine headache.
d. Immune disorder.
e. Bronchial asthma.

For each of the situations/conditions given below, choose the one most appropriate/discriminatory option from above. The options may be used once, more than once, or not at all.

Questions

48. Psychological features of the disorder include immaturity, covertly demanding behavior and sensitivity to the threat of loss.
49. Overly independent as well as overly dependent patients are at higher risk for hospitalization than are those who are psychological "normal".
50. Some studies have shown that patients who react to stress with feelings of hopelessness or depression are at higher risk for this disorder.
51. A behavior pattern that features competitiveness, ambition and impatience is considered to be predisposing.

52. Unresolved grief on the anniversary of the death of a loved one can be precipitating event.
53. The theory that specific psychological conflicts, such as repressed hostility, are casual has not been proved.

THEME: 7
PSYCHIATRIC DIAGNOSIS OF CONDITIONS WHICH MIMIC PHYSICAL DISEASE

Options

a. Conversion disorder
b. Histronic personality disorder.
c. Body dysmorphic disorder
d. Briquet's syndrome
e. Munchausen syndrome

For each of the situations/conditions given below choose the one most appropriate/discriminatory option from above. The options may be used once, more than once, or not at all.

Questions

54. A 40-year-old man insists that his leg is gangrenous and needs to be amputated. On examination, he has normal extremities.
55. A 30-year-old woman presents with a history of multiorgan ailments. She reports that she has always been poorly ever since she was a child. She sees her GP on a regular basis and each time for a different medical symptom. No medical abnormalities can be found. She has multiple surgical scars over her entire body.
56. A 50-year-old man facing redundancy is now paralysed in both legs and wheel chair-bound. The paralysis and sensory loss is inconsistent with anatomical distribution of nerves.
57. A 40-year-old woman after failing her driving test complains of chest pain. No medical cause can be found.
58. A 50-year-old man insists he has throat cancer.He has shopped around and can find no doctor who will concur with him. He visits his GP regularly.

THEME: 8
DIAGNOSIS OF ORGANIC MENTAL DISORDERS

Options

a. Subarachnoid hemorrhage.
b. Huntington's disease.
c. Acute intermittent porphyria.
d. Multi-infarct dementia.
e. Temporal lobe seizures.
f. Parkinson's disease.
g. Chronic subdural hematoma.
h. Korsakoff's psychosis.
i. Alzheimer's disease.
j. Wernicke's encephalopathy.

For each of the situations/conditions given below, choose the one most appropriate/discriminatory option from above. The options may be used once, more than once, or not at all.

Questions

59. A 70-year-old man presents with an abrupt onset of confusion and ataxia. On examination, he also has nystagmus. He is a known drinker.
60. A 65-year-old man presents with gradual deterioration of memory and intellect. His family have noticed a change in personality and behaviour.
61. A 65-year-old alcoholic man presents with persistent headache. His family noted that he is inattentive and becoming more confused. He had a fall a month ago.
62. A 40-year-old man presents with dementia and choreiform movements.
63. A 55-year-old alcoholic man presents with deterioration of both retrograde and anterograde memory. He invents stories.

THEME: 8
DIAGNOSIS OF DEFENCE MECHANISM

Options

a. Reaction formation.

b. Projection.
c. Sublimation.
d. Repression.
e. Displacement.

For each of the situations/conditions given below, choose the one most appropriate/discriminatory option from above. The options may be used once, more than once, or not at all.

Questions

64. Unconscious attribution of one's own unacceptable feelings to another person.
65. Unconscious control of unwanted impulses by behaving in ways opposite to the impulse.
66. Unconscious shift of feelings from the object stimulating the feelings to a more acceptable manner.
67. Satisfaction of an impulse in a related but more socially acceptable manner.

THEME: 9
DIAGNOSIS OF SEXUAL PERVERSIONS

Options

a. Transsexualism.
b. Transvestism.
c. Exhibitionism.
d. Erectile dysfunction.
e. Homosexuality.
f. Voyeurism.
g. Masochism.
h. Fetishism.
i. Pedophilia.

For each of the situations/conditions given below, choose the one most appropriate/discriminatory option from above. The options may be used once, more than once, or not at all.

Questions

68. It often occurs for the first time after overindulgence in alcohol.

69. Most men with this disorder have a history of dressing female clothing before the age of 4 years.
70. Psychologically immature young men with hostile feelings towards their "victims" need this behavior to achieve sexual gratification.
71. Anxiety about sexual performance is the most common psychological cause.
72. The spectrum of psychopathology resembles that of the general population.
73. Men with this disorder have excessively close physical and emotional ties to their mothers and have fathers who were absent during their childhood.
74. Non human object.
75. No physical contact.

THEME: 10
DIAGNOSIS OF PERSONALITY DISORDERS

Options

a. Hysterical personality
b. Schizoid personality
c. Obessional personality
d. Sociopathic personality
e. Affective disorder
f. Manic personality
g. Suicidal personality
h. Immoral personality
i. Asthenic personality

For each of the situations/conditions given below, choose the one most appropriate/discriminatory option from above. The options may be used once, more than once, or not at all.

Questions

76. A 35-year-old lady has a persistent abnormality of mood continually alternating between euphoria and depression.
77. A 36-year-old gentleman who is a perfectionist to a rigid degree.
78. A 45-year-old serial killer who shows no remorse for crimes he has committed.

79. A 24-year-old lady whom has had a number of failed relationships and has a tendency to dramatise limb pains.
80. A shy 27-year-old man who is shy of advances and tends to be aloof.

THEME: 11
DIAGNOSIS OF PERSONALITY DISORDER

Options

a. Paranoid personality disorder.
b. Borderline personality disorder.
c. Narcissistic personality disorder.
d. Antisocial personality disorder.
e. Schizoid personality disorder.
f. Histrionic personality disorder.
g. Passive aggressive personality disorder.
h. Dependent aggressive personality disorder.
i. Sadistic personality disorder.
j. Obsessive compulsive personality.
k. Schizotypal personality.
l. Avoidant personality.
m. Compulsive personality.

For each of the situations/conditions given below, choose the one most appropriate/discriminatory option from above. The options may be used once, more than once, or not at all.

Questions

81. Takes offense quickly and questions the loyalty of others.
82. Has a defective capacity to form social relationships.
83. Fails to plan ahead and is impulsive (e.g., may move without a job).
84. Forms relationships that lack empathy; idealizes or devalues others.
85. Exudes a sense of entitlement with the expectation of special favours but without assuming reciprocal responsibilities.
86. Illness is often perceived as a threat to physical attractiveness.

87. Pleasure, but not sexual arousal, is derived from the suffering of others.
88. Authority is resented, and the efforts of others are obstructed by poor performance.
89. Illness is often perceived as a threat to the control of impulses.
90. Tasks must be performed in certain ways, but delegation of responsibility is all but impossible because of a fear that others will not perform well.
91. A 31-year-old man is shy, socially withdrawn, low in self-esteem, yet eager to please when called on by persons in authority.
92. A 27-year-old man is superstitious, paranoid and believes that he possesses telepathic powers, has no friends.

THEME: 12
DIAGNOSIS OF PSYCHIATRIC DISORDERS

Options

a. Depression
b. Post-traumatic stress disorder
c. Schizophrenia
d. Chronic alcoholism
e. Phobia
f. Anxiety neurosis
g. Mania
h. Obessional neurosis
i. Depersonalisation
j. Hysteria
k. Paranoid state

For each of the situations/conditions given below, choose the one most appropriate/discriminatory option from above. The options may be used once, more than once, or not at all.

Questions

93. A 23-year-old student presents with insomnia, headaches, sweating, palpitations, chest pains and poor appetite.

94. A 35-year-old single woman presents with weight loss, poor appetite, decreased ability to concentrate and guilt feelings.
95. A 19-year-old female student presents with sudden blindness. Neurological examination reveals no abnormality.
96. A 20-year-old man presents with disinhibition, hyperactivity, increased appetite and grandiose delusions.
97. A 30-year-old man presents with auditory hallucinations, social withdrawal and delusions of persecution.
98. A 21-year-old man presents with compulsions and rituals, which he resists.

THEME: 13
DIAGNOSIS OF PSYCHIATRIC DISORDERS

Options

a. Munchausen's syndrome
b. Alcohol withdrawal delirium
c. Extrapyramidal side effect
d. Hypothyroidism
e. Hysterical neurosis
f. Acromegaly
g. Dissociative disorder
h. Malingering disorder
i. Parkinson's disease
j. Cushing's syndrome
k. Autonomic side effect
l. Anticholinergic side effect

For each of the situations/conditions given below, choose the one most appropriate/discriminatory option from above. The options may be used once, more than once, or not at all.

Questions

99. A 28-year-old female presents with lower abdominal pain. On examination she has multiple surgical scars over her abdomen. Her abdominal and pelvic examinations are normal. She insists she needs a laparoscopy.

100. A 50-year-old schizophrenic is started on Haloperidol. A month later he is noted to be drooling salvia and walking with a shuffling gait. He also suffers from involuntary chewing movements.
101. A 40-year-old female complains of a dry mouth, blurry vision and constipation. On examination she had dilated pupils. She was started on Amitriptyline for major depression.
102. A 45-year-old man complains of headaches, excessive thirst, and frequent urination. On examination he is noted to have bad acne, coarse skin and has a goitre. He has moved his wedding band to the 5th finger.
103. A 30-year-old man presents to casualty with a dislocated shoulder. On examination, the shoulder is found not to be dislocated. The patient insists it is dislocated.

THEME: 14
DIAGNOSIS OF PSYCHIATRIC CONDITIONS

Options

a. Bullimia
b. Obsessive compulsive disorder
c. Phobia
d. Acute confusional state
e. Schizophrenia
f. Depression with psychomotor retardation
g. Conversation disorder
h. Cyclothymic disorder
i. Hyperventilation syndrome
j. Anorexia Nervosa
k. Mania
l. Hypomania

For each of the situations/conditions given below, choose the one most appropriate/discriminatory option from above. The options may be used once, more than once, or not at all.

Questions

104. A mother is worried about her 25-year-old son. He seems to jump from one topic to another, make-up words, laugh at inappropriate things and talk to someone imaginary.

He has blacked out his windows and complains that someone else is controlling his thoughts.

105. A 40-year-old man presents to his GP with headaches, insomnia and weight gain. He is slow and sluggish when he speaks. He describes a loss of interest in everything, a feeling of worthlessness and often cries alone.

106. A 23-year-old woman presents with an episode of generalised paraethesia, "flapping" limbs, loss of urinary incontinence and abnormal posturing of the hands. These episodes are preceded by chest tightness and difficulty in swallowing. Recently she has been feeling that parts of her are made of cotton wool.

107. A wife cannot cope with her husband's moods. She says he is very labile. He goes from being full of energy and happy one day to being so pessimistic about everything the next day.

THEME: 15
CAUSES OF HALLUCINATIONS AND DELUSIONS

Options

a. Schizophrenia
b. Psychotic depression
c. Mania
d. Toxic confusional state
e. Delirium tremens
f. Korsakoff's psychosis
g. Paraphrenia
h. Drug-induced
i. Personality disorder
j. Hysteria

For each of the situations/conditions given below, choose the one most appropriate/discriminatory option from above. The options may be used once, more than once, or not at all.

Questions

108. A35-year-old man is agitated and euphoric. He claims to be helping the Prime Minister with economic policy, although he is not true when checked.

109. A 20-year-old man complains that all his movements are being watched. Sometimes he feels as though his actions are being controlled by his radio. At other times he is aware of voices describing what he is doing.
110. A 50-year-old man complains of being pursued by the police for a crime he denies committing. He has poor concentration and impaired short-term memory. He admits to drinking large amounts of alcohol.
111. A 65-year-old woman says that she dies 3 months ago and is very distressed that nobody buried has buried her. When she is outdoors she hears people say that she is evil and needs to be punished.
112. A 40-year-old teetotal woman is recovering from a hysterectomy 2 days ago. At night she becomes agitated and complains of seeing animals and her children walking around the wards.

THEME: 16
DIAGNOSIS OF NEUROTIC DISORDERS

Options

a. Depression
b. Bipolar affective disorder
c. Anxiety neurosis
d. Agoraphobia
e. Obsessive-compulsive disorder
f. Social Phobia
g. Panic attacks
h. Post-traumatic stress disorder
i. Specific phobia

For each of the situations/conditions given below, choose the one most appropriate/discriminatory option from above. The options may be used once, more than once, or not at all.

Questions

113. A 25-year-old woman finds it difficult to leave her home. She becomes very agitated in supermarkets and describes palpitations and difficulty in breathing when in crowds.

114. A 40-year-old man complains of low mood and fatigue. He has a poor appetite and has loss of libido. He wakes up at 2 a.m. and is unable to return to sleep. He feels guilty about the death of his mother two years ago.
115. A 30-year-old man is seen in dermatology outpatients with very sore hands. He has dry, cracked skin on all his fingers. He says he has to wash his hands at least 30 times a day and is unable to sleep until he has done so.
116. A 20-year-old woman attends A&E complaining of sudden breathlessness and anxiety. She describes palpitations and paraesthesia of her hands, feet and lips. ECG shows tachycardia and O_2 saturation is normal.
117. A 35-year-old train driver is on sick leave after an accident in which a child ran onto the tracks. He is unable to go near railways and takes excessively long routes to avoid them. He is troubled by flashbacks of the accident which frequently disturbs his sleep.

THEME: 17
DIAGNOSIS OF PSYCHIATRIC DISORDERS

Options

a. Schizophrenia.
b. Grand mal epilepsy.
c. Alcohol related psychotic disorder.
d. Alcohol related convulsions.
e. Depression.
f. Panic attacks.
g. Dissociative disorder.
h. Dementia.

For each of the situations/conditions given below, choose the one most appropriate/discriminatory option from above. The options may be used once, more than once, or not at all.

Questions

118. 45-year-old female who has been consuming alcohol continuously for the past 1 year and has been drinking alcohol all most all the time for the past 1 week, suddenly

started complaining that her neighbor wanted to kill her and that she could hear him threatening to kill her all the time, although she was in her house.

119. A 25-year-old male presents to A and E with history of sudden palpitations, tremors and difficulty in breathing he is afraid that he will die. He reports of having such an episode lasted for about 30 minutes. On investigations urine VMA is normal and CT scan brain is normal.
120. A 60-year-old female is brought with history of threatening to kill her husband and accusing him of trying to poison her since the last 15 days. It was noticed her since the last 8-10 months, she has had problems recognizing her neighbors, having difficulty naming all her children and would occasionally have problems finding her way around.
121. A 18-year-old male has been brought by his partner with history of collapsing to the floor slowly, followed by tonic clonic movements of the body which lasts for 10-15 minutes after which he recovers and is oriented to surroundings.
122. A 42-year-old female presents with history of hearing voices telling her to kill herself, she has been constantly feeling like killing herself, has lost her job 2 months ago and has become very sensitive to criticism and has been crying constantly and has started feeling that she has committed a lot of sin for which she is going through all these problems.
123. A 23-year-old woman is brought to the emergency department by the police after assaulting her younger sister. She accused the sister of being "a witch" and said that she was ordered by "the voices" to destroy her. She has no friends and has gradually become preoccupied with witchcraft over a period of several years.

THEME: 18
CAUSES OF DEPRESSION

Options

a. Premenstrual syndrome
b. Puerperal affective disorder

c. Major depression
d. Drug induced depression
e. Bereavment reaction
f. Hypothyroidism
g. Cushing's syndrome
h. Hyperthyroidism
i. Porphria
j. Manic depressive disorder.
k. Drug abuse.
l. Vitamin and mineral disorders

For each of the situations/conditions given below choose the one most appropriate/discriminatory option from above. The options may be used once, more than once, or not at all.

Questions

124. A 23-year-old female complains of irritability and constant depression. She has thought about suicide. She has trouble sleeping and has lost her appetite.
125. A 20-year-old female complains of episodes of irritability and depression. She also complains of monthly bloating and tension.
126. A 30-year-old female complains of depression, lethargy, constipation and weight gain. She also suffers from menorrhagia.
127. A 40-year-old woman presents with depression and weight gain. She complains of back pain and excessive thirst. Her menstrual period lasts for 3 days and sometimes she skips a cycle. On examination, she is obese with acne and peripheral oedema.
128. A 30-year-old female on oral contraceptive presents with colicky abdominal pain, vomiting, anxiety, and depression. She is noted to be hypertensive. On standing, the urine turns deep red.

THEME: 18
TREATMENT OF DEPRESSION

Options

a. SSRI
b. St Johns Wort

c. Lithium
d. MAOI
e. Carbamazepine
f. Lorazepam
g. Electroconvulsive therapy
h. Tricyclic depressants
i. Reserpine
j. Sodium Valproate

For each of the situations/conditions given below, choose the one most appropriate/discriminatory option from above. The options may be used once, more than once, or not at all.

Questions

129. A 30-year-old male slides into a severe depression over a number of months for no particular reason. His hobbies and interests are dropped, his social contact diminishes and his mood lower. He visits a psychiatrist for the first time because he is becoming increasingly distressed with disturbed sleep patterns and no appetite. He feels his future his hopeless.
130. A 40-year-old has repeated episodes of depressed mood in response to feeling rejected and a craving for sweets and chocolates. These reactive mood changes are accompanied by hypersomnia, lethargy and increased appetite particularly with a preference to carbohydrates.
131. A 55-year-old woman has mania associated with cyclic and frequent depressive features.
132. An 18-year-old previously healthy girl waiting for her college exam result. The result is arriving that day by post and she is suffering from acute anxiety due to the importance of the results for her future career. Her mother consults her GP.
133. A 30-year-old female patient with suspected manic depression suffers from severe mood swings.

THEME: 19

MANAGEMENT OF PSYCHIATRIC DISORDERS

Options

a. Disulfiram.

b. Haloperidol.
c. Long-term psychotherapy.
d. Prozac.
e. Lithium.
f. Methadone.
g. Donepezil.
h. Carbedopa.
i. Tetrabenazine.

For each of the situations/conditions given below, choose the one most appropriate/discriminatory option from above. The options may be used once, more than once, or not at all.

Questions

134. An 18-year-old man presents with sweating, muscle twitching, and abdominal cramps. On examination, he has dilated pupils.
135. A 75-year-old man presents with progressive forgetfulness and mood changes. He has a shuffling gait. The head CT scan shows cortical atrophy and enlarged ventricles.
136. A 45-year-old man presents with ataxia. His wife states that it runs in her husband's family. He is difficult to live with, very irritable, clumpsy, and suffers from jerky movements of the legs.
137. A 65-year-old man presents with disturbance of voluntary motor function. His face is expressionless. On examination, he has cogwheel rigidity and bradykinesia.
138. A 12-year-old boy presents with brief, repetitive motor tics and is brought in by his parents for shouting obscenities at school.

THEME: 20
MANGEMENT OF PSYCHIATRIC ILLNESS

Options

a. Inform the police
b. Inform social services
c. Refer to a dietician
d. Refer to a psychiatrist

e. Refer to genera medical team
f. Reassure
g. Imipramine
h. Counselling
i. Contact the GP

For each of the situations/conditions given below, choose the one most appropriate/discriminatory option from above. The options may be used once, more than once, or not at all.

Questions

139. A mother brings her child to you with chronic diarrhoea. You have strong grounds to suspect a fractious illness because the nursing staff have found a number of packets of laxatives in her bag.
140. A 25-year-old lady arrives at the local accident and emergency department after ingesting an unknown amount of an unknown drug.
141. You get a call to visit a patient's house. The patient had been missing for the last 4 days. The patient's neighbour tells you that 4 days back the patient's GP had come to visit him.
142. A 30-year-old man presents with dizziness and irritability. In the A&E the patient behaves aggressively and abuses the nursing staff. On examination you find him to be febrile. Mild neck rigidity is present.
143. A young lady who used to be an IV drug abuser has now completely stopped taking drugs. She comes to you saying that her boyfriend is now forcing her to take drugs again.
144. A 32-year-old lady is afraid to go out in the market. Whenever she goes out of the house she comes home running and gasping for breath. She immediately locks her doors and windows after reaching home. She is otherwise normal in the house.

THEME: 21
CHILDHOOD PSYCHIATRIC DISORDERS

Options

a. Childhood depression.

b. Childhood schizophrenia.
c. Conduct disorder.
d. Attention deficit hyperactive disorder.
e. Infantile autism.

For each of the situations/conditions given below, choose the one most appropriate/discriminatory option from above. The options may be used once, more than once, or not at all.

Questions

145. A 9-year-old boy has had persisting difficulties in language and interpersonal relationships since the age of 2 years, and although he can barely read he is able to perform arithmetic calculations at the fifth-grade level.
146. An 11-year-old girl has become uncharacteristically and markedly withdrawn in the past 8 months, staying in her room so that she can "talk to the ghosts in the attic".
147. An 11-year-old girl has become markedly withdrawn in the past 8 months and has complained of persisting abdominal pain and constipation, for which no organic cause has been found.
148. A 5-year-old is reported by his kindergarten teacher to be distractible, impulsive, in need of continual supervision, but not hyperactive.
149. A 3-year-old spends hours rocking in a chair or spinning the blades of a toy windmill; his parents say he never cries when he falls.

THEME: 22
MANAGEMENT OF CHILDHOOD PSYCHIATRIC DISORDERS

Options

a. Thioridazine.
b. Imipramine.
c. Methylphenidate.
d. Phenobarbital.
e. No medication.

For each of the situations/conditions given below, choose the one most appropriate/discriminatory option from above. The options may be used once, more than once, or not at all.

Questions

150. Childhood schizophrenia.
151. Hyperactivity.
152. Enuresis.
153. Autistic disorder.
154. Idiopathic grand mal epilepsy.

THEME: 23
DRUG MANAGEMENT OF PSYCHIATRIC DISEASE

Options

a. Amitriptyline.
b. Carbamazepine.
c. Chlordiazepoxide.
d. Chlorpromazine.
e. Lorazepam.
f. Risperidone.
g. Fluoxetine.
h. Haloperidol.
i. Clozapine.
j. Drug treatment not appropriate.
k. Amphetamines.

For each of the situations/conditions given below, choose the one most appropriate/discriminatory option from above. The options may be used once, more than once, or not at all.

Questions

155. A 65-year-old woman has a three-year history of increasing confusion, loss of mobility and tremor. She has recently developed frequent visual hallucinations and tends to cry out for no reason, particularly at night. There is no evidence of an acute medical cause for her confusion. On examination she is alert but disorientated and quite agitated. She has a coarse resting tremor, increased tone in her limbs and normal reflexes.

156. An 85-year-old man gives a three-month history of increasing insomnia, fatigue and difficulty concentrating. He has lost interest in daily activities and feels a burden on his family.
157. A 20-year-old single woman gave birth to her first child two days ago. Since her birth she has been unable to sleep and is reluctant to hold her baby to feed her. She is very tearful and cries for no reason. She denies any thoughts of harm to herself or her baby. She had been looking forward to having a baby, even though she had no regular partner and was not sure of the father. She lives with her parents.
158. The police bring a 50-year-old man to casualty after threatening staff at a nearby store. He has prominent third-person auditory hallucinations and states that the queen of England, via a radio transmitter implanted in his teeth controls his actions.
159. A 40-year-old man has been brought to casualty after being found in the street acting in bizarre fashion. He was exposing his genitals to passers-by and shouting 'I am the salvation of the world'. In casualty he is very angry and agitated and wants to return to the streets to complete his missionary work. He refuses to have any tests in hospital and says 'the devil will punish you for interfering in his work'.
160. A 28-year-old woman is brought to casualty in an agitated and distractable state. She is in an expansive euphoric mood and will not stop talking. Her friends report that her agitated and excitable behaviour has recently resulted in dismissal from her job.
161. A 65-year-old man presents in an agitated state with confusion and visual hallucinations that terrify him. He has pyrexia, tremor and tachycardia and is sweating profusely. He has previously been admitted repeatedly with symptoms associated with chronic alcoholism .

THEME: 24
MANAGEMENT OF PSYCHIATRIC STATE

Options

a. Lithium
b. Electroconvulsive therapy
c. Cognitive therapy
d. Group therapy
e. Anti-psychotic therapy
f. Anti-depressive medication
g. Emergency care order
h. Benzodiazepine medication
i. Hypnotherapy
j. Behavioural therapy
k. Bereavement counselling
l. Chlorpromazine treatment

For each of the situations/conditions given below, choose the one most appropriate/discriminatory option from above. The options may be used once, more than once, or not at all.

Questions

162. A 54-year-old woman says she sees her deceased husband in and around the house.
163. A 19-year-old university student undertakes hand washing upto 30 times in one day; this is getting in the way of her work.
164. A 50-year-old vagrant thought to be alcoholic is admitted to the ward where he is being unruly and thinks the nurses are going to kill him.
165. A 24-year-old man says that aliens are talking to him and controlling his thoughts.
166. A 40-year-old woman is scared of flying.

Twenty

Ear, Nose and Throat

THEME: 1
INVESTIGATION FOR DEAFNESS

Options

a. Rinne's test
b. Weber's
c. Absolute bone condition.
d. Pure tone audiometry.
e. Speech audiometry.
f. Impedence audiometry.
g. Evoked response audiometry.

For each of the situations/conditions given below,, choose the one most appropriate/discriminatory option from above. The options may be used once, more than once, or not at all.

Questions

1. It is a relative test for sensory neural deafness.
2. Sound is heard in the better ear if there is sensory neural deafness.
3. Diagnostic for otosclerosis.
4. This test checks if the cause of the sensory neural deafness is in cochlea or auditory nerve.
5. This test checks both air conduction and bone conduction.
6. This test predicts if hearing aid will benefit the patient or not.

THEME: 2
DIAGNOSIS OF EARACHE

Options

a. Referred pain

b. Temporo-mandibular joint dysfunction.
c. Bullous myringitis
d. Aerotitis
e. Mastoiditis.
f. Trauma

For each of the situations/conditions given below, choose the one most appropriate/discriminatory option from above. The options may be used once, more than once, or not at all.

Questions

7. A 40-year-old male comes with history of episodes of earache for the last two years. He complains that the pain is in front of tragus and radiates to mandible.
8. A 40-year-old patient with acute rhinitis comes with history of sudden onset earache since morning and complains of sensation of pressure. On examination Rinne's test is negative.
9. A 40-year-old patient comes with 3 day history of earache. On examination there are painful hemorrhagic blisters on ear drum.
10. A 40-year-old patient comes with three day history of earache and low-grade fever. Also complains of noticing foul discharge since this morning.

THEME: 3
OTALGIA

Options

a. Acute otitic barotrauma
b. Acute Otitis externa
c. Acute Otitis media
d. Bell's palsy
e. Cervical spondylosis
f. Furunculosis
g. Malignant Otitis externa
h. Myringitis bullosa
i. Ramsay-Hunt syndrome
j. Squamous cell carcinoma of the ear canal
k. Squamous cell carcinoma of the tongue
l. Temporomandibular joint dysfunction

For each of the situations/conditions given below, choose the one most appropriate/discriminatory option from above. The options may be used once, more than once, or not at all.

Questions

11. A 70-year-old man presents with hearing loss, bloodstained discharge from the ear and facial paralysis.
12. A 6-year-old child complains of severe earache following an upper respiratory tract infection. She is unwell with fever and tachycardia. Examination shows a congested and bulging eardrum.
13. A 60-year-old man complains of sudden onset of right-sided earache with associated right-sided facial weakness. Examination reveals vesicles in the ipsilateral external auditory meatus and pharynx.
14. A 58-year-old woman has generalised discomfort and tenderness around and behind the ear. Movement of the neck is restricted and causes her to experience a similar pain.
15. A 68-year-old male lifelong cigarette smoker complains of worsening right-sided earache, a sore tongue and difficulty talking.

THEME: 4
CASUES OF SWOLLEN/PAINFUL EAR

Options

a. Subperichondrial haematoma
b. Perichondritis
c. Subperichondrial abscess
d. Acute mastoiditis
e. Keloid
f. Infected preauricular sinus
g. Malignant otitis externa
h. Acute otitis externa
i. Ramsay-Hunt syndrome

For each of the situations/conditions given below, choose the one most appropriate/discriminatory option from above. The options may be used once, more than once, or not at all.

Questions

16. A 30-year-old Rugby player presents with a swollen and painful upper pinna after being struck in the side of his head. On palpation, the swelling is boggy and tense.
17. A 70-year-old man is noted to have a collapsed pinna. He states that he has had this for 15 years.
18. A 25-year-old woman presents with intermittent discharge and a swelling in the front of her right ear.
19. A 60-year-old woman presents with unilateral left-sided hearing loss and a painful left ear. On examination, she has skin eruption vesicles in front of her right ear.
20. A 12-year-old boy presents with a painful right ear. He is febrile. On examination, the pinna is pushed forwards and downwards. He is tender on palpation of the concha.

THEME: 5
DIAGNOSIS OF HEARING LOSS AND PAINFUL EARS

Options

a. Acute suppurative otitis media
b. Glue ear
c. Otitis externa
d. Temporo- mandibular joint disease
e. Cholesteatoma
f. Ramsay- Hunt syndrome
g. Wax
h. Chronic otitis externa
i. Ear drum perforation
j. Aerotitis
k. Furunculosis
l. Otosclerosis

Questions

21. A 70-year-old man being treated for cancer of the prostate presents with difficulty in hearing. Examination of his right ear reveals numerous vesicles around the ear and on the meatus.

22. A 40-year-old complains of painful ears and also reports a history of bruxism (teeth grinding) sometimes associated with headaches. His symptoms seem to be worsened by stress and anxiety
23. A 16-year-old girl presents with hearing loss. She admits to a months history of vague right earache associated with a purulent discharge. She now reports no pain.
24. A 40-year-old obese man presents with a painful right ear. Examination reveals a swollen lesion in the external auditory meatus. The pain is so severe and is worsened by jaw movement and traction on the tragus. The man reports no other problem, but is on glibenclamide.
25. A 10-year-old boy diagnosed with acute otitis media 3 weeks ago now presents with hearing loss. There is no ear pain. On ototscopy, the eardrum is concave, lustureless and has superficial radial vessels. Air puffed through the ototscope doesn't move the ear drum

THEME: 6
CAUSES OF HEARING IMPAIRMENT

Options

a. Presbyacusis
b. Otosclerosis
c. Ototoxic drugs
d. Post meningitis
e. Meniere's disease
f. Acoustic Neuroma
g. Excess wad
h. Trauma to the eardrum
i. Otitis media
j. Maternal infection
k. Mumps
l. Glue ear

For each of the situations/conditions given below, choose the one most appropriate/discriminatory option from above. The options may be used once, more than once, or not at all.

Questions

26. A 55-year-old complains of progressive hearing loss. She also suffers attacks of vertigo and tinitus lasting several hours at a time.
27. A 35-year-old woman complains of progressive deafness in both ears. There is a family history of deafness in middle age.
28. A 4-year-old child develops severe hearing loss after a febrile illness with sore throat and painful swollen neck glands. Hearing was normal at 9 months.
29. A 70-year-old man complains of difficulty hearing people talking unless he is face-to-face with them. Examination is otherwise normal.
30. A 6-year-old boy is noticed to have poor attention to detail in school. He was fine until an ear infection 6 months ago. On examination, he has hearing loss in the right ear with a dull, concave eardrum on that side.
31. A 40-year-old woman complains of a 4 month history of hearing loss and tinitus in the left ear. There is also mild left facial weakness that involves the muscles of the forehead.

THEME: 7
DIAGNOSIS OF HEARING PROBLEMS

Options

a. Presbyacusis
b. Cerumen
c. Acute suppurative otitis media
d. Otitis externa
e. Chronic secretory otitis media
f. Barotrauma
g. Chronic suppurative otitis media
h. Dead ear
i. Otosclerosis
j. Temporal bone fracture
k. Ostoegenesis imperfecta

For each of the situations/conditions given below, choose the one most appropriate/discriminatory option from above. The options may be used once, more than once, or not at all.

Questions

32. A 70-year-old man presents with gradual deterioration of hearing in both ears. His Weber tubing fork test is non-lateralising and his Rinne test is positive on both sides. His tympanic membranes are intact.
33. A 60-year-old man presents with unilateral earache, diminished hearing and foul-smelling discharge. The external auditory meatus is edematous, and the canal is stenosed. The discharge is white and creamy in nature.
34. A 40-year-old woman presents with diminished hearing in the right ear. She denies earache or discharge. She is noted to have blue sclarae. The tympanic membrane is normal. The Weber test lateralizes to the right side and the Rinne test is negative on the right side.
35. A 4-year-old girl presents to the GP with diminished hearing noted by the school. On examination she has a bulging yellow tympanic membrane on the right alone.
36. A 70-year-old female presents with longstanding deafness in the left ear. The Weber lateralizes to the right, and the Rinne is negative on the left.

THEME: 8
MANAGEMENT OF HEARING LOSS

Options

a. ENT referral for mastoidectomy
b. ENT referral for stapedectomy
c. ENT referral for grommet insertion
d. Bone anchored hearing aid
e. Aural toilet
f. Betahistidine
g. Insertion of pope wick and sofradex ear drops
h. Amoxycillan suspension
i. ENT referral for tympanoplasty

j. Syringing of the ears
k. In-the-ear hearing aids

For each of the situations/conditions given below, choose the one most appropriate/discriminatory option from above. The options may be used once, more than once, or not at all.

Questions

37. A 4-year-old boy presents with a 4 month history of persistent conductive hearing loss in both ears. On examination, he has a bulging, amber yellow tympanic membrane. He denies pain.
38. A 40-year-old woman presents with persistent, unilateral conductive hearing loss following recurrent ear infections. The hearing loss is confirmed to be severe and on examination the tympanic membrane has a central perforation.
39. A 30-year-old pregnant woman presents with left-sided conductive hearing loss. She states that she can hear well in a noisy surrounding. On examination, the tympanic membrane is normal.
40. A 70-year-old woman presents with unilateral conductive hearing loss. On examination, there is Cerumen in the external auditory meatus.
41. A 5-year-old girl presents with fever, a painful right ear and deafness. On examination, the tympanic membrane is full and red.

THEME: 9
MANAGEMENT OF ENT EMERGENCIES

Options

a. Give Nifedepine 10 mg
b. Obtain a barium swallow
c. Obtain a sialogram
d. Advise patient to drink more and avoid citrus fruits.
e. List for bronchoscopy
f. list for rigid esophagoscopy
g. IM Buscopan

h. Insert 2 large bore IV cannula and run gelofusin
i. Ligate sphenopalantine artery in theatre
j. Consult haematologist
k. Check INR

For each of the situations/conditions given below, choose the one most appropriate/discriminatory option from above. The options may be used once, more than once, or not at all.

Questions

42. A 70-year-old woman presents with severe epistaxis. Her BP is noted to be 205/115. She has no prior history of hypertension. She denies aspirin or Warfarin use. Bloods are taken and IV line is inserted. She continues to bleed profusely through her nose packs.
43. A 60-year-old man on Warfarin 6 m OD for a previous DVT now presents with right-sided epistaxis. His BP is 120/70 with a pulse rate of 90. He has no visible vessels in the Little's area. He continues to bleed through the nose pack.
44. A 60-year-old woman presents with a piece of chicken stuck in her throat. Soft tissue neck X-ray reveals a calcified bolus at the level of cricopharyngeus.
45. A 70-year-old woman complains of mashed potato stuck in her throat since dinner. She is not distressed. She is able to sip water.
46. A 30-year-old man complains of intermittent unilateral cheek swelling while eating. On examination no swelling is palpated and the oral cavity is clear.

THEME: 10
DIAGNOSIS OF EAR DISCHARGE

Options

a. Furunculosis.
b. Mastoiditis.
c. Otitis media.
d. Chronic supurative otitis media.
e. Otitis externa
f. Cholesteatoma

For each of the situations/conditions given below, choose the one most appropriate/discriminatory option from above. The options may be used once, more than once, or not at all.

Questions

47. A 40-year-old male patients with foul smelling ear discharge for last one month. He also complains of vertigo and earache. On examination is also noticed to have same sided VIIth nerve palsy.
48. A 40-year-old male patients present with painless hearing loss and ear discharge for last one month.
49. A 30-year-old male swimmer complains of severe earache and thick discharge.
50. A 30-year-old male presents with a history of earache for last 15 days, since last night he has also noticed ear discharge which is profuse and purulent.
51. A 40-year-old diabetic presents with sudden onset earache for last 2 days but only mild discharge. He also complains of severe pain worse on jaw movement.

THEME: 11
DIAGNOSIS OF FLUID IN THE MIDDLE EAR

Options

a. Acute suppurative otitis media.
b. Serous otitis media.
c. Bullous myringitis.

For each of the situations/conditions given below, choose the one most appropriate/discriminatory option from above. The options may be used once, more than once, or not at all.

Questions

52. Most common cause of hearing loss in children.
53. A 4-year-old child comes with history of rhinitis for last 5 days and since last night complains of ear ache, sensation of pressure in ear and deafness but no discharge.
54. A 4-year-old child presents with painless deafness for last two days. On examination, pneumatic otoscopy is negative.

THEME: 12
DIAGNOSIS OF VERTIGO

Options

a. Labyrinthine disorder
b. Migraine
c. Paroxysmal benign positional vertigo
d. Idiopathic vestibular faliure
e. Ototoxic vestibular faliure
f. Poor vestibular compensation
g. Uncompensated periphral vestibulopathy
h. Vestibular neuronitis

For each of the situations/conditions given below, choose the one most appropriate/discriminatory option from above. The options may be used once, more than once, or not at all.

Questions

55. A 40-year-old female complains of episodic vertigo associated with headache. Her mother also had the same problem.
56. A 40-year-old patient had came to OPD one week ago, when he was treated for UTI as inpatient for five days. Now he has come back with history of vertigo and tendency to fall in dark.
57. A 30-year-old patient presents with recurrent episodes of vertigo lasting days to weeks with gradual resolution.
58. A 40-year-old patient presents with severe vertigo for last one week. On admission his symptoms remarkably improved over four days.
59. An 40-year-old patient presents with clusters of short episodes of vertigo which are not related to head movements.

THEME: 13
CAUSES OF VERTIGO

Options

a. Meniere's disease
b. Benign positional vertigo

c. Acute vestibular neuronitis
d. Acoustic neuroma
e. Multiple sclerosis
f. Iatrogenic
g. Cardiovascular disease
h. Musculoskeletal disease
i. Hyperventilation
j. Migraine

For each of the situations/conditions given below, choose the one most appropriate/discriminatory option from above. The options may be used once, more than once, or not at all.

Questions

60. A 42-year-old woman presents with repeated episodes of fluctuating hearing loss, vertigo and tinnitus lasting hours over the past few months.
61. A 50-year-old man presents with asymmetrical sensory neural hearing loss, dizziness, unilateral tinnitus and facial pain. He is taking Atenolol.
62. A 70-year-old woman presents with vertigo when rolling over in bed. She also notices that she gets dizzy when bending over or reaching for the top of the shelf.
63. A 55-year-old man complains of dizziness ever since he was a passenger in a car involved in an RTA. His hearing is intact.
64. A 20-year-old anxious woman presents with profound vertigo following an upper respiratory tract infection lasting days.

THEME: 14
CAUSES OF VERTIGO

Options

a. Migraine
b. Vestibular neuronitis
c. Multiple sclerosis
d. Lateral medullary syndrome
e. Wernicke's encephalopathy

f. Vertebrobasiliar ischaemia
g. Epilepsy
h. Hypoglycaemia
i. Arrhythmias
j. Meniere's disease
k. Acoustic Neuroma
l. Postural hypotension

For each of the situations/conditions given below, choose the one most appropriate/discriminatory option from above. The options may be used once, more than once, or not at all.

Questions

65. A 40-year-old man presents with vertigo, nausea and weakness. He also complains of tingling sensation down his right arm and double vision in one eye. On examination he has loss of central vision, nystagmus and ataxia.
66. A 50-year-old man presents with severe vertigo, vomiting and left-sided facial pain. On examination he has nystagmus on looking to the left. His soft palate is paralysed on the left side and he has analgesia to pinprick on the left side of his face and right limbs. He also has a left-sided Horner's syndrome.
67. A 50-year-old woman presents with vertigo and unilateral deafness. The attacks of vertigo last for hours and are accompanied by vomiting. On examination she has nystagmus and a low frequency sensory neural hearing loss.
68. A 20-year-old man presents with sudden onset of vertigo and vomiting. He denies tinnitus or hearing loss. He had an upper respiratory tract infection a week prior.
69. A 60-year-old man presents with vertigo brought on by turning his head, ataxia, dysarthria and nystagmus.

THEME: 15
DIAGNOSIS OF NASAL OBSTRUCTIONS

Options

a. Rhinitis medicamentosa

b. Vasomotor rhinitis
c. Deviated nasal septum
d. Allergic rhinitis
e. Nasal obstruction with chronic sinusitis
f. Nasal polyps

For each of the situations/conditions given below, choose the one most appropriate/discriminatory option from above. The options may be used once, more than once, or not at all.

Questions

70. A 30-year-old boxer present with bilateral nasal obstruction for last six months.
71. A 30-year-old male a known patient with allergic rhinitis complains of nasal obstruction. He has been an nasal drops for last five years.
72. A 50-year-old male complains of unilateral nasal obstruction. Record reveal that he has been otherwise well other than some treatments he seeked 20 years ago for his infertility.
73. A 10-year-old boy complains of rhinorrhea and nasal obstruction during every year.

THEME: 16
CAUSES OF HOARSENESS

Options

a. Laryngitis
b. Vocal cord trauma
c. Angioedema
d. Carcinoma larynx
e. Laryngeal nerve palsy
f. Hypothyroidism
g. Acromegaly
h. Vocal cord nodules
i. Wegener's syndrome
j. Sjogren's syndrome
k. Hysterical
l. Foreign body

For each of the situations/conditions given below, choose the one most appropriate/discriminatory option from above. The options may be used once, more than once, or not at all.

Questions

74. A 32-year-old opera singer has developed hoarseness 2 days before a world premiere for which she has been rehearsing extensively. She does not have a sore throat.
75. A 25-year-old man suddenly developed hoarseness, wheeze and stridor whilst eating peanuts in a bar. He has a swollen tongue.
76. A 55-year-old woman develops hoarseness 2 days after a partial thyroidectomy for thyrotoxicosis.
77. A 58-year-old male smoker has a 2-months history of progressive persistent hoarseness and pain in his left ear on swallowing. He has enlarged left cervical lymph nodes.
78. A 40-year-old woman develops a progressively hoarse voice over 6 months. She has also gained 8 kg in weight and complains of constipation. She had a partial thyroidectomy 2 years previously for thyrotoxicosis.
79. A 21-year-old has 3- days history of hoarseness. He has throat pain, which is worse on talking and eating. Throat looks normal on examination.

THEME: 17
CAUSES OF NASAL BLOCKAGE

Options

a. Deviated nasal septum
b. Allergic rhinitis
c. Vasomotor rhinitis
d. Nasal polyps
e. Viral infection
f. Tuberculosis
g. Adenoidal enlargement
h. Foreign body
i. Wegener's granulomatosis
j. Iatrogenic

For each of the situations/conditions given below, choose the one most appropriate/discriminatory option from above. The options may be used once, more than once, or not at all.

Questions

80. A 38-year-old man complains of persistent nasal blockage and runny nose for 2 years. On examination, he has swollen inferior turbinates. Allergy testing is negative.
81. A 6-year-old child suffers recurrent upper respiratory tract infections. She has nasal stuffiness and often has a runny nose. Voice quality is nasal.
82. A 40-year-old man presents with nasal stuffiness and haemoptysis. Examination is normal but tests reveal haematuria and renal impairment.
83. A 15-year-old girl with cystic fibrosis complains of recurrent episodes of nasal obstruction on one or both sides.
84. A 25-year-old woman has a blocked nose along with other symptoms of a viral illness. She used over the counter nasal sprays and although the other symptoms quickly resolved, the nose seems to have become increasingly blocked over the last 6 weeks.

THEME: 18
DIAGNOSIS OF ENT DISEASES

Options

a. Malignant otitis externa
b. Rhinocerebral mucormycosis
c. Lymphoma
d. Quinsy
e. Nasal polyposis
f. Rhinosinusitis
g. Otitis externa
h. Acute otitis media
i. Otitis media with effusion
j. Glandular fever

For each of the situations/conditions given below, choose the one most appropriate/discriminatory option from above. The options may be used once, more than once, or not at all.

Questions

85. A 50-year-old poorly controlled diabetic woman presents with periorbital and perinasal swelling with bloody nasal discharge. On examination, the nasal mucosa is black and necrotic.
86. A 25-year-old man presents with worsening sore throat. On examination he has trismus and unilateral enlargement of his right tonsil.
87. A 60-year-old woman is noted to have unilateral tonsillar enlargement. She denies sore throat.
88. A 30-year-old woman complains of otalgia and purulent discharge from the right ear. On examination, the auditory meatus is swollen and the canal is inflamed and filled with creamy white discharge.
89. A 60-year-old diabetic woman complains of severe otalgia. On examination, she has granulation tissue in her ear canal.

THEME: 19
DIAGNOSIS OF STRIDOR

Options

a. Laryngo tracheobronchitis
b. Acute epiglotitis
c. Laryngomalacia
d. Laryngeal paralysis
e. Acute airway obstruction
f. Retropharyngeal abscess
g. Quinsy

For each of the situations/conditions given below, choose the one most appropriate/discriminatory option from above. The options may be used once, more than once, or not at all.

Questions

90. Stridor most noticeable during sleep or during excitement.
91. A 2-year old boy presents with fever, stridor and barking cough.
92. A 2-month-old infant born by forceps delivery comes with stridor.
93. A 2-year-old boy with stridor , high fever and drooling saliva.

THEME: 20
DIAGNOSIS OF STRIDOR

Options

a. Laryngomalacia
b. Intubation granulomas
c. Bilateral recurrent laryngeal nerve palsies
d. Neck space abscess
e. Laryngeal papillomatosis
f. Acute laryngo-tracheo-bronchitis
g. Subglottic stenosis
h. Angioneurotic edema
i. Acute epiglottis
j. Acute laryngitis
k. Multinodular goitre

For each of the situations/conditions given below, choose the one most appropriate/discriminatory option from above. The options may be used once, more than once, or not at all.

Questions

94. A 4-year-old girl presents to casualty with a sudden onset of pyrexia, stridor and sits with her mouth open and chin forward. She is drooling saliva and is in discomfort.
95. A 2-year-old girl presents to casualty with a week's duration of noisy cough and stridorous breathing. She is lying on her mother's lap.
96. A 40-year-old man presents with fever, stridor, dysphagia and a neck swelling. He admits to a dental procedure the week before.

97. A 16-year-old girl presents to the casualty with a rapid onset of stridorous breathing and a petecchial rash. She is apyrexial. She is noted to have a swollen uvula and tongue.
98. A 6-month-old baby boy presents to the GP with stridorous breathing. The mother reports that this began a few weeks after birth. His breathing improves when he is lying down on his stomach. He is apyrexial. He has always had laboured breathing, worse when feeding.

THEME: 21
DIAGNOSIS OF THROAT PROBLEMS

Options

a. Tonsillitis
b. Scarlet fever
c. Retropharyngeal abscess
d. Quinsy
e. Tonsillar tumor

For each of the situations/conditions given below, choose the one most appropriate/discriminatory option from above. The options may be used once, more than once, or not at all.

Questions

99. A 70-year-old male presents with some throat , dysphagia and otalgia
100. A 7-year-old boy with fever and looking unwell also complains of failure to eat or drink.
101. A 18-month-boy with abdominal pain and cough.
102. A 40-year-old male with difficulty in swallowing and cough, also complains of lock jaw.

THEME: 22
ENT TUMORS

Options

a. Carcinoma of larynx/hypopharynx

b. Nasopharynageal carcinoma
c. Sinus tumor
d. Pharyngeal carcinoma
e. Acoustic neuroma

For each of the situations/conditions given below, choose the one most appropriate/discriminatory option from above. The options may be used once, more than once, or not at all.

Questions

103. A 55-year-old smoker presents with blood stained nasal discharge, nasal obstruction and ptosis .
104. A 55-year-old smoker presents with persistent and progressive hoarseness, stridor and odynophagia.
105. A 55-year-old smoker from China presents with nasal obstruction and neck lumps, also complains of episodic earache.
106. A 55-year-old smoker from China presents with some throat pain for three months and a sensation of a lump in the throat. He also complains of episodic earache.
107. A 55-year-old smoker from China presents with nasal obstruction and neck lumps. Also complains of deafness.

Twenty one

Ophthalmology

THEME: 1
DIAGNOSIS OF SUDDEN LOSS OF VISION

Options

a. Amaurosis fugax.
b. Papilloedema.
c. Ischemic optic neuropathy.
d. Central retinal artery occlusion.
e. Central retinal vein occlusion.
f. CMV infection.
g. Vitreous hemorrhage.
h. Optic neuritis.
i. Retrobulbar neuritis.
j. Cerebral haemorrhage
k. Temporal arteritis

For each of the situations/conditions given below, choose the one most appropriate/discriminatory option from above. The options may be used once, more than once, or not at all.

Questions

1. A 40-year-old male with heart disease and diabetes presents with dramatic visual loss within seconds. On examination, retina appears white with a cherry red spot at macula.
2. A 40-year-old diabetic presents with acute loss of vision. On examination retina is not seen.
3. Temporary loss of vision, like a curtain descending in front of eyes.
4. Blind patient presents with pain in the blind eye. He gives a history acute onset blindness, which happened about three months ago.

5. 40-year-old male presents with blindness in right eye which has developed over four hours, also complains of pain on moving the eye. On examination fundus is normal.
6. A 65-year-old female has had a painful scalp and headache for three weeks and is generally unwell and complains of acute onset of blindness in her right eye.
7. A 75-year-old male noticed sudden worsening of visual acuity. On examination he is found to have homonymous hemianopia.

THEME: 2
RISK FACTORS OF OPHTHALMIC PATHOLOGY

Options

a. Myopia
b. Hypermetropia
c. Astigmatism
d. Hereditary in 30%
e. Hypocalcemia
f. Polycythaemia rubra vera
g. Immunosuppresion
h. Candidiasis
i. Myoxedema
j. Sjogren's syndrome

For each of the situations/conditions given below, choose the one most appropriate/discriminatory option from above. The options may be used once, more than once, or not at all.

Questions

8. A 38-year-old man suddenly notices markedly reduced vision in his right eye. He cannot read the visual chart and can only count fingers.The fundus looks red and intensely hypaeremic.
9. A 57-year-old man complains of sudden loss of vision in his right eye. She describes the incident like "a curtain coming down".

10. A 59-year-old man says he is always running into objects. His vision is blurred and complains of dazzling in bright light.
11. A 39-year-old woman complains of a gritty feeling in her eyes. A Schirmer's test is performed and is found to be positive.

THEME: 3
DIAGNOSIS OF VISUAL LOSS

Options

a. Acute glaucoma
b. Central retinal vein occlusion
c. Central retinal artery occlusion
d. Cranial arteritis
e. Uveitis
f. Occipital lobal infarct
g. Direct trauma
h. Retrobulbar neuritis
i. Retinal detachment

For each of the situations/conditions given below, choose the one most appropriate/discriminatory option from above. The options may be used once, more than once, or not at all.

Questions

12. A 35-year-old man presents with pain in the right eye, vomiting and loss of vision.
13. A 55-year-old known diabetic and hypertensive wakes up in the morning with diminished vision.
14. A 25-year-old man presents to the A&E Department with pain in the right eye associated with backache.
15. An elderly woman presents with a history of visual loss and scalp soreness.
16. An elderly man who is an in-patient (for hypertension) wakes in the morning notes that he can't see his breakfast. He has no other complaint. He has a carotid bruit.

THEME: 4
DIAGNOSIS OF EYE PROBLEM

Options

a. Xanthelesma
b. Optic atrophy
c. Corneal arcus
d. Background retinopathy
e. Hypertensive fundus
f. Proliferative retinopathy
g. Amaurosis fugax
h. Lens opacities
i. Senile cataracts
j. Periorbital abscess
k. Kayser-Fleischer rings

For each of the situations/conditions given below, choose the one most appropriate/discriminatory option from above. The options may be used once, more than once, or not at all.

Questions

17. A 10-year-old boy, following an episode of sinusitis, complains of persistent pain behind the right eye with eyelid swelling and diminished vision.
18. A 35-year-old man is noted to have rubeosis iridis, cotton wool spots and cluster headaches.
19. A 60-year-old man complains of an episode of an episode of visual loss in one eye like a curtain falling down. Of note is the presence of carotid bruits on auscultation.
20. A 65-year-old insulin-dependent diabetic is noted to have a white ring in his cornea surrounding his iris.

THEME: 5
CAUSES OF VISUAL DISTURBANCE

Options

a. Pituitary tumour
b. Chronic glaucoma

c. Temporal lobe tumour
d. Macular degeneration
e. Multiple sclerosis
f. Horner's syndrome
g. Neurosyphilis
h. Oculomotor nerve lesion
i. Abducens nerve lesion
j. Optic atrophy
k. Optic neuritis

For each of the situations/conditions given below, choose the one most appropriate/discriminatory option from above. The options may be used once, more than once, or not at all.

Questions

21. A 60-year-old man complains of very gradual onset of tunnel vision with no other symptoms. Her optic disc shows cupping
22. A 35-year-old man is noted to have small, irregular pupil that is fixed to light but constricts on convergence. His fasting glucose is 5mmol/L
23. A 35-year-old man has gradual onset of tunnel vision, dull constant headache and fatigue. On examination, she has a bitemporal hemianopia.
24. A 45-year-old diabetic man presents with a unilateral complete ptosis. The eye is noted to be facing down and out. The pupil is spared.
25. A 65-year-old woman has gradual loss of vision such that she cannot read, even with glasses. Apart from loss of acuity, eye examination is normal.
26. A 30-year-old man who has sustained head injury in an RTA presents with diplopia on lateral gaze. On examination, he has a convergent squint with diplopia when looking to the left side.
27. A 30-year-old woman presents with unilateral papillary constriction with slight ptosis and enophthalmos. He is noted to have a cervical rib on X-ray.

THEME: 6
DIAGNOSIS OF GRADUAL LOSS OF VISION

Options

a. Retinal detachment.
b. Choroiditis.
c. Malignant melanoma of choroid.
d. Senile macular degeneration.
e. Tobacco amblyopia.
f. Optic atrophy.
g. Optic neuritis.
h. Open angle glaucoma.
i. Retinitis pigmentosa.
j. Retinoblastoma.
k. Amaurosis fugax.

For each of the situations/conditions given below, choose the one most appropriate/discriminatory option from above. The options may be used once, more than once, or not at all.

Questions

28. It is the most common cause of registrable blindness in UK.
29. 40-year-old male presents with generalized weakness, loss of appetite and gradual fundus appears mottled black.
30. 40-year-old presents with gradual blurring of vision. On examination, vitreous opacities are seen and there is grey white raised patch on retina.
31. 40-year-old male presents with painless loss of vision, says he felt as if a curtain was falling down in front of his eyes. On fundoscopy, a grey opalescent retina is seen which is ballooning forward.

THEME: 7
DIFFERENTIAL DIAGNOSIS OF RED EYE

Options

a. Closed angle glaucoma.
b. Acute iritis.

c. Conjunctivitis.
d. Subconjuntival hemorrhage.
e. Episcleritis.
f. Scleritis.
g. Ulcerative keratitis.
h. Dacrocystitis
i. Dacroadenitis
j. Endopthalmitis
k. Foreign body
l. Trachoma
m. Trauma
n. Uveitis
o. Herpes Zoster ulcer
p. Dendritic ulcer
q. Ulcerative keratitis

For each of the situations/conditions given below, choose the one most appropriate/discriminatory option from above. The options may be used once, more than once, or not at all.

Questions

32. A 50-year-old male presents with complaints of blurred vision, night haloes and red eye for last 1 hour after coming out of movie theater. On examination his cornea is hazy and pupils are fixed and dilated.
33. A 20-year-old male presents with acute onset pain and redness in left eye and also complains of blurred vision. On examination there is circumcorneal congestion, cornea is normal but pupil is small and irregular.
34. A 20-year male presents with acute onset pain, redness of both eyes but admits that his vision is normal, complains of photophobia. On examination cornea and pupils are normal.
35. A 40-year-old farmer gives a history of trauma and complains of redness and difficulty seeing in bright light.
36. A 60-year-old patient presented to his GP with sudden onset of redness in the left eye. There was no pain and the vision was unaffected.
37. A seven-year-old North African boy gave a history of two years of discomfort, redness and mucopurulent discharge

affecting both eyes. His two siblings have a similar problem.

38. A 24-year-old man has a history of recurrent attacks of blurring of vision associated with redness, pain and photophobia. Both eyes have been affected in the past. His older brother is currently being investigated for severe backache.
39. A 35-year-old Rugby player sustained facial injuries. Twelve months later he presented with a painful swelling at the left medial canthus associated with a red eye and purulent discharge.
40. A 24-year-old man with a painful red eye has his eye stained with fluorescein drops. Areas of the cornea are stained yellow. Steroid eye drops are given and massive ulceration and blindness results.

THEME: 8
THE MANAGEMENT OF RED EYE

Options

a. No treatment
b. Check blood pressure and do coagulation studies
c. Immediate antibiotic therapy
d. Enucleation
e. 0.5% prednisolone drops 4 hourly
f. 0.55 prednisolone drops 2 hourly and cyclopentolate drops
g. 3% pilocarpine drops and acetazolamide
h. 500 mg acetazolamide
i. Acylovir drops
j. Total iredectomy
k. 5% flourescein drops

For each of the situations/conditions given below, choose the one most appropriate/discriminatory option from above. The options may be used once, more than once, or not at all.

Questions

41. A 69-year-old patient presented to his GP with sudden onset of redness in the right eye. There was no pain and vision was unaffected.

42. A 60-year-old patient complains of severe pain in his left eye with severe deterioration of vision . He had noticed haloes around street lights at night for a few days before the onset of pain.
43. A mother brings her 2-year-old child with a squint. On examination a leucokoric right pupil is seen with an absent red reflex.
44. A 12-year-old Libyan boy gave a two week history of discomfort, redness and mucopurulent discharge affecting both eyes. His two siblings have a similar problem.
45. A 23-year-old man has a history of recurrent attacks of blurring of vision associated with redness, pain and photophobia. Both eyes have been affected in the past . His older is currently being investigated for bowel disease and a severe backache.
46. A 25 year cricket player sustained facial injuries. 10 months later he presented with a painful swelling at the left medial canthus, associated with red eye and purulent discharge.

THEME: 9
LESIONS IN VASCULAR RETINOPATHY

Options

a. Cotton wool spots.
b. Vitreous hemorrhage.
c. Flame shaped hemorrhage.
d. Blots.
e. Hard exudates.
f. Soft exudates.
g. Dots.
h. Papilloedema.
i. A – V nipping.

For each of the situations/conditions given below, choose the one most appropriate/discriminatory option from above. The options may be used once, more than once, or not at all.

Questions

47. Microaneurysm rupture at nerve fiber level.
48. Bleeding from large sized new vessels.
49. Seen in final stage of hypertensive retinopathy.
50. Ischemic nerve fibers.
51. Microaneurysm rupture deep in retina.
52. Unruptured microaneurysms.

THEME: 10
DISORDERS OF THE PUPIL

Options

a. Marcus Gunn pupil.
b. IIIrd cranial nerve palsy.
c. Holmes Adie pupil.
d. Horner's syndrome.
e. Argyl Robertson pupil.
f. Hutchinson pupil.
g. Cavernous sinus thrombosis
h. Syringomyelia

For each of the situations/conditions given below, choose the one most appropriate/discriminatory option from above. The options may be used once, more than once, or not at all.

Questions

53. Irregular, miotic pupil with accommodation reflex present but light reflex absent.
54. Irregular, mydriatic pupil with accommodation reflex present but light reflex absent.
55. Mid dilated and unreactive pupil, pupils with afferent pupillary defect.
56. Miotic pupil with ptosis but normal range of lid movement.
57. On examination of the 42-year-old man, the pupils were fixed, dilated. The patient presented with chemosis and grossly edematous eyelids.
58. A 32-year-old woman presented with wasting and weakness of the hands associated with dissociated sensory

loss over the trunk and arms. The right pupil is miotic and in addition has shows partial ptosis. Her right face is anhydrotic and knees swollen and grossly deformed.

59. A 21-year-old woman reports a sudden onset of blurring of near vision. The pupil is slightly dilated and there is a delayed response to accommodation and especially too. When light is shone in the eye. Her knee and ankle jerks are noted to be absent.

THEME: 11
PUPILS

Options

a. Midposition and unreactive and irregular.
b. Pinpoint and reactive.
c. Small and reactive.
d. Widely dilated and fixed.

For each of the situations/conditions given below, choose the one most appropriate/discriminatory option from above. The options may be used once, more than once, or not at all.

Questions

60. Bilateral hemispheric dysfunction of the cerebrum.
61. Lesion of pons.
62. Tentorial herniation.
63. Lesions in midbrain.

THEME: 12
DIAGNOSIS OF PAIN IN THE EYE

Options

a. Closed angle glaucoma.
b. Hypermetropia.
c. Conjunctivitis.
d. Central retinal vein occlusion.
e. Central retinal artery occlusion.
f. Orbital cellulitis.

g. Retinoblastoma.
h. Trauma.
i. Acute dacrocystitis.
j. Iritis.

For each of the situations/conditions given below, choose the one most appropriate/discriminatory option from above. The options may be used once, more than once, or not at all.

Questions

64. Young male has developed in the eye. He recently started his job as a programmer. He has excessive watering as well.
65. A 25-year-old male comes with severe pain in the left eye with watering and discharge. He looks unwell.
66. A 30-year-old male complains of gradual loss of vision particularly peripheral fields and also complains of dull pain in the both eyes.
67. A 3-year-old body has severe edema of the lids and pain around the eyes.

THEME: 13
CAUSES OF NYSTAGMUS

Options

a. Vestibular neuritis
b. Benign positional vertigo
c. Vertebro-basilar ischemia
d. Phenytoin toxicity
e. Right cerebellar Infarction
f. Left cerebellar Infarction
g. Acoustic neuroma
h. Congenital visual Impairment
i. Wernicke's encephalopathy
j. Multiple sclerosis
k. Meniere's disease
l. Physiological nystagmus

For each of the situations/conditions given below, choose the one most appropriate/discriminatory option from above. The options may be used once, more than once, or not at all.

Questions

68. A 48-year-old woman presents with intermittent vertigo, tinitus and hearing loss in the left ear. On examination she has horizontal nystagmus on right keys.
69. A 65-year-old man with atrial fibrillation presents with left sided tremor and giddiness. He has past pointing of the left hand and nystagmus on looking to the left.
70. A 23-year-old albino male is noticed to have pendular nystagmus.
71. A 43-year-old alcoholic man presents with confusion and falls. On examination he has nystagmus in all directions of keys and ataxic gait.
72. A 53-year-old man presents with intermittent giddiness. On examination he has three beats of nystagmus at the extremes of the left and right keys.
73. An 18-year-old man presents with presents with an acute onset of giddiness and nausea. He is unable to stand upright without vomiting. On examination he has nystagmus on the left keys.

THEME: 14
DIAGNOSIS OF EPIPHORA

Options

a. Ectropion.
b. Refractive error.
c. Entropion.
d. Keratitis.
e. Closed angle glaucoma.
f. Dacrocystitis.
g. Spring catarrh.
h. Conjunctivitis.
i. Phlyctenular conjunctivitis.

For each of the situations/conditions given below, choose the one most appropriate/discriminatory option from above. The options may be used once, more than once, or not at all.

Questions

74. A 5-year-old boy is brought with complaints of severe itching and watering.
75. A 50-year-old male presents with excessive was from the eyes associated with photophobia. He also has caries tooth.
76. A 70-year-old patient with previous history of bell's palsy presents epiphora.
77. A 50-year male presents with progressive loss peripheral vision and has recently also noticed increasing watering from both his eyes, more so after working in dim light.

THEME: 15
MANAGEMENT OF GLAUCOMA

Options

a. Pilocarpine.
b. Betablockers.
c. Enucleation.
d. Steroids.
e. Trabeculectomy.
f. Argon laser trabeculoplasty.
g. Laser peripheral iridectomy.
h. Cyclocryosurgery.
i. Goniotomy.
j. Trabeculotomy.
k. Photocoagulation.

For each of the situations/conditions given below, choose the one most appropriate/discriminatory option from above. The options may be used once, more than once, or not at all.

Questions

78. A 40-year female with a painful blind eye. Patient wants to retain eye for cosmetic reasons.
79. A 70-year man with open angle glaucoma, uncontrolled on medical treatment.
80. A 40-year-old man with medically uncontrolled open angle glaucoma.

81. Normal eye of a 24-year-old female, the other eyeball has an angle closure glaucoma.
82. A 15-year-old boy with joint pain, complaining of pain, redness, photophobia in both eyes. Tonometry shows raised tension in both eyes.
83. A 3-year-old baby with complaints of watering, photophobia. O/E corneal size is enlarged, cup disc ratio is 0.3:1.

THEME: 16
EYE MANIFESTATIONS OF SYSTEMIC DISEASES

Options

a. Hypertension
b. Hyperparathyroidism
c. AIDS
d. Sickle cell anaemia
e. Rheumatoid arthritis
f. Hyperlipidaemia
g. Diabetes mellitus
h. Hyperthyroidism
i. Tuberculosis
j. Wilson's disease
k. Dermatomyositis
l. SLE

For each of the situations/conditions given below, choose the one most appropriate/discriminatory option from above. The options may be used once, more than once, or not at all.

Questions

84. A 55-year-old woman has corneal and conjunctival calcification. She also complains of thirst, polyuria and mild confusion.
85. A 60-year-old woman has a voracious rash on her eyelids with associated orbital oedema and retinal haemorrhages.
86. A 30-year-old man has visual impairment with profuse cotton wool spots on both retina. There are no other retinal abnormalities. He also has a number of painless pigmented lesions on his face.

87. A 52-year-old man has mild visual impairment. On fundoscopy there is evidence of flame haemorrhages, AV nipping and cotton wool spots.
88. A 30-year-old man is being investigated for jaundice. He has a reddish brown ring around the periphery of the iris.
89. A 43-year-old man has visual impairment. On fundoscopy there are microaneurysms, hard and soft exhibits and leaches of new vessels.

Twenty two

Obstetrics

THEME: 1
ANTENATAL CARE

Options

a. Specialized fetal ultrasound.
b. Amniocentesis or CVS.
c. Maternal serum AFP.
d. Fetoscopy
e. Cordocentesis
f. Rhesus status
g. Kleihauer test
h. Chorionic villous sampling
i. Abdominal ultrasound
j. Biophysical profile

For each of the situations/conditions given below, choose the one most appropriate/discriminatory option from above. The options may be used once, more than once, or not at all.

Questions

1. A 27-year-old woman in eighteenth week of her pregnancy; both the patient and her husband are heterogeneous for the sickle cell gene.
2. A 25-year-old woman who is married to her first cousin.
3. A 29-year-old woman who previously had a child with microcephaly.
4. A 22-year-old woman in her tenth week of pregnancy whose husband is a carrier of a familial balanced translocation.
5. A 25-year-old primigravida at 14 weeks, is told after screening that she has a 75% chance of getting a baby with Down's syndrome. She wants to know whether her child actually has the syndrome.

6. A 24-year-old pregnant lady with sickle cell anaemia wants to know whether her baby will have the hemoglobin.
7. A 31-weeks pregnant female had an episode of APH during the current pregnancy. A detailed USG shows a grossly retarted fetus but with no physical abnormality.
8. A 34-year-old Rh negative female has isoimmunisation in her last pregnancy. Biophysical profile shows an odematus fetus.

THEME: 2
DIAGNOSIS OF PLACENTAL DISORDER

Options

a. Abruptio placenta.
b. Placenta previa.
c. Placenta accreta.
d. Monoamniotic monochorionic twin placenta.
e. Diamniotic monochorionic twin placenta.
f. Diamniotic dichorionic twin placenta (fused).
g. Diamniotic dichorionic twin placenta (separate).
h Battledore placenta
i. Velamentous placenta.

For each of the situations/conditions given below, choose the one most appropriate/discriminatory option from above. The options may be used once, more than once, or not at all.

Questions

9. Placenta associated with siamese twins fused at the abdomen.
10. Placenta associated with painful vaginal bleeding in a pregnant woman who is a cocaine addict.
11. Placenta associated with absence of the decidua basalis and severe postpartum bleeding.
12. Placenta associated with painless bleeding and an abnormal implantation site.
13. Umbilical cord inserts into side of the placenta.

THEME: 3
CAUSES OF GENITAL TRACT BLEEDING IN PREGNANCY

Options

a. Placenta praevia
b. Abruptio placenta
c. Vasa praevia
d. Cervical carcinoma
e. Ectopic pregnancy
f. Cervical polyp
g. Vaginal laceration
h. Uterine fibromyomata
i. Hydatiform mole
j. Threatened abortion
k. Unknown etiology

For each of the situations/conditions given below, choose the one most appropriate/discriminatory option from above. The option may be used once, more than once, or not at all.

Questions

14. A 20-year-old nulliparous woman of 30 weeks gestation presents with bright red bleeding. On USG the placenta is found to be lying over the internal os.
15. A 44-year-old multiparous woman of 37 weeks gestation presents with heavy dark vaginal bleeding and uterine pain. The uterus is hypertonic and tender to palpation. The fetal lie is longitudinal and there is an increase in fundal height.
16. A 25-year-old nulliparous woman of 18 weeks gestation presents with uterine pain and mild pyrexia. Pelvic USG reveals an enlarged uterus with smoothly rounded protusions from the uterine wall.
17. A 34-year-old nulliparous woman of 6 weeks gestation presents with painless uterine bleeding. USG shows no fetal echos. The HCG levels are high.
18. A 20-year-old nulliparous woman of 8 weeks gestation presents with severe lower abdominal pain, scant vaginal bleeding and an empty uterus on ultrasound.

THEME: 4
PRENATAL DIAGNOSIS

Options

a. Cordocentesis
b. Rhesus status
c. Kleihauser test
d. Chorionic villus sampling
e. Abdominal ultrasound
f. Biophysical profile
g. Amniocentesis

For each of the situations/conditions given below, choose the one most appropriate/discriminatory option from above. The option may be used once, more than once, or not at all.

Questions

19. A 23-year-old primigravida at 13 weeks is told after screening that she has a 75% chance of getting a child with Down's syndrome. She wants to know whether her child actually has the syndrome.
20. A 25-year-old pregnant sickler wants to know whether her baby will have the hemaglobinopathy.
21. A 30-week pregnant woman had an episode of APH during the current pregnancy. A detailed USG shows a grossly retarded fetus, but with no physical abnormality.
22. A 33-years rhesus negative woman had isoimmunization in her last pregnancy. A biophysical profile shows and edematous fetus.

THEME: 5
METHOD OF DELIVERY

Options

a. Cesarean section.
b. Normal vaginal delivery.
c. Instrumental podalic version.
d. Internal podalic delivery.

e. External cephalic.
f. Destructive procedure.

For each of the situations/conditions given below, choose the one most appropriate/discriminatory option from above. The options may be used once, more than once, or not at all.

Questions

23. Transverse arrest.
24. Cord prolapse during second stage.
25. Occipitoposterior presentation.
26. First twin is in transverse position.
27. Cord presentation.
28. Mento anterior presentation.
29. Second twin is in tranverse position.

THEME: 6
DIAGNOSIS OF DISTENDED UTERUS

Options

a. Multiple pregnancy.
b. Hydramnios.
c. Big baby.
d. Fibroid uterus.
e. Hydatidiform mole.
f. Concealed hemorrhage.

For each of the situations/conditions given below, choose the one most appropriate/discriminatory option from above. The options may be used once, more than once, or not at all.

Questions

30. Primigravida with history of 5 months amenorrhea and hyperemesis. On examination BP 160/90 mm Hg, uterus 26 weeks size and doughy in consistency.
31. A 35-year-old gravida 4 with 7 months amenorrhea. On examination pallor present, BP 150/90 mm Hg, uterus is of 32 weeks size, liquor is excess and 3 fetal poles felt.
32. A 35-year-old gravida 4 who is a known diabetic on irregular treatment presents with 8 months amenorrhea.

On examination, she is found to be having uterus of 36 weeks size, and slightly excess liquor.

33. Primi with 6 months amenorrhea c/o sudden abdominal pain associated with vomiting. On examination, uterus is 28 week size, abdomen is tense and there is difficulty in palpating fetal parts BP is 110/70 and pulse is 92 per minute.
34. A 36-year-old primigravida c/o amenorrhea of 5 months duration. On examination, she is found to be having a uterus of 28 weeks size and fetal heart sounds are heard. Her previous cycles were heavy and painful.

THEME: 7
DIFFERENTIAL DIAGNOSIS OF ECTOPIC PREGNANCY

Options

a. Appendicitis
b. Bacterial vaginosis
c. Crohn's disease
d. Ectopic pregnancy
e. Endometriosis
f. Inevitable miscarriage
g. Irritable Bowel syndrome
h. Missed abortion
i. Normal pregnancy
j. Pelvic inflammatory disease
k. Renal colic
l. Septic abortion
m. Threatened miscarriage
n. Torted ovarian mass
o. Ulcerative colitis

For each of the situations/conditions given below, choose the one most appropriate/discriminatory option from above. The options may be used once, more than once, or not at all.

Questions

35. A 21-year-old woman presents as an emergency with a four hour history of lower abdominal pain and bright red

vaginal blood loss. She has not had a menstrual period for nine weeks and had a positive home pregnancy one week ago. On vaginal examination the uterus is tender and bulky. The cervical os is open.

36. A 16-year-old woman presents with a sudden onset of severe right iliac fossa pain. On vaginal examination a 6 cm diameter echogenic cystic mass is seen in the right fornix.
37. An 18-year-old student due to take her examinations reports that she missed her period and that a pregnancy test is negative. She has worsening abdominal pain which has been troublesome for three months. She is otherwise well.
38. A 22-year-old woman who has two terminations of pregnancy reports that she is pregnant again. She noted a small amount of watery brown discharge and is tender in the right iliac fossa.
39. A 27-year-old woman who conscientiously uses the oral contraceptive pills has experienced intermittent vaginal bleeding and malodorous discharge for several weeks. When examined she has pain all over the lower abdomen, worse on the left. Her temperature is 39°C and her white cell count is elevated.

THEME: 8
DIAGNOSIS OF RECURRENT ABORTIONS

Options

a. Cervical incompetence.
b. Chromosomal abnormalities.
c. TORCH infections.
d. Uterine abnormalities.
e. Fibroid uterus.
f. Rh incompatibility.
g. Diabetes mellitus.
h. Syphilis.
i. Recurrent PIH.
j. Recurrent abruption.
k. Recurrent UTI.

For each of the situations/conditions given below, choose the one most appropriate/discriminatory option from above. The options may be used once, more than once, or not at all.

Questions

40. A 26-year-old gravida 3 para 0 has had 3 abortions between 6-10 weeks of gestation. She is found to be negative for TORCH infections.
41. A 38-year-old gravida 3 at 22 weeks of gestation. First pregnancy got terminated as anencephalic fetus, second pregnancy was intrauterine death at term, in spite of intensive monitoring in hospital.
42. A 30-year-old gravida with history of two abortions at 20 weeks of gestation presents with past history of sudden rupture of membranes and bleeding followed by expulsion of products of conception within 2 hours.
43. A 30-year-old gravida 3 with 7 months amenorrhea presents with past history of spontaneous abortions at 22 week and the next one was a preterm delivery at 30 weeks. On examination, uterus is 26 weeks in size, fetal heart sounds heard and fundus is felt to be brood.

THEME: 9
TERMINATION OF PREGNANCY

Options

a. Medical termination of pregnancy.
b. Dilatation and Curettage.
c. Extra-amniotic prostaglandin.
d. Suction evacuation.
e. Hysterotomy.
f. Enema.
g. Intra-amniotic prostaglandin.
h. None of the above.
i. Advice about contraception.

For each of the situations/conditions given below, choose the one most appropriate/discriminatory option from above. The options may be used once, more than once, or not at all.

Questions

44. A 21-year girl presents to the gynae clinic with eight weeks of amenorrhea. On examination, the uterus is 8 weeks in size and the UPT is + ve. She is still at college and not in a steady relation. She wants to terminate the pregnancy.
45. An 18-year-old girl presents to the gyne clinic with history of being pregnant. She wants termination of pregnancy for social reasons. On examination, the uterus is felt at the umbilicus.
46. A 19-year-old girl presents to the gyne clinic with history of 7 weeks amenorrhea. She wants termination of this pregnancy. This is her third TOP in the last two years.

THEME: 10
CAUSES OF PRE – AND PERINATAL INFECTION

Options

a. Toxoplasma fondii
b. Herpes simplex
c. Herpes zoster
d. Rubella
e. Cytomegalovirus
f. Human immunodefieciency virus
g. Group B *Streptococcus*
h. Listeria monocytogenes
i. Chlamydia trachomatis
j. *Escherichia coli*

For each of the situations/conditions given below, choose the one most appropriate/discriminatory option from above. The option may be used once, more than once, or not at all

Questions

47. The child was initially quite well and was on the 50th centile for weight. From eight months, however she failed to thrice and rapidly fell to the 3rd centile over the next three months. She had severe diarrhoea, recurrent episodes of fever and breathing difficulties. On examination, she has generalised lymphadenopathy and eczema.

48. This child has moderate learning difficulties, cerebral palsy and growth delay. There was prolonged jaundice after birth. There is also severe visual impairment due to choroidorentinitis. The mother was unaware of any illness during pregnancy.
49. This child was well for the first week after birth before rapidly deteriorating. He now refuses to feed, is drowsy and has had apnoea attacks and fits. On examination he appears very unwell and shocked with evidence of neck stiffness.
50. This child developed a blistering rash on his scalp and face 10 days after birth. The conjunctivae are also red and blistered . He has jaundice and hepatomegaly.
51. This child developed a purulent discharge of both conjunctivae eight days after birth. On examination there are corneal ulcers or retinal changes. He was otherwise well, initially, but has now developed a cough, fever and cyanosis.

THEME: 11
CAUSES OF INFECTIONS IN PREGNANCY

Options

a. HIV
b. Gonorrhoea
c. Trichomoniasis
d. Candidiasis
e. Herpes genitalis
f. Listeriosis
g. Rubella
h. Trepnonema pallidum
i. *Streptococcus*
j. Cytomegalovirus
k. Toxoplasmosis

For each of the situations/conditions given below, choose the one most appropriate/discriminatory option from above. The option may be used once, more than once, or not at all.

Questions

52. A nulliparous woman of 12 weeks gestation presents with diarrhoea, pyrexia and premature labour. She reports eating unpasteurized cheese and cooked meat.
53. A multiparous woman of 16 weeks gestation reports an intensely itchy, green-coloured offensive vaginal discharge.
54. A nulliparous woman of 8 weeks gestation is found to have painless ulcers on the labia with regional lymphedeopathy.
55. A nulliparous woman of 10 weeks gestation is found to have shallow painful ulcers on her cervix and labia. She also has associated inguinal lymphedenopathy. She reports recurrent tingling sensation in the affected areas.
56. A nulliparous woman of 12 weeks gestation reports a mild glandular fever like illness. She has 2 cats at home.

THEME: 12
DIAGNOSIS OF ANTENATAL INFECTIONS

Options

a. Cytomegalovirus.
b. Toxoplasmosis.
c. Varicella zoster virus.
d. Syphilis.
e. Rubella virus.

For each of the situations/conditions given below, choose the one most appropriate/discriminatory option from above. The options may be used once, more than once, or not at all.

Questions

57. Causes birth defects when a mother is infected with primary infection versus recurrent infection.
58. Congenital infection very rare before 16 weeks gestation.
59. Has a 24 percent incidence of congenital infection when maternal infection occurs in the last month of pregnancy.
60. Infects all infants, 50 percent of whom will be asymptomatic, born to women with recent infection.

THEME: 13
INVESTIGATIONS IN PREGNANCY

Options

a. 24 hour urine protein excretion
b. Amniocentisis
c. Bile acids
d. Doppler ultrasound of the umbilical artery
e. Glucose tolerance test
f. Kleihauer test

For each of the situations/conditions given below, choose the one most appropriate/discriminatory option from above. The option may be used once, more than once, or not at all

Questions

61. Arhese-negative woman has a significant antepartum haemorrhage at 29-week gestation.
62. A 29-year-old primparous woman presents at 35 weeks with itching.
63. A 35-year-old multiparous woman is admitted with a blood pressure of 160/95 and 1+protein excretion in the urine dipstick test.
64. A 27-year-old woman has a reduced symphsial-fundal height at clinical examination. A subsequently arranged ultrasound scan reveals intrauterine growth restriction.
65. The triple test of a 25-year-old woman has shown that her baby is at increased risk of having a Down's syndrome.

THEME: 14
DIFFERENTIAL DIAGNOSIS OF ABDOMINAL PAIN IN WOMEN

Options

a. Uterine prolapse
b. Ulcerative colitis
c. Twisted ovarian mass
d. Threatened miscarriage
e. Irritable bowel syndrome

f. Pelvic inflammatory disease
g. Renal colic
h. Endometriosis
i. Appendicitis
j. Acute pancreatitis
k. Ectopic pregnancy
l. Septic abortion
m. Break trough bleeding

For each of the situations/conditions given below, choose the one most appropriate/discriminatory option from above. The option may be used once, more than once, or not at all.

Questions

66. A 35-year-old woman complains of abdominal discomfort relieved by passing flatus or stools. Over the past 6 months she has had episodes of diarrhoea and constipation, but denied weight loss. Her mother died of bowel carcinoma.
67. A 31-year-old man reports a 7-week history of gradual onset rectal bleeding associated with constipation. On examination he is found to have red eyes and skin lesions on both his shins. His brother had similar bowel symptoms and back pain.
68. A 17-year-old woman presents with a sudden onset of severe left iliac fossa pain. On vaginal ultrasound examination, 2 cm echogenic masses are seen in the broad ligament. She says this pain seems to come on every month.
69. A 22-year-old has just had an IUCD fitted. She complains of a watery brown vaginal discharge and abdominal pain.
70. A 19-year-old woman presents as an emergency with a 3 hours history of lower abdominal pain and bleeding per vaginum. She has not seen her period of 8 weeks and had a positive home pregnancy test yesterday. On examination, the uterus is tender and bulky. The os is closed.
71. A 32-year-old who conscientious uses OC pill has experienced monthly vaginal bleeding. On abdominal examination she is comfortable. Her temperature is 37°C but is otherwise healthy.

THEME: 15
DIAGNOSIS OF ABDOMINAL PAIN IN PREGNANCY

Options

a. Peptic ulcer disease
b. Fulminating pre-eclampsia
c. Appendicitis
d. Abortion
e. Fibroids
f. Cholecystitis
g. Ectopic pregnancy
h. Urinary infection
i. Ureteric stone
j. Abruption placenta
k. Hydramnios
l. Pyelonephritis

For each of the situations/conditions given below, choose the one most appropriate/discriminatory option from above. The option may be used once, more than once, or not at all.

Questions

72. A 33-year-old multiparous woman of 32 weeks gestation complains of severe back pain. The urinalysis reveals red blood cells. She is apyrexial.
73. A 35-year-old primi gravida of 8 weeks gestation presents with severe lower abdominal cramping, vaginal bleeding and passage of clots. The internal os is open.
74. A 28-year-old primi gravida of 10 weeks gestation presents with sudden severe abdominal pain. Her abdomen is rigid and the uterus tender.
75. A 30-year-old multiparous woman of 12 weeks gestation presents with lower abdominal pain and tenderness. She also complains of urinary frequency. She is apyrexial.
76. A 26-year-old nulliparous woman of 20 weeks gestation presents with headache and epigastric pain. Her BP is noted to be 150/100 and rising.

THEME: 16
DIAGNOSIS OF CHEST PAIN IN PREGNANCY

Options

a. Aortic dissection
b. Massive pulmonary embolism
c. Pulmonary infarction
d. Myocardial infarction
e. Aortic rupture
f. Cardiopathia fantstica
g. Pneumothorax
h. Esophageal spasm
i. Pericarditis
j. Musculoskeletl pain

For each of the situations/conditions given below, choose the one most appropriate/discriminatory option from above. The option may be used once, more than once, or not at all.

Questions

77. A 30-year-old pregnant woman (31 weeks) presents with severe chest pain of acute onset. There is a family history of ischaemic heart disease. Clinical examination demonstrates dyspnoea, cyanosis, and hypertension (90/50) and distended neck veins.
78. A 24-year-old pregnant woman (27 weeks) presents with a 6 hours history of pleuritic chest pain and haemoptysis. She has a family history of ischaemic heart disease.
79. A tall slim 30-year-old pregnant woman (26 weeks) presents with central chest pain, hypertension (90/40) and tachycardia. There is a family history of ischaemic heart disease.
80. A 33-year-old pregnant woman (29 weeks) present with inspiratory chest pain. The pain is much less when she sits up and leans forward. She had an upper respiratory infection a week earlier.

THEME: 17
MANAGEMENT OF ABDOMINAL DISCOMFORT IN PREGNANCY

Options

a. Give 500 mg stat PO of acetazolamide
b. Do emergency cardiotocography
c. Propanolol immediately
d. Induce labour and delivery immediately
e. No treatment observation
f. Abdominal amniocentesis
g. Give diazepam rectally after a period observation
h. 4-5 g IV Magnesium sulphate over 20 min. then 1-3g hr-hypotensive initially

For each of the situations/conditions given below, choose the one most appropriate/discriminatory option from above. The options may be used once, more than once, or not at all.

Questions

81. A 35-year-old gravida 4, para 3-1 presents at 20 weeks with a grossly distended abdomen. She is dyspnoeic and complains of general abdominal discomfort. Abdominal ultrasound shows the deepest pool of amniotic fluid to be 10 cm and a normal fetus
82. A 23-year-old primigravida presents at 36 weeks with abdominal discomfort and on examination her abdomen is found to be larger for dates. She is dyspnoeic and complains of indigestion and claims the abdomen has swollen to this size within aweek.Ultrasound shows the fetus to be normal.
83. A 40-year-old lady 38 weeks pregnant is brought to A&E fitting. Prior to this she had complained of epigastric pain. Her blood pressure is found to be 200/100 mmHg.

THEME: 18
DIAGNOSIS OF ANTEPARTUM HEMORRHAGE

Options

a. Abruptio placenta.

b. Vasa praevia.
c. Placenta praevia.
d. Circumvallate placenta.
e. Cervical polyp.
f. Preterm labor.
g. Cervical cervix.
h. Rupture uterus.
i. Carcinoma cervix.

For each of the situations/conditions given below, choose the one most appropriate/discriminatory option from above. The options may be used once, more than once, or not at all.

Questions

84. A 35-year-old gravida 5 par 4 comes with a history of 8 months amenorrhea and bleeding per vaginum since 3 days. On examination uterus is 32 weeks size, is non-tender and fetal heart sounds are heard.
85. Primigravida with 32 weeks into pregnancy c/o tightening of abdomen and bleeding per vaginum. On examination, uterus is cervix is effaced and there is blood stained mucoid discharge.
86. A 30-year-old gravida 2 at 40 weeks and in labor since 3 hour noticed of fluid per vaginum followed by bleeding per vaginum. On examination, fetal heart sounds are absent.
87. Primigravida at 34 weeks gestation c/o tightening of abdomen and bleeding per vaginum. On examination, uterus is 36 weeks and is tender on palpation and fetal heart sounds are absent. BP is 140/90 mmHg and urine albumin^{++}.
88. Multigravida at 24 weeks gestation c/o bleeding per vaginum since 5 days. On examination, uterus is of 24 weeks size, fetal heart sounds are present and ultrasound revealed that placenta is present in the upper segment. Per speculum examination revealed a soft, friable growth.
89. A woman presents in active labor with significant vaginal bleeding. She is incoherent but does say that has had a previous cesarean section. Fetal heart tones are heard at 60/min.

THEME: 19
DIAGNOSIS AND INVESTIGATION FOR ANTEPARTUM HAEMORRAGE

Options

a. Biophysical profile (e.g. fetal heart monitoring)
b. Cord blood flow studies (doppler)
c. Central venous pressure
d. Coagulation profile
e. Cardiotocography
f. Electronic maternal cardiovascular monitoring
g. Placental localisation (USS ultrasound scan)
h. Haemoglobin
i. Kleihauer test
j. Pulse oximetry
k. Rhesus status
l. Speculum examination
m. Urinalysis

For each of the situations/conditions given below, choose the one most appropriate/discriminatory option from above. The options may be used once, more than once, or not at all.

Questions

90. A 24-year-old gravida 4 para 3 presents unprovoked vaginal bleed of approximately 50 ml at 32 weeks. She is generally well but worried.
91. A 25-year-old nullipara presents at 26 weeks gestation with slight postcoital vaginal bleeding.
92. Following recurrent antepartum haemorrhage, investigaion shows the foetus to be small for dates at 32 weeks. Conservative management is preferred. A 19 week fetal anomaly ultrasound scan confirmed normal placental localisation.
93. A woman whose previous pregnancy was complicated by isoimmunisation has vaginal spotting at 36 weeks in an otherwise normal pregnancy
94. A 31 -year-old woman is anxious about slight per vaginal bleeding. She is 22 weeks pregnant and had similar complaints 2 years ago when she was on pill.

THEME: 20
DIAGNOSIS OF VAGINAL BLEEDING

Options

a. Retention of succenturiate lobe
b. Placenta praevia
c. Uterine rupture
d. Cervical carcinoma
e. Ruptured vasa previa
f. Cervical laceration
g. Thrombocytopenia
h. Implantaion in the uterine segment
i. Endometrial carcinoma
j. Atonic uterus
k. Placenta accreta

For each of the situations/conditions given below, choose the one most appropriate/discriminatory option from above. The option may be used once, more than once, or not at all.

Questions

95. Following a spontaneous vaginal delivery. A 22-year-old woman continues to bleed in spite of the use of oxytocin. The uterus appears to contract well but then relaxes with increased bleeding.
96. A 28-year-old woman has just delivered her second baby in 2 yrs after an oxytocin-induced labour. She is bleeding heavily despite use of oxytocin. The uterus is well contracted and there is no evidence of vaginal or cervical tears. The baby weighs 4.5 kg.
97. A 32-year-old woman is still bleeding heavily 6 hours after having delivered twins vaginally.
98. A 40-year-old woman who has had no antenatal care presents at term with heavy bleeding. Her last pregnancy was 14 years ago. Abdominal USG shows a fetal heart rate of 150/min and a fundal placenta.
99. A 32-year-old woman present in active labour with excessive vaginal bleeding. She has had a previous caesarean section. The fetal heart rate is 65/min.

100. A 28-year-old woman who is 36 weeks pregnant presents with vaginal bleeding, contractions and a tender abdomen.
101. A 31-year-old woman has delivered with a complete placenta praevia by caesarean section. 2 hrs later, she is noted to have significant postpartum haemorrhage.

THEME: 21
MANAGEMENT OF ANTEPARTUM HEMORRHAGE

Options

a. Immediate LSCS.
b. Artificial rupture of membranes.
c. Reassurance.
d. Internal podalic version.
e. Admit and observe.
f. Steroids and ritodine.
g. Oxytocin infusion.

For each of the situations/conditions given below, choose the one most appropriate/discriminatory option from above. The options may be used once, more than once, or not at all.

Questions

102. A 26-year-old woman has had bleeding per vaginum on and off throughout the pregnancy and now at 29 weeks bled and passed a few clots. Her uterus is relaxed and the baby is in transverse lie.
103. A 24-year-old woman with heavy bleeding at 32 weeks soaked her bedsheets. Cardioechogram is fine, baby in breech position and the mother has Hb of 8 gm% . Uterus is non-tender and the bleeding continues.
104. A 40-year-old woman, in her 6th pregnancy c/o bleeding per vaginum one cupful and a steady, small trickle since. Her baby has not moved since morning and per vaginal examination revealed the cervix to be 2 cm dilated and the presenting part at 2 cm above the spine. The uterus is tender on palpation.
105. A 28-year-old woman is in pain for the last 4 hours and now passed some bloody mucus, the contractions are

increasing in duration, coming 3-4 every 10 minutes. She is 39 weeks pregnant and the CTG is reactive.

THEME: 22
BLEEDING IN PREGNANCY

Options

a. Abembryonic pregnancy
b. Abryptio placenta
c. Cancer of the cervix
d. Cervical erosion
e. Ectopic pregnancy
f. Insertio velametosa
g. Molar pregnancy
h. Placenta praevia

For each of the situations/conditions given below, choose the one most appropriate/discriminatory option from above. The option may be used once, more than once, or not at all.

Questions

106. A 20-year-old woman with a 7-week history of amenor–rhoea with lower abdominal pain who fainted twice.
107. A 35-year-old para 5+1 with a painless bleeding of 200 ml at 35 weeks of pregnancy.
108. A woman in advanced labour and normal vital signs with the fetal heart dropping steadily.
109. A woman presents at 16 weeks with the symphysial – fundal height measuring 20 cm and severe nausea, vomiting and heavy vaginal bleeding.
110. A 29-year-old para 3+2 with a history of intercourse the day before and painless dark brown bleeding of a teaspoonful of blood.

THEME: 23
THE TREATMENT OF MENOPAUSAL SYMPTOMS

Options

a. Clonidine.

b. Combined hormone replacement.
c. Therapy (HRT).
d. Dietary modification.
e. Mineral supplements.
f. Oestrogen only HRT.
g. Psychological support.
h. Referral to psychiatrist.
i. Regular exercise.
j. Vaginal lubricants.
k. Vaginal oestrogens.
l. Medroxyprogesterone.
m. Endometrial biopsy.
n. Hysterectomy.

For each of the situations/conditions given below, choose the one most appropriate/discriminatory option from above. The options may be used once, more than once, or not at all.

Questions

111. A 56-year-old woman whose periods stopped five years ago has become increasingly depressed. She now feels life is no longer worth living and threatens suicide.
112. A 72-year-old woman has experienced frequency of micturition intermittently for the last few months. Mid-stream urine (MRU) cultures been persistently negative. She is well otherwise, but would like the symptoms resolved.
113. A married 52-year-old woman who has a family history of breast cancer has been experiencing mild discomfort for a few hours following intercourse for the last month. She is worried about using hormones.
114. A 45-year-old woman who has had a total abdominal hysterectomy (TAH) and bilateral salpingo-oophorectomy (BSO) for fibroids and menorrhagia and complains of hot flushes, night sweats and moos swings. She has no other medical problems.
115. A 55-year-old woman presents with complaints of hot flushes and night sweats. Her last menstrual period was 3 years ago. Her only other medical complaint is migraine headaches. Family history includes breast cancer in her maternal aunt.

116. A 49-year-old woman presents with irregular cycles, intermenstrual bleeding, and hot flashes and insists that she needs medication. She has had the irregular bleeding for 18 months.
117. A 54-year-old woman presents complaining of vaginal spotting, discharge and dyspareunia. She has been menopausal for 3 years. She had an endometrial biopsy 3 months ago, which revealed an atrophic endometrium.

THEME: 24
DIAGNOSIS OF STAGE OF LABOR

Options

a. False labor.
b. Hypertonic uterine dysfunction.
c. Hypotonic uterine dysfunction.
d. Active phase of labor.
e. Latent phase of labor.

For each of the situations/conditions given below, choose the one most appropriate/discriminatory option from above. The options may be used once, more than once, or not at all.

Questions

118. A woman presents to the labor floor complaining of painful contractions that occur every 2 minutes. She is 2 cm dilated. Two hours later, she continues to complain of frequent painful contractions, but she is still only 2 cm dilated.
119. A woman presents to the labor floor 3 cm dilated with contractions every 5-7 minutes. About 2 hours later she is having contractions every 3 minutes and is 6 cm dilated. She is 8 cm dilated 1 hour later.
120. A woman presents to the labor floor with contractions 8-12 minutes apart. She complains of lower abdominal discomfort with her contractions, which last for only 20 seconds each. Sedation causes the contractions to space out to intervals of 15-20 minutes.
121. A woman presents to the floor complaining of painful contractions that occur every 4 minutes. She is 2 cm dilated. Two hours later, she continues to complain of frequent painful contractions and is now 3 cm dilated.

THEME: 25
DIAGNOSIS OF FETAL CONDITION

Options

a. Breech presentation.
b. Oliguria.
c. Occiput posterior position.
d. Transient fetal distress.
e. Hyperreflexia.
f. Cord presentation.
g. Brow presentation.
h. Oligohydramnios.
i. Twins.

For each of the situations/conditions given below, choose the one most appropriate/discriminatory option from above. The options may be used once, more than once, or not at all.

Questions

122. A multiparous woman presents at 33 weeks gestation, complaining of vaginal bleeding in the absence of both contractions and ruptured membranes.
123. A woman at term is admitted with a tender uterus and a tense abdomen and no audible fetal heart tone.
124. A woman presents with moderate vaginal bleeding and uterine contractions that do not completely relax between contractions.
125. A woman presents with over distended abdomen. She conceived after treatment for infertility.
126. A woman presents to the labor floor. Artificial rupture of membranes is done by a junior doctor and CTG shows distress soon afterwards.

THEME: 26
MANAGEMENT DURING LABOR

Options

a. Intravenous hydration.
b. Nasal oxygen.

c. Fetal heart rate (FHR) monitoring.
d. Fetal scalp pH.
e. Cesarean section.
f. Instrumental delivery.
g. Wait and watch.
h. Cardiotocograph.
i. Oxytocin.

For each of the situations/conditions given below, choose the one most appropriate/discriminatory option from above. The options may be used once, more than once, or not at all.

Questions

127. A patient chronic hypertension presents to the labor floor at term in active labor. Her blood pressure is 140/100, and she has 1 + urinary protein. She is 4 cm dilated.
128. FHR monitoring reveals persistent late decelerations in a patient whose cervix is 8 cm dilated.
129. Fetal scalp pH in a patient having late decelerations with slow recovery over a 30-minute period is returned 7.19.
130. A woman presents to the labor floor complaining of painful contractions every 4 minutes. She is 2 cm dilated. Two hours later, she continues to complain of frequent painful contractions and is now 3 cm dilated.
131. A woman presents to the labor floor 3 cm dilated with contractions every 5 -7 minutes. About 2 hours later she is having contractions every 3 minutes and is 6 cm dilated. She is 8 cm dilated 1 hour later.

THEME: 27
MANAGEMENT OF LABOUR AND DELIVERY

Options

a. LSCS
b. Classic caesarean section
c. Mid-forceps rotation
d. Syntocinon IV
e. Admit and perform external cephalic version
f. Spontaneous vaginal delivery

g. External cephalic version in clinic.
h. Intrauterine injection of PG F2 alpha
i. Epidural anaesthesia
j. Epiostomy
k. Vacuum extraction
l. Hysterectomy

For each of the situations/conditions given below, choose the one most appropriate/discriminatory option from above. The option may be used once, more than once, or not at all.

Questions

132. A 10-year-old nulliparous woman continues to bleed heavily following delivery of the baby and intact placenta. Massaging the uterus infusion IV syntocinon and infusion blood fail to stem this postpartum haemorrhage,
133. A 25-year-old multiparous woman is found to carry a fetus with face presentation. There are no signs of fetal distress.
134. A 35-year-old multiparous woman of 39 weeks gestation is found to have a fetus in transverse lie presentation confirmed by ultrasound.
135. A 5 feet high nulliparous woman has prolonged labour lasting 20 hours. On examination her cervix is 8 cm dilated and the vertex is at–1 position. There have been no changes in the past 2 hours. She is still having regular contractions.
136. A 30-year-old primi gravida has prolonged labour lasting 18 hours. The cervix is dilated to 8 cm. Fetal monitoring now shows late decelerations and a scalp ph of 7.2.

THEME: 28
MANAGEMENT OF OBSTETRIC CONDITIONS

Options

a. Elective LSCS
b. Epidural anaesthesia
c. Ventouse extraction
d. Ruptured membranes
e. Bedrest and control BP

f. Crash caesarean section
g. IV Syntocinon
h. Allow vaginal delivery
i. Episotomy

For each of the situations/conditions given below, choose the one most appropriate/discriminatory option from above. The option may be used once, more than once, or not at all.

Questions

137. A 30-year-old female gravida 2, para 1 with one previous LSCS for fetal distress, presents at 38 weeks with regular uterine contractions and with fetal head engaged.
138. A 20-year-old primi gravida presents with uterine contractions for the past 14 hours. On examination the os is 6cm dilated. The membranes are intact. The fetal heart rate is 140/min.
139. A 21-year-old multiparous woman presents with uterine contractions for the past 18 hours. On examination, the os is 9 cm dilated and the presentating part is at the level of the ischial spines. The fetal heart monitor shows a variable deceleration with fetal heart rate of 100/min.
140. A 30-year-old primi gravida of 36 weeks gestation presents with a blood pressure of 160/110.
141. A 35-year-old second para is admitted in labour. However, she suddenly ruptures her membranes with drainage of meconium stained liquor and prolapse of the umbilical cord. The fetal heart monitor shows a fetal heart rate of 100/min.

THEME: 29
MANAGEMENT OF COMPLICATIONS OF PREGNANCY

Options

a. Urgent LSCS
b. Oral methydopa
c. IV labetolol
d. IV fluids

e. Blood transfusion
f. Oral antibiotics
g. Warfarin
h. Heparin
i. Induction of labour
j. Admit for monitoring
k. High concentration oxygen
l. No treatment required

For each of the situations/conditions given below, choose the one most appropriate/discriminatory option from above. The option may be used once, more than once, or not at all.

Questions

142. A 28-year-old woman is 8 weeks pregnant with her first child. She has severe vomiting and is unable to keep foods or fluids down. She has lost 3kg in the last week. Her skin turgor is low. Urinalysis reveals ketones and a trace of blood and protein but no nitrites.
143. A 32-year-old woman is 34 weeks pregnant with her fourth child. She has not had any antenatal check up. She presents with sudden massive vaginal bleeding preceded by a couple of small bleeds. She has no pain or tenderness. Pulse is 110, BP is 80/30 and fetal heart is 140/min.
144. A 40-year-old pregnant woman had an amniocentesis at 16 weeks, as she was concerned about the risk of Down's syndrome. 12hrs later she collapsed at home. She is breathless and cyanoses. She has had a generalized convulsion and is developing a purpuric rash. Pulse is 100 and BP 100/50.
145. A 26-year-old woman is 27 weeks pregnant with her first child. She is complaining of aching of both lower legs, with are swollen. She is also suffering with crampy pains in her left calf at night. On examination there is symmetrical pitting oedema of both calves with no tenderness of either calf. BP is 90/40 and she has proteinuria.
146. A 17-year-old woman is in the 25th week of her first pregnancy and is attending a routine antenatal clinic. Her pulse is 110/min and BP is 150/90. There is proteinuria on urine dipstick.

147. A 36-year-old woman is 34 weeks pregnant with her first child. She has recently received treatment to correct a breech presentation. Recent USG showed the placenta to lying in the normal position. She has collapsed with severe lower abdominal pain and has lost around 100 ml of blood vaginally. Her pulse is 120 and BP is 80/50. The fetal heart rate is 80/min.

THEME: 30
MANAGEMENT OF LABOR PAIN

Options

a. Pudendal block.
b. Spinal anesthesia.
c. Intramuscular morphine.
d. Epidural anesthesia.
e. IV meperidine.
f. GA with intubation.
g. Paracervical block.
h. GA with laryngeal mask.
i. Regional block.

For each of the situations/conditions given below, choose the one most appropriate/discriminatory option from above. The options may be used once, more than once, or not at all.

Questions

148. A woman presents with painful uterine contractions that occur every 2 to 3 minutes. On examination, she is 2-cm dilated and 60 percent effaced. Three hours later, she is even more uncomfortable with the same contraction pattern, but her cervix is still only 2 cm dilated.
149. A woman is in active labor having contractions every 2-3 minutes. She is 3 cm dilated with the vertex at the-1 station. Two hours later, she is 5-6 cm dilated with the vertex at the + 1 station; she requests pain relief.
150. A woman is in the delivery room ready for delivery. She has had no analgesia or anesthesia upto this point. The vertex presents at on the perineum with each push.

151. A 24-year-old woman has been in labor for last 2 hours and tired. She is being taken for foreceps, baby being occipito anterior, station 2 cm below, the ischial spines.
152. A 24-year-old woman is in labor and requires a cesarean section as the baby has been showing late deceleration while the cervix is only 2 cm dilated.
153. This woman has had an abnormal cervical smear and colposcopy shows CIN-III. She requires a biopsy for a procedure, which is both diagnostic as well as therapeutic.
154. A woman is in labor, and her cervix is 2 cm dilated. She is having regular contractions, which occur every 3 minutes. She requests pain relief but is allergic to meperidine. Within 10 minutes of receiving the anesthesia agent the fetal heart tones drop to 60 beats/min.
155. A woman is in active labor, and her cervix is 5 cm dilated. She requests something for pain relief. Within 5 minutes of receiving the anesthesia, she is in respiratory arrests.

THEME: 31
MANAGEMENT OF PAIN IN LABOUR

Options

a. Spinal anaesthesia
b. Epidural anaesthesia
c. Pudendal nerve block
d. General anaesthesia
e. Pethadine injection
f. Nitrous oxide
g. Local anaesthesia

For each of the situations/conditions given below, choose the one most appropriate/discriminatory option from above. The option may be used once, more than once, or not at all.

Questions

156. A 20-year-old primi gravidi at 40 weeks is 6 cm dilated and she request pain relief. She dislikes injections.
157. A 39-year-old gravida 3, para 2, presents at 39 weeks. Her cervix is 8 cm dilated but she complains of severe pain. Her baby is in occipito-posterior position.

158. A 28-year-old woman wants to be able to move around during the labour pain free.
159. A gravida 4, para 2+1, has been in labour for 4 hours. She is 3 cm dilated and has already received 2 injection of pethadine. She still complains of pain.
160. A 31-year-old woman has a retained placenta, following a spontaneous vaginal delivery.

THEME: 32
ANAESTHESIA DURING LABOUR

Options

a. Spinal anaesthesia
b. Epidural anaesthesia
c. General anaesthesia
d. Pudendal block
e. Paracervical block
f. Intravenous meperidine
g. Intramuscular morphine
h. Naloxine
i. Butorphanol

For each of the situations/conditions given below, choose the one most appropriate/discriminatory option from above. The option may be used once, more than once, or not at all.

Questions

161. A 28-year-old woman is in labour. The vertex is on the perineum and the infant's head is visible at the perineum with each push. She has had no analgesia upto this point.
162. A 26-year-old woman presents with painful uterine contraction occurring every three minutes. On examination she is 2 cm dilated and 60% effaced. Three hours later she still had the same contractions pattern but her cervix is still only 2 cm dilated.
163. A 25-year-old woman presents with painful uterine contraction occurring every 2 minutes. She is 3 cm dilated with the vertex at station. 1.2 hours later she is 6 cm dilated with the vertex at +1 station.

164. A 30-year-old woman is in labour. Her cervix is 2 cm dilated. 5 min after being given anaesthesia, she is in respiratory arrest.
165. A 22-year-old woman is in labour. Her cervix is 2 cm dilated and she had regular contraction occurring every 3 minutes. She is allergic to meperidine. 10 minute after being given anaesthesia, the fetal heart rate drops to 50 beats per minute.

THEME: 33
CLINICAL MANAGEMENT OF HYPERTENSION IN PREGNANCY

Options

a. Low-dose asprin
b. A period of observation for blood pressure
c. 24 hour urinary protein
d. Fetal ultrasound
e. Retinoscopy
f. Induction of labour
g. Renal function test
h. Intravenous antihypertensive
i. Intravenous benzodiazepine
j. Magnesium sulphate
k. Oral antihypertensive
l. Oral diuretic
m. Recheck blood pressure in 7 days
n. Complete neurological examination
o. Immediate caeserean section

For each of the situations/conditions given below, choose the one most appropriate/discriminatory option from above. The options may be used once, more than once, or not at all.

Questions

166. A patient in her third pregnancy presents to her GP at 12 weeks of gestation. She was mildly hypertensive in both her previous pregnancies. Her BP is 150/100 mmHg.Two weeks later at the hospital antenatal clinic BP is 150/95 mmHg.

167. A 24-year-old woman has an uneventful first pregnancy to 30 weeks. She is then admitted as an emergency with epigastric pain. During the first 2 hours her BP rises from 150/105 to 170/120 mmHg.On dipstick she is found to have 3+ proteinuria.The fetal cardiotocogram(CTG) is normal.
168. At an antenatal clinic visit at38 weeks gestation a 36-year-old multiparous woman has a BP of 145/92 mmHg.She has no proteinuria and is otherwise well.
169. At 32 weeks, a 24-year-old primigravida is found to have a BP of 150/100mmHg.She has no proteinuria, but she is found to have oedema of knees.
170. At 34 weeks, a 86 Kg woman complains og persistent headaches and "flashing lights".There is no hyperreflexia and her BP is 150/100 mmHg.Urinalysis is negative but she has finger oedema.

THEME: 34
CONVULSION IN PREGNANCY

Options

a. Cerevral infarction
b. Cerebral vein thrombosis
c. Drug and alcohol withdrawal
d. Eclampsia
e. Epilepsy
f. Gestational epilepsy
g. Hypoglycaemia
h. Hypronatraemia
i. Pseudoepilepsy
j. Thrombotic thrombocytopenic purpura

For each of the situations/conditions given below, choose the one most appropriate/discriminatory option from above. The option may be used once, more than once, or not at all.

Questions

171. A 39-year-old hypertensive multiparous woman who smokes 25 cigarettes per day.

172. An 18-year-old primparous woman in early labour who was induced for a sudden rise in blood pressure.
173. A 25-year-old woman who has been on methadone for the past 3 weeks.
174. A 27-year-old woman who has had tow second trimester pregnancy losses in the past and a deep vein thrombosis outside pregnancy.

THEME: 35
DIAGNOSIS OF POSTPARTUM HEMORRHAGE

Options

a. Atonic postpartum hemorrhage.
b. Uterine rupture.
c. DIC.
d. Drug induced postpartum hemorrhage.
e. Vaginal tear.
f. Uterine inversion.
g. Retained placenta.

For each of the situations/conditions given below, choose the one most appropriate/discriminatory option from above. The options may be used once, more than once, or not at all.

Questions

175. A 22-year-old woman has delivered a baby following 2 hours of second stage 11 hours of first stage. She was keen on avoiding an episiotomy. Pulse is 90/m and BP 112/70. Estimated blood loss 700 ml.
176. This fifth gravida has delivered in the car as she had a rapid labor and could not reach the hospital in time. Her pulse is 160/m and BP 106/66 Estimated blood loss is 1200 ml.
177. This 24-year-old lady had an uneventful delivery following which she had to be taken to the theatre for a retained placenta, which was done under spinal anesthesia. Her pulse is 130 p.m. and blood pressure 90/60. Estimated blood loss is 500 ml.

178. This 30-year-old second gravida had an uneventful labor and was hence delivered. She noticed that there was a gush of bleeding and considering that to be due to a retained placenta, she tried to expedite it's delivery. The patient collapsed and now has a BP of 70 systolic and pulse of 40/m. and estimated blood loss is 600 ml.

THEME: 36
MANAGEMENT OF POSTPARTUM HEMORRHAGE

Options

a. IV ergometrine and oxytocin.
b. IV oxytocin drip and im ergometrine.
c. PGE2 injection.
d. PGF alpha 2 injection.
e. Surgical management.
f. Surgical exploration.
g. Supportive management.

For each of the situations/conditions given below, choose the one most appropriate/discriminatory option from above. The options may be used once, more than once, or not at all.

Questions

179. 22-year-old woman has delivered a baby following 2 hours of second stage and 11 hours of first stage. She was keen on avoiding an episiotomy. Pulse is 90/min and BP 112/70 mmHg. Estimated blood loss is 700 ml.
180. A 29-year-old gravida 5 has delivered in the car park as she had rapid labor and could not reach the hospital in time. Her pulse is 106/min and BP 106/66-mm Hg. Estimated blood loss is 1200 ml.
181. A 24-year-old lady had an uneventful delivery following which she had to be taken to the theatre for a retained placenta, which was done under spinal anesthesia. Her pulse is 130/min and BP is 90/60 mmHg. Estimated blood loss is 500 ml.

182. A 30-year-old gravida 2 had an uneventful labor and was hence delivered by a student midwife. Immediately after the delivery she noticed that there was a gush of bleeding and considering that to be due to a retained placenta, she tried to expedite it's delivery. The patient collapsed and now has a BP of 70/30 and pulse of 40/min. Estimated blood loss is 600 ml.

THEME: 37
INTRAUTERINE CONTRACEPTIVE DEVICE (IUCD)

Options

a. Antibiotic therapy and remove IUCD
b. Contraindicated
c. IUCD should be inserted after the next period
d. Remove IUCD and offer alternative contraception
e. Suspect ectopic pregnancy – refer to early pregnancy assessment

For each of the situations/conditions given below, choose the one most appropriate/discriminatory option from above. The option may be used once, more than once, or not at all.

Questions

183. A 25-year-old woman is complaining of persistent lower abdominal pain and irregular vaginal bleeding since the insertion of an IUCD six months ago.
184. A 32-year-old woman who had an IUCD inserted three weeks ago is complaining of severe abdominal pain. On examination: pulse 92/min, temperature 37.7°C, the abdomen is tender but there is no rigidity of guarding.
185. A 27-year-old woman has come to your family planning clinic requesting insertion of IUCD. Her last menstrual period was three weeks ago.
186. A woman in her early twenties presents with left iliac fossa pain and vaginal bleeding for three days. An IUCD was inserted three months ago and her last normal period was 5 weeks ago.

187. A woman in her late twenties with a history of pelvic inflammatory disease was reported to have pelvic adhesions at laparoscopy six months ago and is requesting an IUCD for contraception.

THEME: 38
CHOICE OF CONTRACEPTION

Options

a. Rhythm methods
b. Barrier methods
c. Progesterone-only pill
d. Combined oral contraceptive
e. Progesterone depot injection
f. Postcoital high-dose levonorgestrel
g. Intrauterine contraceptive device
h. Vasectomy

For each of the situations/conditions given below, choose the one most appropriate/discriminatory option from above. The option may be used once, more than once, or not at all.

Questions

188. A couple have had three children and are both sure that they have completed their family. The wife does not wish to take the oral contraceptive, as she is concerned about the possible risks, and they are not keen on using condoms. Both are aged 35.
189. A 25-year-old shift worker wishes to avoid pregnancy for at least the next six months. She suffers with regular classical migraines. Her partner has a latex allergy.
190. A 38-year-old married woman has had two children and would like reliable contraception. She is not absolutely sure that she and her husband will not want a third child at some stage.
191. A 21-year-old woman had unprotected intercourse at a party tow days ago. She does not wish to become pregnant.

192. A 26-year-old Catholic couple attend their GP's surgery asking about contraception. The wife suffers with irregular periods that are painful and heavy.
193. A 28-year-old woman has discovered that her partner has been using intravenous heroin. She wishes to continue a sexual relationship with him.

THEME: 39
CHOICE OF CONTRACEPTION

Options

a. Oral contraceptive pills
b. Condon and OC pills
c. IUCD
d. Rhythm method
e. Bilateral tubal ligaiton
f. Vasectomy
g. The morning after pill
h. Injectable contraceptive
i. Douching
j. Barrier contraception

For each of the situations/conditions given below, choose the one most appropriate/discriminatory option from above. The option may be used once, more than once, or not at all.

Questions

194. An 18-year-old university student would like to start having sexual relationships.
195. A 25-year-old woman living with her boyfriend asks advice regarding contraception.
196. A married 26-year-old healthy nulliparous woman would like to postpone having a family for 2 yrs.
197. A married 36-year-old obese mother of 3 with varicose veins and a 20 cigarette per day smoking habit would like a form of contraception.
198. A married 25-year-old woman with recent glandular fever would like a form of contraception as she would like to postpone starting a family for 1 year.

Twenty three

Gynecology

THEME: 1
HORMONE LEVELS

Options

a. FSH normal, LH normal.
b. FSH low, LH high.
c. FSH high, LH high.
d. FSH high, LH normal.
e. FSH low, LH high.

For each of the situations/conditions given below, choose the one most appropriate/discriminatory option from above. The options may be used once, more than once, or not at all.

Questions

1. Turner's syndrome.
2. Asherman's syndrome.
3. Polycystic ovarian syndrome.
4. Menopause.
5. Sheehan's syndrome.
6. Perimenopause.

THEME: 2
DIAGNOSIS OF MENORRHALGIA

Options

a. Fibroid.
b. Endometrial hyperplasia.
c. DUB.
d. Endometriosis.
e. PCOD.
f. IUCD.

For each of the situations/conditions given below, choose the one most appropriate/discriminatory option from above. The options may be used once, more than once, or not at all.

Questions

7. A 34-year-old lady presents with heavy periods since 3 years. The periods are irregular. On examination, there is no obvious abnormality. Transvaginal scan is normal Hb is 9 gm percent.
8. A 35-year-old lady gives history of heavy periods. She feels weak and tired. Since 6 months, she has noticed slightly increased urinary frequency. On examination,, she is pale; the uterus is 8 weeks in size. Hb is 8 gm percent, urine pregnancy test is negative. She underwent a myomectomy 3 years ago.
9. A 36-year-old lady gives history of recent onset dysmenorrhea and dys/areunia. Her cycles are regular, painful and she c/o excessive bleeding.
10. 30-year-old lady complains of heavy periods needs double protection. She is on oral contraceptive pills since 3 years. On examination, the uterus is normal in size.
11. 15-year-old girl c/o irregular periods with heavy bleeding not associated with pain gives history of recent weight gain. On examination, hirsutism is present and abdomen is soft.

THEME: 3
DIAGNOSIS OF AMENORRHEA

Options

a. Tuberculosis.
b. Sheehan's syndrome.
c. Prolactinoma
d. Premature ovarian failure.
e. Turner's syndrome.
f. Hyperthyroidism.
g. Ashermen's syndrome.
h. Delayed menarche.

i. PCOD.
j. Anorexia nervosa.
k. Rokitansky-Kustner syndrome.
l. Cryptomenorrhea.
m. Obesity.

For each of the situations/conditions given below, choose the one most appropriate/discriminatory option from above. The options may be used once, more than once, or not at all.

Questions

12. A 34-year-old female c/o 6 months history of amenorrhea, associated with hot flushes, palpitations and sweating. General and abdominal examination, is normal.
13. This 18-year-old student has been with her boyfriend for last 2 years and has used condoms for protection. On examination, breast development and axillary hair appear to be normal, the uterus is normal with a fundal fibroid.
14. A 18-year-old girl with amenorrhea. On examination, she is noticed to have a short stature, breasts are underdeveloped, carrying angle of forearm is more.
15. This young lady of 23 has had no periods for the last 4 months. Her past cycles have been normal. She has recently had heartbreak and has put on 14 kilograms since then.
16. A 30-year-old female delivered a boy baby 8 months' back. Comes with c/o periods not yet started. She also gives history of lactational failure and postpartum hemorrhage during her last delivery. Examination, revealed atrophic breasts.
17. This 24-year-old mother of one has noticed increased hair growth on her face and arms since last 2 years. Her periods have been irregular since the beginning. She has been trying for another child for the last 3 years without success.
18. A 26-year-old girl gives history of secondary amenorrhea following D and C after incomplete abortion.
19. A 28-year-old lady presented with history of 6 months amenorrhea and galactorrhea. On examination, uterus is antiverted and antiflexed.

THEME: 4
DIAGNOSIS OF AMENORRHOEA/INFERTILITY

Options

a. Menopause
b. Polycystic ovarian syndrome
c. Hypothyroidism
d. Prolactinoma
e. Premature ovarian failure
f. Anorexia nervosa
g. Hypopituitarism
h. Hyperthyroidism
i. Pregnancy
j. Turner's syndrome
k. Addison's disease

For each of the situations/conditions given below, choose the one most appropriate/discriminatory option from above. The option may be used once, more than once, or not at all.

Quesiotns

20. A 45-year-old woman with 3 months amenorrhoea preceded by 6 months irregular periods. Beta HCG is positive. Normal LH and FSH, normal testosterone. Raised TSH and thyroxine.
21. A 28-year-old woman of short stature: high LH and FSH, normal prolactin and testosterone. Buccal smear examination shows no Barr bodies.
22. A 30-year-old obese woman with heavy periods and infertility: Normal LH and FSH, high prolactin, normal testosterone, high TSH and low throxine.
23. A 25-year-old woman with weight loss and amenorrhoea for 2 years. Beta HCG negative. Low LH and FSH, normal prolactin and testosterone.
24. A 30-year-old obese, hirsute woman with irregular periods and infertility; beta HCG negative, moderately raised LH, normal FSH, normal prolactin and slightly raised testosterone.

25. A 47-year-old woman with 3 months of amenorrhoea preceded by 6 months irregular periods. Beta HCG negative, High LH and FSH, normal prolactin and testosterone.

THEME: 5
INVESTIGATIONS FOR AMENORRHEA

Options

a. Gonadotrophin levels.
b. Serum prolactin levels.
c. Progesterone challenge.
d. Thyroid-stimulating hormone levels.
e. Serum testosterone levels.
f. Triple stimulation test.

For each of the situations/conditions given below, choose the one most appropriate/discriminatory option from above. The options may be used once, more than once, or not at all.

Questions

26. A 24-year-old nulligravida stopped taking birth control pills in order to conceive. After the last pill withdrawal flow, she was amenorrheic for 6 months.
27. A 24-year-old primipara returns 6 months postpartum, complaining of amenorrhea. Her pregnancy terminated with a cesarean section because of abruptio placentae and fetal distress with an estimated blood loss of 2000 ml due to transient coagulation problem.
28. A 24-year-old woman with previously normal menstrual cycles develops irregular cycles and anovulation. Serum prolactin levels are elevated.

THEME: 6
CAUSES OF AMENORRHOEA

Options

a. Prolactinoma
b. Polycystic ovarian disease

c. Hypothyroidism
d. Cushing's syndrome
e. Exercise-induced
f. Kallman's syndrome
g. Gonodal tumor
h. Imperforate hymen
i. Ovarian failure
j. Drugs causing hyperprolactinemia
k. Anorexia.

For each of the situations/conditions given below, choose the one most appropriate/discriminatory option from above. The option may be used once, more than once, or not at all.

Questions

29. A 20-year-old obese woman presents to her GP with amenorrhoea. She is noted to be hirsute and have severe acne.
30. A 16-year-old woman presents to the GP with primary amenorrhoea. She also complains of lack of smell and is notes to be color-blind. Investigation reveal a low FSH.
31. A 20-year-old woman presents with galactorrhoea and amenorrhoea. Her urine pregnancy test is negative. She takes cimetidine for dyspepsia. Her serum prolactin level is 2000 mu/l.
32. A 30-year-old obese hirsute woman presents with amenorrhoea. Her BP is 170/90 and urine dipstick is positive for glucose.
33. A 25-year-old petite ballet dancer presents with amenorrhoea. She is wearing several layers of clothing. She explains that she is sensitive to cold. On examination she has lanugo.

THEME: 7
INVESTIGATIONS OF AMENORRHOEA

Options

a. Measurement of serum prolactin
b. Laparoscopy

c. Measurement of TSH levels
d. Measurement of Gonadotropin
e. Karyotyping
f. Progesterone challenge
g. Measurement of serum testosterone level
h. Skull radiography
i. Hysteroscopy
j. IV pyelography
k. Measurement Of HCG levels over 24 hours
l. Measurement of HCG levels over 1 week.

For each of the situations/conditions given below, choose the one most appropriate/discriminatory option from above. The option may be used once, more than once, or not at all.

Questions

34. A 22-year-old woman with previously normal menstrual cycles begins to have irregular anovulatory cycles. Serum prolactin levels are elevated.
35. A 23-year-old nulliparous stopped her OC pills to conceive. She has a menstrual flow after the last pack of contraceptive pills and then was amenorrhoea for 7 months.
36. A 25-year-old primi para returns 8 months after deliver complaining of amenorrhoea. Her pregnancy terminated with a caesarean section because of abruptio placenta and fetal distress with an estimated blood loss of 1500 ml from a transient coagulation problem.
37. A 27-year-old nulliparous presents with amenorrhoea. Pregnancy test is negative.
38. A 26-year-old woman presents with amenorrhoea for 7 weeks, vaginal spotting and mild right lower abdominal quadrant pain, her periods have always been irregular. On examination the uterus is of normal size and the right lower quadrant is tender. Her HCG levels the day before were 1100 MIU/ML.

THEME: 8
CAUSES OF AMENORRHOEA

Options

a. Drug side effect
b. Imperforate hymen
c. Likely to be premature menopause
d. Postpill amenorrhoea
e. Primary amenorrhoea

For each of the situations/conditions given below, choose the one most appropriate/discriminatory option from above. The option may be used once, more than once, or not at all.

Questions

39. A 34-year-old woman being treated for endometriosis.
40. A 32-year-old woman with a history of hot flushes.
41. A 14-year-old girl who is experiencing cyclical pelvic and vaginal pain but no period.
42. A 17-year-old girl who has had only withdrawal bleeds.
43. A 24-year-old woman has recently discontinued contraceptive precaution.

THEME: 8
CAUSES OF AMENORRHOEA

Options

a. Absent uterus
b. Constitutional
c. Imperforate hymen
d. Prolactinoma
e. Sheehan's syndrome
f. XO-karyotype

For each of the situations/conditions given below, choose the one most appropriate/discriminatory option from above. The option may be used once, more than once, or not at all.

Questions

44. A 16-year-old girl with normal secondary characteristics gives a history of cyclical abdominal pain.
45. An asymptomatic 17-year-old girl with normal secondary characteristics and normal endocrine results has a negative progesterone challenge test.
46. A 35-year-old woman had a normal vaginal delivery followed by a massive postpartum haemorrhage.
47. An 18-year-old woman has a short stature and absent secondary sexual characteristics.

THEME: 9
DIAGNOSIS OF AMENORRHOEA

Options

a. Anorexia nervosa
b. Complete androgen insensitivity
c. Hyperthyroidism
d. Hypogonadal hypogonadism
e. Hypothyroidism
f. Intrauterine synechiae
g. Menopause
h. Polycystic ovarian syndrome
i. Pregnancy
j. Premature ovarian failure
k. Prolactinoma
l. Turner's syndrome
m. Bulimia.

For each of the situations/conditions given below, choose the one most appropriate/discriminatory option from above. The option may be used once, more than once, or not at all.

Questions

48. A 18-year-old dancer presents with secondary amenorrhoea. On examination she is 1m 68 cm tall and weighs 46 kg.
49. A 34-year-old woman presents with an 8-month history of secondary amenorrhoea. On direct questioning she admits to a weight loss of 6 kg despite having a good appetite.

50. A 19-year-old woman presents with an 8-month history of secondary amenorrhoea. Prior to this her period have been irregular since menarche at the age of 12. Her BMI is 32.
51. A 33-year-old woman presents with a 7 – month history of amenorrhoea. She also complains of hot flushes, night sweats and mood swings.
52. A 17-year-old girl with secondary amenorrhoea, is reported to be binge eating. She has a BMI of 16 and is concerned that she is fat and goes to the gym 4 times a day!

THEME: 10
DIAGNOSIS OF INFERTILITY

Options

a. Polycystic ovary disease
b. Endometriosis
c. Adenomyosis
d. Chronic salpingitis
e. Diabetes mellitus
f. Hyperprolactinemia
g. Hypopititarism
h. Hyperthyroidism
i. Hypothyroidism
j. Pulmonary tuberculosis
k. Possible malignancy

For each of the situations/conditions given below, choose the one most appropriate/discriminatory option from above. The option may be used once, more than once, or not at all.

Questions

53. A 41-year-old woman complains of being unable to conceive for 2 years despite having regular unprotected sex. She complains of sweating all the time, frequent defecation and says this explains her loss in weight in recent weeks. She denied starving herself and says she has a very good appetite. HbA1c levels are 5%.
54. A 28-year-old woman complains of infertility for 3 years. She has a low libido and has put on a lot of weight. Her breast are discharging.

55. A 38-year-old complains of infertility and is otherwise healthy. She had been on Haloperidol treatment for schizophreniform illness for last 6 years. She has a healthy 3-year-old daughter.
56. A 31-year-old woman complains of abdominal pain, which seems to increase during her periods. Over the last year she has noticed difficulty in breathing and chest pain associated with occasional haemoptysis, following her periods. Her mother is asthmatic and she has eczema. She has been unable to conceive. On examination she is found to have an enlarge and tender uterus. Her BMI is just 20.

THEME: 11
TREATMENT OF INFERTILITY

Options

a. In vitro fertilization
b. Laparoscopy
c. Ethinyl estradiol from days 1-10
d. Salpingolysis
e. Human menopausal gonadotropins
f. Clomiphene citrate
g. Ligation of varicocoele
h. Artificial insemination from husband
i. Artificial insemination from donor semen

For each of the situations/conditions given below, choose the one most appropriate/discriminatory option from above. The option may be used once, more than once, or not at all.

Questions

57. The plasma progesterone level during the luteal phase of the cycle is absent suggestive that ovulation is not occurring FSH and LH levels are low.
58. The cervical mucus contact tests reveals aggulination of the sperm head to head
59. Sperm antibodies are also noted in the man's plasma.
60. The semen analysis reveals oligospermia. The husband also suffers from premature ejaculation. The wife has patent tubes and a normal uterus.

61. The post-coital test reveals absence of sperm. The husband has a past history of mumps and orchitis. The wife has patent tubes and a normal uterus.
62. A 35-year-old woman is found to have blocked and severely diseased tubes on laparoscopy. The uterus is normal.

THEME: 12
CAUSES OF VAGINAL DISCHARGE

Options

a. Trichomonaisis
b. Gardnerella
c. Chlamydia
d. Gonorrhea
e. Mycobacterium tuberculosis
f. HIV
g. Lymphogranuloma venereum
h. Treponema pallidum
i. Granuloma inguinale
j. Candida albicans
k. *Staphylococci aureus*

For each of the situations/conditions given below, choose the one most appropriate/discriminatory option from above. The option may be used once, more than once, or not at all.

Questions

63. A 22-year-old woman presents with intensely irritating yellowish-green frothy vaginal discharge with severe dyspareunia. The organism is seen best under microscope in a drop of saline.
64. A 30-year-old pregnant woman presents with thick white vaginal discharge associated with irritation of the vulva.
65. A 16-year-old girl who uses tampons presents with cervicitis, urethritis and right knee pain.
66. A 28-year-old woman presents with acute right upper quadrant abdominal pain and watery vaginal discharge. The organism is detected by microimmunoflurescence

67. A 23-year-old woman presents with fishy smelling vaginal odour. Clue cells are found in the smear.

THEME: 13
DIAGNOSIS OF A VAGINAL DISCHARGE

Options

a. Bacterial vaginosis
b. Herpes simplex virus
c. Syphlis
d. Chlamydial pelvic infection
e. Gonorrhea
f. Lymphogranuloma Inguinale
g. Candidiasis
h. Trichomonas Vaginalis
i. Scabies
j. Cervical erosion
k. Endometrial carcinoma
l. Cervical carcinoma

For each of the situations/conditions given below, choose the one most appropriate/discriminatory option from above. The options may be used once, more than once, or not at all.

Questions

68. A 39-year-old woman presents with a malodorous discharge .A wet smear shows 'clue cells'.
69. A 28-year-old woman presents with a white curdy discharge from her vagina. Wet smear shows mycelium growth.
70. A 32-year-old woman presents with painful shallow ulcers around the vulva and an offensive discharge and deep dyspaerunia. She has no gonorrhea.
71. A 28-year-old woman presents with lower abdominal pain, an offensive discharge and deep dyspaerunia.She has no gonorrhea.
72. A 31-year-old woman complains of a chronic nonfoul smelling discharge.She bleeds after sexual intercourse.

THEME: 14
MANAGEMENT OF VAGINAL DISCHARGE

Options

a. Metronidazole.
b. Candid pessary.
c. Oral fluconazole.
d. Augmentin.
e. Dosycycline.
f. Penicillin.
g. Reassure.
h. Tetracycline.
i. Estrogen cream.
j. Vinegar douch.
k. Sulfonamide vaginal cream.

For each of the situations/conditions given below, choose the one most appropriate/discriminatory option from above. The options may be used once, more than once, or not at all.

Questions

73. A woman states that she has been on ampicillin for a week because of urinary tract infection. Upon completing the antibiotics, she noted a thick white vaginal discharge with severe vulvar itching.
74. A patient states that she has a malodorous discharge and intense itching. She adds that her partner also has a slight discharge. Pelvic examination, reveals "strawberry spots" on the cervix.
75. A patient complains of a watery, malodorous discharge with very little itching or burning. A wet mount preparation in saline of the vaginal secretion reveals "clue cells".
76. A 35-year-old lady underwent LSCS 6 months ago. The baby weighed 4.0 kg. Since then she c/o curdy white vaginal discharge.
77. A 29-year-old lady presents to the gyne clinic with history of greyish green colored discharged which has fishy odour.

THEME: 15
DIAGNOSIS OF PELVIC PAIN

Options

a. Urinary tract infection.
b. Twisted ovarian cyst.
c. Ectopic pregnancy.
d. Incomplete miscarriage.
e. Ovulatory pain.
f. Musculoskeletal pain.
g. Endometriosis.
h. Fibroids.
i. PID.
j. Ovarian tumor.
k. Adenomyosis.
l. Ovarian abscess.
m. Corpus luteum hemorrhage.
n. Appendicitis.
o. Cholecystitis.
p. Heterotopic pregnancy.
q. Threatened abortion.

For each of the situations/conditions given below, choose the one most appropriate/discriminatory option from above. The options may be used once, more than once, or not at all.

Questions

78. A 28-year-old woman complains of continuous dull lower abdominal pain. Her last menstrual period (LMP) was 3 weeks age. She feels sick and has no vaginal bleeding. She gives history of similar episodes in the past for which she was given antibiotics.
79. A 23-year-old woman with regular periods and dysmenorrhea. PV findings show tenderness with fixity of uterus in the pouch of Dougles. She has been trying for a baby with her boy friend from 2 years without success.
80. A 34-year-old woman presents with severe right-sided abdominal pain which started suddenly. She feels sick and has noticed some spotting. She gives history of feeling faint and also some discomfort in her shoulders.

81. A 25-year-old lady complains of 20 weeks amenorrhea and pain in her abdomen, mainly in the right hypochondrium. She has a mild temperature but is not feeling too well.
82. A 35-year-old woman presents with lower abdominal pain that started since she returned from shopping. Her LMP was 6 weeks ago and her cycles are of irregular lengths. She does not feel faint and the pain is better since she took some painkillers.
83. A 25-year-old woman whose last menses were 6 weeks ago presents with acute left lower quadrant pain. Serum human chorionic gonadotropin (HCG) beta-subunit levels are positive. Pelvic ultrasound reveals no sac in the uterus and a 3 × 3 cm left adnexal mass.
84. A 30-year-old woman whose last menses were 8 weeks ago presents with heavy vaginal bleeding and lower left quadrant pain. Serum HCG Beta-subunit levels are low for dates. Pelvic ultrasound reveals an intrauterine sac without fetal parts.
85. A 38-year-old woman presents to the gynecology clinic with long standing lower abdominal pain. Painkillers do not seem to help. Her last menstrual period (LMP) was 6 weeks ago and her cycles are of varying lengths. Pain tends to be worse for few days before her periods.
86. 29-year-old woman presents with bleeding per vagina. She gives history of passing clots. Now she is also having lower abdominal pain. Her LMP was 6 weeks ago. Her pulse rate is 110/min and BP 90/60 ands she feels faint.
87. 44-year-old woman has heavy painful periods, has an enlarged uterus which is tender on palpation. Fornices do not show any masses though the right ovary is palpable.
88. This woman with 6 weeks amenorrhea, c/o pain in the abdomen making her feel faint, has pain in her shoulder tips especially when she lies down. Urinary pregnancy test is positive and scan shows hyperechoeic area high in the endometrial cavity with suggestion of fetal heart movements.
89. A 32-year-old woman presents with sudden onset of severe abdominal pain. She feels sick and has vomited few times. The pain is not relieved by analgesics. Her pulse

rate is 110/min and BP 90/60. Her LMP was 4 weeks ago and there is no vaginal bleeding.

90. A 31-year-old woman has stopped taking OC pills for 1 year. Since last 8 months she complains of lower abdominal pain. The pain lasts for about two days. Her last menstrual period (LMP) was 2 weeks ago and she gas regular 28-day cycles.
91. A 35-year-old woman whose last menses were 6 weeks ago presents with acute lower left quadrant pain but no vaginal bleeding. Serum HCG beta-subunit levels are appropriate for dates. Culdocentesis reveals non-clotting blood. There is a tender left 3 × 4 cm adnexal mass on pelvic examination,. Pelvic ultrasound reveals no gestational sac in the uterus.

THEME: 16
INVESTIGATIONS FOR LOWER ABDOMINAL PAIN

Options

a. Urine pregnancy test.
b. Serial BHCG.
c. TVS.
d. FBC.
e. Group and save.
f. Group and crossmatch.
g. Cervical smear.

For each of the situations/conditions given below, choose the one most appropriate/discriminatory option from above. The options may be used once, more than once, or not at all.

Questions

92. 31-year-old lady presents with left sided lower abdominal pain and history of fainting attacks. On examination, P-92/min, BP 100/70, abdomen – non-tender, soft. Vaginal examination - non-conclusive. UPT - + ve.
93. 28-year-old lady was admitted unconscious with ectopic pregnancy is now 2 days post surgery. She feels light headed and giddy. Pulse- 106/min, BP – 90/60, abdomen – soft, non-tender.

94. A 26-year-old lady presents with right sided lower abdominal pain. On examination, P – 80/min, BP – 110/80. Lower abdomen soft, non-tender. UPT +ve shows no e/o pregnancy. She has been admitted for observation.
95. A 38-year-old presents with left sided lower abdominal pain and sickness. On examination, the left side is tender. Pulse – 80/min, BP – 120/80.

THEME: 17
DIFFERENTIAL DIAGNOSIS OF ECTOPIC PREGNANCY

Options

a. Appendicitis
b. Bacterial vaginosis
c. Crohn's disease
d. Ectopic pregnancy
e. Endometriosis
f. Inevitable miscarriage
g. Irritable bowel syndrome
h. Missed abortion
i. Normal pregnancy
j. Pelvic inflammatory disease
k. Renal colic
l. Septic abortion
m. Threatened miscarriage
n. Torsion of ovarian cyst
o. Ulcerative colitis

For each of the situations/conditions given below, choose the one most appropriate/discriminatory option from above. The option may be used once, more than once, or not at all.

Questions

96. A 21-year-old woman presents as an emergency with a 4 hr history of abdominal pain and bright red vaginal blood loss. She has not had a menstrual period for 9 weeks and had a home pregnancy test 1 week ago. On vaginal examination the uterus is tender and bulky. The cervical is open.

97. A 16-year-old woman presents with a sudden onset of severe iliac fossa pain. On vaginal ultrasound examination a 6 cm diameter echogenic cystic mass is seen in right fornix.
98. An 18-year-old student due to take her examination reports that she missed her period and that a pregnancy test is negative. She has worsening abdominal pain, which has been troublesome for 3 months. She is otherwise well.
99. A 22-year-old woman who has had 2 terminations of pregnancy, reports that she is pregnant again. She has noticed a small amount of watery brown discharge and is tender in right iliac fossa.
100. A 27-year-old who conscientiously uses OC pill has experienced intermittent breakthrough vaginal bleeding and malodorous discharge for several weeks. When examined she has pain over the lower abdomen, worse on the left. Her temperature is 39°C and her white cell count is elevated.

THEME: 18
DIAGNOSIS OF PAINFUL INTERCOURSE

Options

a. Genital herpes
b. Human papilloma virus
c. Chancroid
d. Candidiasis
e. Chlamydia trachomatis
f. Prostatis
g. Syphilis
h. *E. coli*
i. Molluscum contagiosum
j. Donovanosis
k. Gardnerella
l. Gonorrhea

For each of the situations/conditions given below, choose the one most appropriate/discriminatory option from above. The option may be used once, more than once, or not at all.

Questions

101. A young woman complains of painful intercourse. She has a mild vaginal discharge and a burning sensation when passing urine.
102. A 28-year-old woman say she finds intercourse painful. She has a vaginal discharge, which is foul smelling.
103. A 33-year-old woman says she must leave off with intercourse because of intense pain. She has a fever, headache, and is generally unwell. On examination you find inguinal lymphedenopathy and small painful genital ulcers.
104. A 45-year-old man presents with pain during intercourse. He says the pain is sharp and stabbing from the tip of the penis. He also complains of a pelvic ache and burning sensation.
105. A young woman complains of painful intercourse. There is mild degree of vaginal pain, but it lies deep within the pelvis and worse with penetration. There are no other symptoms or signs.

THEME: 19
CAUSES OF PELVIC INFLAMMATORY DISEASE

Options

a. *Staphylococcus aureus*
b. Gonococcus
c. Chlamydia trachomatis
d. *E. coli*
e. Actinomyces israelii
f. Mycobacterium tuberculosis

For each of the situations/conditions given below, choose the one most appropriate/discriminatory option from above. The option may be used once, more than once, or not at all.

Questions

106. A 24-year-old sexually active girl with lower abdominal pain.

107. A 42-year-old has had chronic pelvic inflammatory disease and tubo-ovarian abscess has recently been removed.
108. A 30-year-old lady who has an intrauterine device presents with lower abdominal pain.
109. A 25-year-old woman with very mild abdominal pain; laparoscopy reveals a severe inflammatory process.
110. A teenage girl presents with septic shock.

THEME: 20
MANAGEMENT OF DYSFUNCTION UTERINE BLEEDING

Options

a. Hysterectomy
b. Clomiphene citrate
c. Oral contraceptives
d. Measure progesterone level on day 21
e. Pipelle endometrial sampling
f. Ethinyl estradiol
g. Mefanamic acid
h. Provera
i. Hysteroscopy

For each of the situations/conditions given below, choose the one most appropriate/discriminatory option from above. The option may be used once, more than once, or not at all.

Questions

111. A 25-year-old married woman presents with irregular cycles and menorhagia. She would not like to start a family yet.
112. A 50-year-old woman presents with abnormal uterine bleeding.
113. A 14-year-old female complains of heavy periods and pain. She is not sexually active.
114. A 35-year-old married woman presents with intermenstrual spotting. She would like to conceive.

115. A 33-year-old married woman presents with intermenstrual bleeding that is not controlled with oral contraceptives.

THEME: 21
INVESTIGATION OF POSTMENOPAUSAL BLEEDING

Options

a. Full blood count
b. None of the above
c. Pipelle biopsy
d. Referral to gynaecology clinic
e. Transvaginal ultrasound scan
f. Vulval biopsy

For each of the situations/conditions given below, choose the one most appropriate/discriminatory option from above. The option may be used once, more than once, or not at all.

Questions

116. Postmenopausal woman complaining of pruritus vulvae.
117. A 50-year-old woman on cyclical hormone replacement therapy complains of irregular vaginal bleeding.
118. An episode of vaginal bleeding ten years after the menopause.
119. A 60-year-old woman complaining of labial ulceration and bleeding.
120. Is of little value in the management of postmenopausal bleeding.

THEME: 22
TREATMENT OF DYSMENORRHOEA

Options

a. Laser treatment at laparoscopy
b. Danazol
c. Oral contraceptive
d. Mefenamic acid
e. Gonadotropin release hormone agonist

f. Total abdominal hysterectomy
g. No treatment
h. Pelvic sympathectomy
i. Laparotomy

For each of the situations/conditions given below, choose the one most appropriate/discriminatory option from above. The option may be used once, more than once, or not at all.

Questions

121. A 30-year-old woman complains of painful periods and pain during intercourse. She is afebrile and has a firm, tender nodule into the pouch of Douglas. Small foci of endometriosis are found at the time of laparoscopy.
122. A 28-year-old woman is diagnosed with endometriosis. Her symptoms are not incapacitating. She would like to start a family.
123. A 45-year-old woman complains of intractable dysmenorrhoea and menorrhagia. She doesn't want any more children.
124. A 40-year-old woman is diagnosed with endometriosis. The pain is severe and she refuses surgical treatment. She doesn't want any more children.
125. A 20-year-old woman presents with severe left lower abdominal pain, increasing abdominal girth, painful periods and menorrhagiua. USG demonstrates a 20 cm left ovarian cyst.

THEME: 23
MANAGEMENT OF ENDOMETRIOSIS

Options

a. Danazol therapy
b. Estrogen replacement therapy
c. Expectant management
d. Methotrexate
e. Conservative endometriosis surgery
f. GnRH agonists
g. Progestrogens
h. Cylic oral contraceptives

i. NSAIDS
j. Radical endometriosis surgery

For each of the situations/conditions given below, choose the one most appropriate/discriminatory option from above. The option may be used once, more than once, or not at all.

Questions

126. A 27-year-old journalist presents with an established diagnosis of mild endometriosis. She states that she wants to travel for 3 years before considering pregnancy.
127. A 23-year-old woman presents with a 7-month history of infertility. Diagnostic laparoscopy shows evidence of mild endometriosis with scattered cul-de sac implants. She has no other infertility factors.
128. A 33-year-old computer programmer presents with a 4-year history of infertility. A laporoscopic diagnosis of moderate endometriosis is made. Scattered endometrial implants in the pelvis, a 1cm endometrioma on the right ovary and adhesion between the tube and ovary on each side are found.
129. A 37-year-old woman has just undergone radical endometriosis surgery.
130. A 36-year-old woman completed her treatment for endometriosis 6 months ago. During treatment she suffered from bouts of depression, weight gain and metrorrhagia, but there was no dyspareunia. She now complains of amenorrhoea.
131. A 22-year-old student is diagnosed with mild endometriosis and dysmenorrhoea.

THEME: 24
CERVICAL SCREENING

Options

a. Repeat smear.
b. Colposcopy.
c. Colposcopy and biopsy.
d. Repeat smear in 6 months.

e. Follow-up smear in 6 months.
f. Repeat smear in 1 year.
g. Repeat smear in 3 years.
h. Hysterectomy.
i. Radical hysterectomy.
j. Radiotherapy.
k. Cervical conisation.

For each of the situations/conditions given below, choose the one most appropriate/discriminatory option from above. The options may be used once, more than once, or not at all.

Questions

132. Unsatisfactory smear.
133. Mild dyskaryosis.
134. Moderate dyskaryosis.
135. Severe dyskaryosis.
136. Microinvasive.

THEME: 25
INVESTIGATIONS FOR SUSPECTED MALIGNANT DISEASE IN GYNAECOLOGY

Options

a. CT abdomen and pelvis
b. Cytology
c. D and C alone
d. Diagnostic laparoscopy
e. Examination under anaesthesia and representative biopsies
f. Hysteroscopy alone
g. Hsteroscopy and D and C
h. Pelvic ultrasound scan

For each of the situations/conditions given below, choose the one most appropriate/discriminatory option from above. The option may be used once, more than once, or not at all.

Questions

137. A 65-year-old obese, diabetic and hypertensive woman presents with two recent episodes of postmenopausal bleeding.

138. A 59-year-old woman noticed loss of appetite, constipation and a swollen abdomen. She had a pelvic ultrasound scan which showed cystic ovaries.
139. A 38-year-old woman attends for a smear test 10 years after the previous one. On speculum examination the cervix looks irregular in shape and bleeds easily of touch.

THEME: 26
DIAGNOSTIC TESTS IN CANCER

Options

a. Diagnostic curettage.
b. Fractional curettage.
c. Hysteroscopy and directed biopsy.
d. Edge biopsy.
e. Excision biopsy.
f. Wedge biopsy.
g. Brush biopsy.
h. Cytology.
i. Cervical smear.
j. Colposcopy.
k. Cone biopsy.
l. Laparoscopy and biopsy.
m. Laparotomy.
n. U/S scan.
o. Serum AFP.
p. Serum HCG.

For each of the situations/conditions given below, choose the one most appropriate/discriminatory option from above. The options may be used once, more than once, or not at all.

Questions

140. A 70-year-old woman complains of pruritis vulvae and discharge per vaginum. She has noticed a lump on her labia majora.
141. A 40-year-old woman with 5 children and history of tubal ligation complains of bleeding PV following intercourse. She also has continuous bleeding since last 10 days. Her cervical smears done a month ago showed severe dyskaryotosis.

142. 60-year-old woman complains of bleeding PV for the last 2 months. She has one child and had received treatment for breast cancer 10 years ago.
143. 30-year-old woman has had treatment for hydatidiform mole 2 years ago and now c/o bleeding per vaginum and her pregnancy test was positive.
144. 24-year-old woman has a lump in her abdomen. Scan showed a solid tumor, 20 cm in diameter.

THEME: 27
DIAGNOSIS OF OVARIAN TUMORS

Options

a. Gonadoblastoma.
b. Dysgerminoma.
c. Immature teratoma.
d. Solid teratoma.
e. Dermoid cyst.
f. Serous cystoadenocarcinoma.
g. Clear-cell tumor.
h. Granulosa cell tumor.
i. Mucinous cystoadenocarcinoma.
j. Kruckenberg's tumor.
k. Brenner's tumor.
l. Ovarian fibroid.

For each of the situations/conditions given below, choose the one most appropriate/discriminatory option from above. The options may be used once, more than once, or not at all.

Questions

145. 26-year-old patient was found to have an acute abdomen. She is 20 weeks pregnant. Scan showed a single ovarian cyst 10 × 14 cm in size, with an area of echodensity. She needed emergency operation for this condition.
146. This cystic lesion was found in a 55-year-old post-menopausal woman who was bleeding PV for a few days. The tumor was unilateral and found to be lined with cylindrical cells with coffee bean appearance.

147. Predominantly found in persons with genetic abnormalities.
148. Often includes tissue.
149. Most cases of malignant transformation are found in postmenopausal women.
150. Highly radiosensitive tumor.
151. May be associated with a syndrome of hemolytic anemia.
152. This solid tumor was found in a 20-year-old woman. The tumor is typical encapsulated, fragile, yellow in color and was managed by chemotherapy.
153. A 38-year-old woman presented with ascitis and difficulty in breathing. Scan showed a small solid tumor on the one ovary and clear ascitis. Removal of the tumor cured the ascitis and her symptoms.

THEME: 28
DIAGNOSIS OF OVARIAN TUMORS

Options

a. Mucinous cystadenoma
b. Corpus luteum cysts
c. Endometrial cysts
d. Teratoma
e. Primary ovarian carcinoma
f. Serous cystadenoma
g. Retention cysts
h. Arrhenoblastoma
i. Ovarian fibroma
j. Theca cell tumour
k. Polycystic ovaries

For each of the situations/conditions given below, choose the one most appropriate/discriminatory option from above. The option may be used once, more than once, or not at all.

Questions

154. The most common virilizing tumor of the ovary. Secretes androgens.
155. Large multicavity ovarian cyst, filled with thick fluid. It may reach a huge size occupying the whole peritoneal cavity.

156. Single cavity ovarian cyst, filled with watery fluid. Often bilateral. Potentially malignant.
157. Small, solid and hard, white benign tumor. Usually unilateral. May be associated with ascites and pleural effusion.
158. May contain sebaceous fluid, hair and teeth. May be benign or malignant.
159. Causes excessive estrogen production. May occur at any age causing precocious puberty in children, metrorrhagia in adults and postmenopausal bleeding in older women.

THEME: 29
PRINCIPAL MANAGEMENT OF CANCERS

Options

a. Surgery.
b. Radiotherapy.
c. Chemotherapy.
d. None of the above.

For each of the situations/conditions given below, choose the one most appropriate/discriminatory option from above. The options may be used once, more than once, or not at all.

Questions

160. Carcinoma vulva.
161. Carcinoma vagina.
162. Carcinoma cervix.
163. Carcinoma ovary.
164. Carcinoma endometrium.

THEME: 30
DIAGNOSIS IN GYNAECOLOGY

Options

a. Cancer of the endometrium
b. Irratable bowel syndrome
c. Ovarian cancer
d. Pelvic endometriosis

e. Pelvic inflammatory disease
f. Ruptured ovarian cyst
g. Torsion of an ovarian cyst

For each of the situations/conditions given below, choose the one most appropriate/discriminatory option from above. The option may be used once, more than once, or not at all.

Questions

165. An 18-year-old woman who is not sexually active presents at midcycle with acute onset of lower abdominal pain, which resolves 6 hours after admission.
166. A 24-year-old woman in a stable relationship presents in the clinic with a one year history of lower abdominal pain, deep dyspareunia and an inability to conceive.
167. A 49-year-old woman noticed an increase in abdominal girth alongside with constipation and weight loss.
168. A 23-year-old woman had a diagnostic laparoscopy for recurrent lower abdominal pain, which showed normal pelvic organs. High vaginal swab and endocervical swabs were negative.

THEME: 31
TREATMENT OF GYNAECOLOGICAL CONDITIONS

Options

a. Laparoscopy
b. Colposcopy
c. Suction curettage
d. Postcoital pill
e. IV antibiotics
f. Total abdominal hysterectomy with bilateral salpingo oopherectomy
g. Urgent resuscitation and laparotomy
h. PAP smear
i. Hysterectomy alone
j. Excision with diathermy
k. 5-flourouracil
l. Myomectomy
m. Cone biopsy

For each of the situations/conditions given below, choose the one most appropriate/discriminatory option from above. The option may be used once, more than once, or not at all.

Questions

169. A 28-year-old woman is noted to have an abdominal cervical smear that demonstrates condyloma accuminata.
170. A 20-year-old woman presents to the casualty with severe right-sided abdominal pain and left shoulder pain. She stopped taking the pill 2 months ago and has not menstruated since. Her BP is 90/50 and her pulse is 120/min.
171. An 18-year-old primigravida of 12 weeks gestation would like to terminate her pregnancy.
172. A 30-year-old nulliparous woman complains of infertility. She has regular periods that are heavy and last for 8 days. She and her husband have been trying to conceive for over a year now. Her husband has seen an urologist and has been cleared, and she now wonders if she is at fault. Her ovulation test is normal USG reveals uterine fibroids.
173. A 70-year-old woman presents with a 3-month history of vaginal bleeding. Pipelle endometrial sampling and curettage reveal adenocarcinoma.

THEME: 33
DIAGNOSIS OF GYNECOLOGICAL CONDITIONS

Options

a. Follicular cyst.
b. Lesion of the infundibular stalk.
c. Trophoblastic tumor with a 46 XX chromosome pattern.
d. Idiopathic hirsutism.
e. Choriocarcinoma.
f. Weight loss syndrome.
g. Mucinous cystadenoma.

For each of the situations/conditions given below, choose the one most appropriate/discriminatory option from above. The options may be used once, more than once, or not at all.

Questions

174. A 20-year-old woman is competing in long distance running for the olympics. She has been amenorrhic for last 4 months. Her periods prior to her athletic training were regular. Her physical examination, is normal. The serum prolactin and TSH levels are normal. Serum FSH is slightly decreased. The serum beta-HCG is negative. She does not have withdrawal bleeding after being given progesterones.
175. A 24-year-old woman with history of recurrent right lower quadrant pain has a palpable right ovarian mass. An ultrasound of the abdomen confirms the presence of a cystic mass of the ovary. No calcifications noted.
176. Laboratory analysis of an eutypic female patient reveals decreased plasma levels of FSH and LH, but an increased plasma prolactin level. The systemic administration of GnRH results in an increased plasma level of LH and FSH.
177. A 22-year-old asian woman in her first trimester has a uterus that is too large for gestational age. An ultrasound exhibits a "Snow storm appearance" and absence of a fetus in the uterine cavity.
178. A woman with mild hirsutism has a normal total testosterone level, increased free testosterone level, normal DHEA-S, and normal urine for 17-ketosteriods.

THEME: 34
DIAGNOSIS OF VAGINAL BLEEDING

Options

a. Cervical carcinoma
b. Vulval carcinoma
c. Cervical ectorpion
d. Endometrial carcinoma
e. Endometriosis
f. Ectopic pregnancy
g. Ovarian carcinoma
h. Menopause
i. Hyperthyroidism
j. Rhesus incompatibility

k. Von Willebrand's disease
l. Pelvic inflammatory disease
m. Pelvic adhesions

For each of the situations/conditions given below, choose the one most appropriate/discriminatory option from above. The option may be used once, more than once, or not at all.

Questions

179. A 50-year-old woman presents with a 9-month history of prolonged, slightly irregular periods. Clinical examination shows a normal size uterus with no adnexal masses.
180. A 31-year-old nulliparous woman with a history of cyclical pelvic pain, complains of heavy and frequent periods. On vaginal examination a fixed retroverted uterus is found.
181. A 53-year-old woman has had a history of offensive vaginal discharge and intermittent vaginal bleeding over the past 3 months. Her husband died of carcinoma of the penis.
182. A 46-year-old woman who has breast cancer and is on Tamoxifen has had 2 episodes of bright red bleeding. Her last period was when she started Tamoxifen 2 years ago.
183. A 22-year-old woman with a 6-week history of amenorrhoea presents to A&E with vaginal bleeding. An ultrasound shows "empty uterus".
184. An obese 55-year-old woman presents with per vaginal bleeding associated with watery nonfoul smelling discharge. She is nulliparous. Her mother and father died of carcinoma colon.

THEME: 35
TREATMENT OF MENOPAUSAL SYMPTOMS

Options

a. Clonidine
b. Combined HRT
c. Hypnotic preparations
d. Mineral supplements
e. Oestrogen only HRT

f. Psychological support
g. Referral to psychiatrist
h. Regular exercise
i. Vaginal lubricant
j. Vaginal estrogens

For each of the situations/conditions given below, choose the one most appropriate/discriminatory option from above. The option may be used once, more than once, or not at all.

Questions

185. A 59-year-old woman whose periods stopped 5 year ago becomes increasingly depressed. She now feels life is no longer worth living and threatens suicide.
186. A 72-year-old woman has experienced of micturation intermittently for the last few months. Midstream urine cultures have been persistently negative. She is otherwise well, but would like her symptoms to be resolved.
187. A married 52-year-old woman who has a family history of breast cancer has been experiencing mild discomfort for a few hours following intercourse for last month. She is worried about using hormones.
188. A 45-year-old woman who has had a total abdominal hysterectomy and bilateral salingo oopherectomy for fibroids and menorrhagia complains of hot flushes, night sweats and mood swings. She has no other medical problems.

THEME: 36
CAUSES OF PELVIC INFLAMMATORY DISEASE

Options

a. Chlamydia.
b. Streptococcus.
c. Anaerobes.
d. Tuberculosis.
e. Actinomyces.

For each of the situations/conditions given below, choose the one most appropriate/discriminatory option from above. The options may be used once, more than once, or not at all.

Questions

189. Blood borne infection.
190. Follows instrumentation.
191. Sexually acquired.
192. Follow IUCD insertion.

THEME: 37
INVESTIGATIONS FOR INFERTILITY

Options

a. Hysterosalpingo graphy.
b. MRI.
c. Serum LH/FSH.
d. Laparoscopy and dye.
e. Basal body temperature.
f. Hysteroscopy.
g. CT scan.
h. Semen analysis.
i. Serum oestrogen.
j. Serum prolactin.

For each of the situations/conditions given below, choose the one most appropriate/discriminatory option from above. The options may be used once, more than once, or not at all.

Questions

193. Male 25-year, female 23-year, infertility for 3-year cycles 4/20-25, irregular and painless. C/O occasional discharge from the nipple. BMI 32 and has excessive hair growth on her face.
194. Male and female both 35-year with infertility for 5-year Cycles 4/27 regular. BMI 29. The man has had a surgery for hernia in the past.
195. Male 31-year, female 24-year with infertility of 2-year. BMI 26. Cycles 4/33 regular, normal has dysmenorrhea, c/o excessive hair growth on her arms compared to her friends. Has been treated for chlamydia in the past. Male has no significant history.

196. Male 30-year, female 32-year, infertility for 5-year. Cycles 4/30, with dysmenorrhea. They had a child 5-year ago, without any problem. HSG normal. Semen analysis is normal.

THEME: 38
DIAGNOSIS OF POSTMENOPAUSAL BLEEDING

Options

a. Endometrial cancer.
b. Endometrial polyp.
c. Atrophic vaginitis.
d. HRT.
e. Cervical cancer.

For each of the situations/conditions given below, choose the one most appropriate/discriminatory option from above. The options may be used once, more than once, or not at all.

Questions

197. A 76-year-old lady presents to the gyne clinic with history of dryness in the vagina. Intercourses are very uncomfortable and occasionally she bleeds after that.
198. A 58-year-old lady presents to the gyne clinic with history of copious offensive blood stained discharge. She gives history of cervical conisation for abnormal smears, 8 years ago.
199. A 78-year-old lady presents to the gynecology clinic with history of spotting. She also gives history of offensive blood stained vaginal discharge. She is taking HRT. On examination, the uterus is 6 weeks size and there is no other abnormality. Her smears have been done regularly and were normal.
200. A 88-year-old lady referred by her GP because of bleeding. She gives history of occasional non-offensive white discharge. On examination, there is no abnormality.
201. A 60-year-old lady presents to the gyne clinic with history of minimal, but irregular bleeding. She is on HRT since 6 months. On examination apart from minimal cystocele, there is no obvious abnormality.

THEME: 39
CAUSES OF VAGINAL BLEEDING

Options

a. Normal menstruation
b. Cervical polyps
c. Cervical carcinoma
d. Cervical ectropion
e. Atrophic vaginitis
f. Endometrial carcinoma
g. Exogenous estrogens
h. Ectopic pregnancy
i. Spontaneous abortion
j. Bleeding disorder
k. Foreign body

For each of the situations/conditions given below, choose the one most appropriate/discriminatory option from above. The option may be used once, more than once, or not at all.

Questions

202. A 20-year-old has a very heavy period and passes several clots. Her last period was 45 days ago. She normally has a regular 30 day cycle with light periods. She is otherwise well.
203. A 22-year-old woman has been on the OC pill for 6 months. She has developed intermenstrual and postcoital bleeding. Speculum examination show visible part of cervix to be red.
204. A 78-year-old woman who had treatment for uterine prolapse. She has recently developed vaginal bleeding which is increasing in severity. She is frail but otherwise well. Uterine curettage reveals no histological abnormality.
205. A 34-year-old woman present with dark vaginal bleeding. Prior to this she has had colicky left sided pain for days. She has a history of pelvic inflammatory disease and irregular periods.

206. A 55-year-old postmenopausal woman has developed post-coital bleeding. She also describes dyspareunia and urinary stress incontinence.

THEME: 40
INVESTIGATION OF VAGINAL BLEEDING

Options

a. Cervical inspection
b. Cervical smear
c. Endocervical swab
d. Endometrial sampling
e. Full blood count
f. Gonadotrophin levels
g. Hysteroscopy
h. Kleihauer count (fetal cells in maternal circulation)
i. Pregnancy test
j. Thyroid function tests
k. Ultrasound scan

For each of the situations/conditions given below, choose the one most appropriate/discriminatory option from above. The options may be used once, more than once, or not at all.

Questions

207. A 52-year-old woman has had a history of offensive vaginal discharge and intermittent vaginal bleeding over past three months. Her last cervical smear was taken four years ago.
208. A 23-year-old woman has a new sexual partner .She has been on combined oral contraceptive pill for the last six years.She presents with a two month history of breakthrough bleeding.
209. A 47-year-old woman who has breast cancer and is on Tamoxifen has two episodes of bright bleeding. Her last period was when she started Tamoxifen two years ago.
210. A 26-year-old woman with a six week history of amenorrhoea presents to the A&E dept. with vaginal blleeding, ultrasound scan report shows an empty uterus

211. A 49-year-old woman presents with a nine month history of prolonged, slightly irregular periods. Clinical examination shows a normal size uterus with no adnexal masses.

THEME : 41
MANAGEMENT OF TROPHOBLASTIC DISEASE

Options

a. Chemotherapy.
b. Hysterectomy.
c. Chemotherapy and hysterectomy.
d. Suction dilatation and evacuation.
e. Suction dilatation and curettage.
f. No treatment.

For each of the situations/conditions given below, choose the one most appropriate/discriminatory option from above. The options may be used once, more than once, or not at all.

Questions

212. A 20-year-old nullipara presents with irregular vaginal bleeding. She gives a history of abortion at 3 months, last year. On investigating. Her beat HCG levels are high but her chest X-ray, abdominal scan and pelvic examination is normal. Dilation and curettage revealed gestational trophoblastic neoplasia.
213. A 30-year-old multigravida comes with uterine bleeding and raised HCG titres. She gives a history of therapeutic abortion and tubal ligation 3 months back. Her pelvic examination, pelvic scan and chest X-ray are normal. Dilation and curettage revealed gestational trophoblastic neoplasm.
214. A 43-year-old grand multipara who had a tubal ligatation test year comes 12 weeks after her last menstrual period with complaints of vaginal bleeding. On examination, her uterus is enlarged to the level of the umbilicus and very light HCG titres. Flat plate of the abdomen reveals no fetal skeketon. ultrasound reveals no gestational sac or fetus.

THEME: 42
MANAGEMENT OF ENDOMETRIOSIS

Options

a. Expectant management.
b. Danazol therapy.
c. Conservative endometriosis surgery.
d. Cyclic oral contraceptives.
e. Radical endometriosis surgery.
f. Goserelin.
g. Progesterone.

For each of the situations/conditions given below, choose the one most appropriate/discriminatory option from above. The options may be used once, more than once, or not at all.

Questions

215. A 26-year-old medical student presents with an established diagnosis of mild endometriosis. She states that she wants to finish a residency program before even thinking of a pregnancy.
216. A 24-year-old woman presents with a 6 months history of infertility. A laparoscopic diagnosis of mild endometriosis with scattered cul-de-sac implants is made. There are no other infertility factors involved with this woman.
217. A 32-year-old lawyer presents with a 5 year history of infertility. A laparoscopic diagnosis of moderate endometriosis is made. Scattered endometrial implants in the pelvis, a 2 cm endometrioma on the left ovary, and adhesions between the tube and ovary on each side are found.
218. Suppresses ovulation.
219. Pseudo pregnancy.
220. Pseudo menopause.

THEME: 43
MANAGEMENT OF UTERINE FIBROIDS

Options

a. Oral iron therapy.
b. Hormone suppression.

c. Dilatation and curettage.
d. Myomectomy.
e. Hysterectomy.

For each of the situations/conditions given below, choose the one most appropriate/discriminatory option from above. The options may be used once, more than once, or not at all.

Questions

221. 47-year-old lady came with vague lower abdominal pain. Routine ultrasound revealed a small fundal fibroid. In examination, she was found to have mild pallor.
222. A 50-year-old woman with a known myomatous uterus presents with the complaint of irregular bleeding. She states that her menses are heavy and occur every 5-6 weeks. She also mentions that she has had 5-7 days of intermenstrual spotting over the past three cycles.
223. A 32-year-old black woman with known myomas returns to the office after 3 years, complaining of mild left lower quadrant pain. Three years ago she had a tubal ligation. Physical examination reveals a 14-week, irregular uterus with an apparent 4 cm left fundal myoma.
224. A 28-year-old primipara presents with a 14 week uterine mass, pain and hypermenorrhea. On physical examination, she has a prominent posterior fundal mass, which seems to make up the bulk of the uterine mass.

THEME: 44
THE MANAGEMENT OF MENOPAUSAL SYMPTOMS

Options

a. Transdermal oestrogen patch
b. Raloxifene
c. Oestrogen implants
d. Oestrogen pessaries
e. Thyroid function tests
f. Vaginal lubricant
g. Regular exercise
h. Prophylactic hormone replacement therapy

i. Endometrial sampling
j. Cervical inspection
k. Cervical smears
l. High protein diet
m. Referral to psyciatrist

For each of the situations/conditions given below, choose the one most appropriate/discriminatory option from above. The options may be used once, more than once, or not at all.

Questions

225. A 34-year-old woman is worried about the menopause and wants advice on how best to reduce the incidence of osteoporosis.
226. An obese 59-year-old post menopausal woman presents with a two week history of per vaginal bleeding . which is becoming more frequent. She had previously been on Tamoxifen.
227. An obese 40-year-old woman with a two hour history of postcoital bleeding associated with a foul smelling vaginal discharge.
228. An obese 50-year-old pre-mensopausal woman presenta with menorrhagia. She complains of constipation and says she cant stand cold weather.
229. A 56-year-old woman complains of nights sweats and mood swings. She had a fracture neck of femur which is being treated. She deniedd a history of hot flushes. She has a family history of breast and endometrial carcinoma.She wants relief from her symptoms.
230. A 53-year-old who has a family history of breast cancer has been experiencing mild discomfort for a few hours following intercourse for the last month. She is worried about using hormones.
231. A 59 -year-old woman whose period stopped 5-year ago has become increasingly depressed. She now feels life is no longer worth living and threatens suicide.
232. A 72-year-old woman has experienced of micturition intermittently for the last few months. Midstream urine (MSU) cultures have been persistently negative. She is

otherwise well but would like her symptoms to be resolved.

233. A married 52-year-old woman has a family history of breast cancer has been experiencing mild discomfort for a few hours following intercourse for the last month. She is worried about using hormones.

Twenty four

Renal Diseases

THEME: 1
DIAGNOSIS OF GLOMERULAR DISEASE

Options

a. Focal segmental glomerulosclerosis.
b. Type I membranoproliferative glomerulo nephritis.
c. Rapidly progressive crescentic nephritis.
d. Membranous glomerulosclerosis.
e. Type II membrano proliferative glomerulonephritis.
f. Minimal change disease.
g. Hereditary nephritis.

For each of the situation/condition given below, choose the one most appropriate/discriminatory option from above. The options may be used once, more than once, or not at all.

Questions

1. A 49-year-old male with colon cancer develops generalised anasarca. He has massive proteinuria and fatty casts in his urine. Renal biopsy reveals diffuse glomerular disease and a granular immunofluorescent pattern. Electron microscopy shows the presence of subepithelial deposits.
2. A 35-year man with AIDS has moderately severe proteinuria and hypertension. Renal biopsy reveals focal glomerular disease as well as focal detachment of epithelial cells from the glomerular basement membrane. Electron microscopy shows fusion of podocytes.
3. A 20-year-old man, who initially presented to the hospital with hemoptysis has progressed to renal failure. The urine

contains RBC casts. Renal biopsy reveals a linear immunofluorescent pattern in the glomeruli and no electron dense deposit.

4. A 16-year old girl presents with generalised pitting edema and hypertension. Renal biopsy reveals diffuse glomerular disease with a granular immunofluorescent pattern. Electron microscopy shows sub-endothelial deposits.
5. A 45-year-old woman has moderate proteinuria, hypertension and fatty casts in urine. Renal biopsy reveals eosinophilic nodular lesions in the mesangium, hyaline arteriosclerosis of the afferent and efferent arterioles and increased thickness of the basement membranes of the tubules.

THEME: 2
DIAGNOSIS OF RENAL CYSTIC DISEASE

Options

a. Childhood polycystic kidney disease.
b. Juvenile medullary cystic disease.
c. Simple cysts.
d. Cystic renal dysplasia.
e. Medullary sponge kidney.
f. Adult onset medullary cystic disease.
g. Adult polycystic kidney disease.

For each of the situation/condition given below, choose the one most appropriate/discriminatory option from above. The options may be used once, more than once, or not at all.

Questions

6. Sporadic childhood cystic disease characterised by the presence of cartilage, primitive mesenchymal tissue and immature collecting ducts in the renal parenchyma.
7. Autosomal recessive childhood cystic disease that is bilateral and associated with polyuria, growth retardation, the presence of corticomedullary cysts, and cortical atrophy of the tubules.

8. Most common cause of a palpable abdominal mass in a newborn.
9. Cystic disease that most commonly manifests as an incidental finding on an IVP that exhibits dilated collecting ducts in the medulla, often containing small calcium stones.

THEME: 3
INVESTIGATION OF URINARY TRACT SYMPTOMS

Options

a. Urine microscopy
b. Urine microscopy and culture
c. KUB X-ray
d. Renal tract ultrasound
e. Urodynamic studies
f. Urine cytology
g. Flexible cystoscopy
h. Barium enema
i. Prostate specific antigen
j. Blood glucose
k. Serum calcium
l. Urethral swab culture

For each of the situation/condition given below, choose the one most appropriate/discriminatory option from above. The options may be used once, more than once, or not at all.

Questions

10. A 26-year-old woman was admitted 2 days ago with high fevers, rigors and left loin pain. She has received 6 doses of IV Cefuroxime. Urine culture has grown coliform organisms, which is sensitive to cephalosporins. Her loin pain is getting worse and she continues to spike very high fevers.
11. A 30-year-old man complains of sharp pain on passing urine. He has also noticed a thick discharge after micturition. He has a number of sexual partners and does not use condoms.

12. A 65-year-old carpenter complains of urinary frequency and urgency, fatigue and thirst. He has lost one stone in weight over the past 3 months.
13. A 58-year-old tyre-factory worker has noticed a number of episodes of fresh haematuria. He has no pain on passing urine and otherwise feels well.
14. A 68-year-old woman presents with a short history of passing foul urine with green-brown discolouration. She has also noticed bubbles in her stream of urine. She was treated for carcinoma cervix in the past.

THEME: 4
DIAGNOSIS OF UROLOGICAL CONDITIONS

Options

a. Carcinoma bladder
b. Carcinoma kidney
c. Carcinoma prostate
d. Acute pyelonephritis
e. Testicular torsion
f. Acute epididymo-orchitis
g. Testicular tumour
h. Inflamed hydatid cysts of Morgani
i. Acute tubular necrosis
j. Chronic renal failure
k. Ureteric colic
l. Hydrocoele

For each of the situation/condition given below, choose the one most appropriate/discriminatory option from above. The options may be used once, more than once, or not at all.

Questions

15. A 26-year-old man presents with a painless lump in his left testis of 6 weeks duration. On examination he has no inguinal lymphadenopathy. He has an elevated serum alpha-fetoprotein.
16. A 6-year-old boy presents with a painless haematuria and scrotal oedema for 2 days duration. His urine demonstrates granular casts.

17. A 70-year-old man presents with poor stream and nocturia. On examination he has a lemon tinge to his skin, ascites, a palpable bladder and an enlarged prostate gland. His blood pressure is 170/95 mmHg.
18. A 75-year-old man presents with increased micturition and backache. On examination he has a palpable bladder and an enlarged prostate. His serum acid and phosphatase and alkaline are both elevated.
19. A 12-year-old boy presents to casualty with a red, painful, swollen scrotum. His midstream urine is normal.

THEME: 5
DIAGNOSIS OF RENAL DISEASE

Options

a. Acute hypothyroidism
b. Type 4 renal tubular acidosis
c. Acute adrenal insufficiency
d. Central nervous lesion with panhypopituitarism
e. Cytomegalovirus disease
f. Type 1 renal tubular acidosis
g. Syndrome of inappropiate ADH secretion (SIADH) with nephrotic syndrome
h. None of the answers
i. Membranous nephropathy
j. Type 2 renal tubular acidosis

For each of the situation/condition given below, choose the one most appropriate/discriminatory option from above. The options may be used once, more than once, or not at all.

Questions

20. A 30-year-old man with AIDS presented in shock. Serum biochemistry reveals
    Potassium 6.7 mmol/L
    Bicarbonate 20 mmol/L
    Chloride 84 mmol/L
    Creatinine 160 umol/L

21. A 41-year-old Londoner developed a temperature of 41°C five weeks after cadaveric transplantation
    WBC 2.1+1,000,000,000 L
    Hb 8.8 g dl
    Creatinine 177 umol/L
    Aspartate aminotransferase (AST)82UL
    Alanine Aminotransferase (ALT)132UL
22. A 36-year-old woman with leukemia has been treated with amphotericin B for a fungal pneumonia. She presents with muscle weakness
    Sodium 137 mmol/L
    Potassium 2.7 mmol/L
    Bicarbonate 19 mmol/L
    Chloride 110 mmol/L
    Creatinine 84 umol L
    Urine pH 6.8 mmol/L
23. An 83-year-old woman with small cell cancer presents with ankle oedema and is found to have 8g/day. Urine proteinuria. He is started on Frusemide. 10 days later his Blood Pressure is 115/75 mmHg lying and 85/65 mmHg standing. Serum biochemistry was:
    Sodium 121 mmol/L
    Bicarbonate 24 mmol/L
    Potassium 3.6 mmol/L
    Creatinine 113umol L
    Chloride 95 mmol/L
    Urea 11.5 mmol/L
    Glucose 5.7 mmol/L
    Albumin 27 g
    Osmolality 263 mOsm/L
    Urine Osmolality 417 mOsm/L
24. A 50-year-old man is prescribed oral Acetazolamide by an Opthalmologist for suspected glaucoma. He presents with lethargy and shortness on exertion.
    Sodium 140 mmol/L
    Potassium 3.2 mmol/L
    Bicarbonate 18 mmol/L
    Chloride 115 mmol/L
    Urea 6.7 mmol/L
    Creatinine 114 umol/L

THEME: 6
INVESTIGATION OF URINARY TRACT INFECTION(UTI)

Options

a. Abdominal X-ray
b. Intravenous urogram
c. Isotope renal scan
d. Laprotomy
e. Lumbosacral spine X-ray
f. Micturating cysto-urethrogram
g. Mid-stream specimen of urine
h. Serum creatinine
i. Suprapubic aspiration of urine for culture
j. Urinary glucose test
k. Urodynamics

For each of the situation/condition given below, choose the one most appropriate/discriminatory option from above. The options may be used once, more than once, or not at all.

Questions

25. A 10-day-old girl has developed fever and jaundice and is not feeding as well as normal. A bag of urine specimen showed red and white cells and a culture of mixed organisms. Abdominal examination is normal.
26. A one-year-old boy had a severe urine infection complicated by *E.coli* septicemia one month ago. Urine is now sterile. He is on prophylactic antibiotics. Ultrasound examination of the abdomen during the acute infection was normal.
27. A five-year-old boy has a persistent history of diurnal and nocturnal enuresis and soiling. Abdominal examination is normal. A proteus urinary tract infection (UTI) has been confirmed on culture. He has had a series of orthopedic operations for talipes equino varus.
28. An eight-year-old girl presents with a 12 hour history of nausea and central abdominal pain now radiating to the right ilaic fossa. She has urinary frequency.

29. A 14-year-old girl has a pseudomonal urinary tract infection and her blood pressure is 140/95 mmHg persistently. She has a past history of recurrent urinary tract infections and an abdominal ultrasound at the age of two was normal.

THEME: 7
INVESTIGATION OF URINARY TRACT OBSTRUCTION

Options

a. Excretion urography
b. USG renal tract
c. Dynamic scintigraphy
d. Cystourethroscopy
e. Plain KUB film
f. Pressure flow studies
g. Retrograde urethrography
h. Antegrade urethrography
i. Serum urea and electrolytes
j. Urinanalysis
k. Midstream urine culture

For each of the situation/condition given below, choose the one most appropriate/discriminatory option from above. The options may be used once, more than once, or not at all.

Questions

30. A 65-year-old diabetic man presents with painless distended bladder. On digital rectal examination, his prostrate is not enlarged.
31. A 40-year-old man presents with severe colicky loin pain radiating to his testicle. Plain abdominal X-ray is unremarkable. He has microscopic haematuria.
32. A 50-year-old man presents with severe oliguria, post kidney transplant.
33. A 60-year-old man post-thyroidectomy presents with painful urinary retention. There is some difficulty in catheterisation, with 900 ml of residual urine. Digital rectal examination reveals a smooth enlarged prostate.

34. A 60-year-old man presents with malaise, back pain, normochromic anaemia, uraemia and a high ESR. He has known carcinoma of the colon.

THEME: 8
DIAGNOSIS OF HEMATURIA

Options

a. Urinary tract infection.
b. Glomerulonephritis.
c. Nephrotic syndrome.
d. Henoch-Schonlein purpura.
e. Nephroblastoma.
f. Grawitz tumor.
g. Adult polycystic kidney disease.

For each of the situation/condition given below, choose the one most appropriate/discriminatory option from above. The options may be used once, more than once, or not at all.

Questions

35. A 10-year-old boy brought to A and E at 6 p.m. with history of sudden onset abdominal pain, vomiting and red coloured urine. On examination, there is tenderness over right iliac fossa and rashes over the buttocks and extensor surfaces.
36. An 8-year-old boy presents in the OPD with history of pedal edema and "tea coloured" urine. On examination BP is raised, pedal edema present. Rest of examination is normal.
37. A 3-year-old child with fever for 1 week and two episodes of hematuria. On examination, there is a mass in left flank with flank tenderness.
38. A 50-year-old man with painless hematuria, abdominal mass and fever. On examination pallor present, left sided varicocoele present.
39. A 35-year-old man with history of hematuria, dysuria, abdominal pain for 2 weeks. On examination renal masses felt, CVS—systolic murmur at apex and his BP is found to be 150/110 mm of Hg.

THEME: 9
DIAGNOSIS OF HEMATURIA

Options

a. Aniline dye.
b. Uretheral stones.
c. Buerger's disease.
d. Uretheritis.
e. Ureteric stones.
f. Cystitis.
g. Renal infarcts.
h. Rapidly progressive glomerulonephritis.
i. Minimal change glomerulonephritis.
j. Focal segmental glomerulonephritis.
k. Renal tuberculosis.

For each of the situation/condition given below, choose the one most appropriate/discriminatory option from above. The options may be used once, more than once, or not at all.

Questions

40. A 55-year-old woman who underwent mastectomy about 2 months back and now undergoing chemotherapy presenting with gross hematuria.
41. A 10-year-old child presents with history of bee sting presents with swelling around the eye. On urine examination, he had urine proteins of +4, BP–120/80 mm of Hg.
42. A 35-year-old male who is a known IV during abuser, presents with hematuria.
43. A 25-year-old male suffering from URI presents with gross hematuria. He has had 2 similar episodes in the last 18 months.
44. A 65-year-old male, who is a known hypertensive has developed left hemiparesis in last 24 hours, urine examination reveals microscopic hematuria.

THEME: 10
DIAGNOSIS OF HEMATURIA

Options

a. UTI
b. Transitional cell carcinoma of ureter
c. Renal adenocarcinoma
d. Ureteric calculus
e. Prostrate carcinoma
f. Prostatic hyperplasia
g. Urinary bladder calculus
h. Hemorrhagic cystitis
i. Glomerulonephritis
j. Polycystic kidney disease
k. Vasculitis

For each of the situation/condition given below, choose the one most appropriate/discriminatory option from above. The options may be used once, more than once, or not at all.

Questions

45. A 51-year-old man presents with 2 month history of haematuria and pain in the right flank. Urine microscopy confirms haematuria (HB 19, WCC 1300/mm3, hematocrit 59%)
46. A 20-year-old woman presents with urinary frequency, haematuria and lower abdominal pain.
48. A 75-year-old man presents with haematuria and backache. Plain radiographs show sclerotic areas in the lumbosacral spine.
49. A 46-year-old worker in rubber factory presents with haematuria and renal colic. A plain abdominal radiograph shows no abnormality.
49. A 35-year-old surgeon presents with severe flank plain, nausea and vomiting. Urine microscopy shows red cells and crystals (HB 14, WCC 1500/mm3).

THEME: 11
DIAGNOSIS OF HEMATURIA

Options

a. Anticoagulant therapy
b. Bladder tumour
c. Pregnancy
d. Inflammatory bowel disease
e. Wilm's tumour
f. Renal calculi
g. Acute glomerulonephritis
h. Angioneurotic edema
i. Cystitis
j. Prostatic enlargement
k. Chronic pyelonephritis
l. Papilloma
m. Carcinoma kidney

For each of the situation/condition given below, choose the one most appropriate/discriminatory option from above. The options may be used once, more than once, or not at all.

Questions

50. A 12-year-old boy has a sore throat for the past month with headache, malaise and a persistent low-grade fever. You notice some fullness in the face and very dark urine.
51. A 41-year-old man complains of recurrent abdominal pains especially on the left side. He says the pain travels down to his scrotum. And he says his urine has been dark for months.
52. A 50-year-old diabetic complains of feeling unwell, frequency, dysuria and dark urine. Over the past 3 months he has felt feverish.
53. A 32-year-old woman complains of sudden onset of frequency, nocturia and vomiting. She does not have a fever and she has missed a period. Her urine is dark.
54. A 62-year-old woman complains of feeling unwell and weight loss. She looks pale and unwell and on palpation you discover a mass in her left flank. She has had painless haematuria for 3 months.

THEME: 12
CAUSES OF HEMATURIA

Options

a. Ureteric calculus
b. Acute pyelonephritis
c. Benign prostatic hypertrophy
d. Acute cystitis
e. Malaria
f. Carcinoma kidney
g. Bladder carcinoma
h. Bilharzia
i. Prostrate carcinoma
j. Renal vein thrombosis
k. Acute intermittent porphyria

For each of the situation/condition given below, choose the one most appropriate/discriminatory option from above. The options may be used once, more than once, or not at all.

Questions

55. An 18-year-old woman started on oral contraceptive pills complains of colicky abdominal pain, vomiting and fever. Her urine is positive for red cells and protein. She develops weakness in her extremities.
56. A 60-year-old presents with intermittent colicky loin pain and night sweats. He has profuse haematuria with passage of blood clots. He is noted to have varicocele and peripheral edema. He admits of having loss of energy and weight loss.
57. A 25-year-old woman presents with fever and tachycardia. On examination the renal angle is very tender. Her urine is cloudy and blood stained.
58. A 40-year-old man complains of severe colicky loin pain that radiates to his scrotum. He is noted to have microscopic haematuria. No masses are palpated.
59. A 60-year-old man complains of increased frequency of micturition with suprapubic ache. The urine is cloudy and brown in colour.

THEME: 13
INVESTIGATION OF HEMATURIA

Options

a. Midstream urine microscopy & culture.
b. Midstream urine microscopy for casts.
c. Ultrasound of kidney, ureters & bladder
d. Isotope scanning
e. Micturating cystourethrography.
f. Intravenous urography.
g. Computed tomography of the abdomen.
h. Ultrasound of the abdomen.
i. Cystoscopy.

Questions

60. A young woman complains of painful hematuria
61. A 43-year-old man complains of severe right loin pain and hematuria.
62. A 22-year-old university student is found to have microscopic hematuria on routine investigations
63. A 50-year-old man complains of painless hematuria.

THEME: 14
DIURETICS

Options

a. Mannitol.
b. Frusemide.
c. Thiazides.
d. Spironolactone.
e. Dopamine.

For each of the situation/condition given below, choose the one most appropriate/discriminatory option from above. The options may be used once, more than once, or not at all.

Questions

64. Acts on the cortical diluting segment and reduced Na reabsorption.
65. Diuretic with highest efficiency.
66. Acts on site IV of the nephron and is usually used in combination with other diuretics.
67. Causes osmotic diuretics.
68. Potassium sparing diuretic.
69. Ineffective if GFR < 20 ml/min.

THEME: 15
SIDE EFFECTS OF DIURETICS

Options

a. Mannitol.
b. Ethacrynic acid.
c. Hydrochlorothiazide.
d. Acetazolamide.
e. Triamterene.
f. Spironolactone.

For each of the situation/condition given below, choose the one most appropriate/discriminatory option from above. The options may be used once, more than once, or not at all.

Questions

70. A patient presents with weakness and a swollen and a painful big toe. Laboratory tests reveal elevated glucose and uric acid levels.
71. A patient complains of tinnitus, heaving loss and vertigo after several days of diuretic therapy.
72. An elderly man reports the development of tender and enlarged breasts.
73. After several weeks of therapy, a patient reports numbers and tingling in her toes and fingers. Laboratory tests reveal a mild metabolic acidosis.

THEME: 16
AZOTEMIA

Options

a. Associated with prerenal azotemia but not intrinsic renal azotemia.
b. Associated with intrinsic renal azotemia but not prerenal azotemia.
c. Associated with both prerenal and intrinsic renal azotemia.
d. Associated with neither prerenal nor intrinsic renal azotemia.

For each of the situation/condition given below, choose the one most appropriate/discriminatory option from above. The options may be used once, more than once, or not at all.

Questions

74. Hyaline casts.
75. Oliguria is helpful in determining the cause.
76. Urine sodium concentration < 10 m mol/L.
77. Urine specific gravity < 1.012.
78. Fractional excretion of sodium is a sensitive test.
79. Plasma BUN/creatinine ratio (mg/dL) < 10.

THEME: 17
DIAGNOSIS OF PROTEINURIA

Options

a. Acute nephritis.
b. Nephrotic syndrome.
c. Acute renal failure.
d. Chronic renal failure.
e. Urinary tract infection.
f. Tubular defects.
g. Hypertension.
h. Nephrolithiasis.
i. Isolated proteinuria.

For each of the situation/condition given below, choose the one most appropriate/discriminatory option from above. The options may be used once, more than once, or not at all.

Questions

80. Urine protein < 1.0 gm/24 hr, normal creatinine clearance and RBC casts in urine.
81. Urine protein > 3.5 gm/24 hr, variable creatinine clearance and variable urinary casts.
82. Urine protein < 1.0 gm/hr, normal creatinine clearance and WBC casts in urine.
83. Urine protein 0.5–1.5 gm/hr, normal creatinine clearance and no casts in urine.

THEME: 18
CAUSES OF PROTEINURIA

Options

a. Alport's syndrome
b. Minimal change disease
c. Lupus nephritis
d. Focal glomerulosclerosis
e. Membranoproliferative glomerulonephritis
f. Mesangial Proliferative glomerulonephritis
g. Membrane glomerulonephritis
h. Idiopathic crescenteric GN
i. Diabetic nephropathy
j. Henoch-Schonlein purpura
k. Goodpasture's syndrome
l. Post infectious glomerulonephritis

For each of the situation/condition given below, choose the one most appropriate/discriminatory option from above. The options may be used once, more than once, or not at all.

Questions

84. A 40-year-old man presents with proteinuria, haematuria and progressive renal failure. He is noted to have a high frequency sensorineural deafness. He has a sister who was noted to have microscopic haematuria but is asymptomatic.

85. A 7-year-old boy presents with generalised edema and proteinuria. Electron microscopy reveals fusion of epithelial foot processes and normal appearing capillary and basement membranes.
86. A 30-year-old heroin addict presents with hypertension, edema, oliguria and is noted to have heavy proteinuria. Renal biopsy confirms loss of glomerular cellularity and collapse of loops. Adhesions between portions of glomerular tuft and Bowman's capsule are also seen.
87. A 12-year-old boy presents with sudden onset haematuria and edema. Further investigations reveal proteinuria and hypocomplementemia (C3). Sub-epithelial humps and foot process fusion are seen on microscopy.
88. A 4-year-old boy presents with a faint leg rash, bloody diarrhoea and oliguria. Further investigations reveal heavy proteinuria and an elevated serum IgA.

THEME: 19
DIALYSIS

Options

a. Hemodialysis.
b. Hemofiltration.
c. Intermittent peritoneal dialysis.
d. Continuous ambulatory peritoneal dialysis.

For each of the situation/condition given below, choose the one most appropriate/discriminatory option from above. The options may be used once, more than once, or not at all.

Questions

89. Used continuously for treatment of acute renal failure and has the advantage of fever hypotensive episodes.
90. Used as an alternative to hemodialysis and has the advantage of less risk of development of uremic anemia.
91. Can cause dialysis arthropathy due to amyloid formation especially in shoulders and wrists.

THEME: 20
ELECTROLYTE IMBALANCE

Options

	A	*B*	*C*	*D*	*E*
Sodium	142	138	138	138	122
Potassium	5.7	2.2	4.2	5.7	5.7
Chloride	100	112	112	112	76
Bicarbonate	16	16	16	16	16

For each of the situation/condition given below, choose the one most appropriate/discriminatory option from above. The options may be used once, more than once, or not at all.

QUESTIONS

92. Diabetic ketoacidosis.
93. Type IV Renal tubular acidosis.
94. Distal renal tubular acidosis.
95. Proximal renal tubular acidosis.
96. Uremic acidosis but no hyponatremia.

THEME: 21
MEDICATION THAT EFFECTS CONTINENCE

Options

a. Polyuria.
b. Urinary retention.
c. Stress incontinence.
d. Anuria.

For each of the situation/condition given below, choose the one most appropriate/discriminatory option from above. The options may be used once, more than once, or not at all.

Questions

97. Anticholinergics.
98. Alcohol.

99. Vincristine.
100. Opioids.
101. ACE inhibitors.

THEME: 22
MORPHOLOGY OF RENAL STONES

Options

a. Spiky and radio opaque.
b. Smooth, big and radio opaque.
c. Smooth, brown and soft and radiolucent.
d. Big, horny and radio opaque.
e. Yellow and crystalline and semilucent.

For each of the situation/condition given below, choose the one most appropriate/discriminatory option from above. The options may be used once, more than once, or not at all.

Questions

102. Triple phosphate stones.
103. Calcium oxalate stones.
104. Cystine stone.
105. Calcium phosphate stones.
106. Urate stones.
107. Xanthine stones.

THEME: 23
PREVENTION OF RENAL STONE FORMATION

Options

a. Bendro fluazide.
b. Allopurinol.
c. D–penicillemine.
d. Antibiotics.
e. Pyridoxine.
f. Thiazides.
g. Isoniazid.
h. Fibrates.

For each of the situation/condition given below, choose the one most appropriate/discriminatory option from above. The options may be used once, more than once, or not at all.

Questions

108. Oxalate stone.
109. Cystine stone.
110. Hypercalciuria.
111. Calcium phosphate stones.
112. Urate stones.
113. Triple phosphate stones.

THEME: 24
DIFFERENTIAL DIAGNOSIS OF WILM'S TUMOR

Options

a. Wilm's tumor.
b. Hydronephrosis.
c. Neuroblastoma.
d. Polycystic disease.
e. Teratoma.

For each of the situation/condition given below, choose the one most appropriate/discriminatory option from above. The options may be used once, more than once, or not at all.

Questions

114. Abdominal mass whose share is not well defined, irregular, nodular and crosses mid line.
115. Abdominal mass of variable size, usually hard in consistency and arises from the mid line of the body.
116. Cystic mass felt on right side only which is tense.
117. Abdominal mass which has oblong shape, is firm in consistency and rounded and does not extend beyond mid line and is usually painless.

THEME: 25
INTRAVENOUS UROGRAPHY

Options

a. Intense nephrogram phase.
b. Prolonged nephrogram phase.
c. Absent nephrogram phase.
d. Delayed nephrogram phase.

For each of the situation/condition given below, choose the one most appropriate/discriminatory option from above. The options may be used once, more than once, or not at all.

Questions

118. Renal artery stenosis.
119. Ureteric obstruction.
120. Acute renal failure.
121. Glomerulo nephritis.

THEME: 26
INTRAVENOUS UROGRAPHY

Options

a. Chronic pyelonephritis.
b. Chronic glomerulo nephritis.
c. Normal kidney.
d. Polycystic kidney.
e. Renal tumour.
f. Papillary necrosis.

For each of the situation/condition given below, choose the one most appropriate/discriminatory option from above. The options may be used once, more than once, or not at all.

Questions

122. Clubbed calyces.
123. Spidery calyces.
124. Ring shadows.
125. Stretched calyces.

126. Small kidney.
127. Linear breaks at papillary basis.

THEME: 27
DIAGNOSIS OF DIFFICULTY IN MICTURITION

Options

a. Detrusor muscle paralysis
b. Meningioma
c. Crushed vertebrae
d. Overflow incontinence
e. Fractured pelvis
f. Exposure to cold
g. Alcohol excess
h. Adenoma
i. Carcinoma
j. Abscess
k. Prostatitis
l. Urethral stricture
m. Urethral calculus
n. Ureteric stone

For each of the situation/condition given below, choose the one most appropriate/discriminatory option from above. The options may be used once, more than once, or not at all.

Questions

128. An elderly man has some difficulties with micturition. Last night he put off going to the toilet and has been unable to pass urine since. He thinks he has ruptured his bladder although he feels no pain.
129. A 58-year-old man complains of increasing frequency, especially at night. He finds himself straining and passing very little urine. On per rectal examination you find the prostate to be enlarged, smooth, elastic and moveable.
130. A young man has difficulties with micturition. Over a period of months he has found his stream to be increasingly narrow and on finishing he dribbles. A year ago he was treated for gonorrhoea.

131. A 32-year-old man presents with acute retention of urine. Over a period of weeks he had noticed some dribbling and pain on passing urine and just before arriving in A&E he felt a sudden pain on micturition and his stream stopped with a few drops of blood. The pain is still very sharp.
132. An overnight office worker complains that he cannot pass urine. He was playing football with his mates the previous day and injured his lower back. Aspirin has helped him with the pain and he is confident he soon will be up and about as normal, but he cannot urinate.

THEME: 28
DIAGNOSIS OF DIFFICULTY IN MICTURITION

Options

a. Parkinson's disease
b. Multiple sclerosis
c. Cerebrovascular accident
d. Transient ischaemic attack
e. Stress incontinence
f. Urge incontinence
g. Functional incontinence
h. Senile vaginitis
i. General paralysis of insane
j. Dementia
k. Carcinoma prostate
l. Prostatism
m. UTI
n. Diabetes

For each of the situation/condition given below, choose the one most appropriate/discriminatory option from above. The options may be used once, more than once, or not at all.

Questions

133. An elderly man wets himself uncontrollably. He says he has had back pain for a few weeks and he thinks his urine is much darker than normal. While watching television

he suddenly had to go for urination. The sofa on which he was sitting was wet already.

134. An elderly woman wets herself. Whenever she goes out she has to make certain she knows where the toilets are because she fears an embarrassing moment.
135. A 78-year-old woman is waiting in reception. Suddenly she passes a very large quantity of urine down her legs. She knew she had to go, but felt there was no chance of her going to the toilet on time.
136. A 76-year-old woman complains about wetting herself. Whenever she coughs or bends over or lifts something she pees and she finds this very irritating. She says she has always had excellent control in the past.
137. An 83-year-old retired professor complains of being unable to control the passage of urine. He also complains of numbness in his legs and falling. Finally when he talks he has to do so in a very deliberate fashion or he slurs his words.

THEME: 29
DIAGNOSIS OF DIFFICULTY IN MICTURITION

Options

a. Pregnancy
b. Infection
c. Glycosuria
d. Congenital abnormalities
e. Bladder tumour
f. Childbirth
g. Crohn's disease
h. Urge incontinence
i. Stress incontinence
j. True incontinence
k. Vesico-vaginal fistula
l. Urethral syndrome
m. Gonorrhoea
n. Tuberculosis

For each of the situation/condition given below, choose the one most appropriate/discriminatory option from above. The options may be used once, more than once, or not at all.

Questions

138. An overweight woman complains of having to go to the toilet more frequently. She says she does drink a lot of tea but that she is always thirsty and tired.
139. A young mother with chronic bronchitis says that every time she coughs she passes urine and she would like you to do something about it. She is on a course of antibiotics at the moment.
140. A middle-aged woman complains of having to urinate frequently. She says that unless she rushes to the toilet she wets herself and she finds wetting herself most embarrassing.
141. A 36-year-old sales executive says that she wets herself without warning. Before the birth of her third child she had no complaints but now she has no control whatsoever.
142. A 27-year-old travel guide wants something done about the pains she feels on micturition, especially when its cold. Repeated urine cultures have all been negative. Sometimes, she says, going to the toilet is very painful for her.

THEME: 30
INVESTIGATION FOR INCONTINENCE

Options

a. Midstream urine examination.
b. Transrectal USG.
c. X-ray KUB.
d. Ultrasound scan abdomen.
e. Prostatic specific antigen.
f. Intravenous urography.
g. Cystometry/urine flow rate measurement.

h. Per rectal examination.
i. Trans rectal prostatic biopsy.

For each of the situation/condition given below, choose the one most appropriate/discriminatory option from above. The options may be used once, more than once, or not at all.

Questions

143. An 80-year-old man complaining of incontinence of urine and the urge to pass urine frequently. Ultrasound pelvis revealed Grade I prostatic enlargement, which is the next investigation you would like to do.
144. An 75-year-old man with history of frequency, urgency, hesistency and occasional incontinence. Pre-rectal examination, revealed a hard nodule in one of the lobes of the prostate. Which other test will confirm your diagnosis?

THEME: 31
TREATMENT OF URINARY INCONTINENCE

Options

a. Trimethoprim
b. Oxybutinin
c. Ring pessary
d. Oral hypoglycaemic agent
e. Pelvic floor exercises
f. Vaginal estrogens
g. Adjust diuretics
h. Transurethral resection of prostrate
i. Laxatives
j. Imipramine

For each of the situation/condition given below, choose the one most appropriate/discriminatory option from above. The options may be used once, more than once, or not at all.

Questions

145. A 55-year-old menopausal woman complains of urinary incontinence, frequency and nocturia. The midstream urine culture is negative.

146. A 33-year-old woman complains of leaking small amounts of urine when coughing. This began following childbirth.
147. An 80-year-old woman presents with urinary incontinence and is found to have a uterine prolapse. The midstream urine culture is negative.
148. A 55-year-old diabetic presents with urge incontinence and an enlarged prostrate glad. The midstream urine culture is negative.
149. A 50-year-old newly diagnosed hypertensive complains of urinary frequency and dysuria. The urinanalysis reveals the presence of white cells and protein.

THEME: 32
MANAGEMENT OF PROSTATIC INFECTIONS

Options

a. Trimethoprim–sulfamethoxazole 160/800 mg orally, once daily for 12 weeks.
b. Cephalexin, 500 mg orally, twice daily for 2 weeks.
c. Ciprofloxacin, 500 mg orally, twice daily for 2–4 weeks.
d. Ibuprofen, 600 mg orally, four times daily as needed for pain.
e. Cefpodoxime, one dose of 200 mg orally.

For each of the situation/condition given below, choose the one most appropriate/discriminatory option from above. The options may be used once, more than once, or not at all.

Questions

150. The patient is 45 years of age and complains of urinary urgency, fever, and arthralgias. His prostate is extremely tender.
151. The patient is 53 years of age and presents to the Emergency Department (ED) with suprapubic pain and a boggy, non-tender prostate on examination.
152. The patient is 49 years of age and comes to the ED because of nocturia, dysuria prostatitis. A rectal examination and urinalysis are unremarkable.

THEME: 33
MANAGEMENT OF CYSTITIS

Options

a. Computed tomography(CT)scan
b. Cystoscopy
c. Intravenous urogram(IVU)
d. Longterm trimethoprim
e. Midstream urine culture in three months
f. Midstream specimen of urine for culture and trimethoprim
g. Monthly midstream urine culture
h. No action
i. Nuclear medicine scan
j. Potassium citrate
k. Ultrasound of kidneys and bladder

For each of the situation/condition given below, choose the one most appropriate/discriminatory option from above. The options may be used once, more than once, or not at all.

Questions

153. An 18-year-old woman became sexually active one month ago. She has had frequency dysuria and one episode of haematuria.
154. A three-year-old boy has a first confirmed urinary tract infection.
155. A 70-year-old man with prostate symptoms develops dysuria and frequency. Urine testing reveals microscopic haematuria.
156. A previously uninvestigated 25-year-old woman has her third attack of frequency and dysuria. Midstream specimen of urine grows E.coli on each occasion.
157. A 25-year-old man has his first proven episode of urinary tract infection. The intravenous urogram is normal.

THEME: 34
PRESCRIBING IN RENAL FAILURE

Options

a. Aluminium hydroxide
b. Aspirin
c. Bendrofluazide
d. Calcitriol
e. Calcium
f. Captopril
g. Diamorphine
h. Enalapril
i. Frusemide
j. Insulin-increased dosage
k. Insulin-reduced dosage
l. Magnesium
m. Mefenemic acid
n. Metoprolol
o. Metformin
p. Paracetamol
q. Spironolactone

For each of the situation/condition given below, choose the one most appropriate/discriminatory option from above. The options may be used once, more than once, or not at all.

Questions

158. A 30-year-old man with diabetes mellitus and severe renal failure (serum creatinine 700 mmol/l) has a blood glucose concentration of 24 mmol/l .
159. A 43-year-old woman with severe renal failure (serum creatinine concentration 750 mmol/l) presents with markedly swollen ankles.
160. A 21-year-old man with a failing renal transplant(serum creatinine concentration 600 mmol/l) has a blood pressure of 220/142mmHg.
161. A 62-year-old man with chronic renal failure (serum creatinine concentration 800 mmol/l) and known renal calculi presents with left sided renal colic.

162. A 20-year-old man with severe renal failure (serum creatinine concentration 700 mmol/l presents with proximal myopathy.

THEME: 35
CAUSE OF RENAL IMPAIRMENT

Options

a. Renal vein thrombosis
b. Medullary cystic disease
c. Bartter's syndrome
d. Berger's disease
e. Renal tubular acidosis
f. Nephrotic syndrome
g. Alport's syndrome
h. Cystinuria
i. Renal artery stenosis
j. Rhabdomyolysis
k. Fanconi's syndrome

For each of the situation/condition given below, choose the one most appropriate/discriminatory option from above. The options may be used once, more than once, or not at all.

Questions

163. A 10-year-old boy presents with nocturnal enuresis, easy fatigability and poor progress at school. On examination he looks short and is normotensive. Blood tests show hypokalemic hypochloremic acidosis.
164. A 62-year-old epileptic was found unconscious at home. Blood tests showed evidence of renal failure. Urine dipstick shows blood +++. Ammonium sulphate test shows coloured supernatant.
165. A 12-year-old girl presents with marked edema. Blood tests show Hypoalbuminaemia. Urine shows heavy proteinuria.
166. A 16-year-old student presented with a 4 month history of urinary frequency. Examination showed no abnormalities, apart from a mild hearing impairment. Blood tests showed evidence of mild impairment.

167. A 35-year-old man presented with acute abdominal pain. He had been fit till a month ago when he noticed increasing swelling of both legs, up to his pelvis. On examination there was dullness at the right base with decreased air entry. The rest of the examination was normal, apart from tenderness at the right iliac fossa. His blood tests showed evidence of renal failure.
168. A 40-year-old insurance broker presented with backache and pelvic pain. Radiography of the spine showed osteoporotic changes and medullary calcification of the kidney.

THEME: 36
CAUSE OF RENAL IMPAIRMENT

Options

a. Medullary sponge kidney
b. Renal tubular acidosis
c. Renal vein thrombosis
d. Acute interstitial nephritis
e. Bartter's syndrome
f. Idiopathic hypercalciuria
g. Diabetic nephropathy
h. Cystinuria
i. Renal artery stenosis
j. Lupus nephritis
k. Minimal change nephropathy

For each of the situation/condition given below, choose the one most appropriate/discriminatory option from above. The options may be used once, more than once, or not at all.

Questions

169. A 19-year-old mechanic was started on Flucoxacillin for an infected wound. Blood tests done 3 days later showed evidence of renal failure. Urine was positive for blood and protein. Abdominal USG showed normal kidneys with no evidence of obstruction.

170. A 35-year-old woman presented with a blood pressure of 190/110 and impaired renal function. Urine microscopy showed scanty red cells and granular casts. Renal biopsy showed linear IgG on glomerular basement membrane.
171. A 40-year-old man presented with renal colic. He has had several similar episodes in the past which were sometimes associated with passing small stones. Abdominal radiography showed calcified opacities in both kidneys. All blood and urinary tests were normal.
172. A 27-year-old woman presented with renal colic. She was previously fit and had not family history of renal problems. Blood tests were all normal but urinary calcium was elevated.
173. A previously fit 17-year-old porter presented with renal colic. On examination, his left flank was tender. Blood tests were normal. Urine microscopy showed hexagonal crystals. Intravenous pyelography showed faintly opaque staghorn calculus in the left renal pelvis.
174. A 65-year-old diabetic woman was investigated for hyperkalemia. She was on Indomethacin and Glibenclamide. Blood tests showed evidence of renal impairment, hyperkalemia and hyperchloremia.

THEME: 37
DIAGNOSIS OF RENAL FAILURE

Options

a. Goodpasture's syndrome
b. Amyloidosis
c. SLE
d. Polyarteritis nodosa
e. Wegener's granulomatosis
f. Systemic sclerosis
g. Post streptococcal glomerulonephritis
h. Multiple myeloma
i. Diabetic glomerulosclerosis
j. Drug induced nephrotic syndrome
k. Haemolytic uraeamic syndrome
l. Acute tubulo-interstitial nephritis

For each of the situation/condition given below, choose the one most appropriate/discriminatory option from above. The options may be used once, more than once, or not at all.

Questions

175. A 4-year-old boy presents to the GP with bloody diarrhoea and haematuria. His full blood count reveals leukocytosis, haemolytic anaemia and thrombocytopenia.
176. A 50-year-old woman presents with fever, polyarthralgia, a skin rash and oliguria. She is a diabetic and suffers from arthritis. She takes insulin and allopurinol.
177. A 50-year-old man with a history of heart failure now presents in renal failure. On examination, he has an enlarged tongue hepatosplenomegaly and peripheral oedema. He has heavy urinary protein loss and low serum albumin.
178. A 55-year-old man presents in acute renal failure. He suffers from rhinitis. Round lung shadows are noted on chest X-ray.
179. A 20-year-old man presents with rapidly progressive renal failure. He describes a recent history of cough, fatigue and occasional haemoptysis. His chest X-ray reveals blotchy shadows.

THEME: 38
INVESTIGATION OF RENAL DISEASE

Options

a. Urinary protein
b. Rectal examination
c. Cystoscopy
d. Renal USG
e. Urine microscopy and culture
f. Renal angiography
g. KUB X-ray
h. Renal function tests
i. Urinary electrolytes
j. Cyclosporin levels

k. Chest X-ray
l. Intravenous urography

For each of the situation/condition given below, choose the one most appropriate/discriminatory option from above. The options may be used once, more than once, or not at all.

Questions

180. A 64-year-old man develops urinary hesitancy and dribbling. He is frustrated that he has to wake up to pass urine infrequently, especially since his back has been very sore.
181. A 30-year-old woman presents with ankle swelling and frothy urine. Examination is normal.
182. A 4-year-old girl presents with abdominal pain, dysuria and fever.
183. A 22-year-old man presents with abdominal pain and raised blood pressure. He thinks his father and brother have the same thing.
184. A 45-year-old is admitted with excruciating left sided pain radiating from his back to his groin. He says it is the worst pain he has ever had.

THEME: 39
MANAGEMENT OF RENAL FAILURE

Options

a. Intravenous fluids
b. Fluid restriction
c. Hemodialysis
d. Hemofiltration
e. Peritoneal dialysis
f. Insulin and dextrose
g. Urinary catheter
h. Calcium gluconate
i. Calcium resonium
j. Venesection
k. Intravenous dopamine
l. Intravenous frusemide
m. Intravenous nitrate

For each of the situation/condition given below, choose the one most appropriate/discriminatory option from above. The options may be used once, more than once, or not at all.

Questions

185. A 65-year-old woman receives CPAD for chronic renal impairment due to hypertensive nephropathy. She is on no medications likely to cause hyperkalemia but her potassium level is persistently in the range of 6-6.4 mmol/l. She doesn't feel unwell and her ECG is normal.
186. A 72-year-old man is admitted with increasing breathlessness and anuria for 3 days. His clinical signs are consistent with pulmonary edema with small pleural effusions. He has a distended abdomen, which is dull to percussion between the umbilicus and symphysis pubis. His K is 5.9, urea 62 and his creatinine 110.
187. A 36-year-old presents with one-week history of breathlessness, haemoptysis and oliguria. He has widespread crackles and wheezes in his chest. He has a pericardial rub and S3. K+ is 5.5, urea is 53 and creatinine 620. His chest X-ray shows pulmonary oedema, bilateral pleural effusions and diffuse pulmonary infiltrates. Urinanalysis reveals red cells and casts. ECG shows widespread ST elevation. You have full renal facilities available at your hospital.
188. A 42-year-old woman had a hysterectomy 3 days ago for fibroids. Since the operation she has been vomiting profusely and is now complaining of thirst and malaise. Na is 148, K 3.1, urea 24 and creatinine 118. Her pre-operative blood tests were normal.
189. A 51-year-old man presents with severe breathlessness. Clinically he is in severe pulmonary oedema and looks moribund. His ECG shows no acute changes. His K is 5.5, urea 48, creatinine 520. He has received 2 intravenous boluses of 100mg Frusemide, with no improvement in his clinical condition. His BP is 80/40 despite IV Dopamine. No urine has been passed since he was catheterised. Your ITU has no beds and cannot provide Hemofiltration. The nearest renal unit is 2 hrs away.

THEME: 40
TREATMENT OF RENAL DISEASE

Options

a. Cyclophosphamide
b. Bendrofluazide
c. Hemodialysis
d. Renal transplantation
e. Immunosuppressants and plasmapharesis
f. Fluid and protein restriction
g. Continuous hemofiltration
h. Withdrawal of the offending drug
i. Albumin Infusion with mannitol
j. Salt restriction with frusemide
k. Peritoneal dialysis
l. Corticosteroids

For each of the situation/condition given below, choose the one most appropriate/discriminatory option from above. The options may be used once, more than once, or not at all.

Questions

190. A 20-year-old man presents with dyspnoea, haemoptysis and acute renal failure. He has serum anti-glomerular basement membrane antibodies.
191. A 55-year-old man is noted to have a nasal septal perforation, hypertension and Glomerulonephritis. The chest X-ray reveals multiple nodules.
192. A 60-year-old man presents with fits, confusion, pulmonary edema and anuria. His serum urea is 50 mmol/l and his potassium is 8 mmol/l . He has a history of MI and previous bowel resection.
193. A 5-year-old boy presents with generalised edema. On examination he is noted to have facial edema, ascites and scrotal edema. His urine is frothy with presence of proteins and hyaline casts. His serum albumin is 25 g/l and the serum cholesterol is raised.
194. A 7-year-old boy presents with bright red urine and edema of the eyelids. His BP is noted to be high. The urine reveals white cells, red cells, granular casts and protein.

Twenty five

Miscellaneous

THEME: 1
CAUSES OF FINGER CLUBBING

Options

a. Bronchial carcinoma
b. Bronchiaectasis
c. Lung abscess
d. Empyema
e. Cryptogenic fibrosing alveolitis
f. Mesothelioma
g. Cyanotic heart disease
h. Subacute bacterial endocarditis
i. Cirrhosis
j. Inflammatory bowel disease
k. Coeliac disease
l. Gastro-intestinal lymphoma

For each of the situation/condition given below, choose the one most appropriate/discriminatory option from above. The option may be used once, more than once, or not at all.

Questions

1. A 35-year-old heroin addict presents with fever, night sweats and haematuria. On examination, he is noted to have a heart murmur and finger clubbing.
2. A 50-year-old farmer is noted to have a dry cough, exert ional dyspnoea, weight loss, arthralgia and finger clubbing. On X-ray there are bilateral diffuse reticulonodular shadowing at the bases.

3. A 60-year-old man presents with sever chest pain, dyspnoea, and finger clubbing. He admits to asbestos exposure 20 yrs ago. He denies smoking. The chest X-ray reveals a unilateral pleural effusion
4. A 30-year-old woman presents with fever, diarrhoea and crampy abdominal pain. She is noted to have finger clubbing, anal fissures and a skin tag.
5. A 50-year-old man presents with haematemesis. He is noted to have finger clubbing, gynaecomastia and spider naevi.

THEME: 2
CAUSES OF CLUBBING

Options

a. Squamous cell carcinoma lung
b. Mesothelioma
c. Cystic fibrosis
d. Cronchiectasis
e. Fibrosing alveolitis
f. Celiac disease
g. Hepatic cirrhosis
h. Crohn's disease
i. Infective endocarditis
j. Cyanotic congential heart disease
k. Hyperthyroidism
l. Axillary artery aneurysm

For each of the situation/condition given below, choose the one most appropriate/discriminatory option from above. The option may be used once, more than once, or not at all.

Questions

6. A 75-year-old man is admitted with fever and breathlessness. He recently had a TURP but was otherwise well until 3 weeks ago. On examination his temperature was 37.7, pulse 96/min and regular, BP was 180/80. he has an early diastolic murmur. His chest is clear. He has evidence of early clubbing.

7. A 27-year-old woman suffers with recurrent chest infections and has a chronic productive cough. She remembers having had whooping cough as a child. She is not febrile or cyanosed but has marked clubbing.
8. A 68-year-old man presents with a 3-month history of cough and weight loss. On examination, he is cachetic. He has a hyper-expanded quiet chest with no abnormal breath sounds heard. He has left-sided ptosis and bilateral clubbing. He recently stopped smoking and gives a history of asbestos exposure in the 80's.
9. A 15-year-old boy under investigation for weight loss. He gives a history of intermittent abdominal pain and diarrhoea. His stools are often pale and hard to flush away. On examination he is thin and pale-skinned with fair hair but with no specific abnormalities apart from clubbing.
10. A 53-year-old man has clubbing in the left hand only. He has a history of hypertension and angina, with a 3-vessel coronary artery disease shown on angiography 2 yrs ago. His hypertension and angina are well controlled on medication.

THEME: 3
APPROPRIATE INVESTIGATIONS

Options

a. CSF examination
b. Barium studies
c. Skull X-ray
d. Full blood count
e. Audiometry
f. Syphilis serology
g. Glucose tolerance test.
h. Sputum culture
i. EEG
j. Abdominal X-ray
k. Urine analysis

l. Laparotomy
m. Chest X-ray
n. Funoscopy

For each of the situation/condition given below, choose the one most appropriate/discriminatory option from above. The option may be used once, more than once, or not at all.

Questions

11. A 26-year-old housewife developed recurrent attacks of dizziness. Each attack lasted about 1 – 2 min. During her attacks everything around moved, but did not rotate.
12. A 74-year-old printer complains of left sided abdominal pain, bloody diarrhoea and vomiting which began 8 hrs previously. At first the pain varied in intensity then became constant.
13. A 45-year-old bank manager presents with a history of increasing shortness of breath over the past 2 yrs. He had noticed his exercise tolerance declining over a long period.
14. A middle-aged gardens has had left sided abdominal pain for the past 5 months. The pain is colicky and associated with constipation. It is relieved by defecation.
15. A 38-year-old businessman has become impotent over the past 5 months. He is also dizzy on getting up in the morning. He is happily married.

THEME: 4
DIAGNOSIS OF FATIGUE

Options

a. Fluid retention
b. Chronic blood loss
c. Alcoholic cardiomyopathy
d. Hiatus hernia
e. Constrictive pericarditis
f. Bronchogenic carcinoma
g. Hypertension
h. Congestive cardiac failure

i. Liver
j. Financial worries
k. Duodenal ulceration
l. Narcolepsy
m. Gastric ulceration
n. Angina

For each of the situation/condition given below, choose the one most appropriate/discriminatory option from above. The option may be used once, more than once, or not at all.

Questions

16. A retired company director has chronic fatigue. He is a heavy drinker and smoker. On physical examination you find pedal oedema.
17. A middle-aged man complains of no enthusiasm for his work. He also complains of recurrent indigestion following ever the lightest of meals.
18. A 50-year-old Greek businessman feels his health has declined. Over the past year he has lost all of his energy and required more and mores sleep. A chest X-ray shows a very dense and relatively small heart shadow.
19. A 60-year-old woman complains of breathlessness and ankle swelling. She says walking to the shops causes her chest pain, particular on the left side.
20. An obese woman with a protuberant abdomen present to the GP and wants him to do something about her lethargy. She is pale with normal blood pressure and pulse rate. Protoscopy shows presence of haemorrhoids.

THEME: 5
APPROPRIATE INVESTIGATIONS

Options

a. Cholecystography
b. Full blood count
c. Liver biopsy
d. Ultrasound

e. EEG
f. Endoscopy
g. Chest X-ray
h. Laparoscopy
i. Liver function tests
j. Cholangiography
k. Blood glucose
l. ECG
m. Barium enema

For each of the situation/condition given below, choose the one most appropriate/discriminatory option from above. The option may be used once, more than once, or not at all.

Questions

21. An overweight woman of 40 yrs complains of right-sided upper abdominal pain. She feels sick and wants to vomit. Previously she had celebrated her birthday in a restaurant and had a very rich meal.
22. A 23-year-old man complains of pain in the lower right abdomen. He was feeling perfectly well, he developed a stomach pain, which disappeared and was replaced by a sharper pain lower down and to one side.
23. A middle-aged man complains of loss of body hair and mild confusion. Physical examination reveals mild hepatosplenomegaly. He says that he is a moderate drinker.
24. A 45-year-old vegetarian complains of chronic breathlessness and fatigue. She has always been fit but recently had a child and feels under pressure at work.
25. A 60-year-old market trader collapses while working on his market stall. He is brought in with soiled trousers and bleeding at the mouth.

THEME: 6
INVESTIGATION OF CHRONIC FATIGUE

Options

a. Chromosomal analysis

b. Full blood count
c. Blood film
d. Barium meal
e. Bone marrow biopsy
f. Gastroscopy
g. Abdominal X-ray
h. Fractional test meal
i. Serum B12
j. Stool examination
k. Hb estimation
l. Liver function tests
m. Lymphangiogram
n. Lymph node biopsy

For each of the situation/condition given below, choose the one most appropriate/discriminatory option from above. The option may be used once, more than once, or not at all.

Questions

26. A 46-year-old lecturer complains of being chronically tired. She says that the 2-year-old is just too much for her and that she and her husband have trouble getting him at accept vegetarian diet. On physical examination you find the patient to be pale and off colour.
27. A 30-year-old programmer complains of fatigue and intermittent fever. On physical examination you find him to have swollen lymph nodes and upper left sided abdominal distension. He has a high ESR.
28. A 63-year-old man complains soft tiredness and indigestion. He has been treated with antacids 5 weeks ago and the treatment has helped out but the pains in his abdomen have returned and become more or less constant.
29. A 48-year-old man complains of tiredness and abdominal pain. He says his gums bleed when he brushes his teeth. On physical examination you find an enlarged spleen and bruises of various ages.
30. A 53-year-old physical education instructor complains of malaise, fatigue, sore tongue and diarrhoea. On physical examination you find some atrophy of the tongue and a very high pulse rate.

THEME: 7
INVESTIGATION OF OBESITY

Options

a. Chest X-ray
b. Abdominal X-ray
c. IV unography
d. Dexamethasone suppression test
e. Assessment of visual fields
f. CAT scan of the skull
g. Waer deprivation test
h. Sleeping pulse rate
i. T3, T4 and TSH
j. Serium corisol
k. Abdominal ultrasound
l. Hormone assay
m. Basal body temperature

For each of the situation/condition given below, choose the one most appropriate/discriminatory option from above. The option may be used once, more than once, or not at all.

Questions

31. A 14-year-old girl presents with lethargy and weight gain. She is depressed and sensitive to cold/She would like something to be done about the excessive weight. The other children abuse her.
32. An obese 12-year-old is brought in by his mother who complains about his weight and lack of energy. He also has polyuria and polydipsia. His height I normal for his age.
33. A 52-year-old man has been gaining weigh. He complains of chronic cough acne and bruising. On physical examination you find his legs and arms to abnormally thin.
34. A teenage boy presents with obesity, greasy skin and acne. His face is found and his cheeks are red. In the past year he has suffered recurrent bouts of bronchitis.

35. An 18-year-old girl complains of her appearance. She is much too fat, she says. She also complains of missed periods and excess hair growth in the wrong places. On physical examination you find her to be 10kg overweight.

THEME: 8
CONFIRMATION OF DIAGNOSTIC SUSPICIONS

Options

a. ESR
b. Haemoglobin
c. Full blood count
d. Diazepan trial
e. Amitriptyline trial
f. Dexamethasone trial
g. Ergotamine trial
h. Chest X-ray
i. Throat swab
j. Serology
k. CT scan
l. Lumbar puncture
m. Angiography
n. ECG

For each of the situation/condition given below, choose the one most appropriate/discriminatory option from above. The option may be used once, more than once, or not at all.

Questions

36. A 60-year-old complains of severe headache. She says she rarely gets headaches and an aspirin is usually enough but this headache is so severe it makes her take to her bed.
37. A middle-aged man complains of severe headaches behind the eyes one side. He says he has been getting the headaches 3–4 times a day and that his left eye sells with pain. He says it has been getting worse in the evening.
38. A 32-year-old sales executive says that he cannot enjoy his dinner. On getting home from work he suffers an awful

headache and must for to bed immediately. Someti
he feels the pain in the day as well but it is worse in the evening.

39. An obese young woman complains of recurrent headaches. She has no other neurological symptoms and signs, although on physical examination you note mild papilloedema.
40. A young man falls over on leaving the pub in the evening. Since then he has had a steadily worsening headache. He finds it unbearable. Aspirin has not really helped and he feels drowsy.

THEME: 9
CAUSES OF FATIGUE

Options

a. Anaemia
b. Hypothyroidism
c. Hyperthyroidism
d. Addison's disease
e. Crohn's disease
f. Menopause
g. Viral illness
h. Post-viral infection
i. AIDS
j. Tuberculosis
k. Depression
l. Chronic fatigue syndrome

For each of the situation/condition given below, choose the one most appropriate/discriminatory option from above. The option may be used once, more than once, or not at all.

Questions

41. A 40-year-old woman complains of fatigue, weight loss and intermittent abdominal pain. She looks well tanned, although it is winter. She has postural hypertension and buccal pigmentation.

42. A 30-year-old homeless man complains of increasing fatigue and night sweats. He has a chronic cough and has recently noticed haemoptysis.
43. A 21-year-old woman complains of fatigue and intermittent abdominal pain. She has severe mouth ulcers, anal skin tags and painful raised lesions on her shins. Colonoscopy is normal.
44. A 25-year-old man presents with fatigue for approximately 1 yr. This is worse after exercise, which he rarely does as his muscles hurt after a few minutes. He says he needs at least 10 hrs of sleep a day to keep going.
45. A 52-year-old woman complains of fatigue and weight gain. She also describes irritability, hot flushes and sweats, but no night sweats.
46. A 35-year-old man complains of fatigue, poor appetite, and loss of libido and poor concentration. He no longer enjoys going out with friends. He gets tearful for no reason. He is unable to sleep for more that 3 hrs at a time.

THEME: 10
TYPES OF RESPIRATION

Options

a. Chyne stokes respiration.
b. Kussmaul's breathing.
c. Biot's respiration.
d. Sighing respiration.
e. Prolonged inspiratory phase.
f. Prolonged expiratory period.

For each of the situation/condition given below, choose the one most appropriate/discriminatory option from above. The options may be used once, more than once, or not at all.

Questions

47. Meningitis.
48. Anxiety.
49. Left ventricular failure.

50. Diabetic ketoacidosis.
51. Emphysema.

THEME: 11
INVESTIGATION OF ALLERGIES

Options

a. Skin prick testing
b. Patch testing
c. Serum IgE levels
d. RAST
e. Oral challenge testing
f. Measure C1 and C4 levels
g. IM adrenaline 1:1000 + piriton
h. Inspect for nasal polyps

For each of the situation/condition given below, choose the one most appropriate/discriminatory option from above. The option may be used once, more than once, or not at all.

Questions

52. A 30-year-old man presents with nasal blockage and watery nasal discharge. He states that the symptoms are worse at work. The floors are carpeted, and there is central heating. On examination he was edematous and pale nasal inferior turbinates.
53. A 20-year-old female is started on penicillin for acute tonsillitis. She develops stridor and a generalised rash.
54. A 10-year-old boy presents with abdominal pain and bloating after eating shellfish.
55. A 12-year-old boy with cystic fibrosis complains of bilateral nasal blockage and mouth breathing.
56. A 30-year-old woman presents with recurrent attacks of cutaneous swelling of the face. These episodes seen to be triggered by stress. There is no associated urticaria or pruritus.

THEME: 12
OROFACIAL MANIFESTATION OF SYSTEMIC DISEASE

Options

a. ACE inhibitor therapy
b. Beta blocker therapy
c. Bulimia nervosa
d. C1 esterase deficiency
e. Chronic alcohol abuse
f. Crohn's disease
g. Dietary allergy
h. HIV disease
i. Mumps
j. Nifedipine therapy
k. Sarcoidosis
l. Sjörgren's syndrome

For each of the situation/condition given below, choose the one most appropriate/discriminatory option from above. The option may be used once, more than once, or not at all.

Questions

57. A 65-year-old man with hypertension develops gingical hyperplasia.
58. An otherwise healthy 13-year-old boy presents with recurrent episodes of facial and tongue swelling and abdominal pain. His father has had similar episodes.
59. A 70-year-old woman presents with recurrent episodes of parotid swelling. She complains of difficulty talking and speaking and her eyes feel gritty on waking in the morning.
60. A thin 18-year-old girl has bilateral parotid swelling with thickened calluses on the dorsum of her hand.
61. A 40-year-old man with marked weight loss over the preceding 6 months has bilateral white. Vertically corrugate lesions on the lateral surfaces of the tongue.

Answers

Cardiovascular System

1. B
2. E
3. C
4. D
5. A
6. B
7. C
8. A
9. E
10. D
11. F
12. B
13. E
14. A
15. A
16. A
17. D
18. G
19. C
20. B
21. F
22. C
23. E
24. F
25. B
26. C
27. D
28. G
29. I
30. B
31. J
32. C
33. D
34. A
35. F
36. G
37. H
38. A
39. D
40. I
41. K
42. A
43. H
44. G
45. C
46. J
47. B
48. K
49. E
50. H
51. D
52. A
53. F
54. J
55. H
56. I
57. K
58. F
59. C
60. B
61. A
62. N
63. B
64. H
65. J
66. C
67. L
68. K
69. C
70. F
71. H
72. B
73. F
74. A
75. J
76. I
77. K
78. F
79. B
80. D
81. C
82. F
83. B
84. K
85. N
86. C
87. L
88. B
89. K
90. A
91. H
92. E
93. C
94. L
95. E
96. B
97. A
98. H
99. F
100. D
101. H
102. E
103. A
104. F
105. K
106. C
107. E
108. H
109. I
110. N
111. F
112. E
113. D
114. E
115. D
116. E
117. K
118. E
119. D
120. J
121. D
122. C
123. B
124. A
125. C
126. B
127. A
128. D
129. C
130. E
131. B
132. D
133. A
134. I
135. J
136. A
137. B
138. K
139. E
140. A
141. I
142. C
143. G
144. F
145. G
146. F
147. K
148. B
149. J
150. K
151. O
152. E

153. B
154. G
155. M
156. M
157. G
158. F
159. K
160. E
161. B
162. G
163. F
164. B
165. G
166. H
167. K
168. I
169. H
170. A
171. D
172. E
173. G
174. B
175. L
176. J
177. K
178. H
179. F
180. A
181. E
182. B
183. I
184. K
185. J
186. M
187. C
188. G
189. D
190. B
191. B
192. B
193. A
194. E
195. B
196. D
197. F
198. J
199. I
200. G
201. I
202. H
203. A
204. H
205. F
206. I
207. K
208. D
209. G
210. I
211. B
212. A
213. E
214. A
215. C
216. C
217. G
218. M
219. I
220. K
221. B
222. E
223. A
224. H
225. F
226. D
227. C
228. H
229. J
230. A
231. F
232. I
233. B
234. A
235. B
236. B
237. A
238. D
239. A
240. B
241. C
242. I
243. D
244. H
245. E
246. F
247. G
248. B
249. A
250. E
251. C
252. F
253. J
254. D
255. G
256. A
257. L
258. H
259. A
260. G
261. D
262. F
263. C
264. E
265. B
266. F
267. E
268. G
269. D
270. H
271. B
272. G
273. A
274. C
275. F
276. G
277. E
278. B
279. F
280. A
281. H
282. D
283. J
284. K
285. F
286. K
287. A
288. B
289. I
290. E
291. C
292. B
293. D
294. A
295. B
296. D
297. C
298. C
299. A
300. B
301. C
302. B
303. E
304. A
305. A
306. C
307. A
308. C
309. B

Respiratory Diseases

1. H
2. G
3. E
4. D
5. B
6. A
7. F
8. M
9. I
10. B
11. J
12. E
13. G
14. B
15. C
16. D
17. A
18. A
19. E
20. C

21. B
22. A
23. D
24. A
25. D
26. C
27. B
28. E
29. E
30. H
31. G
32. D
33. A
34. C
35. A
36. B
37. E
38. F
39. C
40. A
41. D
42. B
43. A
44. C
45. B
46. D
47. A
48. E
49. B
50. C
51. D
52. F
53. B
54. A
55. C
56. E
57. B
58. H
59. A
60. F
61. E
62. C
63. A
64. B
65. D
66. F
67. C
68. B
69. B
70. A
71. C
72. D
73. A
74. B
75. E
76. E
77. F
78. B
79. I
80. K
81. C
82. K
83. J
84. L
85. I
86. E
87. K
88. F
89. I
90. J
91. M
92. C
93. J
94. B
95. F
96. D
97. J
98. A
99. K
100. I
101. H
102. A
103. I
104. F
105. G
106. H
107. A
108. B
109. D
110. E
111. C
112. C
113. A
114. E
115. D
116. B
117. K
118. I
119. E
120. H
121. D
122. K
123. D
124. C
125. M
126. L
127. H
128. J
129. I
130. C
131. E
132. J
133. G
134. L
135. D
136. F
137. E
138. A
139. D
140. I
141. C
142. J
143. L
144. H
145. F
146. F
147. C
148. A
149. H
150. G
151. D
152. E
153. A
154. I
155. H
156. D
157. E
158. E
159. J
160. A
161. D
162. B
163. E
164. A
165. C
166. E
167. D
168. J
169. G
170. B
171. I
172. F
173. D
174. E
175. A
176. C
177. B
178. B
179. A
180. C
181. D
182. B
183. H
184. J
185. K
186. G
187. D
188. E
189. D
190. A
191. L
192. G
193. I
194. F
195. E
196. B
197. K
198. I
199. L
200. I
201. A
202. A
203. B
204. C
205. D
206. E
207. F
208. G
209. H
210. I
211. A
212. D

213. A
214. D
215. E
216. A
217. D
218. E
219. B
220. C
221. H
222. D
223. B
224. F
225. I
226. F
227. G
228. B
229. D
230. A
231. I
232. E
233. J
234. C
235. H

Neurology

1. E
2. C
3. A
4. F
5. B
6. D
7. B
8. E
9. L
10. C
11. H
12. H
13. F
14. C
15. K
16. J
17. H
18. D
19. A
20. K
21. I
22. F
23. C
24. H
25. A
26. G
27. B
28. D
29. E
30. E
31. D
32. C
33. A
34. B
35. A
36. D
37. C
38. F
39. D
40. A
41. G
42. F
43. I
44. B
45. H
46. F
47. G
48. I
49. E
50. H
51. C
52. E
53. G
54. I
55. E
56. B
57. D
58. A
59. D
60. G
61. I
62. F
63. J
64. D
65. B
66. C
67. D
68. D
69. D
70. B
71. D
72. L
73. H
74. N
75. E
76. D
77. B
78. C
79. A
80. D
81. A
82. F
83. B
84. E
85. D
86. B
87. A
88. E
89. C
90. C
91. D
92. B
93. E
94. A
95. D
96. E
97. G
98. E
99. E
100. I
101. D
102. F
103. G
104. E
105. E
106. C
107. B
108. F
109. F
110. J
111. H
112. G
113. A
114. K
115. D
116. E
117. F
118. B
119. C
120. A
121. B
122. D
123. C
124. E
125. A
126. D
127. B
128. C
129. B
130. E
131. D
132. A
133. N
134. J
135. H
136. K
137. O
138. B
139. L
140. G
141. A
142. I
143. B
144. B
145. M
146. L
147. B
148. C
149. F
150. I
151. G
152. B
153. C
154. E
155. A
156. D

157. A
158. K
159. E
160. B
161. D
162. C
163. I
164. E
165. D
166. A
167. C
168. B
169. F
170. E
171. C
172. D
173. B
174. A
175. C
176. A
177. B
178. E
179. D
180. B
181. G
182. C
183. L
184. D
185. E
186. C
187. H
188. G
189. A
190. D
191. H
192. A
193. N
194. G
195. F
196. E
197. J
198. A
199. H
200. C
201. E
202. B
203. I
204. G
205. D
206. C
207. A
208. B
209. E
210. M
211. D
212. G
213. H
214. J
215. B
216. E
217. B
218. D
219. A
220. C
221. D
222. C
223. B
224. E
225. A
226. E
227. A
228. G
229. D
230. B
231. F
232. D
233. H
234. A
235. J
236. D
237. C
238. F
239. B
240. G
241. E
242. H
243. F
244. K
245. C
246. J
247. B
248. E
249. C
250. A
251. D
252. C
253. A
254. D
255. G
256. D
257. H
258. L
259. G
260. K
261. I
262. B
263. E
264. D
265. K
266. H
267. B
268. A
269. D
270. E
271. I
272. G
273. H
274. L
275. E
276. F
277. E
278. N
279. H
280. A
281. B
282. C
283. H
284. G
285. E
286. C
287. B
288. I
289. F
290. B
291. C
292. G
293. A
294. D
295. J
296. C
297. G
298. K
299. H
300. C
301. F
302. B
303. D
304. H
305. E
306. H
307. C
308. J
309. F
310. A
311. E
312. C
313. B
314. E
315. F
316. K
317. N
318. M
319. I
320. A
321. N
322. H
323. L
324. C
325. A
326. H
327. B
328. G
329. F
330. J
331. B
332. I
333. A
334. H
335. K
336. A
337. E
338. B
339. F
340. D
341. I
342. H
343. C
344. C
345. H
346. I
347. D
348. C

349. L
350. L
351. H
352. I
353. G
354. B
355. D
356. G
357. A
358. A
359. G
360. I
361. A
362. C
363. G
364. F
365. D
366. E
367. F
368. H
369. A
370. B
371. G
372. C
373. E
374. D
375. L
376. M
377. H
378. B
379. M
380. E
381. F
382. G
383. B
384. K
385. I
386. L
387. J
388. A
389. B
390. E
391. H
392. F
393. I
394. A
395. B
396. K
397. J

Hematology

1. C
2. E
3. E
4. F
5. H
6. B
7. J
8. A
9. B
10. C
11. D
12. B
13. C
14. A
15. B
16. A
17. A
18. D
19. G
20. H
21. I
22. J
23. K
24. F
25. B
26. D
27. G
28. I
29. B
30. I
31. A
32. F
33. G
34. B
35. D
36. C
37. A
38. B
39. A
40. D
41. I
42. C
43. E
44. C
45. D
46. K
47. B
48. G
49. C
50. C
51. B
52. F
53. I
54. L
55. G
56. C
57. B
58. C
59. B
60. A
61. E
62. H
63. D
64. H
65. A
66. F
67. G
68. D
69. E
70. C
71. C
72. J
73. F
74. H
75. D
76. K
77. I
78. H
79. G
80. D
81. B
82. C
83. D
84. B
85. F
86. G
87. E
88. D
89. I
90. A
91. J
92. B
93. A
94. C
95. F
96. L
97. H
98. C
99. B
100. D
101. A
102. F
103. G
104. E
105. A
106. B
107. A
108. C
109. E
110. G
111. E
112. C
113. A
114. G
115. B
116. A
117. D
118. B
119. D
120. A
121. A
122. D
123. C
124. B
125. C
126. D
127. C
128. C

129. A	133. H	137. B	141. B
130. D	134. B	138. B	142. A
131. E	135. E	139. E	143. D
132. C	136. G	140. A	

Endocrinology

1. A	34. C	67. C	100. J
2. B	35. E	68. A	101. C
3. E	36. F	69. C	102. H
4. D	37. J	70. D	103. G
5. C	38. I	71. B	104. D
6. D	39. A	72. A	105. E
7. A	40. K	73. B	106. C
8. B	41. E	74. H	107. K
9. E	42. C	75. G	108. G
10. C	43. A	76. F	109. E
11. A	44. M	77. F	110. B
12. D	45. D	78. E	111. C
13. H	46. C	79. A	112. A
14. G	47. A	80. D	113. D
15. E	48. E	81. A	114. B
16. K	49. D	82. A	115. B
17. C	50. A	83. E	116. A
18. G	51. C	84. B	117. D
19. F	52. B	85. D	118. C
20. E	53. B	86. C	119. B
21. A	54. A	87. D	120. A
22. C	55. C	88. A	121. B
23. B	56. A	89. E	122. C
24. E	57. B	90. C	123. D
25. F	58. C	91. B	124. E
26. A	59. B	92. C	125. C
27. F	60. D	93. B	126. C
28. C	61. A	94. D	127. D
29. H	62. A	95. A	128. B
30. B	63. D	96. A	129. A
31. D	64. B	97. D	130. C
32. B	65. E	98. K	131. D
33. G	66. B	99. H	

Gastroenterology

1. C	6. A	11. A	16. B
2. D	7. B	12. G	17. D
3. A	8. D	13. H	18. I
4. E	9. E	14. I	19. F
5. B	10. F	15. J	20. A

21. G
22. H
23. C
24. D
25. A
26. F
27. G
28. B
29. H
30. A
31. E
32. C
33. D
34. H
35. F
36. A
37. C
38. J
39. B
40. B
41. C
42. C
43. G
44. A
45. E
46. A
47. D
48. C
49. B
50. B
51. C
52. I
53. H
54. D
55. I
56. I
57. C
58. A
59. B
60. A
61. C
62. B
63. D
64. H
65. I
66. C
67. B
68. F
69. K
70. G
71. A
72. H
73. I
74. A
75. D
76. B
77. F
78. A
79. D
80. B
81. C
82. A
83. J
84. E
85. B
86. F
87. E
88. A
89. B
90. G
91. I
92. D
93. E
94. G
95. H
96. A
97. F
98. C
99. D
100. E
101. H
102. L
103. E
104. M
105. C
106. A
107. D
108. E
109. G
110. B
111. A
112. C
113. D
114. H
115. D
116. J
117. F
118. H
119. K
120. G
121. I
122. J
123. L
124. C
125. B
126. M
127. K
128. F
129. D
130. K
131. L
132. C
133. D
134. M
135. L
136. N
137. E
138. J
139. L
140. F
141. E
142. D
143. A
144. E
145. F
146. K
147. L
148. D
149. B
150. B
151. I
152. E
153. F
154. C
155. J
156. H
157. A
158. D
159. F
160. M
161. L
162. I
163. E
164. F
165. H
166. E
167. G
168. A
169. A
170. F
171. B
172. G
173. E
174. I
175. F
176. D
177. B
178. G
179. J
180. H
181. C
182. F
183. L
184. E
185. K
186. A
187. B
188. D
189. E
190. B
191. K
192. C
193. L
194. J
195. J
196. K
197. I
198. B
199. B
200. H
201. G
202. F
203. B
204. C
205. A
206. I
207. F
208. J
209. D
210. E
211. G
212. A

213. C
214. A
215. G
216. B
217. K
218. E
219. C
220. M
221. D
222. G
223. E
224. A
225. F
226. E
227. C
228. H
229. B
230. D
231. K
232. C
233. E
234. F
235. I
236. B
237. A
238. E
239. H
240. D
241. I
242. A
243. J
244. B
245. B
246. G
247. H
248. J
249. L
250. G
251. D
252. J
253. I
254. A
255. E
256. B
257. J
258. G
259. C
260. A
261. G
262. F
263. E
264. J
265. L
266. G
267. H
268. K
269. E
270. I
271. H
272. L
273. A
274. B
275. K
276. A
277. C
278. F
279. G
280. L
281. A
282. E
283. C
284. B
285. G
286. A
287. E
288. H
289. K
290. B
291. C
292. D
293. F
294. H
295. J
296. A
297. B
298. C
299. G
300. A
301. J
302. B
303. I
304. L
305. G
306. D
307. I
308. C
309. A
310. F
311. H
312. N
313. G
314. J
315. M
316. G
317. H
318. D
319. L
320. A
321. D
322. C
323. B
324. B
325. G
326. I
327. E
328. K
329. J
330. F
331. G
332. B
333. I
334. E
335. G
336. J
337. K
338. L
339. D
340. F
341. A
342. L
343. J
344. B
345. K
346. E
347. F
348. D
349. I
350. B
351. B
352. E
353. A
354. B
355. E
356. C
357. D
358. E
359. B
360. J
361. F
362. A
363. E
364. F
365. J
366. B
367. E
368. F
369. B
370. D
371. G
372. K
373. H
374. J
375. B
376. H
377. I
378. C
379. A
380. K
381. E
382. F
383. A

Rheumatology

1. O
2. H
3. F
4. C
5. K
6. A
7. P
8. A
9. Q
10. C
11. R
12. S

13. J
14. C
15. A
16. B
17. A
18. C
19. A
20. D
21. B
22. B
23. D
24. A
25. G
26. E
27. C
28. M
29. K
30. L
31. A
32. E
33. A
34. C
35. A
36. B
37. A
38. B
39. J
40. G
41. L
42. I
43. K
44. A
45. C
46. E
47. E
48. B
49. F
50. D
51. K
52. H
53. F
54. A
55. E
56. I
57. D
58. G
59. G
60. D
61. I
62. L
63. D
64. A
65. H
66. G
67. C
68. C
69. B
70. D
71. E
72. A
73. A
74. C
75. D
76. F
77. C
78. B
79. E
80. A
81. G
82. B
83. D
84. H
85. G
86. F
87. E
88. K
89. J
90. C
91. L
92. E
93. C
94. J
95. F
96. A
97. G
98. B
99. F
100. I
101. A
102. H
103. J
104. F
105. E
106. D
107. C
108. B
109. A
110. D
111. F
112. E
113. B
114. C
115. A
116. H
117. K
118. C
119. A
120. E
121. F
122. G
123. A
124. B
125. D
126. E
127. C
128. B
129. D
130. A
131. E
132. G
133. A
134. B
135. F
136. D
137. D
138. F
139. I
140. H
141. J

Infectious Diseases

1. E
2. F
3. B
4. A
5. C
6. G
7. D
8. G
9. G
10. J
11. C
12. C
13. B
14. G
15. F
16. A
17. C
18. A
19. E
20. B
21. H
22. C
23. A
24. F
25. G
26. E
27. D
28. B
29. H
30. J
31. A
32. G
33. C
34. D
35. N
36. B
37. D
38. G
39. H
40. I
41. B
42. H
43. B
44. E
45. J
46. F
47. E
48. B

49. I
50. A
51. F
52. D
53. C
54. I
55. A
56. A
57. K
58. I
59. N
60. H
61. G
62. E
63. B
64. B
65. A
66. F
67. A
68. G
69. J
70. O
71. M
72. D
73. K
74. B
75. C
76. C
77. E
78. F
79. I
80. F
81. I
82. A
83. G
84. H
85. E
86. C
87. D
88. A
89. I
90. H
91. A
92. D
93. E
94. B
95. G
96. I
97. C
98. C
99. P
100. M
101. E
102. S
103. C
104. D
105. A
106. B
107. I
108. D
109. D
110. N
111. R
112. F
113. A
114. D
115. N
116. J
117. H
118. A
119. K
120. F
121. A
122. H
123. K
124. B
125. F
126. E
127. D
128. H
129. F
130. C
131. C
132. E
133. G
134. A
135. B
136. F
137. D
138. I
139. C
140. F
141. A
142. B
143. B
144. A
145. C
146. D
147. B
148. E
149. H
150. G
151. J
152. A
153. D
154. C
155. A
156. F
157. B
158. C
159. A
160. E
161. D
162. C
163. D
164. B
165. G
166. A
167. E
168. A
169. D
170. E
171. B
172. A
173. C
174. G
175. F
176. F
177. I
178. A
179. L
180. C
181. H
182. F
183. D
184. B
185. A
186. A
187. G
188. C
189. E
190. I
191. G
192. D
193. A
194. A
195. E
196. C
197. F
198. J
199. F
200. D
201. A
202. B
203. D
204. A
205. C
206. D
207. A
208. C
209. E
210. A
211. D
212. B
213. B
214. E
215. E
216. B
217. A
218. D
219. C
220. B
221. C
222. E
223. D
224. A
225. G
226. H
227. D
228. B
229. C
230. J
231. H
232. E
233. B
234. F
235. B
236. A
237. J
238. F
239. I
240. I

241. A
242. E
243. F
244. J
245. I
246. B
247. G
248. D
249. L
250. E
251. H
252. I
253. D
254. J
255. G

Oncology

1. B
2. F
3. J
4. M
5. I
6. K
7. H
8. O
9. A
10. C
11. E
12. K
13. I
14. A
15. D
16. I
17. H
18. F
19. A
20. C
21. E
22. K
23. I
24. A
25. D
26. I
27. H
28. F
29. R
30. P
31. Q
32. L
33. K
34. G
35. J
36. A
37. K
38. E
39. D
40. D
41. A
42. C
43. B
44. F
45. G
46. I
47. L
48. M
49. F
50. I
51. G
52. L
53. I
54. J
55. I
56. A
57. K
58. D
59. B
60. D
61. A
62. E
63. B
64. A
65. B
66. J
67. D
68. H
69. H
70. K
71. F
72. G
73. D
74. E
75. B
76. A
77. I
78. J
79. C
80. A
81. A
82. C
83. D
84. B
85. B
86. A
87. A
88. F
89. E

Emergencies

1. D
2. A
3. C
4. E
5. F
6. C
7. B
8. I
9. E
10. A
11. C
12. D
13. H
14. I
15. F
16. B
17. C
18. C
19. J
20. F
21. A
22. B
23. A
24. D
25. E
26. M
27. L
28. D
29. F
30. I
31. P
32. C
33. F
34. H
35. A
36. C
37. D
38. C
39. F
40. C
41. A
42. D
43. B
44. C
45. A
46. B
47. I
48. H
49. C
50. I
51. I
52. C
53. G
54. M
55. I
56. K
57. E
58. B
59. C
60. A

61. D
62. A
63. D
64. G
65. H
66. I
67. I
68. B
69. L
70. E
71. C
72. F
73. B
74. C
75. I
76. E
77. H
78. G
79. K
80. F
81. D
82. J
83. C
84. D
85. A
86. B
87. E
88. D
89. A
90. C
91. C
92. A
93. E
94. B
95. D
96. C
97. E
98. A
99. B
100. K
101. B
102. M
103. L
104. D
105. H
106. K
107. C
108. D

Ethics

1. B
2. F
3. E
4. I
5. K
6. A
7. H
8. N
9. D
10. E
11. D
12. K
13. J
14. F
15. H
16. A
17. N
18. C
19. L
20. D
21. A
22. F
23. H
24. B

Pharmacology

1. B
2. B
3. H
4. J
5. D
6. H
7. C
8. B
9. C
10. M
11. G
12. D
13. A
14. H
15. K
16. G
17. F
18. L
19. B
20. G
21. H
22. L
23. L
24. K
25. H
26. K
27. A
28. F
29. M
30. C
31. A
32. L
33. H
34. B
35. A
36. F
37. G
38. E
39. C
40. D
41. H
42. I
43. K
44. G
45. L
46. A
47. C
48. I
49. K
50. K
51. M
52. B
53. E
54. G
55. K
56. A
57. H
58. G
59. E
60. I
61. D
62. E
63. C
64. J
65. E
66. D
67. F
68. F
69. C
70. I
71. G
72. H
73. E
74. H
75. G
76. A
77. B
78. L
79. B
80. D
81. D
82. E
83. H
84. L
85. E
86. M
87. B
88. N
89. E
90. E
91. P
92. E

93. C
94. F
95. C
96. H
97. E
98. J
99. F
100. D
101. H
102. I
103. B
104. A
105. D
106. G
107. B
108. H
109. F
110. A
111. G
112. J
113. K
114. I
115. C
116. A
117. G
118. I
119. D

Dermatology

1. G
2. A
3. I
4. A
5. H
6. C
7. J
8. D
9. C
10. A
11. D
12. B
13. E
14. H
15. G
16. J
17. L
18. I
19. M
20. L
21. F
22. A
23. G
24. I
25. D
26. C
27. E
28. F
29. E
30. B
31. I
32. I
33. C
34. A
35. C
36. F
37. D
38. H
39. A
40. L
41. C
42. F
43. A
44. G
45. H
46. A
47. E
48. J
49. C
50. F
51. H
52. G
53. F
54. C
55. B
56. E
57. C
58. B
59. A
60. B
61. G
62. L
63. K
64. H
65. D
66. C
67. H
68. A
69. G
70. A
71. G
72. E
73. H
74. F
75. A
76. B
77. K
78. F
79. B
80. K
81. I
82. B
83. C
84. D
85. G
86. E
87. H
88. J
89. L
90. I
91. J
92. D
93. C
94. G
95. E
96. B
97. A
98. N
99. F
100. K
101. I
102. H
103. F
104. B
105. G
106. D
107. F
108. B
109. A
110. C
111. E
112. H
113. F
114. D
115. A
116. C
117. D
118. B
119. E
120. F
121. D
122. A
123. C
124. B
125. J
126. C
127. C
128. B
129. D
130. K
131. K
132. L
133. J
134. H
135. A
136. B
137. A
138. C
139. E
140. B
141. I
142. G
143. D
144. F
145. A
146. K
147. B
148. D
149. I
150. O
151. J
152. D

153. G
154. A
155. M
156. L
157. E
158. A
159. B
160. N
161. E
162. F
163. G
164. J

Surgery

1. F
2. C
3. D
4. E
5. A
6. B
7. F
8. F
9. F
10. F
11. F
12. H
13. G
14. E
15. D
16. L
17. D
18. E
19. F
20. K
21. I
22. J
23. H
24. E
25. J
26. F
27. A
28. E
29. H
30. F
31. J
32. B
33. I
34. K
35. J
36. K
37. C
38. A
39. I
40. A
41. D
42. B
43. C
44. D
45. K
46. E
47. I
48. H
49. G
50. C
51. A
52. E
53. D
54. B
55. D
56. B
57. D
58. E
59. A
60. C
61. C
62. H
63. C
64. E
65. L
66. A
67. I
68. B
69. N
70. M
71. A
72. A
73. E
74. C
75. F
76. B
77. D
78. A
79. A
80. B
81. C
82. D
83. F
84. A
85. G
86. C
87. E
88. B
89. D
90. G
91. C
92. B
93. J
94. I
95. J
96. H
97. B
98. D
99. I
100. C
101. A
102. G
103. A
104. C
105. E
106. B
107. F
108. G
109. B
110. D
111. A
112. E
113. E
114. B
115. C
116. F
117. D
118. A
119. C
120. D
121. E
122. B
123. A
124. A
125. B
126. F
127. G
128. D
129. G
130. H
131. I
132. F
133. D
134. B
135. A
136. C
137. B
138. G
139. I
140. A
141. D
142. H
143. H
144. E
145. A
146. F
147. B
148. H
149. G
150. C
151. D
152. E
153. A
154. C
155. F
156. F
157. H
158. G
159. D
160. E
161. I
162. F
163. H
164. I
165. J
166. C
167. D
168. G

169. C
170. B
171. E
172. G
173. B
174. C
175. F
176. D
177. G
178. E
179. B
180. H
181. A
182. G
183. G
184. B
185. D
186. A
187. C
188. F
189. C
190. D
191. F
192. E
193. A
194. A
195. D
196. C
197. B
198. F
199. B
200. F
201. E
202. G
203. C
204. I
205. K
206. A
207. G
208. E
209. M
210. J
211. A
212. G
213. I
214. B
215. C
216. A
217. A
218. C
219. A
220. E
221. D
222. B
223. E
224. F
225. C
226. G
227. A
228. C
229. A
230. E
231. B
232. F
233. B
234. D
235. G
236. A
237. F
238. F
239. E
240. B
241. A
242. D
243. G
244. I
245. N
246. F
247. K
248. B
249. D
250. B
251. C
252. A
253. B
254. A
255. C
256. E
257. D
258. G
259. A
260. I
261. M
262. D
263. I
264. G
265. H
266. C
267. B
268. A
269. J
270. H
271. I
272. A
273. B
274. E
275. G
276. J
277. A
278. B
279. E
280. I
281. K
282. D
283. G
284. H
285. E
286. A
287. J
288. I
289. A
290. E
291. G
292. F
293. C
294. D
295. L
296. E
297. G
298. G
299. H
300. A
301. D
302. L
303. K
304. A
305. G
306. H
307. B
308. J
309. C
310. D
311. F
312. A
313. J
314. J
315. E
316. A
317. G
318. F
319. L
320. C
321. F
322. D
323. J
324. E
325. A
326. B
327. C
328. E
329. A
330. F
331. B
332. G
333. E
334. C
335. I
336. B
337. J
338. A
339. M
340. E
341. H
342. I
343. N
344. F
345. E
346. C
347. A
348. D
349. A
350. E
351. G
352. F
353. H
354. B
355. G
356. D
357. H
358. K
359. D
360. B

361. E
362. C
363. A
364. G
365. H
366. E
367. A
368. B
369. C
370. D
371. A
372. F
373. E
374. A
375. H
376. K
377. G
378. B
379. D
380. C
381. F
382. E
383. B
384. B
385. D
386. D
387. D
388. E
389. C
390. A
391. F
392. D
393. K
394. I
395. E
396. I
397. B
398. E
399. C
400. D
401. G
402. I
403. D
404. B
405. A
406. A
407. H
408. G
409. H
410. B
411. A
412. C
413. D
414. E
415. D
416. B
417. A
418. C
419. B
420. C
421. E
422. F
423. B
424. A
425. D
426. B
427. F
428. D
429. E
430. C
431. A
432. I
433. D
434. F
435. A
436. B
437. E
438. I
439. D
440. A
441. J
442. K
443. C
444. F
445. E
446. H
447. I
448. F
449. B
450. E
451. J
452. H
453. F
454. C
455. B
456. M
457. K
458. G
459. B
460. C
461. A
462. E
463. B
464. A
465. D
466. C
467. F
468. G
469. D
470. E
471. A
472. A
473. D
474. F
475. A
476. I
477. E
478. G
479. J
480. F
481. C
482. K
483. J
484. C
485. A
486. F
487. B
488. A
489. C
490. E
491. H
492. C
493. A
494. D
495. B
496. B
497. G
498. D
499. A
500. I
501. C
502. A
503. E
504. F
505. G
506. H

Radiology

1. F
2. A
3. D
4. E
5. C
6. A
7. D
8. E
9. B
10. G
11. F
12. C
13. A
14. D
15. B
16. B
17. C
18. A
19. A

Biochemistry

1. D
2. F
3. A
4. D
5. B
6. B
7. B
8. A
9. C
10. A
11. C
12. G
13. C
14. D
15. A
16. C
17. B
18. E
19. A
20. C
21. D
22. B
23. H
24. E
25. F
26. C
27. C
28. A
29. D
30. B
31. D
32. G
33. F
34. B
35. I
36. F
37. E
38. F
39. B
40. D
41. C
42. A
43. H
44. G
45. E
46. C
47. A
48. B
49. H
50. J
51. I
52. A
53. L
54. F
55. I
56. B
57. G
58. B
59. E
60. C
61. D
62. B
63. G
64. C
65. F
66. A

Pediatrics

1. G
2. C
3. F
4. I
5. B
6. C
7. B
8. E
9. A
10. C
11. H
12. A
13. D
14. F
15. B
16. G
17. E
18. B
19. C
20. C
21. F
22. K
23. E
24. A
25. C
26. G
27. H
28. A
29. C
30. H
31. G
32. E
33. E
34. C
35. F
36. A
37. B
38. G
39. A
40. B
41. C
42. E
43. C
44. A
45. D
46. B
47. D
48. B
49. E
50. A
51. C
52. D
53. B
54. E
55. C
56. Q
57. C
58. H
59. K
60. T
61. R
62. P
63. G
64. C
65. D
66. F
67. C
68. A
69. E
70. F
71. G
72. A
73. F
74. D
75. B
76. H
77. E
78. F
79. B
80. G
81. A
82. A
83. G
84. B
85. E
86. J
87. H
88. E
89. F
90. D
91. H
92. L
93. C
94. D
95. H
96. D
97. A
98. A
99. D
100. F

101. G
102. B
103. I
104. E
105. A
106. D
107. H
108. G
109. E
110. J
111. E
112. A
113. A
114. J
115. D
116. G
117. E
118. J
119. I
120. K
121. G
122. A
123. D
124. J
125. J
126. C
127. G
128. H
129. D
130. F
131. H
132. L
133. G
134. C
135. A
136. G
137. I
138. G
139. C
140. C
141. H
142. D
143. G
144. I
145. B
146. A
147. D
148. G
149. F
150. E
151. C
152. F
153. H
154. A
155. F
156. E
157. C
158. I
159. A
160. E
161. B
162. D
163. C
164. B
165. A
166. F
167. J
168. I
169. C
170. L
171. D
172. B
173. E
174. F
175. K
176. B
177. D
178. I
179. L
180. P
181. G
182. F
183. A
184. C
185. D
186. E
187. B
188. D
189. A
190. C
191. E
192. B
193. A
194. C
195. F
196. D
197. G
198. B
199. J
200. K
201. E
202. A
203. D
204. J
205. A
206. D
207. B
208. F
209. A
210. G
211. F
212. A
213. B
214. D
215. B
216. A
217. F
218. F
219. H
220. A
221. G
222. J
223. B
224. G
225. A
226. C
227. E
228. I
229. F
230. E
231. H
232. G
233. B
234. I
235. H
236. C
237. A
238. J
239. E
240. F
241. E
242. B
243. D
244. G
245. C
246. B
247. C
248. D
249. E
250. B
251. F
252. A
253. B
254. I
255. I
256. C
257. F
258. B
259. G
260. I
261. F
262. C
263. A
264. K
265. F
266. A
267. C
268. D
269. I
270. A
271. B
272. C
273. G

Orthopedics

1. C
2. G
3. L
4. E
5. D
6. K
7. J
8. A
9. H
10. I
11. M
12. F
13. D
14. H
15. K
16. J
17. H
18. A
19. C
20. B
21. L
22. O
23. B
24. F
25. I
26. D
27. K
28. D
29. L
30. H
31. A
32. G
33. C
34. D
35. B
36. E
37. A
38. E
39. D
40. F
41. H
42. G
43. B
44. J
45. E
46. G
47. H
48. I
49. A
50. D
51. H
52. A
53. I
54. B
55. H
56. B
57. C
58. G
59. I
60. H
61. D
62. E
63. B
64. D
65. G
66. B
67. B
68. H
69. C
70. E
71. D
72. C
73. A
74. E
75. D
76. B
77. B
78. A
79. C
80. C
81. I
82. A
83. C
84. D
85. A
86. G
87. B
88. J
89. K
90. E
91. I
92. B
93. F
94. A
95. C
96. F
97. D
98. C
99. A
100. G
101. E
102. E
103. A
104. H
105. F
106. B
107. D
108. G
109. C
110. I
111. H
112. K
113. C
114. A
115. E
116. G
117. A
118. H
119. A
120. E
121. A
122. H
123. C
124. E
125. I
126. B
127. F
128. C
129. A
130. B
131. F
132. A
133. E
134. C
135. B
136. B
137. A
138. F
139. D
140. C
141. D
142. G
143. G
144. A
145. C
146. B
147. A
148. F
149. E
150. H
151. C
152. B
153. D
154. K
155. F
156. I
157. H
158. E
159. G
160. H
161. J
162. H
163. A
164. J
165. K
166. D
167. C
168. F
169. G
170. D
171. H
172. E
173. B
174. A
175. F
176. G
177. A
178. C
179. F
180. H
181. K
182. J
183. K
184. G

185. D
186. A
187. G
188. F
189. C
190. E
191. F
192. F
193. G
194. A
195. B
196. D

Psychiatry

1. H
2. B
3. D
4. F
5. C
6. A
7. B
8. A
9. A
10. C
11. B
12. A
13. A
14. E
15. C
16. F
17. A
18. H
19. H
20. A
21. G
22. D
23. E
24. A
25. B
26. D
27. A
28. B
29. D
30. B
31. A
32. E
33. C
34. L
35. O
36. K
37. M
38. N
39. F
40. G
41. I
42. H
43. J
44. C
45. A
46. D
47. B
48. A
49. E
50. D
51. B
52. A
53. C
54. C
55. D
56. A
57. G
58. F
59. J
60. I
61. G
62. B
63. H
64. B
65. A
66. E
67. C
68. D
69. A
70. C
71. D
72. E
73. A
74. H
75. F
76. E
77. C
78. D
79. A
80. B
81. A
82. E
83. D
84. C
85. C
86. F
87. I
88. G
89. J
90. J
91. L
92. K
93. F
94. A
95. J
96. G
97. C
98. H
99. A
100. C
101. L
102. F
103. H
104. E
105. F
106. I
107. H
108. C
109. A
110. F
111. B
112. H
113. D
114. A
115. E
116. C
117. H
118. C
119. F
120. H
121. G
122. E
123. A
124. C
125. A
126. F
127. G
128. I
129. H
130. D
131. J
132. F
133. C
134. F
135. G
136. I
137. H
138. B
139. B
140. E
141. I
142. E
143. A
144. G
145. E
146. B
147. A
148. D
149. E
150. A
151. C
152. B
153. E
154. D
155. F
156. A
157. J
158. D
159. H
160. E
161. C
162. K
163. J
164. H
165. E
166. J

Ear, Nose and Throat

1. C
2. B
3. F
4. E
5. D
6. E
7. B
8. D
9. C
10. E
11. J
12. C
13. I
14. E
15. K
16. A
17. B
18. F
19. I
20. D
21. F
22. D
23. I
24. K
25. B
26. E
27. B
28. K
29. A
30. L
31. F
32. A
33. D
34. I
35. E
36. H
37. C
38. I
39. B
40. J
41. H
42. A
43. K
44. F
45. G
46. D
47. F
48. D
49. E
50. C
51. A
52. B
53. A
54. B
55. B
56. E
57. F
58. A
59. D
60. A
61. D
62. B
63. H
64. C
65. C
66. D
67. J
68. B
69. F
70. C
71. A
72. F
73. D
74. H
75. C
76. E
77. D
78. F
79. A
80. C
81. G
82. I
83. D
84. J
85. B
86. D
87. C
88. G
89. A
90. C
91. A
92. D
93. B
94. I
95. F
96. D
97. H
98. A
99. E
100. C
101. A
102. D
103. C
104. A
105. D
106. B
107. B

Ophthalmology

1. D
2. G
3. A
4. E
5. I
6. K
7. J
8. F
9. A
10. E
11. J
12. D
13. I
14. E
15. D
16. F
17. J
18. F
19. G
20. C
21. B
22. G
23. A
24. H
25. D
26. I
27. F
28. D
29. C
30. B
31. A
32. A
33. B
34. C
35. D
36. D
37. E
38. N
39. I
40. P
41. A
42. G
43. D
44. C
45. F
46. C
47. C
48. B
49. H
50. A
51. D
52. G
53. E
54. C
55. A
56. D
57. G
58. H
59. G
60. C
61. B
62. D
63. A
64. B

65. F
66. A
67. G
68. K
69. F
70. H
71. I
72. L
73. A
74. H
75. I
76. A
77. E
78. H
79. F
80. E
81. G
82. B
83. J
84. B
85. K
86. L
87. A
88. J
89. G

Obstetrics

1. B
2. C
3. A
4. B
5. H
6. E
7. G
8. G
9. D
10. A
11. C
12. B
13. H
14. A
15. B
16. H
17. I
18. E
19. D
20. A
21. F
22. C
23. A
24. C
25. B
26. A
27. A
28. D
29. D
30. E
31. A
32. C
33. D
34. D
35. F
36. N
37. G
38. D
39. J
40. B
41. G
42. A
43. D
44. A
45. H
46. I
47. F
48. E
49. G
50. B
51. I
52. F
53. C
54. H
55. E
56. K
57. A
58. D
59. C
60. D
61. F
62. C
63. A
64. D
65. B
66. E
67. B
68. H
69. F
70. D
71. M
72. I
73. D
74. G
75. E
76. B
77. B
78. C
79. A
80. I
81. F
82. D
83. H
84. C
85. F
86. B
87. A
88. I
89. H
90. G
91. J
92. K
93. I
94. L
95. A
96. C
97. J
98. D
99. C
100. K
101. H
102. E
103. A
104. A
105. G
106. E
107. H
108. F
109. G
110. D
111. H
112. K
113. J
114. F
115. L
116. M
117. K
118. B
119. D
120. A
121. E
122. A
123. B
124. D
125. H
126. F
127. C
128. D
129. E
130. I
131. G
132. H
133. F
134. E
135. D
136. A
137. H
138. D
139. C
140. E
141. F
142. D
143. A
144. K
145. L
146. I
147. H
148. C
149. D
150. A
151. D
152. F

153. G
154. G
155. D
156. F
157. C
158. B
159. B
160. D
161. D
162. G
163. B
164. B
165. E
166. K
167. H
168. B
169. M
170. O
171. A
172. D
173. C
174. B
175. B
176. A
177. E
178. F
179. E
180. A
181. F
182. G
183. D
184. A
185. C
186. E
187. B
188. H
189. E
190. G
191. F
192. D
193. B
194. B
195. A
196. A
197. C
198. J

Gynecology

1. C
2. A
3. E
4. C
5. B
6. D
7. C
8. A
9. D
10. B
11. E
12. D
13. H
14. E
15. M
16. B
17. I
18. G
19. C
20. I
21. J
22. C
23. F
24. B
25. A
26. B
27. A
28. D
29. B
30. F
31. A
32. D
33. K
34. C
35. A
36. D
37. F
38. K
39. A
40. C
41. B
42. E
43. D
44. C
45. A
46. E
47. F
48. A
49. C
50. H
51. J
52. M
53. H
54. F
55. F
56. C
57. F
58. A
59. H
60. I
61. A
62. A
63. A
64. J
65. D
66. C
67. B
68. A
69. C
70. D
71. I
72. F
73. B
74. A
75. A
76. B
77. A
78. A
79. G
80. C
81. I
82. F
83. M
84. Q
85. G
86. D
87. A
88. C
89. B
90. E
91. M
92. C
93. D
94. B
95. A
96. F
97. N
98. G
99. D
100. J
101. L
102. K
103. A
104. F
105. E
106. B
107. D
108. E
109. C
110. A
111. C
112. E
113. G
114. H
115. I
116. B
117. D
118. D
119. F
120. A
121. A
122. G
123. F
124. B
125. I
126. H
127. C
128. E

129. B
130. G
131. H
132. A
133. B
134. B
135. B
136. C
137. G
138. A
139. E
140. C
141. K
142. B
143. N
144. M
145. I
146. K
147. A
148. C
149. E
150. B
151. E
152. A
153. L
154. H
155. A
156. F
157. I
158. D
159. J
160. A
161. B
162. B
163. C
164. A
165. F
166. D
167. C
168. B
169. B
170. G
171. C
172. A
173. F
174. G
175. A
176. D
177. C
178. D
179. H
180. E
181. A
182. D
183. F
184. D
185. G
186. J
187. I
188. E
189. D
190. B
191. A
192. E
193. C
194. I
195. D
196. G
197. C
198. E
199. A
200. D
201. B
202. I
203. D
204. K
205. H
206. E
207. A
208. C
209. D
210. I
211. F
212. A
213. B
214. C
215. D
216. A
217. C
218. B
219. G
220. F
221. A
222. C
223. E
224. D
225. G
226. I
227. J
228. E
229. B
230. F
231. N
232. D
233. F

Renal Diseases

1. D
2. A
3. C
4. B
5. E
6. D
7. B
8. A
9. E
10. D
11. L
12. J
13. G
14. H
15. G
16. I
17. J
18. C
19. E
20. C
21. E
22. F
23. H
24. J
25. I
26. F
27. B
28. D
29. C
30. F
31. A
32. C
33. A
34. A
35. B
36. G
37. E
38. F
39. A
40. F
41. I
42. J
43. C
44. G
45. C
46. A
47. E
48. B
49. D
50. G
51. F
52. K
53. C
54. M
55. K
56. F
57. B
58. A
59. D
60. A
61. A
62. A
63. I
64. C
65. B
66. D
67. A
68. D
69. C
70. C
71. B
72. F

73. D
74. A
75. D
76. A
77. B
78. C
79. B
80. H
81. B
82. E
83. I
84. A
85. B
86. D
87. L
88. J
89. B
90. D
91. A
92. E
93. D
94. B
95. C
96. A
97. B
98. A
99. B
100. B
101. C
102. D
103. A
104. E
105. B
106. C
107. C
108. E
109. C
110. A
111. F
112. B
113. D
114. C
115. E
116. B
117. A
118. D
119. B
120. C
121. A
122. A
123. D
124. F
125. E
126. B
127. F
128. H
129. H
130. L
131. M
132. A
133. M
134. G
135. F
136. E
137. B
138. C
139. I
140. H
141. J
142. L
143. G
144. E
145. F
146. E
147. C
148. H
149. A
150. C
151. A
152. D
153. F
154. K
155. B
156. C
157. H
158. J
159. I
160. F
161. G
162. E
163. C
164. J
165. F
166. G
167. A
168. E
169. D
170. J
171. A
172. F
173. H
174. B
175. K
176. L
177. B
178. E
179. A
180. B
181. A
182. E
183. D
184. G
185. I
186. G
187. C
188. A
189. J
190. E
191. A
192. G
193. L
194. F

Miscellaneous

1. H
2. E
3. F
4. J
5. I
6. I
7. D
8. A
9. F
10. L
11. E
12. B
13. M
14. J
15. G
16. C
17. K
18. E
19. H
20. I
21. D
22. H
23. B
24. I
25. E
26. K
27. N
28. F
29. C
30. I
31. I
32. F
33. D
34. D
35. K
36. A
37. G
38. E
39. F
40. K
41. D
42. J
43. E
44. L
45. F
46. K
47. C
48. D
49. A
50. B
51. F
52. A
53. G
54. E
55. H
56. F
57. J
58. D
59. L
60. C
61. H